Nursing Care of the General Pediatric Surgical Patient

Edited by

Barbara V. Wise, RN, PhD
Clinical Nurse Specialist
Pediatric Surgery
Johns Hopkins Children's Center
Baltimore, Maryland

Chris McKenna, MSN, RN, CRNP
Pediatric Nurse Practitioner
Division of Pediatric Surgery
Pediatric Trauma Nurse Coordinator
Mercy Hospital
Pittsburgh, Pennsylvania

Gail Garvin, RN, MS, ET
Independent USANA Distributor
Former Pediatric Surgical Clinical Nurse Specialist
Oakland Children's Hospital
Oakland, California

Bethany J. Harmon, MSN, MSPH, RN, CPNP
Pediatric Nurse Practitioner
Maine Children's Cancer Program
Barbara Bush Children's Hospital
Maine Medical Center
Portland, Maine
Formerly, Pediatric Surgery
Children's Hospital at Dartmouth
Lebanon, New Hampshire

AN ASPEN PUBLICATION®
Aspen Publishers, Inc.
Gaithersburg, Maryland
2000

The author has made every effort to ensure the accuracy of the information herein. However, appropriate information sources should be consulted, especially for new or unfamiliar procedures. It is the responsibility of every practitioner to evaluate the appropriateness of a particular opinion in the context of actual clinical situations and with due considerations to new developments. The author, editors, and the publisher cannot be held responsible for any typographical or other errors found in this book.

Library of Congress Cataloging-in-Publication Data

Nursing care of the general pediatric surgical patient / editors, Barbara Wise ... [et al.]
p. ; cm.
Includes bibliographical references and index.
ISBN 0-8342-1170-X
1. Children—Surgery—Nursing. I. Wise, Barbara Vollenhover, 1953–
[DNLM: 1. Pediatric Nursing. 2. Perioperative Nursing. WY 161 N97413 2000]
RD137 .N87 2000
610.73′677—dc21
00-023254

Orders: (800) 638-8437
Customer Service: (800) 234-1660

About Aspen Publishers • For more than 40 years, Aspen has been a leading professional publisher in a variety of disciplines. Aspen's vast information resources are available in both print and electronic formats. We are committed to providing the highest quality information available in the most appropriate format for our customers. Visit Aspen's Internet site for more information resources, directories, articles, and a searchable version of Aspen's full catalog, including the most recent publications: **www.aspenpublishers.com**
    Aspen Publishers, Inc. • The hallmark of quality in publishing
    Member of the worldwide Wolters Kluwer group.

Editorial Services: Denise Hawkins Coursey
Library of Congress Catalog Card Number: 00-023254
ISBN: 0-8342-1170-X

Printed in the United States of America

1 2 3 4 5

To the children, families, and colleagues
it has been our privilege to know throughout
our careers in pediatric surgical nursing

To my family—Jonathan, Matthew, Thomas,
and Kate—for their love and support in my life
that makes anything possible

Barbara V. Wise

To my family and Pete, for their constant love
and support, and to my friend and colleague Mike
Hirsh, who has taught me so much about caring
for pediatric surgical children and families

Chris McKenna

To my husband, Victor, for his unconditional
love and support of this endeavor and to
the memory of Robby Fambrini and
his devoted family for teaching me
the meaning of courage and resilience

Gail Garvin

To my parents, David and Joyce, for their love
and support, and to my colleague Nick Shorter,
who taught me about the care of surgical patients

Bethany J. Harmon

Contents

Contributors

Caroline Brass, BSN
Renal Transplant Coordinator
Department of Nephrology
Saint Christopher's Hospital
Philadelphia, Pennsylvania

Allen F. Browne, MD, FACS, FAAP
Pediatric Surgeon
Pediatric Surgery
Barbara Bush Children's Hospital
Portland, Maine

Kelli M. Burns, MSN, CRNP, CCRN
Advanced Practice Nurse
Pediatric General, Thoracic, and Fetal Surgery
The Children's Hospital of Philadelphia
Philadelphia, Pennsylvania

Jennifer Chamberlain, BSN, MS
Clinical Care Coordinator
Department of Pediatric Surgery
C. S. Mott Children's Hospital
Ann Arbor, Michigan

Teri Crawley-Coha, RN, MSN
Children's Memorial Hospital
Chicago, Illinois

Jeannette A. Diana-Zerpa, MSN, ARNP
Clinical Nurse Specialist
Advanced Registered Nurse Practitioner
Pediatric Surgery
Miami, Florida

Barbara S. Ehrenreich, RN, MS, CPNP
Certified Pediatric Nurse Practitioner
Department of Pediatric Surgery
Memorial Sloan-Kettering Cancer Center
New York, New York

Lynn Fagerman, RN, MSN, CS, PNP
DeVos Children's Hospital
Grand Rapids, Michigan

Kathleen Falkenstein, MSN, CPNP, PhD
Assistant Professor
Drexel University
Transplant Nurse Coordinator
Department of Surgery
Saint Christopher's Hospital
Philadelphia, Pennsylvania

Laura M. Flanigan, RN, MSN, PNP
Nurse Clinician
Division of Pediatric Surgery
Babies and Children's Hospital of New York
New York, New York

Marti Fledderman, MS, RN, CS, PNP
Nurse Practitioner
Pediatric Surgery
University of California, Davis Health System
Sacramento, California

Louise Flynn, RN, MSN
Liver Transplant Coordinator
St. Christopher's Hospital for Children
Philadelphia, Pennsylvania

M. Elizabeth Foster, RN, MS, CPN, CWOCN
Enterostomal Therapist
Clinical Nurse Specialist
Pediatric Surgery
Children's Medical Center of Dallas
Dallas, Texas

Gail Garvin, RN, MS, ET
Independent USANA Distributor
Former Pediatric Surgical Clinical Nurse Specialist
Oakland Children's Hospital
Oakland, California

Kathleen O'Connor Guardino, RN, MSN, CNS
Clinical Nurse Specialist
Pediatric Surgery
Schneider Children's Hospital
New Hyde Park, New York

Lori J. Howell, RN, MS
Coordinator
The Center for Fetal Diagnosis and Treatment
Director
Surgical Advanced Practice Nurse Program
Division of General, Thoracic, and Fetal Surgery
The Children's Hospital of Philadelphia
Clinical Associate
University of Pennsylvania, School of Nursing
Philadelphia, Pennsylvania

Kelly A. Jedlicki, RNC, MSN, CCRN, CPNP
Pediatric Clinical Instructor
Bellarmine College
Louisville, Kentucky

Betty R. Kasson, RN, MS, CNS, PNP
Clinical Nurse Specialist
Pediatric Surgery
Lucile Packard Children's Hospital at Stanford
Palo Alto, California

Katherine E. Keener, BSN, MS, ARNP
Department of Pediatrics
Section of Neonatology
Children's Hospital at Dartmouth—Hitchcock Medical Center
Lebanon, New Hampshire

Beverly B. Kelleher, RN, MSN, APN
Cardinal Glennon Children's Hospital
St. Louis, Missouri

Melanie A. Kenney, RN, MA, CPNP
Pediatric Central Line Nurse
University of Iowa Hospitals and Clinics
Iowa City, Iowa

Kimberly D. Knoerlein, BSN, MSN, ARNP
Department of Pediatrics
Section of Neonatology
Children's Hospital at Dartmouth—Hitchcock Medical Center
Lebanon, New Hampshire

Kathleen M. Leack, RN, BSN
Surgical Nurse Clinician
Children's Hospital of Wisconsin
Milwaukee, Wisconsin

Wendy Lord Mackey, RN, MSN
Clinical Nurse Specialist
Pediatric Surgery and Pediatrics
Yale New Haven Children's Hospital
Department of Nursing
Section of Pediatric Surgery
Yale University School of Medicine
New Haven, Connecticut

Renee C.B. Manworren, RN, MS, WOCN
Pediatric Clinical Nurse Specialist of Perioperative Services
Children's Medical Center of Dallas
Dallas, Texas

Carmel A. McComiskey, MS, RN, CS, PNP
Pediatric Nurse Practitioner
University of Maryland Medical System
Baltimore, Maryland

Kimberly Haus McIltrot, MS, RN, CPNP
Johns Hopkins Hospital
Baltimore, Maryland

Annie McKenna, MS, RD, CNSD
Pediatric Clinical Nutritionist
Pediatric Nutrition Support Service
Pediatric Gastroenterology and Nutrition
The Johns Hopkins Children's Center
Baltimore, Maryland

Wendy M. McKenney, BSN, MS, ARNP
Department of Pediatrics
Section of Neonatology
Children's Hospital at Dartmouth—Hitchcock Medical Center
Lebanon, New Hampshire

Linda Miranda McNamara, BSN, MSN, ARNP
Department of Pediatrics
Section of Neonatology
Children's Hospital at Dartmouth—Hitchcock Medical Center
Lebanon, New Hampshire

Lisa Meadows, MSN, RN
Clinial Nurse Specialist
Pediatric Surgery/Burns
St. Louis Children's Hospital
St. Louis, Missouri

Margaret Meyer, MSN, PNP
Children's Hospital at Dartmouth—Hitchcock Medical Center
Lebanon, New Hampshire

Joanna Joyce Morganelli, RN, MSN, PNP
Pediatric Nurse Practitioner
Department of General Surgery
Children's Hospital
Boston, Massachusetts

Robin Moushey, MSN, RN
Clinical Nurse Specialist
Pediatric Surgery/Burns
St. Louis Children's Hospital
St. Louis, Missouri

Dorothy M. Mullaney, BS, MHSc, ARNP
Department of Pediatrics
Section of Neonatology
Children's Hospital at Dartmouth—Hitchcock Medical Center
Lebanon, New Hampshire

Danuta E. Nowicki, RN, MN, CPNP
Pediatric Nurse Practitioner
Department of Pediatric Surgery
Children's Hospital of Los Angeles
Los Angeles, California

Susan E. Olsen, MS, RN, CPNP
Certified Pediatric Nurse Practitioner
University Hospital Medical Center
Division of Pediatric Surgery
State University of New York at Stony Brook
Stony Brook, New York

Joanne Palmer, RN, MSN
Renal Transplant Coordinator
Department of Nephrology
Saint Christopher's Hospital
Philadelphia, Pennsylvania

Luanne Pelosi, RN, MS, PNP
Department of Surgery
The Children's Hospital
Boston, Massachusetts

Laura Phearman, RN, BSN, CPNP
University of Iowa Hospital and Clinics
Iowa City, Iowa

Pam Pieper, MSN, ARNP-CS
Pediatric Trauma Coordinator
Pediatric Surgery NP/CNS
Clinical Assistant Professor
Univeristy of Florida College of Nursing
University of Florida Health Science Center—Jacksonville
Jacksonville, Florida

Frances N. Price, RN, MS, CPNP
Pediatric Surgery
The Children's Hospital
Denver, Colorado

Susan M. Quinn, BSN, MS, ARNP
Department of Pediatrics
Section of Neonatology
Children's Hospital at Dartmouth—Hitchcock Medical Center
Lebanon, New Hampshire

Nancy Rabin, RN, MN, CPNP
Clinical Training and Development Specialist
Texas Children's Hospital
Houston, Texas

Jose M. Saavedra, MD
Associate Professor of Pediatrics
Division of Gastroenterology and Nutrition
Johns Hopkins University School of Medicine
Baltimore, Maryland

Laura San Miguel, RNCS, MSN, PNP
Pediatric Nurse Practitioner
Department of Pediatric Surgery
Memorial Sloan-Kettering Cancer Center
New York, New York

Tina Shapiro, MSN, ARNP, CNS
Clinical Nurse Specialist
Advanced Registered Nurse Practitioner
Pediatric Surgery
Miami, Florida

Maureen Smith, RN, MSN
Clinical Nurse Specialist
The Children's Hospital Burn Program
Denver, Colorado

Elaine Stashinko, PhD, RN
Assistant Professor
Johns Hopkins University
Baltimore, Maryland

Judith J. Stellar, MS, CS, CRNP
Nurse Manager
PACU/Day Surgery/Sedation Center
Formerly, Advanced Practice Nurse
Pediatric General and Thoracic Surgery
The Children's Hospital of Philadelphia
Philadelphia, Pennsylvania

Marilyn Miller Stoops, RN, MSN, CRNP
Certified Pediatric Nurse Practitioner
Divisions of Pediatric Surgery and Patient Services
Children's Hospital Medical Center
Cincinnati, Ohio

Jeanette M. Teets, RN, MSN, CPNP
Pediatric Nurse Practitioner
The Cardiac Center at The Children's Hospital of Philadelphia
Philadelphia, Pennsylvania

Daniel H. Teitelbaum, MD
Associate Professor of Surgery
Section of Pediatric Surgery
University of Michigan Medical School
Ann Arbor, Michigan

Nancy J. Tkacz, MS, RN, PNP
Pediatric Nurse Practitioner
Pediatric Surgery
Barbara Bush Children's Hospital
Portland, Maine

Susan K. Von Nessen, MSN, CRNP
Advanced Practice Nurse
Pediatric General, Thoracic, and Fetal Surgery
The Children's Hospital of Philadelphia
Philadelphia, Pennsylvania

Beth Zimmermann, RN, MS
Clinical Nurse Specialist
Enterprise Case Manager
Section of Pediatric Surgery
University of Chicago Children's Hospital
Chicago, Illinois

Preface

Managed care has changed the way health care is financed and administered in the last decade. The practice of pediatric surgery, similar to other pediatric subspecialties, has responded by looking for creative measures that reduce costs without negatively influencing the quality of care provided. One noticeable change is a reduction in hospital length of stay. Because children spend less time in the hospital, nurses now provide services for pediatric surgery patients in a variety of settings, including surgicenters and posthospital care, the community, schools, the child's home, rehabilitation centers, and in long-term care facilities. The goal of this care is to provide quality nursing care throughout the continuum by means of coordinated services, health education, and discharge planning that promotes a positive outcome and eliminates or reduces readmissions.

Nursing Care of the General Pediatric Surgical Patient is a textbook aimed at providing nurses with an understanding of embryology, pathophysiology, surgical treatment, and nursing care of children with common and complex surgical conditions. Readers will find up-to-date information on the nursing care of children with common pediatric surgical conditions and the latest innovations in fetal surgery, minimally invasive surgery, and thoracic and abdominal transplants. Patterns of health and illness experienced by many children with chronic conditions and the necessary follow-up are also addressed.

This text is designed to provide useful information for nurses regardless of practice setting. Part I is devoted to topics that have an impact on all children who are undergoing surgery by providing information about pain management, nutrition, and preparation of the child and family for surgery. These chapters will be valuable to the student nurse, staff nurse, clinical specialist, and home care nurse seeking to master the complex physiology of pediatric surgical care. Part II reviews the nursing care for the child and mother who undergo fetal surgery or a minimally invasive procedure. Emphasis is on early referral to select centers for families who choose fetal surgery. Minimally invasive surgery is a new modality being used in both thoracic and abdominal procedures. Part III covers surgical lesions of the head, neck, and thoracic cavity. Parts IV and V provide information on congenital and acute abdominal problems found in children. Issues specific to the care of injured children are addressed in the chapters on trauma and burns. The final part of this book highlights research efforts that look at the future of the science of pediatric surgical nursing. A caremap that reflects a structured, multidisciplinary approach to care is found at the conclusion of each chapter that focuses specifically on a pediatric surgical problem. Diagnostic and therapeutic interventions performed by the health care team are sequenced in a time frame of hours, days, or weeks required to reach a specific discharge outcome.

This book is endorsed by the American Pediatric Surgical Nurses Association (APSNA). An individual who is actively engaged in the care of pediatric surgical patients has prepared each of the chapters. The editors would like to thank the contributing authors for their expertise and APSNA for its commitment and support in the development of this project.

Barbara V. Wise
Chris McKenna
Gail Garvin
Bethany J. Harmon

Introduction

The goal of pediatric nursing practice is a healthy, happy child. Those of us who practice where we care for children undergoing surgery often meet children and their families at a time of crisis. This includes treatment after an injury related to trauma, an acute appendicitis, or after the birth of an infant with a congenital anomaly. Whether the surgical procedure occurs in a same-day surgery center or involves an inpatient hospitalization, it is viewed by the family as a disruption in their usual lives. Nurses are expected to support the physical, emotional, and developmental needs of the child and family while providing cost-effective quality care in a managed care environment. This introduction discusses the impact of managed care on pediatric surgical nursing and includes sections on case management, critical pathways, and standards of clinical practice. It concludes with innovations for the future in the practice of pediatric surgical nursing.

MANAGED CARE

Nurses have seen many changes in nursing practice during the last decade. The development of managed care over the last several years has had a direct impact on the practice of pediatric nursing and specifically the practice of pediatric surgical nursing. Managed care is a systematic method used to coordinate the financing and delivery of health care. The objective is to provide consumers with prepaid access to high-quality care at low cost. Managed care emphasizes communication and coordination of care. Managed care strategies are used to manage use of hospital care, physician specialty services, and referral for health services (Grimaldi, 1996). Managed care relies on utilization review, prospective payment methods (diagnosis-related groups), case management, and critical pathways. Often the interventions proposed by managed care organizations to control costs overlap and include peer review, audit, standardized orders, and performance improvement activities (Anders, Tomai, Clute, & Olson, 1997). Managed care models are driven by a capitation payment system that requires careful analysis of health services. In a capitated system the potential for conflict exists between providing care to "well" children versus children with chronic health needs. Children with chronic health needs or those who require specialty services are more expensive to treat. In the past they have been denied access to managed care organizations. In 1997 approximately 15.4 million children were recipients of care from managed care organizations (U.S. Department of Health and Human Services, 1999).

Several models of managed care that reflect different practice patterns have evolved. Frequently, two or more models are mixed within one organization, reflecting regional or organizational differences. The models loosely defined as health maintenance organizations (HMOs) offer or arrange for the provision of health care to their members for a fixed prepaid amount. The HMO takes responsibility for the reimbursement and coordination of health services. The following provides a description of the four basic HMO models: group, independent practice association, network, and staff. A group model HMO contracts with a large physician practice to provide medical care to all the members. An independent practice association (IPA) contracts individually with a physician or group practice to provide care for members. In an IPA model, the HMO is able to reach members in a wide geographic area. A network model HMO contracts with several large multidisciplinary physician groups to provide care to members. The last model, a staff model, uses the services of staff physicians employed by the HMO to provide medical care. Physicians are salaried and receive a bonus if they meet performance standards (Grimaldi, 1996).

CASE MANAGEMENT

Case management developed from these physician models to address the coordination of nursing care for patients with complex or extraordinarily costly medical problems (Grimaldi, 1996; Zander, 1988). What is the role or function of nursing within the complex web of health care that often focuses first on cost-effective strategies and second on quality care? Case management describes a process of providing health care to individuals with routine and complex health problems. Pediatric nurse case managers are individuals who use the skills of autonomy, decision making, and guidance to manage care for a selected population of children with a particular condition. Case managers are employed by hospitals, insurance companies, long-term care facilities, and organizations that direct the care of children with complex needs. The case manager determines the human and material resources required for care of the child and family. For example, the case manager anticipates the need for home equipment. Often, this intervention facilitates earlier discharge and family-centered care. The case manager is responsible for coordinating the services of the multidisciplinary team in the care of a child with complex health needs. This includes, but is not limited to, the pediatrician, home care nurse, durable medical equipment company, multiple pediatric subspecialists, referral to an early intervention program, or the school nurse (Norris & Hill, 1991). The goals of the case manager are to prevent duplication of services, fragmentation of services, or barriers to effective care (Smith, 1994). Nursing case management involves providing care within the framework of a planned blueprint. Critical pathways are the written format for a blueprint to care.

CRITICAL PATHWAYS

Critical pathways or caremaps represent an innovation in care planning. Critical pathways are a multidisciplinary tool that is either diagnosis specific or procedure specific and focus on diagnostic and therapeutic interventions provided within an episode of illness. The pathway defines daily expected outcomes or short-term goals and long-term goals necessary to reach discharge criteria. The purpose of the pathway is to identify variations in practice, minimize delays in treatment, and efficiently use resources with a goal of decreasing cost without sacrificing quality. In essence the critical pathway is a decision tree for the care provider. It does not replace clinical judgment or the individual needs of a patient but guides usual or predictable patterns of care. Patients are assisted in meeting subgoals. When the goals are not met, the practitioner analyzes variances and alters the plan of care for the individual patient (Ireson, 1997). Critical pathways classify data or interventions into categories, such as consultations, laboratory tests, activities, treatments, medications, nutrition, teaching and learning, and patient outcomes.

Critical pathways cover a scope or specified period of care that varies from an inpatient hospitalization to an ambulatory experience, such as same-day surgery or outpatient dialysis, to a complete episode of care or life management of a chronic condition. Pathways are developed for common or specialized procedures. Examples of pathways for both common procedures, such as hernia repair, and specialized procedures, such as laparoscopic splenectomy, are found at the end of specific chapters in this text. If patients with the same diagnosis but comorbid conditions are expected to have different outcomes, a separate pathway is needed (Coffey et al., 1992). Often, this is the case in a child with perforated appendicitis versus a child with nonperforated appendicitis. Children with an uncomplicated appendectomy may be ready for discharge within 24 hours. In contrast, children with a perforated appendectomy may require delayed wound closure and intravenous antibiotics for longer than 1 week. These two different scenarios require different approaches or "blueprints," but the goal is the same.

Critical pathways reduce length of hospitalization and therefore costs in many populations (Metcalf, 1991; Zander, 1991). However, this reduction in length of stay often does not equate with improved quality. Developing clear, easily measurable subgoals and predefined interventions for each day provides nurses with a standard to evaluate patient progress. An essential aspect of every critical pathway is review and evaluation of outcomes (Zander & McGill, 1994). The outcomes from critical pathways improve patient and family satisfaction, assist providers in measuring clinical outcomes and performance improvement through variance analysis, decrease costs and patient readmissions, and assist in the administration of managed care contracts.

Nurses can individualize the plan of care if a patient is unable to progress toward a specific subgoal. This is known as a variance, a detour or deviation from the critical pathway. A variance can be positive or negative. Variances are generated from four potential sources: patients and families, clinicians, system barriers, and community issues. For example, if a patient is unable to ambulate because pain was not relieved, the plan can be altered by consulting the pain team. Analysis of variances leads to a change in practice. However, often health care activities or progress is delayed from multiple sources. An integral part of critical pathway development, use, and evaluation is planned revisions. Many institutions review and revise pathways every 6 months, yearly, or on an as-needed basis to reflect current practice standards within the institution.

SETTING STANDARDS IN PEDIATRIC SURGERY PRACTICE

The specialty of pediatric surgery is affected by the goals of managed care and managed competition. In the last several years, pediatric surgery providers (nurses and surgeons) have seen children with benign surgical conditions cared for by general surgeons in their local community hospital. If this trend continues, it is important that appropriate education be provided for the nursing staff and parents.

Few standards of clinical practice have been established. Most standards or pathways reflect current practice rather than a thoughtful analysis comparing two alternative approaches to care. It is imperative that pediatric providers have a positive influence on the health of children. We must advocate for our patients by understanding the social structure that influences health care outcomes and costs. One avenue for influencing the health care of children is the development of standards of practice and critical pathways for surgical disease in children. Other factors that influence the health of children involve developing referral guidelines and evaluating pediatric surgical practice (Grosfeld, 1996).

Few standards of clinical practice have been established in randomized controlled studies. Most studies report standard practice without establishing a scientific basis for algorithms used to guide care. Several studies have attempted to establish criteria for practice in the management of common pediatric surgery problems. Fallat and Casale (1997) reported on pediatric surgeon management of blunt solid organ injury. They surveyed pediatric surgeons at 87 children's hospitals or units involved in trauma care of children. They found that 78% of the children were observed in an intensive care setting for 1 to 2 days with serial monitoring of hematocrit and hemoglobin. Computed tomographic scans to evaluate the extent of injury remain the "gold standard" (98%). Stable hematocrit is used to establish criteria for increasing activity (78%) and discharge home (83%) in the nonoperative management of children with blunt injuries.

In another study, Adolph and Falterman (1996) reviewed the management of children with acute appendicitis in a managed care environment. The authors hypothesized that patients enrolled in a managed care insurance program would have increased incidence of morbidity and mortality. This study actually demonstrated that patients enrolled in a managed care organization had a lower rate of complications after appendicitis compared with children who had indemnity plans ($P < .01$). In a similar study, O'Toole et al. (1996) reported that the greatest incidence in delay of referral to a surgeon in children with acute appendicitis occurred in children with Medicaid. The major cause of delay in treatment occurred because of delay in seeking medical attention. This resulted in an increased incidence of perforation and had an impact on the length of stay after acute appendicitis.

FUTURE DIRECTIONS

The future of health care for children requires us to look for unique solutions to the problem of providing quality care while holding spiraling costs to a manageable level. We must use the resources of managed care and critical pathways and begin to analyze "standards" of practice that have been accepted and challenge traditional practice. The following examples describe two departments of pediatric surgery that have begun to explore changes in traditional practice patterns and patient satisfaction. One solution proposed by Tagge et al. (1999) is "one-stop surgery" as a mechanism to simplify outpatient procedures for the patient and family. In a pilot study, clinical visits were compressed from the usual three visits (preoperative, operative, and postoperative) into one visit. The advantages of one-stop surgery included decreased economic hardships for the family related to transportation costs and lost time from work and increased cooperation among the team members (pediatric surgery, anesthesia, operating room nurses). Success of this program requires close communication between referring physicians and surgeons, follow-up phone calls, and careful screening for appropriate candidates for one-stop surgery. In another study, Dinsmore et al. (1997) challenged the use of nasogastric decompression after abdominal procedures in children. They reported that 89% of the children in their study avoided routine nasogastric decompression. Two subgroups that required decompression were children less than 2 years of age and children who underwent an endorectal pull-through. Nurses in pediatric surgery practices, schools, and home care situations need to support efforts that challenge traditional approaches to care, revise current practices after carefully analyzing pathway variances, and consider patient and family satisfaction with care provided. Additional investigations of these and other standard practices are required in prospective, randomized studies.

Nurses who care for children with surgical needs have positions that are both rewarding and challenging. The reward comes from the privilege of caring for and supporting a child and family through a stressful time. One of the challenges is to provide this care and support with limited resources. As nurses, we must work within the constraints of the growing managed care system to provide cost-effective, quality care to children and families. The use of case management and critical pathways, the establishment of standards of clinical practice, and the development of innovative and research-based patterns will help us as we strive to meet this goal in the changing health care environment.

REFERENCES

Adolph, V.R., & Falterman, K.W. (1996). Appendicitis in children in the managed care era. *Journal of Pediatric Surgery, 31*(8), 1035–1037.

Anders, R.L., Tomai, J.S., Clute, R.M., & Olson, T. (1997). Development of scientifically valid coordinated care path. *Journal of Nursing Administration, 27*(5), 45–51.

Coffey, R.J., Richards, J.S., Remmaert, C.S., LeRoy, S.S., Schoville, R.R., & Baldwin, P.J. (1992). An introduction to critical paths. *Quality Management in Health Care, 1*(1), 45–54.

Dinsmore, J.E., Maxson, R.T., Johnson, D.D., Jackson, R.J., Wagner, C.W., & Smith, S.D. (1997). Is nasogastric tube decompression necessary after major abdominal surgery in children? *Journal of Pediatric Surgery, 32*(7), 982–985.

Fallat, M.E., & Casale, A.J. (1997). Practice patterns of pediatric surgeons caring for stable patients with traumatic solid organ injury. *The Journal of Trauma, 43,* 820–823.

Grimaldi, P.L. (1996). Medicare's point-of service. *Nursing Management Special Supplementation, 14,* 16–17.

Grosfeld, J.L. (1996). Economics and education: Impact on pediatric surgery in the next decade. *Journal of Pediatric Surgery, 31*(1), 3–11.

Ireson, C.L. (1997). Critical pathways: Effectiveness in achieving patient outcomes. *Journal of Nursing Administration, 27*(6), 16–23.

Metcalf, E.M. (1991). The orthopedic critical pathway. *Orthopedic Nursing, 10*(6), 25–31.

Norris, M.K.G., & Hill, C. (1991). The clinical nurse specialist: Developing the case management role. *Dimensions of Critical Care Nursing, 10*(6), 346–353.

O'Toole, S.J., Karamanoukian, H.L., Allen, J.E., Caty, M.G., O'Toole, D., Azizkhan, R.G., & Glick, P.L. (1996). Insurance-related differences in the presentation of pediatric appendicitis. *Journal of Pediatric Surgery, 31*(8), 1032–1034.

Smith, L.D. (1994). Continuity of care through nursing case management of the chronically ill child. *Clinical Nurse Specialist, 8*(2), 65–68.

Tagge, E.P., Hebra, A., Overdyk, F., Burt, N., Egbert, M., Wilder, A., William, A., Roland, P., & Othersen, H.B. (1999). One-stop surgery: Evolving approach to pediatric outpatient surgery. *Journal of Pediatric Surgery, 34*(1), 129–132.

U.S. Department of Health and Human Services, Health Care Financing Administration. (1999). "Child care and Medicaid: Partners for healthy children." http://www.hcfa.gov/medicaid/ch%2Dguide.htm.

Zander, K. (1988). Nursing case management resolving the DRG paradox. *Nursing Clinics of North America, 23*(3), 503–520.

Zander, K. (1991). Case management in acute care: Making the connections. *The Case Manager, 2*(2), 40.

Zander, K., & McGill, R. (1994). Critical and anticipated recovery paths: Only the beginning. *Nursing Management, 25*(8), 34–40.

PART I

Special Considerations in the Care of the Pediatric Surgical Patient

CHAPTER 1

Preparation of the
Child and Family for Surgery

Renee C.B. Manworren and Marti Fledderman

INTRODUCTION

Children have surgery in pediatric and general hospitals, specialty centers, and outpatient surgery centers. Those charged with the care of these children may be pediatric experts or providers who rarely care for children. Each year, almost 2 million children have surgery in the United States, and 9.5% of patients cared for in ambulatory surgery centers are less than 15 years of age (*1998 Health Care Almanac & Yearbook;* Schittroth, 1994). These statistics demand that health care providers have a thorough understanding of surgical preparation and the impact of surgery on children and their families.

Whether the child is having a minor outpatient surgery or an emergency lifesaving procedure, it is an extraordinary stressor for the child and family (Lynch, 1994; Mansson, Fredrikzon, & Rosberg, 1992; Wolfer & Visintainer, 1975; Ziegler & Prior, 1994). The patient and family bring their expectations of the procedure and their fears and concerns regarding anesthesia, pain, surgical success, possible complications, and competence of those caring for their child to the surgical experience. Families are also influenced by their own experiences with hospitalization and surgery, those depicted on television and in the movies, and information and anecdotes from friends and relatives. Those who provide surgical care for children must be prepared to provide care for the child's entire family.

In many surgical units, child life specialists are responsible for the psychological and emotional preparation of children before surgery. Nurses are typically responsible for

Acknowledgments: We wish to thank Earline Robinson for her assistance in the preparation of this manuscript, and Ellen Hollon, MS, CCLS, Frances Morriss, MD, and Stan Davis, MD, for commenting on earlier drafts of this chapter.

physical preparation of children for surgery. Surgical preparation of children and families cannot be divided by health care provider or body system. Children and families will seek information as they are ready to address their fears and concerns. Therefore, all members of the health care team must be comfortable addressing surgical preparation. The trusted primary care provider is often the first member of the health care team asked to address family fears. At the surgical evaluation, the family may ask questions and seek clarification about the necessary procedure or they may be too shocked with the realization that surgery is needed to process the information provided by the surgeon. When the family has had time to formulate surgical questions, a nurse in the surgeon's office or the perioperative nurses may be approached for information. If a child life specialist's services are used in preparing the patient for surgery, the specialist is also in a key position to provide developmentally appropriate information for the child. Home care nurses may be asked to clarify the surgical process if additional care is needed on returning home. Consistency in the information being provided reinforces teaching and secures patient and family trust in the health care team during this time of stress.

The purpose of this chapter is to provide general recommendations for surgery preparation and inform health care team members about the psychological and physical needs of children who require surgery. These needs are addressed in the context of the family. For additional procedure or diagnosis-specific information, please refer to appropriate chapters in this text.

PSYCHOLOGICAL PREPARATION: THE PATIENT

Cognitive development, psychological development, coping styles, and temperament all influence children's responses to surgery and hospitalization. The surgical experience is stressful for children and families. Surgery is a planned injury and includes separation from trusted adults; involves uncertainty about rules, expected behavior, and events; and has the potential for loss of control and autonomy. Children need assistance to cope adaptively during times of distress, anxiety, and pain. In the era of family-centered care, a significant support person (usually a parent) accompanies the child through most of the hospital experience. Parents are encouraged to participate in the care of their child. This necessitates that parents and children are provided with adequate information, guidance regarding their role, coping instructions, and support (Shelton & Stepanek, 1994). When parents and children are provided with this level of support at specific stress points during the hospitalization, they are less anxious, more cooperative, and more satisfied with the hospital experience (Wolfer & Visintainer, 1975). The limitations of managed care and cost containment have altered the timing of stress points. Admission often occurs on the morning of surgery for both inpatients and outpatients. The child no longer has time to become familiar with the hospital environment before going to the operating room (OR). Many hospital practices have changed to facilitate the reduction of stress at previously identified stress points. Preoperative injections are not routinely used, and parents often accompany the child into the OR and the recovery room. At present, the stress points are more likely to occur at admission, any time the child is separated from the parent, and during invasive procedures such as starting an intravenous (IV) line. The current literature continues to support the need for provision of information, role cues, coping skills instruction, and support for both the parent and the child (LaMontagne, Hepworth, Johnson, & Cohen, 1996; Thompson, 1994).

Psychosocial Assessment of the Child

Preparation must be tailored to the child's developmental level, coping style, and temperament. Child development theories developed by Piaget (1968) and Erikson (1964) describe cognitive and personality development that follows a predictable course. Table 1–1 demonstrates the developmental sequence with developmentally appropriate interventions to facilitate the child's transition through the surgical experience.

Coping Styles

Coping strategies vary from child to child, and each child can develop a greater repertoire of strategies with maturity. How the child defines the stress of the surgical experience is integral to facilitating adaptive coping. For younger children and children who adapt gradually, separation from parents may be the greatest stressor. Other children fear the painful

or unknown aspects of the experience. Preparation programs help the child who seeks information develop a better understanding of the surgical experience (Thompson, 1994). Programs that include parents in the OR or provide preoperative sedation are advantageous to children who fear separation. LaMontagne (1984, 1985, 1987) has described three coping styles in children relative to surgical preparation. Table 1–2 defines these coping styles. Children who use an avoidant style of coping prefer not to know extensive details about the surgery and rely on a support person to assist them in coping. Providing these children with more detailed information increases their anxiety. Children who use an active coping style want detailed information about the surgery. The children who use a combination of styles prefer general information. Children who prefer limited information are no more anxious without the information. However, other support mechanisms must be ensured (e.g., parental presence). Individual coping styles can be observed during the child's initial visit to the surgeon or by questioning the parent about the child's response to previous stressful encounters. It is important to assess the child's interest in preoperative information and to provide only the amount of preparation that the child needs.

Temperament

Temperamental attributes can greatly influence the child's response to the surgical experience. The degree to which a child approaches or withdraws in the face of a new experience and the child's level of adaptability can predict how the child will cope with the surgical experience (Chess & Thomas, 1987). Preparations can be altered for the "gradual adapter" (Carey & McDevitt, 1995) by telling the child what will happen next and giving the child time to prepare for the change. Many authors identify shy or quiet children to be more disruptive or more likely to have postoperative behavior disturbances when separated from their parents (Kain, Mayes, O'Connor, & Ciccheti, 1996; McGraw, 1994; Quinonez, Santos, & Boyar, 1997). Ask parents how the child handles new situations, such as starting a new school. Children who adapt slowly to everyday events are likely to need supportive interventions (extra time, parental presence, presedation) when coping with the surgical experience.

Assessing individual differences in children's coping styles and temperament are essential for appropriate preparation. Interventions directed at facilitating individual coping styles can greatly reduce the anxiety and postoperative behavior disturbances experienced by children having surgery.

PSYCHOLOGICAL PREPARATION: THE PARENTS

In most cases, the presence of parents in the hospital is beneficial to the child in terms of normalizing the environ-

Table 1–1 Developmental Influences in Children's Coping

Age	0–1 yr	1–3 yr	3–6 yr	6–12 yr	12–18 yr
Cognitive	Dependent on senses[a] Developing motor skills[a]	Egocentric thought[a] Language comprehension better than verbal skills[a]	Very inquisitive[a] Still egocentric[a]	Logical thought[a] Can consider other points of view[a] Understands body functioning at age 9	Mature reasoning[a] Deductive and hypothetical thought[a]
Psychosocial	Developing trust[b] Relies on consistent, appropriate response to needs[b]	Developing ability to control own body and emotions[b]	Increasing independence[b] Active imagination[b] Mixes fantasy and reality[b]	Achievement oriented[b] Developing mastery and self-esteem[b]	Development of identity and autonomy[b]
Specific fears	Separation from primary caregivers[c] Strangers	Separation[c] Abandonment[c] Dark Threats to body boundary[c]	Separation[c] Loss of control[c] Bodily injury[c] Imagined threats	Loss of bodily or emotional control[c] Bodily harm[c] Separation from family and peers	Loss of self-control Loss of autonomy Disfigurement[c] Disability
Coping ability	Depends on parental presence[c]	Depends on parental presence[c] Decreases in unfamiliar environment[c]	Depends on parental presence[c] Developing some internal coping skills[c]	Has small repertoire of coping skills; can be taught skills Preparation useful	Greater number of coping skills
Interventions	Ensure parental presence Limit strangers Keep normal routine	Parental presence Opportunities to control own body Therapeutic play Security objects	Parental presence Explain what they will experience (sensation) Participate in care	Parental support Peer or other adult support Preparation Teach coping skills Ensure privacy Participation in care	Parental and peer support Preparation Teach coping skills Ensure privacy Participation in care

[a] Piaget, 1968. [b] Erickson, 1964. [c] Stevens, 1981.

ment, providing support, and reducing stress. To decrease the stress and anxiety of parents whose children are having surgery, specific stressors and coping styles must be identified. The most stressful aspects of a child's hospitalization for the parent are related to the loss of the familiar parental role and uncertainty regarding both the outcome of the medical situation and predictability of events (LaMontagne, Hepworth, Pawlak, & Chiafery, 1992; LaMontagne, Johnson, & Hepworth, 1995; Mishel, 1983; Savedra, Tesler, & Ritchie, 1987; Wolfer & Visintainer, 1975). Parents need to negotiate their parental role with staff caring for their child and can be supported in their attempts to advocate for their child. Encourage parents to perform their usual caregiving tasks. Anticipatory guidance decreases anxiety (Schepp, 1991, 1992). Parents desire comprehensive information (Kain, Wang, Cramrico, Hofstader, & Mayes, 1997), especially during waiting periods (Savedra et al., 1987). Parental coping is greatly enhanced by timely updates from the OR or recovery room while waiting for their child in surgery (Mitiguy, 1986). Interventions aimed at reducing the stress of parents during their children's surgeries directly influence the children's coping and response to the surgical experience.

PREPARATION STRATEGIES

Many factors influence children's reactions to anesthesia, surgery, and hospitalization. Children's reactions result from their fears and misconceptions. There are five categories of children's fears: fear of (a) physical harm or bodily injury, including pain, mutilation, or death; (b) separation from or absence of a trusted adult, such as the child's parent; (c) the unknown or the possibility of surprise; (d) not behaving in the expected "acceptable" manner; and (e) loss of control (Wolfer & Visintainer, 1975). Of great concern is the evidence of emotional distress and behavioral disturbances after surgery and hospitalization (LeVieux-Anglin & Sawyer,

Table 1–2 Coping Styles of Children Preparing for Surgery

Behaviors	Interventions
Avoidant coping	
• Limits or avoids detailed information	• Information should not be too complex. Avoid details.
	• Reinforce what the child knows. Be aware of misconceptions about the illness or surgery and clarify with minor details.
• Focuses on Nature and reason for surgery Length of hospital stay	• Reassure child about his or her condition. • Express confidence in staff's skill in caring for children with this type of operation. • Assure the child that the surgery has been done many times without problems. • Introduce minor details about what the child will feel and be expected to do postoperatively.
• Is hesitant or unwilling to talk about feelings associated with the event	• Provide play as a vehicle of self-expression. • Provide books that deal with children overcoming obstacles. • Engage in play activity with the child to establish trust and encourage questions. • Encourage play with peers for support.
• Denies worry or is not specific as to what causes worry	• Accept denial as temporary coping. • Provide reassurance with supportive communication.
• Focuses on benefits of surgery	• Emphasize benefits (e.g., better vision, better health, ability to play sports, new friends in hospital).
• Uses parents as major support	• Encourage parents or supportive adults to be present before the child is anesthetized and to be waiting in the child's room when he or she returns. • Encourage parents to visit frequently and to be present during stressful procedures.
Active coping	
• Seeks detailed information	• Determine child's understanding of the problem and surgery. Focus on clarifying and modifying information.
• Focuses on How surgery will be performed Procedures involved Complications Benefits	• Encourage questioning and active participation in teaching. Use models or diagrams to illustrate explanation.
• Eagerly talks about the surgery and associated feelings	• Provide opportunities to explore and express feelings (e.g., child-nurse conversations, talks with other patients, play activities with peers).
• Acknowledges worry and is specific as to what causes worry	• Relieve worry when possible (e.g., clarify misconceptions, express confidence in well-trained staff).
• Focuses on benefits of surgery	• Emphasize benefits (e.g., better vision, better health, ability to play sports, new friends in hospital).
• Expresses concern about the negative postoperative outcomes Restrictions Pain Nausea and vomiting	• Focus on the reason for negative aspects (e.g., eye patches help keep the eye clean and protected). • Familiarize the child with ways nurses can help (e.g., helping the child to relax, giving medicine to relieve pain).
Avoidant-active coping	
• Seeks minor details: nature of surgery, how surgery will correct the problem	• Determine the child's understanding of the problem and surgery. Based on the child's answers, an appropriate explanation can be offered.
• Is willing to talk about the operation and feelings associated with the event	• Encourage the child to ask questions and provide clarification. • Check back frequently with the child for questions and concerns.
• Denies any worry or acknowledges one worry or fear	• Accept denial as temporary coping. • Clarify any concerns. • Teach positive thinking and relaxation techniques.
• Focuses on benefits of surgery	• Emphasize benefits (e.g., better vision, better health, ability to play sports, new friends in the hospital).
• Is aware of some negative postoperative outcomes Pain Fluid restrictions	• Elicit what the child knows and clarify information (e.g., tell the child why pain is expected and why fluid restrictions are necessary). • Familiarize child with ways nurses can help (e.g., providing medicine for pain, back rubs, helping to relax).

1993; Schmidt, 1990; Wolfer & Visintainer, 1975; Ziegler & Prior, 1994). Specific adverse reactions include preoperative agitation requiring physical restraint and postoperative psychological upset, such as bedwetting, nightmares, and disturbances in children's eating and sleeping patterns (Watcha, 1997; Wolfer & Visintainer, 1975). Preoperative preparation programs reduce or eliminate children's fears and anxiety and decrease the incidence of postoperative emotional distress and behavioral disturbances in children having both inpatient and outpatient day surgery (Ellerton & Merriam, 1994; Lynch, 1994; Schmidt, 1990; Ziegler & Prior, 1994). A review of specific strategies follows.

Providing Information

An increasing number of surgical procedures are being performed on an outpatient basis (Ellerton & Merriam, 1994; *1998 Health Care Almanac & Yearbook*). This shift demands that parents assume more responsibility for the psychological preparation of children experiencing surgery. Regardless of where the surgery takes place, parents are instrumental in providing and reinforcing information for thorough preparation of the child (Lynch, 1994).

Parents need to be well informed about the anticipated surgery so that they can accurately respond to their children's surgical questions and concerns (Coté, Todres, & Ryan, 1993). Ensure that parents have all the information they need. Information must be available to parents and reinforced throughout the surgical experience to reduce their anxiety and distress. Identify for parents appropriate sources for the information they seek.

Determine the child's and family's previous experience with surgery and hospitalization (Ziegler & Prior, 1994). Ask the family and child what they know about the upcoming surgery. Studies indicate that children and parents with previous surgical experience report greater levels of preoperative anxiety than those families who have no experience with surgery; thus preparation must be individualized in an attempt to correct misconceptions based on prior experiences (Ellerton & Merriam, 1994; Vetter, 1993). A child's preoperative anxiety may be merely a reflection of the parent's anxiety, and therefore it is essential to prepare both parent and child for surgery (Ellerton & Merriam, 1994; Lynch, 1994; Schmidt, 1990; Steward, 1995; Wolfer & Visintainer, 1975).

The child needs honest answers to questions (Mansson et al., 1992; Watcha, 1997; Ziegler & Prior, 1994). The child needs an accurate description of what, when, how, who, where, and why. Specifically, address with the child: Why do I need this operation? Who will be with me? What will happen? Will I hurt? Will I have a scar? When will I go home?

Provide the child with concrete information. Use descriptive and simple comparisons; specifically detail colors, sounds, feelings and sensations, size, and shapes. Avoid words the child may not understand or define a word for the child when a suitable synonym does not exist. For example "surgery" is another word for an "operation." "Anesthesia" is a medicine you will get by breathing into a mask; the medicine will make you sleep and make it so you cannot feel the operation; it is not a "nap." Many children are fearful that they will awaken in the middle of surgery (Coté et al., 1993). Include in the explanation of anesthesia that the child will be monitored closely and will not awaken until after the operation is completed. Avoid words that may have negative implications, such as "shot" or "put to sleep," or emotionally charged words; use "make an opening" rather than "cut you open" (Coté et al., 1993; Ziegler & Prior, 1994). The language of the OR can be easily misinterpreted by both children and their families. Try to use terms consistent with those the family uses to reinforce explanations. For example, if the family calls the procedure "surgery," the child and family may be confused when the words "surgery," "operation," and "procedure" are interchanged during explanations or by different members of the surgical team.

Provide children with both procedural and sensory information (Lynch, 1994; Wolfer & Visintainer, 1975). Preoperative procedural information should detail the sequence of operative events. Sensory information focuses on the sights, sounds, smells, taste, and feel of the operative experience. Descriptions, pictures, and videos provide some information about the look of the OR but lack the multisensory information children use to explore new experiences (Ziegler & Prior, 1994).

Active Participation

Provide the child with opportunities to practice his or her surgical role. Allow the child to be an active participant in the surgical process. For example, ask the child to help hold the mask over his or her mouth and nose, rather than just placing the mask on the child's face (Watcha, 1997). Provide the child with a genuine choice if and when there is one. For example, "do you want to walk or ride in the wagon to surgery?" rather than "are you ready to go to surgery?" Suggest positive coping strategies. For example, "you can squeeze my hand until it's over."

Role Cues

In new or stressful experiences, the child needs a role model. The child may be unable to determine what is socially acceptable or unacceptable behavior during a surgical or hospital experience (Wolfer & Visintainer, 1975; Ziegler & Prior, 1994). Research supports the effectiveness of using a filmed model to reduce children's preoperative anxiety (Robinson & Kobayashi, 1991). Videos, books, and slide presentations that support preparation programs typically include an appropriate patient role model. Build on these models. Examine books, videos, and other sources of information not prepared by the surgical site for developmental appropriateness of content, content accuracy, and applicability to the institution's surgical process (Manworren & Woodring, 1998).

Therapeutic Play

Children use play both to express their understanding of the world and to learn more about the world. They can master stressful situations through play (LeVieux-Anglin & Sawyer, 1993). Structured play activities that are designed to facilitate self-expression, develop coping mechanisms, and promote psychological well-being of children undergoing medical procedures and hospitalization are termed therapeutic play (Ziegler & Prior, 1994). Make use of therapeutic play activities in preoperative preparation programs to facilitate children's understanding of surgery and to provide a means to address fears and clarify misconceptions related to the surgical equipment and procedures. The tools of therapeutic play are similar to the tools of child's play. Examples of therapeutic play tools include stuffed animals, anatomically correct dolls, puppets, drawings, toy medical equipment, and real medical equipment (Ellerton & Merriam, 1994; Lynch, 1994; Ziegler & Prior, 1994).

PREPARATION PROGRAM DEVELOPMENT GUIDELINES

Preoperative preparation programs provide information, familiarize the family with the surgical process, encourage emotional expression, and teach coping strategies. Despite the reported positive impact of preoperative preparation, these programs are poorly attended (Agency for Health Care Policy and Research, 1992; Lynch, 1994; Vetter, 1993). Design preoperative preparation programs to accommodate the patient population. Consider the following elements when developing a preoperative program.

Attendance

Timing of a surgical preparation program depends on the child's interest and on the family's availability. Children 3 years of age and older benefit from surgical preparation regardless of the complexity of the procedure. Use the individual child's age as a guide. Schedule the program on the basis of a direct proportion between the number of days before surgery and the child's developmental age (e.g., prepare a 7-year-old up to 7 days before surgery). Older children and adolescents may need more time to cognitively and emotionally process the information provided and to formulate questions to clarify the information and their concerns (Ziegler & Prior, 1994). Participation in a preoperative preparation program is important for older children, adolescents, and children who have had previous surgeries because these children may be reluctant to express concerns or ask questions of their parents about surgery for fear of upsetting their parents. Unfortunately, older children and children who have had previous surgeries are less likely to attend preoperative preparation programs (Vetter, 1993).

Educators

Preoperative programs are facilitated by nurses, child life specialists, or both. Child life specialists strive to reduce the impact of stressful life events that affect the development, health, and well-being of children and families (Child Life Council, 1997). The child life specialist focuses preparation efforts on the child's point of view. The nurse or child life specialist clarifies medical information and terminology for the child and family. Hospital volunteers support preoperative preparation programs by assisting program educators.

Individualized versus Group Preparation: The Audience as the Guide

Preoperative preparation may occur individually or in a group setting. See Table 1–3 for a comparison of advantages and disadvantages of individual and group preparation programs.

Table 1–3 Advantages and Disadvantages of Group and Individual Preparation Programs

Group Preparation	Individual Preparation
• Less than 100% participation	• Increased time and cost for 100% participation
• OR needed less frequently for tour	• Availability of OR for tour may be limited
• Large groups can be disruptive	• Able to be sensitive and respond to child's cues
• Focus on information	• Focus on individual family
• Preset pace	• Pace set by family and family's needs
• Role models, surgery not unique	• Preserves patient confidentiality

Touring the Operating Room

The OR has unique sights, sounds, and smells that are difficult to describe and may be frightening to children having surgery. For children who are not sedated before surgery, preoperative tours of the OR should be included in the preparation when possible. Limited availability of the OR restricts OR access for a preoperative preparation tour. Infection control concerns are also cited for not allowing a tour of the OR; however, institutions have successfully adopted this practice without an increased incidence of operative infections.

Preoperative Sedation in Addition to Preparation

Historically, children were restrained to facilitate necessary medical procedures. Pharmaceutical agents are now available as an adjunct to psychological preparatory interventions. Most clinicians selectively recommend pharmaceutical agents in addition to psychological preparation (Mansson et al., 1992; Steward, 1995; Vetter, 1993). The pharmacologic agent must be carefully selected by weighing the preanesthetic benefits with the agent's postoperative side effects (Haber, 1990; Mansson et al., 1992; Steward, 1995; Vetter, 1993).

The primary goal of preoperative sedation is the quiet induction of anesthesia. Most pediatric patients are cooperative with anesthesia induction; therefore, routine use of preanesthetic sedatives is a costly practice that may be clinically unnecessary (Vetter, 1993). Children less than 6 years of age, however, are more likely to act distressed on parental separation for anesthesia induction than older children (Liu & Ryan, 1993; Vetter, 1993). If the child and parent must be separated before anesthesia induction, consider preoperative sedation for children less than 6 years of age and for children who are "gradual adapters" (Carey & McDevitt, 1995), children who have not had preoperative preparation, or children who have had previous negative surgical experiences (Steward, 1995; Vetter, 1993; Watcha, 1997).

PHYSICAL PREPARATION

Essential elements of a presurgical history and physical examination are reviewed in this section. The anesthetic and surgical implications of specific findings are presented. General laboratory testing and dietary restrictions are outlined. Painless induction strategies are also presented.

Preoperative Medical History and Physical

Obtain a thorough medical history and physical examination before any surgical procedure (American Academy of Pediatrics, Section on Anesthesiology, 1996). Essential elements of a routine examination include allergies, recent illnesses and illness exposure, current medications, birth history, anesthetic history, family medical history, review of body systems, and complete physical examination (American Academy of Pediatrics, Section on Anesthesiology, 1996; Coté et al., 1993; Haber, 1990) (see Table 1–4).

Allergies

A history of allergic reactions to medications and latex should be obtained (American Academy of Pediatrics, Section on Anesthesiology, 1996). One in every 5,000 to 25,000 anesthetic inductions is complicated by an allergic reaction, with a mortality rate of 3.4% (Green & McNiece, 1992). Common causes of anaphylactic reactions include antibiotics (especially penicillins), radiographic contrast agents, and latex products.

There has been increased awareness of the risk of allergic reactions from latex gloves and other latex-containing products. Reactions to latex can range from contact urticaria to bronchial asthma to anaphylactic shock and death (Blanco, Carillo, Castillo, Quiralte, & Cuevas, 1994; Green & McNiece, 1992). Latex products should, therefore, be avoided or used cautiously in all patients with a history of spina bifida or urologic problems requiring repeated surgeries (Porri et al., 1997). Healthy children with a latex allergy may give a history of urticaria or swelling of the lips and face after contact with latex balloons or foods that share common antigenic determinants to latex such as papayas, bananas, kiwi, raw potatoes, chestnuts, and avocados (Blanco et al., 1994).

Recent Illnesses or Illness Exposure

Children with a recent history of bronchitis, cough, or cold, and children with asthma are at a greater risk for irritable airway, laryngospasm, bronchospasm, cough, postoperative hypoxemia, and atelectasis with anesthesia (American Academy of Pediatrics, Section on Anesthesiology, 1996; Haber, 1990). Therefore, a recent history of an upper respiratory infection may necessitate canceling surgery.

Current Medications

By reviewing the medications the child has taken in the last two weeks, the examiner develops a picture of the child's health. Clarify for the parent that antipyretics and other over-the-counter medications, such as antihistamines, decongestants, antacids, and analgesics, should be included in the patient's list of current medications (American Academy of Pediatrics, Section on Anesthesiology, 1996). Discuss administration of routine medications on the day of surgery. Bronchodilators taken by nebulizer or inhaler should be administered just before anesthesia induction (American

Table 1–4 Review of Body Systems and Physical Examination

Conditions	Anesthetic/Surgical Implications
Head, eyes, ears, nose, throat	
• Hearing or vision loss	• Affects staff's ability to communicate with child. • Remove and secure glasses, contact lenses, or hearing aids.
• Loose or broken teeth	• Avoid unintentional loss or injury during intubation.[a,b]
Respiratory	
• Airway disturbances	• May affect intubation (laryngomalacia, micrognathia). • Increase the risk of postanesthetic apnea (sleep apnea).
• History of asthma, bronchopulmonary dysplasia, or cystic fibrosis	• Describe severity, symptoms, triggers, and last exacerbation. • Optimize medical management in anticipation of surgery.[a,c]
Cardiovascular	
• Cardiac murmurs	• Identify any cardiac condition before surgery.[d] • May require subacute bacterial endocarditis prophylaxis.[e]
Gastrointestinal	
• Gastroesophageal reflux	• Dietary restrictions may need to be modified.
• History of vomiting or diarrhea	• May be dehydrated and/or have an electrolyte imbalance.[a] • Consider laboratory confirmation and fluid and electrolyte restoration.
Genitourinary	
• Urinary frequency	• May indicate infection or diabetes.
• Routine intermittent catheterization	• Communicate care requirements to the perioperative staff.
Neurologic	
• Intracranial hypertension risk	• Anesthesia can alter intracranial and cerebral perfusion pressures.[f]
• Seizures	• Assess frequency, duration, and characteristics of seizures.[c] • Evaluate any recent change in the patient's seizure pattern. • Anesthesia and preoperative anxiolytics may alter seizure threshold.[b]
• Developmental delays?	• Anesthetic implications of degenerative neuromuscular disorders.[a] • Consider referring the child for further evaluation.
Endocrine	
• Diabetes	• Surgery often scheduled as the first case in the morning.[b] • Know child's insulin requirements and acceptable serum glucose range.
• Adolescent females	• Determine menarche, menstrual cycle, and last menstrual period. • Rule out pregnancy with laboratory screening.[c]
Musculoskeletal	
• Contractures, plegias	• Prevent intraoperative injury.
Dermatologic	
• Alterations in skin integrity	• Prevent further injury.
• Contagious skin conditions	• Prevent transmission of infections and wound infections.
Hematologic/oncologic	
• Anemias or other blood disorders	• Require further laboratory evaluation.
• Receiving chemotherapy	• Chemotherapy can alter both cardiac and pulmonary functions.[c]
• Mediastinal masses	• Increased risk during anesthesia induction.

[a] Haber, 1990. [b] Coté et al., 1993. [c] American Academy of Pediatrics, Section on Anesthesiology, 1996. [d] Green & McNiece, 1992. [e] American Heart Association, 1997. [f] Watcha, 1997.

Academy of Pediatrics, Section on Anesthesiology, 1996). Medications that influence electrolyte status and cardiovascular function should be reviewed with the anesthesiologist to determine the appropriate time of administration or the need for laboratory evaluation.

Birth History

Obtain a prenatal and neonatal history. Conditions associated with prematurity such as apnea, subglottic stenosis, bronchopulmonary dysplasia, patent ductus arteriosus, and intraventricular hemorrhage may complicate the anesthetic plan (American Academy of Pediatrics, Section on Anesthesiology, 1996; Green & McNiece, 1992). Inquire about the child's birth weight, length of hospital stay, and length of time on ventilatory support after birth.

Anesthetic History

Inquire about the child's previous anesthetic experiences. Specifically, did the child have any problems with anesthesia, such as nausea, vomiting, prolonged recovery, or awareness during the procedure (American Academy of Pediatrics, Section on Anesthesiology, 1996)?

Family Medical History

It is unnecessary to obtain a full family medical history. Instead, the examiner focuses on information that assists in the development of the anesthetic and surgical plan. Specifically address family reactions to anesthetic agents, family history of neurodegenerative conditions, and a family history of inherited blood disorders. Families may recall a relative that required a prolonged hospitalization to "wake up" after anesthesia. This type of reaction to anesthesia is suspicious for a family history of atypical pseudocholinesterase. In patients with atypical pseudocholinesterase, succinylcholine is not metabolized and prolonged muscle relaxation results. The incidence of atypical pseudocholinesterase is 1 in 2,800 patients (Green & McNiece, 1992). If the family history indicates the possibility of this inherited condition, the anesthetic plan can be modified to avoid the use of succinylcholine.

The incidence of malignant hyperthermia is 1 in 15,000 anesthetics in children (Byers & Krishna, 1992). A malignant hyperthermia reaction consists of an unexplained increase in end-tidal CO_2, followed by tachycardia, tachypnea, and muscle rigidity. The reaction is finally defined by a rapid increase in temperature. Any history of a high or unexplained fever related to anesthesia administration in a family member requires further investigation. Malignant hyperthermia–susceptible individuals include those with a first-degree relative with the condition and those with neurodegenerative conditions, such as Duchenne muscular dystrophy, myotonic dystrophy, and myotonia congenita. Therefore, it is also important to screen for a family history of inherited neuromuscular degenerative conditions. A malignant hyperthermia reaction requires that a triggering agent, such as the volatile anesthetic agents halothane, isoflurane, sevoflurane, and the depolarizing muscle relaxant succinylcholine, be administered. If a strong suspicion of malignant hyperthermia susceptibility exists, the anesthetic plan can be altered to avoid these agents.

Finally, screen for inherited blood disorders, such as sickle cell anemia and hemophilia. These conditions are typically diagnosed through neonatal screenings and routine health maintenance examinations. However, a strong family history of such diseases requires that documentation of negative laboratory screening of these conditions be obtained before surgery.

Laboratory Testing

Routine laboratory testing of pediatric surgical patients is no longer recommended. Laboratory testing should be determined by the medical condition of the child and the nature of the surgery (Haber, 1990) (see Table 1–5).

DIETARY RESTRICTIONS

Children have a higher potential for fluid loss than do adults (Steward, 1995). Prolonged preoperative fasting may cause dehydration, hypoglycemia, ketosis, and discomfort from hunger (Gleghorn, 1997; Steward, 1995). Therefore, periods of fluid restriction must be minimized and closely monitored so that significant dehydration is avoided before anesthetic induction. Statistically, the risk of aspiration during anesthesia administration in healthy children is 1 in 10,000 anesthetics (Gleghorn, 1997). Recent studies conclude that in healthy children no increase in gastric volume or decrease in gastric pH occurs when the child is allowed apple juice 2 hours before surgery compared with children fasted for longer periods of time preoperatively (American Academy of Pediatrics, Section on Anesthesiology, 1996; Gleghorn, 1997; Phillips, Daborn, & Hatch, 1994). Therefore, abstinence from clear liquids longer than 2 hours before surgery is unnecessary (Gleghorn, 1997; Watcha, 1997). Current preoperative fasting recommendations for healthy children, developed by the Society of Pediatric Anesthesiologists and the American Academy of Pediatrics, are presented in Table 1–6. Institutional dietary restriction recommendations may vary (Green & McNiece, 1992).

TRANSITION TO THE OPERATING ROOM

Preoperative Medications

Several goals exist for the use of preoperative medications, including (1) reduction of secretions, (2) preventing autonomic reflex response, (3) antiemetic effect, (4) reduction of gastric volumes, (5) increased gastric pH, (6) anxiety reduction, (7) amnesia, and (8) sedation (Haber, 1990; Hoffer, 1995; Liu & Ryan, 1993; Morris, 1990; Steward, 1995). Intraoperative medication administration for management of secretions to prevent autonomic reflex response and control nausea and vomiting are currently recommended (Green & McNiece, 1992).

Histamine receptor (H_2) blocking agents, such as cimetidine, ranitidine, and famotidine, have been used to increase

Table 1–5 Preoperative Laboratory Screening Recommendations and Indications

Laboratory Test	Indication
Hemoglobin[a–e]	Very young children, especially those with a history of prematurity. Children with chronic illnesses. Children with a history of recent blood loss. Children having surgeries in which a significant blood loss is expected.
Type and crossmatch	Obtain whenever extensive blood loss caused by the operative procedure is expected. If time is sufficient for donation processing and the child is appropriate for directed donor transfusions or autologous transfusions, the risks and benefits of these procedures should then be addressed with the family.
Electrolytes, kidney and liver function	Determine hydration and electrolyte status. Further evaluate children with renal or hepatic problems.
Platelet counts, prothrombin time (PT), partial thromboplastin time (PTT)	Should be obtained for patients with a history of bleeding disorders.
Blood gas analysis	May be desired in patients with chronic lung disease or congenital heart disease.
Chest radiograph[e,f]	Evaluate a child with a recent history of pneumonia or severe respiratory infection.
Urinalysis (UA)	Suspected urinary tract infection.
Beta human chorionic gonadotrophin (HCG)	Postmenarche females.

[a] Green & McNiece, 1992. [b] Watcha, 1997. [c] Steward, 1995. [d] American Academy of Pediatrics, Section on Anesthesiology, 1996. [e] Coté et al., 1993. [f] Haber, 1990.

gastric pH preoperatively (Green & McNiece, 1992; Hoffer, 1995). Metoclopramide has been used with mixed results to reduce preoperative gastric volumes. As previously noted, the risk of aspiration during anesthesia administration in healthy children and the morbidity from anesthesia-related aspiration are minimal (Gleghorn, 1997). Therefore, routine use of preoperative medications to decrease gastric volume and neutralize gastric pH is not recommended. Patients with delayed gastric motility or needing emergency surgery may, however, benefit from an H_2 antagonist (Haber, 1990).

Midazolam provides for preoperative anxiety reduction, amnesia, and sedation effects (American Academy of Pediatrics, Section on Anesthesiology, 1996; Feld, Negus, & White, 1990; Hoffer, 1995; Steward, 1995). Because anxiety reduction is the primary purpose of preoperative sedatives, the oral route is considered superior to the IV, intramuscular (IM), or rectal route in children (Feld et al., 1990; Haber,

Table 1–6 Preoperative Fasting Recommendations for Healthy Infants and Children

	Age	Recommendation
Milk/solids	< 6 months	Up until 4 hr before surgery
	6–36 mo	Up until 6 hr before surgery
	> 36 mo	Up until 6–8 hr before surgery
Clear liquids	< 6 months	Up until 2 hr before surgery
	6–36 mo	Up until 3 hr before surgery
	> 36 mo	Up until 3 hr before surgery

1990; Hoffer, 1995; Steward, 1995). Significant sedation is achieved after 30 minutes at a dose of 0.25 mg/kg to 1 mg/kg (maximum dose of 20 mg) midazolam given orally (Feld et al., 1990; Watcha, 1997). The high-dose requirements necessary to achieve sedation and the anxiolytic effect is due to the limited bioavailability, incomplete absorption, and first-pass metabolism after oral administration (Feld et al., 1990; Liu & Ryan, 1993). The IV preparation of midazolam has a bitter taste (if given orally) and has been routinely sweetened by mixing it in a sweetened solution, including acetaminophen or ibuprofen suspension for oral administration (Coté et al., 1993; Steward, 1995; Watcha, 1997). In October 1998, Roche pharmaceuticals introduced an oral preparation of midazolam.

Other anxiolytic or sedative agents may be selected on the basis of the experience of the patient, the anesthesiologist, and the institution's policies (Haber, 1990; Watcha, 1997). Regardless of the agent administered, sedation guidelines from the American Academy of Pediatrics, Committee on Drugs (1992) or other protocols consistent with professional standards should be followed for all sedated patients (Joint Commission, 1996). These guidelines address minimal monitoring requirements for children receiving sedatives and general anesthetic agents (American Academy of Pediatrics, Committee on Drugs, 1992).

Painless Induction

Anesthesia induction of the pediatric patient is commonly accomplished by administering inhalation agents in combination with nitrous oxide and oxygen by mask technique (Watcha, 1997). This is the preferred method of initial anesthesia delivery because of children's universal fear of needles (Agency for Health Care Policy and Research, 1992; Liu & Ryan, 1993; Watcha, 1997). Pediatric anesthesia masks come in flavors or can be altered with flavored cooking oils or lip balm to encourage placement directly on the child's face while detracting from the unpleasant smell of the inhalation agents (Haber, 1990). Children enjoy sampling the variety of smells and being able to select their favorite mask. If intravenous induction is necessary, pharmacologic agents can be used to minimize the pain of starting an IV line. Three topical agents are successfully and routinely used for this purpose: ethyl chloride, EMLA, and Numby Stuff (American Academy of Pediatrics, Section on Anesthesiology, 1996; *AHFS Drug Information*, 1997; Ashburn et al., 1997; Astra USA, Inc., 1993; Gebauer Company, 1994; IOMED, Inc., 1996; Watcha, 1997).

Parental Presence

Several studies indicate that parents wish to be present when their child is in the induction phase of general anesthesia (Blesch & Fisher, 1996; Braude, Ridley, & Sumner, 1990; Donnelly, 1991; McMahon, 1989). Most parents surveyed believed they could comfort and reassure their child during this stressful time (McMahon, 1989). Those parents who wished to be present for anesthesia induction cited the child's anxiety, parental duty, parental anxiety, and concerns about the child's memories of the experience as their motivation for wanting to be present (Braude et al., 1990; Donnelly, 1991). Parents who had participated in their child's anesthesia induction believed that it was appropriate for them to be with their child and that they would want to be present again if their child needed subsequent anesthesia (Donnelly, 1991). Parents who did not wish to be present stated that concern about interfering in the induction and their own anxiety had influenced their decision (Braude et al., 1990).

Conflicting evidence exists as to whether parental presence for anesthesia induction actually benefits the child (Liu & Ryan, 1993; Steward, 1995; Watcha, 1997). Some studies conclude that anxious parents may increase the anxiety of the child during anesthesia induction (Johnston, Bevan, Haig, Kirnon, & Tousignant, 1988; Steward, 1995). However, allowing a parent to be present during anesthesia induction has been shown in several studies to decrease children's emotional distress, decrease children's postoperative pain, and reduce the incidence of psychological sequelae (Agency for Health Care Policy and Research, 1992; Hannallah & Rosales, 1983; Johnston et al., 1988; Schulman, Foley, Vernon, & Allan, 1967). Refer to Exhibit 1–1 for guidelines about parental inclusion at the time of anesthesia induction.

CONCLUSION

Preoperative preparation encompasses cognitive, psychological, and physical preparation of the child for surgery. Just as each child's physical presentation is unique, so are the psychological needs of each child. Preparation of the child and family for surgery must be focused on their unique needs and must include a holistic approach to the physical and psychological preparation of the child for surgery. Parental presence facilitates a more positive coping response from the child, and parents must be included as much as possible in the child's surgical experience. Attempts to individualize preoperative preparation are highly beneficial to the child's overall surgical experience.

Exhibit 1–1 *Parental Inclusion for Anesthesia Induction*

1. Parents must want to be present. No parent is forced to be with his or her child for anesthesia induction; however, a suitable substitute may by sought.[a,b]
2. Patient safety is of the utmost importance. Therefore, children with airway problems and young children are excluded from the program.[c,d]
3. The parent is prepared preoperatively for the experience and supported emotionally after the experience by a familiar nurse.[e]
4. The parent should be informed about the sequence of events, how the child will look during anesthesia induction, and how the child may react, as well as what the parents role will be.[a,c–f]
5. The parent may sit next to the child or the child is comforted in the parent's lap as inhalation anesthesia commences.[d,g]
6. Parents are encouraged to touch, sing, tell stories, and reassure their children during anesthesia induction.[g]
7. The parent should be escorted from the induction area when the child is no longer aware of his surroundings.[a,c,e,f]

[a] Murphy, 1992. [b] Johnston et al., 1988. [c] Hannallah & Rosales, 1983. [d] Lewyn, 1993. [e] Gauderer, Lorig, & Eastwood, 1989. [f] Steward, 1995. [g] Isaacs, 1988.

14 NURSING CARE OF THE GENERAL PEDIATRIC SURGICAL PATIENT

REFERENCES

1998 Health care almanac & yearbook (1998). New York: Faulkner and Gray.

Agency for Health Care Policy and Research. (1992). *Acute pain management: Operative or medical procedures and trauma* (pp. 37–55). Rockville, MD: U.S. Department of Health and Human Services.

AHFS drug information 97. (1997). Ethyl chloride (pp. 2747–2748).

American Academy of Pediatrics, Committee on Drugs. (1992). Guidelines for monitoring and management of pediatric patients during and after sedation for diagnostic and therapeutic procedures. *Pediatrics, 89*(6), 1110–1115.

American Academy of Pediatrics, Section on Anesthesiology. (1996). Evaluation and preparation of pediatric patients undergoing anesthesia. *Pediatrics, 98*(3), 502–508.

American Heart Association, Committee on Rheumatic Fever, Endocarditis, and Kawasaki Disease. (1997). Prevention of bacterial endocarditis: Recommendations by the American Heart Association. *JAMA, 277*, 1794–1801.

Ashburn, M.A., Gauthier, M., Love, G., Basta, S., Gaylord, B., & Kessler, K. (1997). Iontophoretic administration of 2% lidocaine HCl and 1:100,000 epinephrine in humans. *The Clinical Journal of Pain, 13*, 22–26.

Astra USA, Inc. (1993*). Bibliography and abstracts or research studies.* Westborough, MA: Author.

Blanco, C., Carrillo, T., Castillo, R., Quiralte, J., & Cuevas, M. (1994). Latex allergy: Clinical features and cross-reactivity with fruits. *Annals of Allergy, 73*, 309–314.

Blesch, P., & Fisher, ML. (1996). The impact of parental presence on parental anxiety and satisfaction. *AORN Journal, 63*(4), 761–768.

Braude, N., Ridley, S.A., & Sumner, E. (1990). Parents and paediatric anaesthesia: A prospective survey of parental attitudes to their presence at induction. *Annals of the Royal College of Surgeons of England, 72*(1), 41–44.

Byers, D.J., & Krishna, G. (1992). Malignant hyperthermia. *Seminars in Pediatric Surgery, 1*(1), 88–95.

Carey, W.B., & McDevitt, S.C. (1995). *Coping with children's temperament: A guide for professionals.* New York: Basic Books.

Chess, S., & Thomas, A. (1987). *Know your child: An authoritative guide for today's parents.* New York: Basic Books.

Child Life Council. (1997). Mission statement of the child life profession. *Child Life Council Bulletin, 14*(4).

Coté, C.J., Todres, I.D., & Ryan, J.F. (1993). Preoperative evaluation of pediatric patients. In C.J. Coté, J.F. Ryan, I.D. Todres, & N.G. Goudsouzian (Eds.). *A practice of anesthesia for infants and children* (pp. 39–54). Philadelphia: W.B. Saunders Company.

Donnelly, J. (1991). A question of parent in the anaesthetic room. *The British Journal of Theatre Nursing 28*(3), 4–5.

Ellerton, M.L., & Merriam, C. (1994). Preparing children and families psychologically for day surgery: An evaluation. *Journal of Advanced Nursing, 19*, 1057–1062.

Erikson, E. (1964). *Childhood and society* (Rev. ed.). New York: W.W. Norton & Company.

Feld, L.H., Negus, J.B., & White, P.F. (1990). Oral midazolam preanesthetic medication in pediatric outpatients. *Anesthesiology, 73*(5), 831–834.

Gauderer, M.W.L., Lorig, J.L., & Eastwood, D.W. (1989) Is there a place for parents in the operating room? *Journal of Pediatric Surgery, 24*(7), 705–707.

Gebauer Company. (1994). Ethyl chloride package insert. Cleveland, OH: Author.

Gleghorn, E.E. (1997). Preoperative fasting: You don't have to be cruel to be kind. *Journal of Pediatrics, 131*(1), 12–13.

Green, M.C., & McNiece, W.L. (1992). Preoperative evaluation and preparation of the pediatric patient. *Seminars in Pediatric Surgery, 1*(1), 4–10.

Haber, D. (1990). Preanesthetic assessment of the pediatric patient. *Anesthesiology Clinics of North America, 8*(4), 759–784.

Hannallah, R.S., & Rosales, J.K. (1983). Experience with parents presence during anaesthesia induction in children. *Canadian Anaesthesia Society Journal, 30*(3), 286–289.

Hoffer, J.L. (1995). Anesthesia. In M.H. Meeker & J. C. Rothrock (Eds.). *Alexanders' care of the patient in surgery* (pp. 143–181). St. Louis, MO: Mosby.

IOMED, Inc. (November 13, 1996). Needle-free, local dermal anesthesia in minutes now available. Press release.

Isaacs P.J. (1988). Crises prevention in an outpatient surgery center. *Maternal Child Nursing, 14*, 352–354.

Johnston, C., Bevan, J.C., Haig, M.J., Kirnon, V., & Tousignant, G. (1988). Parental presence during anesthesia induction. *AORN Journal, 47*(1), 187–194.

Joint Commission on Accreditation of Healthcare Organizations. (1996). *1997 Hospital accreditation standards.* Oakbrook Terrace, IL: Author.

Kain, Z., Mayes, L.C., O'Connor, T.Z., & Ciccheti, D.V. (1996). Preoperative anxiety in children: Predictors and outcomes. *Archives for Pediatric Adolescent Medicine, 150*, 1238–1245.

Kain, Z., Wang, S.M., Cramico, L.A., Hofstader, M., & Mayes, L.C. (1997). Parental desire for perioperative information and informed consent: A two-phase study. *Anesthesia and Analgesia, 84*, 299–306.

LaMontagne, L.L. (1984). Three coping strategies used by school-age children. *Pediatric Nursing, 10*(1), 25–28.

LaMontagne, L. (1985). Facilitating children's coping: Preoperative assessment interviews. *AORN Journal, 42*(5), 718–723.

LaMontagne, L. (1987). Children's preoperative coping: Replication and extension. *Nursing Research, 36*(3), 163–167.

LaMontagne, L., Hepworth, J.T., Johnson, B.D., & Cohen, F. (1996). Children's preoperative coping and its effects on postoperative anxiety and return to normal activity. *Nursing Research, 45*(3), 141–147.

LaMontagne, L., Hepworth, J.T., Pawlak, R., & Chiafery, M. (1992). Parental coping and activities during pediatric critical care. *American Journal of Critical Care, 1*, 76–80.

LaMontagne, L., Johnson, B.D., & Hepworth, J.T. (1995). Evolution of parental stress and coping processes: A framework for critical care practice. *Journal of Pediatric Nursing, 10*(4), 212–218.

LeVieux-Anglin, L., & Sawyer, E.H. (1993). Incorporating play interventions into nursing care. *Pediatric Nursing, 19*(5), 459–463.

Lewyn, M.J. (1993). Legal Q & A: Should parents be present while their children receive anesthesia? *Anesthesia Malpractice Protector, May,* 56–57.

Liu, L.M.P., & Ryan, J.F. (1993). Premedication and induction of anesthesia. In C.J. Coté, J.F. Ryan, I.D. Todres, & N.G. Goudsouzian (Eds.). *A practice of anesthesia for infants and children* (pp. 135–149). Philadelphia: W.B. Saunders Company.

Lynch, M. (1994). Preparing children for day surgery. *Children's Health Care, 23*(2), 75–85.

Mansson, M.E., Fredrikzon, B., & Rosberg, B. (1992). Comparison of preparation and narcotic: Sedative premedication in children undergoing surgery. *Pediatric Nursing, 18*(4), 337–342.

Manworren, R.C.B., & Woodring, B. (1998). Evaluating children's literature as a source for patient education. *Pediatric Nursing, 24*(6), 548–553.

McGraw, T. (1994). Preparing children for the operating room: Psychological issues. *Canadian Journal of Anaesthesia, 41*(11), 1094–1103.

McMahon, K. (1989). Parents in the anaesthetic room. *Nursing Standard, 3*, 9–11.

Mishel, M. (1983). Parents' perception of uncertainty concerning their hospitalized child. *Nursing Research, 32*(6), 324–330.

Mitiguy, J. (1986). A surgical liaison program: Making the wait more bearable. *MCN, 11*, 388–392.

Morris, F.C. (1990). Anesthesia: Perioperative principles. In D.L. Levin & F.C. Morris (Eds.). *Essentials of pediatric intensive care* (pp. 434–452). St. Louis, MO: Quality Medical Publishing, Inc.

Murphy, E.K. (1992). OR nursing law: Issues regarding parents in the operating room during their children's care. *AORN Journal, 56*(1), 120–124.

Phillips, S., Daborn, A.K., & Hatch, D.J. (1994). Preoperative fasting for paediatric anaesthesia. *British Journal of Anaesthesia, 73*, 529–536.

Piaget, J. (1968). *Psychological studies.* D. Elkind (Ed). (A. Tenzer, Trans). New York: Random House.

Porri, F., Pradal, M., Lemiere, C., Birnbaum, J., Mege, J.L., Lanteaume, A., Charpin, D., Vervloet, D., & Camboulives, J. (1997). Association between latex sensitivity and repeated latex exposure in children. *Anesthesiology, 86*(3), 599–602.

Quinonez, R., Santos, R.G., & Boyar, R. (1997). Temperament and trait anxiety as predictors of child behavior prior to general anesthesia for dental surgery. *Pediatric Dentistry, 19*(6), 427–431.

Robinson, P.J., & Kobayashi, K. (1991). Development and evaluation of a presurgical preparation program. *Journal of Pediatric Psychology, 16*(2), 193–212.

Savedra, M., Tesler, M., & Ritchie, J. (1987). Parents' waiting: Is it an inevitable part of the hospital experience? *Journal of Pediatric Nursing, 2*(5), 328–332.

Schepp, K. (1991). Factors influencing the coping effort of mothers of hospitalized children. *Nursing Research, 40*(1), 42–46.

Schepp, K. (1992). Correlates of mothers who prefer control over their hospitalized children's care. *Journal of Pediatric Nursing, 7*(2), 83–89.

Schittroth, L. (Ed.). (1994). *Statistical record of children* (p. 424). Detroit, MI: Gale Research, Inc.

Schmidt, C.K. (1990). Pre-operative preparation: Effects on immediate pre-operative behavior, post-operative behavior and recovery in children having same day surgery. *Maternal-Child Nursing Journal, 19*(4), 321–330.

Schulman, J.L., Foley, J.M., Vernon, D.T.A., & Allan, D. (1967). A study of the effect of the mother's presence during anesthesia induction. *Pediatrics, 39*(1), 111–114.

Shelton, T.L., & Stepanek, J.S. (1994). *Family-centered care for children needing specialized health and developmental services.* Bethesda, MD: Association for the Care of Children's Health.

Stevens, K.R. (1981). Humanistic nursing care for critically ill children. *Nursing Clinics of North America, 16*(4), 611–622.

Steward, D.J. (1995). New thoughts on preparation and premedication of children. *Current Reviews for Post Anesthesia Care Nurses, 17*(2), 11–15.

Thompson, M. (1994). Information-seeking coping and anxiety in school-age children anticipating surgery. *Children's Health Care, 23*(2), 87–97.

Vetter, T. (1993). The epidemiology and selective identification of children at risk for preoperative anxiety reactions. *Anesthesia Analgesia, 77*, 96–99.

Watcha, M.F. (1997). Anesthesia. In D.L. Levin & F.C. Morris (Eds.). *Essentials of pediatric intensive care* (2nd ed., pp. 587–603). New York: Churchill Livingstone.

Wolfer, J.A., & Visintainer, M.A. (1975). Pediatric surgical patient's and parents' stress responses and adjustment. *Nursing Research, 24*, 244–255.

Ziegler, D.B., & Prior, M.M. (1994). Preparation for surgery and adjustment to hospitalization. *Nursing Clinics of North America: Pediatric Surgical Nursing, 29*(4), 655–669.

CHAPTER 2

Perioperative Management
of the Child

Kathleen M. Leack

INTRODUCTION

Those who care for the pediatric surgical patient recognize that multiple factors make this population challenging and unique. Perioperative care of the pediatric surgical patient includes not only general knowledge of the proposed surgical procedure and care of a patient in the operating room suite. It also includes the specific understanding of a child's airway and physiologic responses to surgery and anesthesia, an understanding of child development, and care of the child and family (Fairchild, 1996; Noble, Micheli, Hensley, & McKay, 1997). This chapter discusses the care of the pediatric surgical patient in the preoperative holding room, the operating room suite, and transfer to the postanesthesia care unit (PACU).

PREOPERATIVE CARE

A child may come into the care of the pediatric general surgeon electively or emergently. After the referring physician suspects the child has a surgical condition, that child is referred to the surgeon for evaluation and treatment. After diagnosis, the surgeon explains the surgical procedure, its risks and benefits, expectations of surgical recovery (inpatient vs. outpatient status), and timing of the proposed procedure. Consent is obtained from the parents. For children who reside in foster care or in other situations without their legal guardian, appropriate efforts must be made to contact and obtain informed consent from the legal guardian, whether that means the biologic parents or a state agency (Crawley & Gourville, 1994). The support services of an interpreter should be obtained to explain the surgical procedure for families whose primary language is not English (Mooney, 1997).

Once the emergency or elective procedure is scheduled, the family should be given preoperative instructions explaining nothing by mouth (NPO) guidelines and other required preoperative evaluation and testing. Depending on the nature of the proposed surgical procedure and the patient status at that time, the surgeon may request that the patient have a type and crossmatch completed with blood prepared and available for surgery. The surgeon explains the risks and benefits of blood transfusion to the parents. If circumstances allow, directed blood donation by a family member or friend is arranged. In those instances in which blood transfusion is likely and the parents have religious or cultural beliefs that preclude this intervention, the surgeon needs to discuss the use of alternative blood volume–expanding products, if applicable. In some cases, the surgeon may obtain a court order to transfuse the child as medically necessary (Reed, 1996). These issues need to be handled preoperatively with care and sensitivity.

A urine pregnancy test may be ordered preoperatively in the adolescent girl (Dunn, 1997). Unexpected positive results need to be dealt with in a judicious manner.

In addition to meeting with the surgeon preoperatively, the child is also seen by the anesthesiologist. This may occur several days before the proposed procedure or on the day of the procedure. The anesthesiologist obtains a health history, an evaluation of the patient's response to a previous anesthetic, and any family history of anesthetic experiences. A determination of intraoperative and postoperative anesthetic risk is made. The anesthesiologist explains anesthesia and postoperative pain control (Landsman & Cook, 1998). Preoperative opportunities for the parents to discuss their questions and concerns with the physicians that will be caring for their child in the operating room increases their comfort.

For those children who have an electively scheduled procedure, many pediatric institutions have a preoperative education day or tour. The aim of this tour is to prepare the child for the experience of surgery and anesthesia (LaRosa-Nash,

Murphy, Wade, & Clasby, 1995). Further information regarding preoperative preparation can be found in Chapter 1 of this text.

Before sending a child to surgery, the unit nurse prepares the patient and the appropriate paperwork. A preoperative checklist is completed before the child leaves the unit. Items for review include, but are not limited to, NPO status, assessment of other medical diagnoses, allergies, operative consent, completed laboratory work, and radiologic testing (Dunn, 1997; Stellar, 1991). As part of the preoperative care, the nurse on the inpatient or day surgery unit may be the person to premedicate the patient (e.g., midazolam [Versed]) (Mooney, 1997). The goal of premedication is to allay anxiety, provide analgesia, or both (Landsman & Cook, 1998). All efforts are made to have the child and family ready for surgery at the prearranged time to maintain the flow of the operating room schedule. In the event of a delay in the preoperative preparation, the surgeon and the operating room charge nurse need to be informed (Dunn, 1997).

PREOPERATIVE: HOLDING ROOM

The holding room nurse reviews the paperwork after the child and family arrive in the holding room. The holding room nurse monitors the patient for adverse reactions to preoperative medication (Dunn, 1997). A calm environment provides an easy transition into the operating room. Efforts are made to promote patient comfort and to minimize anxiety (Dunn, 1997). Distraction techniques, such as toys and videos, aid in decreasing anxiety (Noble et al., 1997).

A family's perioperative experience can be anxiety provoking. Nursing interventions geared toward alleviating those fears include timely introductions and explanation of the holding room routine, providing opportunities for parents to be involved in their child's care, and reassuring the parents that the child will be safe (Dunn, 1997; Noble et al., 1997). All parents should be assessed for the need for extra supportive care, whether the proposed surgical procedure is planned or an emergency. The child life specialist or chaplain may be called in at this time (Noble et al., 1997). In addition to providing an environment that minimizes anxiety, opportunities for privacy should also be provided, whether that is for discussion or physical examination (Dunn, 1997).

The family meets again with the surgeon and anesthesiologist to review the plan of care and to address questions or concerns. The family also meets with the operating room nurse who will be caring for the child. The operating room nurse discusses his or her role and the manner in which the family will be updated during the surgical procedure (Dunn, 1997; Mooney, 1997).

When parents are present at anesthesia induction, the parent, in appropriate attire, accompanies the child into the operating room suite (Larosa-Nash & Murphy, 1997). If parents are not present for anesthesia induction, the child is transferred by cart or carried into the operating room. Parents should be directed to the waiting area and it should be explained when and where the parents will be able to see their child after the surgical procedure is completed.

INTRAOPERATIVE ROLES

Institutional differences alter the roles of the operating room nursing personnel. The scrub nurse prepares the equipment on the instrument table specific to the surgical procedure to be performed. Current and accurate surgeon preference cards are essential for pediatric surgical cases. These cards list the surgeon's preference for suture material and instruments specific to the anticipated procedure. The preference card should be updated whenever a routine changes (Fuller, 1994).

The circulating nurse advocates for the patient, assists with anesthesia induction, assists in positioning the patient for the procedure, completes the surgical preparation, and assists the surgical team by obtaining equipment during the procedure (Mooney, 1997). The circulating nurse assists the scrub nurse in keeping a correct count of items used (e.g., sponges and needles) (McConnell, 1987). In addition, the circulating nurse is responsible for documenting the nursing interventions occurring in the operating room and updating the family during the surgical procedure (Mooney, 1997).

GENERAL NURSING CONSIDERATIONS OF THE PEDIATRIC PATIENT IN THE OPERATING ROOM

Although standards of nursing practice are followed in the operating room, it is necessary to tailor care to the pediatric surgical patient. Issues that can affect patient status in the operating room and postoperatively include, but are not limited to, temperature regulation, fluid and electrolyte balance, positioning, and skin integrity (Fairchild, 1996).

Patient safety is the underlying theme of all nursing interventions. Interventions to promote patient safety while the child is awake include not leaving the child's side and keeping harmful objects out of the child's reach. After anesthesia induction, safety measures include placement of restraint devices that do not impede the cardiorespiratory status of the child and proper placement of monitoring devices and electrocautery grounding devices (Fairchild, 1996; Wahoff-Stice, 1995).

INDUCTION OF ANESTHESIA

After the child enters the operating room, monitoring leads are placed on the child's chest and a pulse oximetry probe is placed on a digit. Other monitoring devices include a blood pressure cuff, a temperature probe, and an end-tidal CO_2 probe (Mooney, 1997). Arterial or venous monitoring devices required for patient assessment during the surgical procedure are usually placed after induction.

The role of the anesthesiologist is to provide adequate anesthesia in correlation to the proposed duration and specific surgical procedure. The care of the child at anesthesia induction requires knowledge of child development and the ability to calm the fearful child (Landsman & Cook, 1998). For induction, it is necessary to provide a quiet, soothing environment where those present are focused on the child and not on other preparations for the planned procedure.

Anesthesia induction occurs with either an inhalation agent (e.g., halothane, desflurane, sevoflurane) or an intravenous (IV) agent (e.g., propofol) (Burns, 1997). Inhalation is the preferred route of induction because many children enter the operating room without an IV line in place. Inhalation agents have a smell that the pediatric patient finds unpleasant. Children who are frightened of the mask required to provide the anesthetic agent are more willing to participate in induction if given the opportunity to choose an aromatic oil to place on their mask (LaRosa-Nash & Murphy, 1997). Preoperative preparation also plays a role in decreasing a child's anxiety by increasing understanding and voluntary cooperation.

Inhalation agents are fast acting, thus decreasing the time that the child is awake and anxious in the operating room environment. Assess the patient for hypotension, bradycardia, and laryngospasm, the most common adverse effects of inhalation induction (Landsman & Cook, 1998).

Knowledge of the structural differences of the pediatric airway is necessary at the induction of anesthesia. The pediatric airway is more anterior and cephalad compared with adults (Yaster & Wetzel, 1997). More head extension is necessary to properly align the airway for endotracheal intubation (Fontana, 1993). The pediatric airway is more prone to obstruction. The tongue may fall back and obstruct the airway or neck flexion can obstruct the pliable pediatric airway (Hedman-Dennis, 1991; Noble et al., 1997). The narrow pediatric airway requires a loosely fitting endotracheal tube. Compression of the tracheal mucosa by a large endotracheal tube can lead to edema formation. Tracheal edema can lead to glottic spasm at the time of extubation (Noble et al., 1997; Yaster & Wetzel, 1997).

In addition to specific issues regarding the pediatric airway, chest wall pliability and diaphragmatic function also affect ventilation. Tightly placed safety straps restrict chest wall expansion that occurs with respiration/ventilation. An overdistended stomach alters diaphragmatic function, which impedes diaphragmatic lengthening and lung expansion. Passage of a nasogastric tube at the time of intubation allows for gastric decompression. This intervention relieves excess air from the stomach that occurred with preinduction crying and air swallowing, with air entry into the stomach occurring with bag and mask ventilation, and with air entry into the stomach after esophageal intubation (Noble et al., 1997).

SURGICAL PREPARATION AND POSITIONING

While the child is being prepared for the surgical procedure, maintenance of the patient's temperature is crucial. Infants and children are sensitive to their environment, and changes in core body temperature can occur rapidly (Noble et al., 1997). Temperature regulation is more difficult because a child has a higher body surface/weight ratio than an adult does (Fontana, 1993). A thermoneutral environment should be provided. Interventions include adjustment of the temperature of the operating room (a minimum of 10 minutes before the child is expected to enter), warming lights, and warming pads (Fairchild, 1996). Other methods to protect against heat loss include plastic covering or loosely wrapping areas that will not be in the surgical field (Cunningham, 1995; Noble et al., 1997).

Continuous temperature monitoring is essential throughout the entire operative procedure. Temperature instability occurs with heat loss through evaporative or convective losses (Fontana, 1993; Noble et al., 1997). Evaporative heat losses occur through prolonged exposure of the viscera to the environment. Efforts should be made to cover exposed viscera with warmed moist gauze pads. Instilled irrigant should also be warmed (Stellar, 1991). Convective losses occur when a child lies in a pool of fluid (e.g., bodily fluids or preparation solution). To avoid convective heat loss, the nurse should intervene by using careful technique with surgical preparation and by using gauze sponges and suction devices to absorb excess drainage (Fairchild, 1996). The result of hypothermia causes the child's metabolism to increase, which leads to an increase in oxygen consumption and potential hypoxemia.

After anesthesia induction and placement of necessary IV lines and tubes (nasogastric tubes, Foley catheters, etc.), position the patient appropriately for the planned procedure. Positioning goals include proper body alignment, avoidance of skin breakdown and nerve damage, adequate pulmonary expansion, adequate circulation and tissue perfusion, and optimal surgical exposure (Noble et al., 1997). Young infants and children are more flexible than their older counterparts. Hyperextension and/or hyperflexion should be avoided when positioning the pediatric patient (Fairchild, 1996). In addition, modified positioning supports that complement the size of the child should be used to maintain proper body alignment. Padding devices include folded blankets, foam pads cut to size, or gel pads (Stellar, 1991). It is necessary to prevent skin breakdown by adequately padding pressure points (i.e., bony prominences) (Fairchild, 1996). The child should be positioned for the specific surgical procedure and the correct body part or limb included in the surgical procedure should be verified.

Electrosurgery cautery, a high-frequency current, is frequently used for hemostasis during the operative procedure. A dispersive electrode/grounding pad is placed to allow the current to safely pass though the patient's body (Wahoff-Stice, 1995). The patient's skin integrity should be examined before placing the electrocautery-grounding device. The device is placed on an area with sufficient muscle mass nearest to the surgical site (Mooney, 1997). Inappropriately placed dispersive pads can lead to burns where the energy exits the body (Wahoff-Stice, 1995).

The circulating nurse completes the surgical preparation after positioning the patient. The goal of the surgical preparation is to remove superficial skin soil and flora (Kneedler & Dodge, 1991; McConnell, 1987). Attention should be paid to the manner in which the preparation is completed.

After the surgical preparation is completed, the patient is draped, leaving the surgical field exposed. The purpose of surgical draping is to establish a sterile field. The drapes are resistant to liquid penetration, which prevents pooling of secretions under the patient (McConnell, 1987).

DURING THE OPERATION

For further information regarding a specific pediatric surgical procedure, refer to the appropriate chapter in this text.

During the operation, the placement of heavy instruments on the patient should be avoided. Prolonged accidental pressure caused by instruments placed on the sterile field or scrubbed personnel leaning on the patient can cause an alteration in skin integrity (Noble et al., 1997).

During the surgical procedure, the child's fluid and electrolyte and hemodynamic status should be assessed. Intraoperative IV fluid rates are calculated to include fluid replacement from the time that the child was NPO for the procedure in addition to maintenance fluid rate. Most patients receive lactated Ringer's solution intraoperatively. The electrolyte composition of this fluid is similar to that of serum (Landsman & Cook, 1998). Urine output needs to be monitored intraoperatively, especially for longer cases. A fluid shift from intracellular and extracellular spaces into the interstitial spaces occurs during the surgical procedure. The patient may exhibit signs of hypovolemia despite correctly calculated fluid replacement. Intravenous fluid boluses for decreased urine output should be provided (Landsman & Cook, 1998). In addition to fluid shifts, fluid imbalances occur with insensible fluid losses. One method to decrease these fluid losses is to cover the exposed viscera with warmed moist gauze pads (Fuller, 1994).

The nursing team assists the surgeon and anesthesiologist with evaluation of blood losses by weighing gauze pads and surveying drainage in the suction collection canister (Fairchild, 1996; Landsman & Cook, 1998). For excessive fluid or blood losses, transfusion with blood or its components may be necessary. The team considers the patient's current age, underlying medical conditions, preoperative hematocrit and platelet count, and nature of operation when determining the need for blood replacement (Landsman & Cook, 1998). If the patient is to be transfused, the blood should be warmed to prevent hypothermia.

The surgical team may request assessment of laboratory work during the procedure. These laboratory tests may include hemoglobin and hematocrit, serum electrolytes, and blood gases. In addition, serum glucose may be monitored in the young infant. Infants have high glucose requirements and are at high risk for hypoglycemia when stressed (Hedman-Dennis, 1991). Infants do not have sufficient glycogen stores to meet the increased metabolic needs caused by the stress of surgery. To support this need, IV dextrose is provided to maintain serum glucose (Fontana, 1993).

The goals of the proposed procedure may be exploratory or diagnostic, curative or palliative. The case may be considered to be minor or major, elective or emergent. Parents should be kept updated during the procedure. The circulating nurse will have talked with the family before the case to discuss methods (phone call vs. face-to-face update) and timing of updates (Mooney, 1997). In the case of unexpected findings or intraoperative death, the family needs honest information, provided by the circulating nurse or the surgeon, as the patient's status warrants (Onstott, 1998).

Wound closure at the end of the procedure is determined by the nature of the surgery (Ballard, 1991). The surgeon determines the specific type of suture and method of wound closure. A nonabsorbable suture may be used when a wound is anticipated to heal slowly; conversely, absorbable suture material may be used when a wound is expected to heal rapidly (Rout, 1991a). For a "clean" case without contamination, the wound will be closed primarily. A suturing technique in which the suture material is buried under the skin may be the chosen method for wound closure. This avoids the need for suture removal, a procedure that most children find painful and anxiety provoking (Noble et al., 1997). The wound may then be covered with Steri Strips. Another choice for wound coverage is a transparent liquid dressing (Collodion) that lasts 3 to 6 days before peeling off. The advantage to this type of dressing is that it protects the wound from moisture, specifically those incisions that fall below the diaper line of a young child (Gruendemann & Meeker, 1987).

Some wounds are closed with staples rather than sutures. Staples provide a quick method for wound closure, particularly when the patient is unstable. Staples are removed after 5 to 7 days (Wahoff-Stice, 1995).

If the case is considered "dirty," the surgeon may leave the skin open and allow it to heal by secondary intention. Montgomery straps are placed when frequent wound dressing changes are anticipated (Gruendemann & Meeker, 1987).

Depending on the nature of the case, surgical drains or tubes are placed. The drain acts as a route for fluid to exit the site where it is prone to collect. A Penrose drain is the most common type of drain used to establish a drainage tract. Other systems may be used if closed suction is required. Most drains are brought out through a separate stab wound because an increase in wound infection is noted when the drain is brought through the primary incision (Rout, 1991b). All external drainage devices need to be secured to prevent accidental dislodgment of the device. Other considerations at the end of the surgical procedure include placement of a dressing over an implanted device (central venous line or gastrostomy tube) or placement of ostomy pouches (over stomas).

When the surgical procedure has been completed, anesthesia reversal occurs and the child emerges from anesthesia. During emergence from anesthesia, the child's respiratory efforts are assessed. Children are generally extubated when they have awakened from anesthesia because they are more susceptible to laryngospasm and upper airway obstruction if not fully awake (Mooney, 1997).

Before transfer to the postanesthesia care unit (PACU), a head-to-toe assessment of the patient is made, looking for changes from the preoperative state. This patient assessment focuses on inspection of the skin to assess for alterations in skin integrity, temperature (skin and core temperature), and hydration (Mooney, 1997; Stellar, 1991). Variances from baseline can alter metabolism, oxygenation, and comfort.

TRANSFER TO THE POSTANESTHESIA CARE UNIT

Once the child has been transported to the PACU, the operating room nurse gives a verbal report to the PACU nurse. Items included in this report include current status of the child (vital signs, assessment of comfort), surgical procedure, the child's response to surgery and anesthesia, and assessment of the surgical wound and drains (Stellar, 1991).

Continuous monitoring of a child's cardiopulmonary status is essential in the immediate postoperative period. Maintaining a patent airway and maximizing ventilation are the main priorities of the PACU nurse (Meyer-Pahoulis, 1994). Pediatric patients are prone to postanesthesia complications that include apnea, airway obstruction, aspiration, postextubation croup, laryngospasm, and bronchospasm. These postoperative issues reflect the fact that a child's airway is

reactive and easily obstructed. Postoperative airway obstruction results from incorrect positioning, pooling of secretions, or airway edema caused by intubation. Interventions to promote ventilation include assisting with airway positioning until the child is awake enough to maintain his or her own airway, administering oxygen, and suctioning the patient as needed (Meyer-Pahoulis, 1994). Despite short transport times, a child's oxygen saturation can be affected by length of transport from the operating room suite to the PACU. This is due to hypoventilation, suboptimal airway positioning, and the breathing of room air. The patient's oxygen saturation should be monitored on entering the PACU and intervention with supplemental oxygen should be used as needed for decreased oxygen saturation (Fossum & Knowles, 1995).

Apnea can occur postoperatively. The incidence of postoperative apnea in preterm infants is higher than in term infants. Infants less than 52 weeks postconception have an increased risk of postanesthesia apnea. This is most commonly due to the increased airway reactivity of the preterm infant. Although these effects are short lived, the infant must be observed carefully for a minimum of 12 hours before discharge or for 12 hours after the last apneic event (Sims & Johnson, 1994). Postoperative laryngospasm, bronchospasm, and croup are due to irritation of the airway by inhalation agents or secondary to edema caused by a tightly fitting endotracheal tube (Meyer-Pahoulis, Williams, Davidson, McVey, & Mazurek, 1993).

In addition to maximizing optimal ventilation, other goals of the PACU nurse include promoting fluid and electrolyte balance, maintaining adequate perfusion, maintaining body temperature, and promoting comfort (Hedman-Dennis, 1991). For the child who enters the PACU hypothermic, warmed thermal blankets and warming lights are used to restore the child's body temperature (Hershey, Valenciano, & Bookbinder, 1997).

Minimizing anxiety and controlling postoperative pain is another role of the PACU nurse. Postoperative pain is managed with intermittent narcotics or initiation of patient-controlled analgesia, epidural infusions, or acetaminophen. For further information about postoperative pain management, refer to Chapter 6 in this text.

Developmentally focused comfort activities aid in decreasing pain and anxiety. Activities such as allowing an infant to suckle on a pacifier, holding the inconsolable toddler, and using distraction techniques, such as toys, music, or videos for the preschooler, help the postoperative child settle. Older children and adolescents may have questions about their surgical procedure and current status. These questions should be answered honestly (Meyer-Pahoulis, 1994). Because of the success of parental presence at anesthesia induction, many institutions are now implementing a program that allows parental presence in the PACU (Smith & Bassett, 1996).

MISCELLANEOUS PERIOPERATIVE CARE ISSUES

Latex Allergy

One significant issue affecting perioperative care is latex allergy. With the recent increase in the practice of universal precautions, more patients have come in contact with latex. When some patients come in contact with latex, an immunoglobulin E–mediated allergic response occurs. The symptoms and severity vary in each patient. Some children experience mild symptoms, such as urticaria and wheezing, whereas others experience anaphylaxis with associated bronchospasm and hypotension. Many of the early reported cases of adverse effects related to latex allergies occurred in the operating room suite. Direct contact of latex with the airway or the thoracic or abdominal cavity may elicit a life-threatening event (Young & Meyers, 1997). Since the correlation has been made between latex and direct patient exposure, many institutions now have policies to protect patients from latex exposure. Some interventions include a latex-free cart and a frequently updated and easily accessible listing of institutionally used products and their latex content. Other institutions are developing a latex-free environment to decrease exposure for patients and health care workers.

An example of formatting a latex-free chart for institutional use is shown in Table 2–1. Table 2–2 provides a list of latex products and their latex-free alternatives.

Care must be taken preoperatively to assess the patient for environmental allergies. Certain foods, such as bananas and avocados, have been linked with latex allergy, although the cross-reactivity is not fully understood. A correlation between children with spina bifida or genitourinary anomalies and latex allergy has also been made (Young & Meyers, 1997). Latex allergy increases in populations that have frequent exposure to latex, such as bladder catheterizations or operative procedures with anesthesia. The allergic reaction occurs when the patient is exposed to an allergen to which he or she is sensitized.

Whether children have had an allergic response to latex or are in a high-risk group, latex precautions should be implemented. These children should be identified as such in the medical record and by allergy banding (Young & Meyers, 1997).

Trauma

One role of the pediatric general surgeon is that of trauma team member. Some traumatically injured children require immediate surgical intervention. Occasionally, an unstable traumatically injured child requires immediate surgical intervention before parents are available to give their consent. An attempt should be made to notify the family by phone. When the family is unavailable and urgent surgical intervention is required, the surgeon must document the need to proceed without parental consent (Davis & Klein, 1994).

In the event of an urgent trip to the operating room, the child's full trauma workup may not be completed. Cervical spine precautions need to be maintained at all times (Pokorny & Haller, 1991). Members of the trauma team may request that specific laboratory work be sent because the child's history may be unclear or unknown. Laboratory screening includes urine human chorionic gonadotropin and serum and urine toxicologic screens. The results of these tests should be shared with the operating trauma team. Positive results need postoperative follow-up.

In the event that the child was injured as the result of a crime (e.g., gunshot wound, motor vehicle crash), the child's clothing or bullet fragments are evidence for the police (Weigel, 1991). The evidence for the police should be clearly labeled. Specifics about evidence that was removed and given to the police should be documented in the patient's medical record. Further information on evidence gathering can be obtained from institutional and community policies.

Pediatric Human Immunodeficiency Virus

Because of the current medical advancements in the care of pediatric human immunodeficiency virus (HIV) and acquired immune deficiency syndrome (AIDS), opportunities for the HIV-positive child to enter into the surgical domain

Table 2–1 Master Latex List by Description

Hospital Item Number	Description	Manufacturer	Manufacturer's Item Number	Latex Content	Description of Latex Content
	Airway NP Robertazzi 20 Yellow	Rusch International	1230-20F	Latex	Entire product is made of latex
	Cannula nasal pediatric	Salter Labs	1602	No latex	
	Catheter Foley 10 F, w/ temp probe	Medtronic Inc.	2442	Awaiting response	

Table 2–2 Commonly Used Products and Latex-Free Alternatives

Products Containing Latex	Latex-Free Alternatives
Nipple—brown latex or Nuk Orthodontic (Ross Pediatrics)	Nipple—latex free (Evenflo) or Nipple Twist on Premature (Abbott)
Tape—adhesive (Johnson & Johnson) or Perma-Pink Tape	Tape—Durapore (3M) or Transpore (3M)
Catheter—Pezzer (Bard) or Red Rubber (Baxter)	Catheter—Mentor (Mentor Urology) or Silicone Foley (Sherwood Medical)
Gloves—Brown milled/sterile (Professional Medical) or Glove Surgeon/sterile (Ansell Perry)	Gloves—Sensicare Exam/clean (Maxxim Medical) or Tactylon/sterile (Tactyl Technologies)
IV Bags—most IV solutions—medication port contains latex	May use IVF—place tape over medication port—do not puncture
Chest drain—Pleur-Evac (Deknatel)—suction tubing contains latex	May use product—wrap parts containing latex with gauze to prevent patient contact

are increased. Some children require surgical access for nutritional support (i.e., enteral or venous). Special considerations of the patient include management of pulmonary issues/chronic lung processes (e.g., lymphocytic interstitial pneumonitis), cardiac issues (e.g., left ventricular hypertrophy), and hematologic problems (e.g., anemia). Considerations pertaining to the specific surgical procedure include universal precautions, double gloving, and avoidance of direct passage of sharps (Crawley & Gourville, 1994). Contaminated instruments are soaked, prerinsed, washed, rinsed, and sterilized with various enzymatic and detergent agents. The surgical suite is cleaned, again using various enzymatic and detergent agent, with specific attention to spilled body fluid (Groah, 1996).

Care of the Family When Intraoperative Death Occurs

Often the pediatric surgical team cares for critically ill children. Intraoperative death is usually a rare occurrence in a nontrauma situation. The family needs open and honest communication as the information is available on the status

of their child. One role of the perioperative nurse in this situation is to prepare the body for viewing and to assist the family with their emotional needs for closure. Special care of the family also includes enabling their religious and cultural beliefs. A chaplain can be very helpful at this time (Onstott, 1998). For further information on the death of a child, refer to Chapter 8 of this text.

CONCLUSION

Caring for the pediatric patient in the perioperative period requires knowledge of surgical procedures, a child's physiologic response to surgery and anesthesia, and child development. A child is a unique individual with physiologic responses different than the adult. Although it is important to understand pediatric physiology and the pediatric airway, it is also necessary to understand the developmental stages the child moves through. The child is part of a family unit, and parents need to be included in their child's surgical experience.

REFERENCES

Ballard, A.G. (1991). Sutures: An overview of wound closure. *Point of View, 28*(3), 8–13.

Burns, L.S. (1997). Advances in pediatric anesthesia. *Nursing Clinics of North America, 32*(1), 45–67.

Children's Hospital of Wisconsin. (March 1998). *Master latex list.*

Crawley, T., & Gourville, L.S. (1994). Surgical intervention in children with HIV infection. *Nursing Clinics of North America, 29*(4), 631–643.

Cunningham, S.M. (1995). Positioning of infants and children for surgery. *Seminars in Perioperative Nursing, 4*(2), 112–116.

Davis, J.L., & Klein, R.W. (1994). Perioperative care of the pediatric trauma patient. *AORN Journal, 60*(4), 559–565.

Dunn, D. (1997). Responsibilities of the preoperative holding area nurse. *AORN Journal, 66*(5), 820–844.

Fairchild, S.S. (1996). *Perioperative nursing: Principles and practice* (2nd ed.). Boston: Little, Brown and Company.

Fontana, J.L. (1993). Anesthetic considerations for neonatal and infant patients. *Seminars in Perioperative Nursing, 2*(1), 33–37.

Fossum, S.R., & Knowles, R. (1995). Perioperative oxygen saturation levels of pediatric patients. *Journal of Post Anesthesia Nursing, 10*(6), 313–319.

Fuller, J.R. (1994). *Surgical technology: Principles and practice* (3rd ed.). Philadelphia: W.B. Saunders Company.

Groah, L.K. (1996). *Perioperative nursing* (3rd ed.). Stamford, CT: Appleton & Lange.

Gruendemann, B.J., & Meeker, M.H. (1987). *Alexander's care of the patient in surgery.* St. Louis, MO: Mosby.

Hedman-Dennis, S. (1991). Stabilization of the sick infant or child. *Journal of Post Anesthesia Nursing, 5*(3), 165–169.

Hershey, J., Valenciano, C., & Bookbinder, M. (1997). Comparison of three rewarming methods in a postanesthesia care unit. *AORN Journal, 65*(3), 597–601.

Kneedler, J.A., & Dodge, G.H. (1991). *Perioperative patient care: The nursing perspective* (2nd ed.). Boston: Jones & Bartlett Publishers.

Landsman, I.S., & Cook, D.R. (1998). Pediatric anesthesia. In J.A. O'Neill, M.I. Rowe, et al. (Eds.), *Pediatric Surgery* (5th ed., pp. 197–228). St. Louis, MO: Mosby.

LaRosa-Nash, P.A., & Murphy, J.M. (1997). An approach to pediatric perioperative care: Parent-present induction. *Nursing Clinics of North America, 32*(1), 183–199.

LaRosa-Nash, P.A., Murphy, J.M., Wade, L.M., & Clasby, L.L. (1995). Implementing a parent-present induction program. *AORN Journal, 61*(3), 526–531.

McConnell, E.A. (1987). *Clinical considerations in perioperative nursing.* Philadelphia: J.B. Lippincott Company.

Meyer-Paholis, E. (1994). Pediatric postanesthesia care. *Plastic Surgical Nursing, 14*(2), 92–107.

Meyer-Paholis, E., Williams, S.L., Davidson, S.I., McVey, J.R., & Mazurek, A. (1993). The pediatric patient in the post anesthesia care unit. *Nursing Clinics of North America, 28*(3), 519–530.

Mooney, K.M. (1997). Perioperative management of the pediatric patient. *Plastic Surgical Nursing Journal, 17*(2), 69–73.

Noble, R.R., Micheli, A.J., Hensley, M.A., & McKay, N. (1997). Perioperative considerations for the pediatric patient: A developmental approach. *Nursing Clinics of North America, 32*(1), 1–16.

Onstott, A.T. (1998). Perioperative nursing care when sudden patient death occurs in the OR. *AORN Journal, 67*(4), 829–836.

Pokorny, W.J., & Haller, J.A. (1991). Pediatric trauma. In E.E. Moore, K.L. Mattox, & D.V. Feliciano (Eds.), *Trauma* (2nd ed., pp. 689–702). Stamford, CT: Appleton & Lange.

Reed, D.A. (1996). *Blood on the altar: Confessions of a Jehovah's Witness minister.* Buffalo, NY: Prometheus Books.

Rout, W.R. (1991a). Closure of wound. In G.D. Zuidema (Ed.), *Shackelford's surgery of the alimentary tract* (3rd ed., pp. 333–348). Philadelphia: W.B. Saunders Company.

Rout, W.R. (1991b). Drainage of abdominal wounds. In G.D. Zuidema (Ed.), *Shackelford's surgery of the alimentary tract* (3rd ed., pp. 327–330). Philadelphia: W.B. Saunders Company.

Sims, C., & Johnson, C.M. (1994). Postoperative apnea in infants. *Anaesthesia and Intensive Care, 22*(1), 40–45.

Smith, L., & Bassett, C. (1996). Introducing change to the post-anaesthetic care unit. *Nursing Standard, 11*(9), 36–38.

Stellar, J.J. (1991). Pediatric surgery. In M.H. Meeker & J.C. Rothrock (Eds.), *Alexander's care of the patient in surgery* (9th ed., pp. 980–1003). St. Louis, MO: Mosby.

Wahoff-Stice, D. (1995). Surgical wound management. In R.A. Roth (Ed.), *Perioperative nursing core curriculum* (pp. 312–340). Philadelphia: W.B. Saunders Company.

Weigel, C.J. (1991). Medicolegal aspects of trauma. In E.E. Moore, K.L. Mattox, & D.V. Feliciano (Eds.), *Trauma* (2nd ed., pp. 839–846). Stamford, CT: Appleton & Lange.

Yaster, M., & Wetzel, R. (1997). Pediatric anesthesia. In K.T. Oldham, P.M. Colombani, & R.P. Folgia (Eds.), *Surgery of infants and children: Scientific principles and practice* (pp. 327–357). Philadelphia: Lippincott-Raven.

Young, M.A., & Meyers, M. (1997). Latex allergy: Considerations for the care of pediatric patients and employee safety. *Nursing Clinics of North America, 32*(1), 169–182.

CHAPTER 3

Fluid and Electrolyte Management of the Pediatric Surgical Patient

Nancy Rabin

INTRODUCTION

The fluid management of the pediatric surgical patient is a critical element of pediatric care (Rice, Caty, & Glick, 1998). Fluid and electrolyte management of pediatric patients must be extremely precise if these patients are to maintain homeostasis (Helikson & Wolfson, 1993). This chapter reviews considerations in maintaining the fluid and electrolyte status in the pediatric surgical patient in the preoperative, intraoperative, and postoperative phases. It includes a review of deficits, maintenance, and replacement calculations, as well as fluids used in the pediatric surgical patient.

BODY FLUID COMPARTMENTS AND COMPOSITION

Three key factors influence fluid and electrolyte balance and are different in infants and small children than in adults: internal distribution of water, insensible water losses, and kidney function (O'Donnell & Lathrop, 1993). The first major concern is how infants and small children distribute and regulate water. The newborn is made up of approximately 75% to 80% total body water. This falls to about 60% by the time the child reaches 1 year of age. Not only is there more water in the child's body but it is also distributed slightly differently than in an adult. Body fluids are distributed in two main functional compartments: intracellular fluid (ICF) and extracellular fluid (ECF). The primary intracellular cation is potassium, and the primary electrolyte in the ECF is sodium. In the neonate most of the body water is distributed in the extracellular space. Less body water is in the extracellular space in the adult. The ECF is the fluid located outside the cells and includes the intravascular (plasma) and interstitial fluid. The extracellular space is located within the blood vessels, around the cells, and around the brain and spinal cord. The ICF is that located within the cell (Hazinski, 1988). Approximately half of a child's ECF is exchanged every 24 hours. This means that the infant has a greater daily fluid requirement with little fluid volume reserve. Thus, any increase in fluid loss rapidly leads to dehydration (O'Donnell & Lathrop, 1993). Infants and small children also have larger body surface areas than adults. This causes increased fluid losses from evaporation (Fann, 1998). Changes in the ECF volume are the most frequent and important abnormalities encountered in the surgical patient (Schwartz, 1999).

The next important factor contributing to the child's fluid status is that of insensible water loss. Insensible water loss is the invisible, continuous, passive loss of water from the skin (evaporation), lungs (respiration), and metabolism (Statter, 1992). One can estimate daily insensible water losses by multiplying 300 ml by the child's body surface area. In addition to insensible water losses being normally greater in children, they are often increased because of illness or medical treatment (Hazinski, 1988). Fever increases insensible water losses by about 10 ml/kg/°C for each degree above 37°C (Radhakrishnan & Geissler, 1996). Radiant warmers and phototherapy lights also increase insensible losses and should be considered a source of potential increased output (Fann, 1998). Insensible fluid losses from the skin and lungs do not contain salt (Schwartz, 1999); thus, they are electrolyte free (Hellerstein, 1993).

The final physiologic factor affecting a small child's fluid status is the maturity of the kidneys (O'Donnell & Lathrop, 1993). During the first 2 years of life, the kidneys are functionally immature and unable to effectively concentrate or dilute urine, and the mechanisms for sodium regulation are not yet mature. They are also inefficient at excreting waste products of metabolism. Because of this, if infants or small children receive too much fluid, they are not able to increase their urine output and hypervolemia quickly develops and signs of fluid overload are seen. As a result, fluid and electrolyte imbalances may develop and progress quickly (O'Donnell & Lathrop, 1993).

For all the preceding reasons, infants and small children are prone to electrolyte imbalances developing because of the pediatric surgical patient's changing physiology (Rice et al., 1998).

NORMAL EXCHANGE OF FLUID AND ELECTROLYTES

Osmosis is the movement of a fluid through a semipermeable membrane from a solution that has a lower solute concentration to one that has a higher solute concentration. Osmolality refers to the number of particles (proteins and electrolytes) per liter of water. A solution with the same osmolality as blood plasma is called isotonic (Fecteau, 1999). Serum osmolality is maintained at approximately 272 to 300 mOsm/L. Acute changes in serum osmolality produce free water shifts. Free water moves from an area of low osmolality to an area of higher osmolality (Headrick, Hazinski, & Alexander, 1999). A decreased serum osmolality usually indicates low sodium concentration, whereas an increased serum osmolality usually indicates a high concentration of sodium caused by hypernatremia or dehydration (O'Donnell & Lathrop, 1993).

PREOPERATIVE CONSIDERATIONS

A critical part of assisting the pediatric surgical patient to maintain fluid and electrolyte balance is preoperative assessment and identification of risk factors for fluid and electrolyte imbalances. Preoperative laboratory analysis of electrolyte levels should be checked if indicated by the history and physical examination and any abnormalities corrected to within normal limits before any surgical procedure, unless surgery is needed to correct a life-threatening problem (Letton & Chwals, 1997). Preexisting conditions, such as diabetes mellitus, liver disease, or renal insufficiency may be aggravated by surgical stress, increasing a child's risk of fluid and electrolyte imbalances. Preoperative medications may affect the excretion of water and electrolytes. Preoperative surgical regimens, such as administration of enemas or laxatives, may act to increase fluid loss from the gastrointestinal tract. Medical management of preexisting conditions can affect fluid and electrolyte balance (Fecteau, 1999).

Preoperative fluid restrictions are used to reduce nausea, vomiting, and aspiration risk in the surgical patient. Yet, for the neonate or young infant who is accustomed to eating on an every-3-hour basis and whose maintenance volume requirement is significantly greater than the volume requirements of an adult, this type of restriction can lead to significant dehydration. Infants require no more than 3 or at the most 4 hours to empty their stomachs of clear liquids (Filston, 1992). Because infants and toddlers have a greater relative body surface area and higher metabolic rate, "nothing by mouth" status places them at increased risk for fluid loss. It is recommended that they be scheduled as the first surgical cases of the day (Horne, Heitz, & Swearingen, 1997) or clear fluids be allowed up to 3 to 4 hours before surgery (Aker & O'Sullivan, 1998).

Preoperatively, the ECF volume must be restored. The emergency nature of the surgical intervention may preclude the correction of ICF composition or even a near-complete correction of the ECF composition. However, beginnings of such correction should be initiated in the preoperative phase, maintained throughout the operative course, and concluded in the postoperative phase (Finberg, Kravath, & Hellerstein, 1993).

CALCULATING FLUID AND ELECTROLYTE REQUIREMENTS

Fluid therapy should be approached by categorizing water and electrolyte requirements into deficit, maintenance, and replacement therapy (Hellerstein, 1993). Fundamental to any system of fluid management is an accurate determination of the current volume and hydration status of the patient. Deficit therapy refers to the evaluation and management of the losses of fluid and electrolytes that occurred before the patient's presentation. There are three essential components to deficit therapy: an accurate estimation of the severity (degree) of dehydration; determination of the type of deficit that has occurred; and development of an approach to repair the deficit (Rice et al., 1998). Infants and children are relatively sensitive to small degrees of dehydration. Regardless of the management approach adopted to guide therapy, flexibility should take into account the changing physiology of the pediatric surgical patient (Rice et al., 1998).

The most common patient problems associated with fluid and electrolyte balance during surgery include fluid volume deficit, sodium and water imbalances, and potassium imbalances. Fluid volume deficit is an imbalance in isotonic body fluids related to either abnormal fluid loss or decreased oral intake. Children with acute surgical illnesses may have significant fluid and electrolyte deficits from poor oral intake, vomiting, diarrhea, peritonitis, sepsis, burns, or hemorrhage (Helikson & Wolfson, 1993).

The effect of fluid loss on the surgical patient depends on the amount of fluid lost and the speed at which the fluid is lost. A patient who loses fluid rapidly or who loses a large amount of fluid exhibits symptoms of shock (Fecteau, 1999). Extremities will be cool or cold, capillary refill time will be very sluggish, and metabolic acidosis will be present. The child will be oliguric or anuric, and tachycardia, tachypnea, and hypotension will be noted (Hazinski, 1988). The clinical signs and symptoms of classic dehydration are the result of ECF volume depletion: hypovolemia, decreased cardiac output, and decreased tissue perfusion. When approximately one third of ECF volume has been lost, marked physiologic disturbances become evident (Hellerstein, 1993). Intravascular volume must be rapidly restored to maintain adequate tissue perfusion for normal organ function, particularly if the child requires an urgent operation (Helikson & Wolfson, 1993). Dehydration often is characterized as mild, moderate, or severe (Fann, 1998). The degree of severity of dehydration is estimated from the patient's history and physical condition at the time of presentation (O'Donnell & Lathrop, 1993) (see Table 3–1). No single piece of laboratory data can predict the severity of dehydration. In children with mild dehydration (1% to 5% body fluid volume), the findings are largely historical. Children with moderate dehydration (6% to 10%) have a history of abnormal fluid and electrolyte losses, plus physical findings that include tenting of the skin, weight loss, sunken eyes and fontanel, slight lethargy, and dry mucous membranes. With severe dehydration (11% to 15%), the child has cardiovascular instability and neurologic involvement develop (Rice et al., 1998).

Treatment of the dehydrated child is based in large part on the degree of dehydration. To determine the degree of dehydration, it is necessary to calculate the percentage of weight loss (four steps): (1) determine baseline and current weight in kg, (2) determine weight loss (subtract current weight from baseline), (3) determine percentage weight loss (divide weight loss by baseline weight), and (4) determine dehydration status (compare percentage of weight loss to chart). The

degree of dehydration guides treatment. It is important to determine how much fluid has been lost to replace it correctly (Fann, 1998).

The child's fluid deficit refers to the estimated measurement of fluids lost during the illness before the initiation of treatment. This calculation is essential to accurate replacement of fluids because fluids lost during the illness must be replaced during the treatment. For each 1% weight loss, it is known that 10 ml/kg of fluid has been lost. By multiplying the number of milliliters per kilogram by the preillness weight, the fluid deficit can be determined (O'Donnell & Lathrop, 1993). ECF volume deficit is the most common fluid disorder in the surgical patient. The most common causes include loss of gastrointestinal fluids from vomiting, nasogastric suction, diarrhea, and fistula drainage (Schwartz, 1999).

The type of deficit that has occurred can be estimated from the child's electrolyte values. In large part, the type of dehydration is defined by the tonicity of the patient's serum. On this basis, states of dehydration are commonly referred to as isotonic (serum osmolality 270 to 300 mOsm/L, serum sodium 130 to 150 mEq/L), hypotonic (serum osmolality <270 mOsm/L, serum sodium <130 mEq/L), and hypertonic (serum osmolality >310 mOsm/L, serum sodium >150 mEq/L). Patients with hypertonic dehydration must be given special attention because of serious complications, such as central nervous system (CNS) changes from cerebral edema, which may occur during rehydration if plasma sodium levels are reduced by more than 10 mg/day. The period for repair of the deficit is 48 hours or longer in hypertonic dehydration

Table 3–1 Clinic Assessment Data

| Area of assessment | Degrees of Dehydration | | |
	Mild	Moderate	Severe
	Infant 5% loss	Infant 10% loss	Infant 15% loss
	Children 3% loss	Children 6% loss	Children 9% loss
Thirst	Slight	Moderate	Intense
Anterior fontanel	Flat	Depressed	Very sunken
Skin	Pale, cool	Grayish	Cool, pale, mottled[a]
Blood pressure	Normal	Decreased	Low[a]
Pulse	Slightly increased	Increased, weak	Tachycardia[a] (rapid, thready, feeble)
Skin turgor	Decreased	Loss of elasticity	Very poor (pinch retracts very slowly)
Mucous membranes	Normal to dry	Dry	Dry, cracked
Eyes	Normal	Somewhat depressed	Grossly sunken
Tears	Present	Decreased	Absent
Urine output	Decreased	Oliguria	Prerenal azotemia[a]
Behavior	Normal, alert, possibly some restlessness	Irritable, restless or lethargic	Hyperirritable to lethargic, limp

[a] Key symptoms of circulatory shock.

(Hellerstein, 1993). However, initial rehydration is rapid (within 24 hours) in isotonic and hypotonic dehydration.

There are many approaches to the repair of fluid deficits. Regardless of the approach, certain principles should be followed. First, the restoration and preservation of cardiovascular function, the CNS, and renal perfusion are the primary initial concerns. Therapy should be initiated with a volume expander of isotonic fluid that causes rapid expansion of the ECF. The solution of choice usually contains saline in some form, either lactated Ringer's (LR) or normal saline (NS) and is given in a bolus of 10 to 20 ml/kg (Hazinski & Barnard, 1999). Second, total body repair of the fluid deficit may require a considerable period of time. Third, potassium losses cannot be replaced immediately because this is a predominantly intracellular ion. After renal function has been confirmed and the child is producing urine, potassium should be added to the fluid infusion. Potassium is not administered to the oliguric child because the primary site for secretion of potassium is the kidney, resulting in hyperkalemia in the event of kidney damage (Hunsberger, 1994). Maximum concentration of potassium in replacement fluids is 40 mEq/L (Helikson & Wolfson, 1993). Fourth, the adequacy of deficit therapy needs to be constantly reevaluated by continuous monitoring of the clinical condition, urine output, and urine specific gravity (Rice et al., 1998). Therefore, it is essential that the surgical team assess the fluid needs of the patient throughout the entire period of surgical management. Fluids and electrolytes are provided in all three phases, beginning with the preoperative resuscitation phase if there is one; then the intraoperative management phase, tailoring the fluid and electrolyte administration to the degree of deficiencies created by the surgical procedure and the underlying disease state; and finally the postoperative recovery phase until the child has regained the normovolemic state and is back to baseline maintenance fluid requirements (Filston, 1992).

INTRAOPERATIVE MANAGEMENT

The goal of intraoperative fluid management is to replace the fasting fluid deficit, maintenance and third-space fluid losses, and blood loss to maintain fluid homeostasis (Aker & O'Sullivan, 1998). During the operative procedure, the fluid choice reflects the most dominant fluid loss. For simple elective procedures, insensible loss is the dominant fluid deficit, and appropriate hypotonic fluids are used to replace free water and minimal electrolytes. For procedures in which significant blood loss occurs or in which major prolonged invasion of the abdominal or thoracic cavity is involved, volume restoration fluids of the balanced salt (lactated Ringer's) or blood products variety are chosen. It is best to base this volume restoration on a combination of the assessment of the preoperative volume restoration state and the intraoperative

and postoperative fluid requirements. If the patient arrives in the operating room fully volume restored, this estimate can be based on the intraoperative and postoperative requirements alone (Filston, 1992).

To avoid postoperative fluid and electrolyte abnormalities, the operative staff report the type and duration of anesthesia, untoward events, blood loss, and intake and output during surgery to the postanesthesia care unit staff (Nachtsheim, 1999). Induction of anesthesia may lead to the development of hypotension in the patient with preoperative hypovolemia because of the loss of compensatory mechanisms such as tachycardia or vasoconstriction (Horne et al., 1997).

DAILY MAINTENANCE FLUID AND ELECTROLYTE REQUIREMENTS

Maintenance intravenous fluids and electrolytes are the amounts of fluids and solutes required for basal needs. They also replace physiologic losses that occur as a result of normal body processes such as metabolism, insensible fluid loss from the skin (evaporation) and lungs (respiration), and urine losses (Letton & Chwals, 1997). The aim of maintenance therapy is to replace water and electrolytes that are lost under ordinary conditions. Maintenance fluids are designed to maintain water and electrolyte homeostasis with minimal renal compensation. In addition, maintenance fluids should provide 20% of caloric needs as protein-sparing calories for short-term nutritional support (Rice et al., 1998). The addition of 5% to 10% glucose to the maintenance fluid for the usual brief period of parenteral therapy in the child who is not malnourished provides sufficient calories to suppress severe ketosis. However, infants and children who will be maintained on parenteral fluids for longer than 72 hours should receive parenteral alimentation until oral intake is reestablished (Nachtsheim, 1999).

The calculation of a patient's specific maintenance fluid requirement can be based on weight or surface area. The most commonly applied formula is maintenance requirement based on body weight (assuming normal renal function, gastrointestinal status, and temperature) (Klotz, 1998) (see Table 3–2; O'Donnell & Lathrop, 1993). Exceptions to the preceding formula include the following conditions: in

Table 3–2 Scale: Daily Maintenance Fluid Needs

Weight	Fluid Needs/24 hr
Newborn (0–72 hr)	60–100 ml/kg
0–10 kg (0–22 lb)	100 ml/kg
11–20 kg (24–44 lb)	1,000 ml plus 50 ml/kg >10 kg
>20 kg (>44 lb)	1,500 ml plus 20 ml/kg >20 kg

premature infants, during the first few days of life, and during fever and various disease states such as sepsis when the metabolic rate is elevated and fluid needs are increased (Helikson & Wolfson, 1993). The use of mathematical formulas to calculate the patient's fluid requirement is extremely beneficial, but clinicians must follow this by closely monitoring the patient's hydration status. Imbalances of serum electrolytes result from overhydration or underhydration. Close laboratory monitoring of serum electrolytes, hemoglobin, and hematocrit is essential. It is also essential to measure the total fluid intake and output. The total fluid input must consider all sources of fluid administered enterally and parenterally (Klotz, 1998). If the estimate of maintenance needs is correct, the patient's electrolytes remain stable and the child is clinically euvolemic (Rice et al., 1998); the child has sufficient intravascular volume to maintain effective systemic perfusion (Hazinski & Barnard, 1999).

Once the volume of maintenance fluid a child needs in a 24-hour period is calculated, the daily sodium and potassium maintenance requirements may be calculated. Electrolyte maintenance requirements are based on the patient's weight or body surface area. The traditional pediatric approach is to use a per kilogram/per day approach (Klotz, 1998). Daily requirements for electrolytes are sodium, 3 mEq/kg/day, and potassium, 2 mEq/kg/day (Helikson & Wolfson, 1993).

Once the child's maintenance fluid requirements are calculated, the child's actual fluid requirements must be determined by modifying maintenance fluid requirements with consideration of the child's clinical condition. Fluid requirements can be expected to increase if the child has excessive fluid losses. The child can be expected to require reduced fluid administration if cardiorespiratory failure, renal failure, or increased intracranial pressure is present (Hazinski, 1988).

REPLACEMENT OF ONGOING ABNORMAL LOSSES

Replacement fluid therapy is designed to replace ongoing abnormal fluid and electrolyte losses that continue during therapy to reduce persistent vomiting, diarrhea, nasogastric tube drainage, ileostomy, stoma output, wound drainage, pleural fluid, and fistula losses (O'Donnell & Lathrop, 1993). The loss of water and electrolytes in stool is usually negligible unless diarrhea is present (Letton & Chwals, 1997). These losses are not accounted for in the calculation of deficit or maintenance requirements and must be added to fluid therapy. Because the constituents of these losses are frequently quite different from the composition of maintenance fluids, it may be hazardous to simply increase the volume of maintenance fluids in an attempt to compensate for those losses. Table 3–3 represents the average loss of elec-

Table 3–3 Electrolytes in Body Fluids (mEq/L)

Fluid	Na+	K+	Cl-
Gastric	20–80	5–20	100–150
Pancreatic	120–140	5–15	90–120
Small intestine	100–140	5–15	90–130
Bile	120–140	5–15	80–120
Ileostomy	45–135	3–15	20–115
Diarrhea	10–90	10–80	10–110
Sweat[a]			
Normal	10–30	3–10	10–35
Cystic fibrosis	50–130	5–25	50–110
Burns	140	5	110

[a] Sweat sodium concentrations progressively increase with increasing sweat flow rates.

trolytes from various sites (electrolytes in body fluids) (O'Donnell & Lathrop, 1993). In most circumstances, it is preferable to actually measure and analyze the electrolyte content of these losses and replace them milliequivalent for milliequivalent and milliliter for milliliter (Rice et al., 1998). Samples may be sent to the laboratory as needed for exact determinations of electrolyte content of different body fluids (O'Donnell & Lathrop, 1993).

These continuing abnormal measured losses are the fluids that are lost directly from the body in volumes significant enough to be collected and measured. The typical loss of this type is that from a nasogastric tube and consists of gastric aspirate. The composition of such fluid varies somewhat depending on whether it is primarily a gastric aspirate or fluid from beyond the pylorus. Gastric losses from above the pylorus contain sodium, chloride, potassium, and hydrogen ions. Losses from beyond the pylorus are essentially ultrafiltrates of the plasma or serum (Filston, 1992). These losses should be replaced by using fluids similar in composition to those being lost. Solutions suitable for replacing some common ongoing fluid losses are presented in Table 3–4 (O'Donnell & Lathrop, 1993). The rate at which an abnormal loss is replaced depends on the rate at which fluid is being lost and the size of the patient. In the case of an infant, even modest abnormal losses should be replaced every 2 to 4 hours. In the case of a larger patient, abnormal fluid expenditures may be replaced every 4 to 8 hours. In all cases, large ongoing fluid losses should be replaced promptly to avoid the pathophysiologic effects of such depletions (Hellerstein, 1993).

TYPES OF INTRAVENOUS SOLUTIONS

Numerous commercial parenteral solutions and salts used for maintenance or replacement therapy are available (Klotz, 1998). All intravenous (IV) solutions are not created equal.

Table 3–4 Composition and Tonicity of Parenteral Fluids Frequently Used in Pediatrics

Solution	Na+ mEq/L	K+ mEq/L	Cl− mEq/L	Osmolality mOsm/L[a]
5% dextrose in 0.2% sodium chloride	34	—	34	321
5% dextrose in 0.33% sodium chloride	56	—	56	365
5% dextrose in 0.45% sodium chloride	77	—	77	406
5% dextrose in 0.9% sodium chloride	154	—	154	560
Ringer's lactate	130	4	109	261
0.45% sodium chloride	77	—	77	280
0.9% sodium chloride	154	—	154	292
3% sodium chloride	513	—	513	969

[a] Normal physiologic isotonicity range is approximately 280–310 mOsm/L.

The choice depends on the patient's condition (Gasparis, Murray, & Ursomanno, 1989) and the patient's volume status and electrolyte balance (Schwartz, 1999). An isotonic IV solution, which has the same osmolality as serum and other body fluids, expands the intravascular compartment only. One indication for choosing this type of IV fluid is hypotension caused by hypovolemia. Common isotonic solutions include LR and NS. A hypotonic solution shifts fluids and electrolytes out of the intravascular compartment, hydrating intracellular and interstitial compartments and depleting the circulatory system. A hypotonic solution like 0.45% saline or dextrose 5% in water (D5W) is appropriate for patients who need cellular hydration because of conditions such as diabetic ketoacidosis or as a result of diuretic therapy. A hypertonic solution draws fluid and electrolytes into the intravascular compartment, dehydrating the intracellular and interstitial compartments. An example of this solution is 5% dextrose in 0.45% normal saline, D5NS, and D5LR. This is commonly used in postoperative patients to help reduce edema, stabilize blood pressure, and maintain urinary output (Gasparis et al., 1989).

Normal saline/physiologic saline contains 154 mEq/L of sodium and chloride. The solution contains no energy/caloric source because it has no glucose (dextrose). It is isotonic (280 to 300 mOsm/L). Dextrose 5% in half-normal saline contains 170 calories/L and 77 mEq/L of sodium and chloride. It generally is used as a replacement solution for losses caused by gastrointestinal drainage (Klotz, 1998). Gastric juice contains sodium, potassium, chloride, and hydrochloric acid in amounts that are similar to a solution of 5% dextrose in half-normal saline (Filston, 1992). Dextrose 5% in 0.2% sodium chloride provides 170 calories/L and 34 mEq/L of sodium and chloride. This solution generally is used as a maintenance fluid in pediatric patients. LR mimics the normal plasma, is isotonic (273 mOsm/L), and can be used as a replacement or maintenance solution. Losses from beyond the pylorus are ultrafiltrates of plasma and are best replaced by balanced salt solutions such as LR (Filston,

1992). Dextrose 5% in LR is commonly used in patients with hyperemesis because it also provides 170 calories. D5W is an isotonic solution containing no electrolytes. It provides a source of calories. An appropriate indication for administration would be for short-term use in patients with hypernatremia (sodium >150 mEq/L) (Klotz, 1998).

Oral Rehydration Solutions

Intravenous fluids remain the treatment of choice for fluid volume deficit in children. The ability to select from different types of fluids and customize the infusion prescription to the patient's needs is a large part of ensuring positive patient outcomes. However, there is an alternative therapy for some patients after their conditions have been stabilized with IV treatments (Fann, 1998).

Although parenteral fluid therapy remains the traditional treatment for the surgical patient, oral rehydration solutions have recently gained a role in the treatment of dehydration, particularly for the child with gastroenteritis (Rice et al., 1998). Oral solutions are successful in treating many children with mild isotonic, hypotonic, or hypertonic dehydration. Vomiting is not a contraindication. Give the child who is vomiting frequent, small doses of oral rehydration solutions. After successful IV rehydration, oral rehydration solutions are used during the maintenance fluid therapy phase. Alternating an IV solution with a low-sodium fluid such as water, breast milk, lactose-free formula, or half-strength lactose–containing formula is an effective treatment plan (Fann, 1998).

Adequacy of Intravenous Fluid Therapy/Clinical Response to Fluid Replacement Therapy

Dynamic fluid and electrolyte management requires ongoing assessment and adjustment of dextrose, electrolytes, and fluid rates (Statter, 1992). It is essential that careful hourly monitoring assess the results of the volume restoration, ensuring that an adequate urine output has been achieved, and demonstrate adequate volume restoration in the patient. By the same token, excessive urine output demonstrates an overabundance of volume restoration and requires a reduction in the volume of fluid being administered (Filston, 1992). Good assessment skills help the surgical nurse recognize subtle clues before an infant or child progresses into serious fluid and electrolyte problems. The optimal state of resuscitation is determined by the clinical parameters of normal skin turgor, moist mucous membranes, and a urine output of >1 ml/kg/hr. The most important laboratory parameters that determine the safety of anesthesia are serum electrolytes (Rice et al., 1998). Assessing physical data, the results of laboratory tests, body weight, and intake and output are important aspects of care to monitor (Fann, 1998). Serial physical examinations should include inspection and palpation of the skin for the presence and absence of edema, palpation of the peripheral pulses, and auscultation of the heart and lungs. In addition, the parameters of body weight; net fluid intake; urine output; blood glucose; and serum sodium, chloride, and potassium are useful to monitor. An appropriate urine output is 1 to 2 ml/kg/hr (Statter, 1992). Overhydration must be avoided just as aggressively as underhydration (Klotz, 1998). The administration of excessive free water may result in water intoxication, which can lead to death (Klotz, 1998). Carefully tracking all the patient's intake and output is critical to safe and effective fluid and electrolyte therapy. A nasogastric tube should be irrigated with isotonic sodium chloride solution only because plain water increases the loss of electrolytes (Horne et al., 1997). Checking mucous membranes, skin, fontanels in infants, and urine specific gravity can give the clinician an idea of the patient's fluid status. A well-hydrated child demonstrates good skin turgor, and the skin does not remain "tented" when pinched. Mucous membranes are moist and tearing is noted. The infant's fontanel is flat, not sunken or bulging. Urine specific gravity usually ranges from 1.005 to 1.020, serum osmolality is approximately 272 to 290 mOsm/L, and blood urea nitrogen ranges from 5 to 22 mg/dl (Hazinski, 1988).

Adequate intravascular volume is necessary to ensure adequate systemic perfusion. It is essential that this volume be maintained to prevent hypovolemic shock. Adequate systemic perfusion is present when the heart rate is normal, extremities are warm, and capillary refill is brisk (within 1 to 2 seconds). The child's color is consistent, not mottled, and mucous membranes are pink. Peripheral pulses are strong and blood pressure is normal for age (Hazinski, 1988). The child's weight is measured on the same scale at the same time of day. Significant weight changes should be discussed with the health care team and attempts should be made to determine the source of the child's fluid gain or loss (Hazinski, 1988).

THIRD-SPACING

The ECF is composed of the intravascular fluid (plasma) and the interstitial fluid compartments. At times, because of increases in capillary permeability, plasma proteins diffuse from the intravascular fluid compartment into the interstitial spaces, making the fluid physiologically useless. This movement of fluids, electrolytes, and proteins outside of their normal boundaries in the vascular system and into the interstitial spaces is called "third-space shifting." Shifts to the third space may occur after abdominal surgery, trauma, burns, and infection, when fluid shifts into such nonfunctional and nonvisible compartments as the peritoneum and bowel wall. Because of the systemic effects, fluid shifts to the third space may be life threatening. Third-spacing traps fluid away from the normal fluid compartments and results in a deficit in ECF volume (O'Donnell & Lathrop, 1993). In children with surgical diseases, such fluid can accumulate in the gastrointestinal tract from obstruction and inflammation, in body cavities as ascites and pleural effusions, and diffusely as edema from leaky capillary syndrome that accompanies shock (Helikson & Wolfson, 1993).

Signs and symptoms of fluid shift to the third space include reduction in urinary output, increase in specific gravity, rapid increase in hemoglobin and hematocrit, tachycardia, hypotension, sluggish capillary refill time, and decrease in the intensity of the peripheral pulses. In addition, if fluid is shifted into the peritoneum and bowel, the weight and abdominal girth increase. Also, edema is present in the eyes, hands, feet, and genitalia. The surgical nurse must be constantly alert for early signs of third-space shifting. Meticulous measurements and monitoring of intake and output, specific gravity, abdominal girth, weight, and vital signs are mandatory. Third-space losses cannot be directly measured (Radhakrishnan & Geissler, 1996), and their intravenous replacement must be approximated. Sequestered fluid is almost always isotonic, and its replacement may be given as a crystalloid balanced salt solution such as LR (Helikson & Wolfson, 1993).

As the causative inflammation or infection decreases, the permeability of the cell membranes and the intracellular osmotic pressure return to normal. The third-spacing phenomenon then resolves itself. This begins another critical time for fluid balance in the infant or child. During this recovery phase, the fluids that were trapped in the interstitial spaces shift back into the vascular space. Unless fluid administration is reevaluated, fluid overload may result. This recovery phase is marked by dramatically decreased urine specific gravity and increased urinary output. Fluid administration during this phase, as in the other phases, needs to be monitored and adjusted frequently in light of clinical signs and serum electrolytes to ensure adequate blood pressure and to avoid dehydration or overhydration (O'Donnell & Lathrop, 1993).

CONCLUSION

Fluid and electrolyte therapy requires a knowledge of normal basic requirements, preexisting deficits, and continuing losses (deLorimier, Harrison, & Adzick, 1994). The surgical procedure itself, as well as the postoperative phase, is associated with major losses of fluid and electrolytes. The goal of the management of the pediatric surgical patient is not only to correct the abnormality that required surgical intervention but also to maintain normal growth and development (Finberg et al., 1993). Administering IV fluids and maintaining fluid and electrolyte homeostasis is essential for successful outcomes in the pediatric surgical patient (Aker & O'Sullivan, 1998).

REFERENCES

Aker, J., & O'Sullivan, C. (1998). The selection and administration of perioperative intravenous fluids for the pediatric patient. *Journal of PeriAnesthesia Nursing, 13*(3), 172–181.

deLorimier, A., Harrison, M., & Adzick, S. (1994). Pediatric surgery. In L. Way (Ed.), *Current surgical diagnosis and treatment* (10th ed.). East Norwalk, CT: Appleton & Lange.

Fann, B. (1998). Fluid and electrolyte balance in the pediatric patient. *Journal of Intravenous Nursing, 21*(3), 153–159.

Fecteau, D. (1999). Patient and environmental safety. In M. Meeker & J. Rothrock (Eds.), *Alexander's care of the patient in surgery* (11th ed.). St. Louis, MO: Mosby.

Filston, H. (1992). Fluid and electrolyte management in the pediatric surgical patient. *Surgical Clinics of North America, 72*(6), 1189–1205.

Finberg, L., Kravath, R., & Hellerstein, S. (1993). *Water and electrolytes in pediatrics: Physiology, pathophysiology, and treatment* (2nd ed.). Philadelphia: W.B. Saunders Company.

Gasparis, L., Murray, E., & Ursomanno, P. (1989). I.V. Solutions. *Nursing 89, April,* 62–64.

Hazinski, M. (1988). Understanding fluid balance in the seriously ill child. *Pediatric Nursing, 14*(3), 231–236.

Hazinski, M., & Barnard, J. (1999). Gastrointestinal disorders. In M. Hazinski (Ed.), *Manual of pediatric critical care.* St. Louis, MO: Mosby.

Headrick, C., Hazinski, M., & Alexander, J. (1999). Renal disorders. In M. Hazinski (Ed.), *Manual of pediatric critical care.* St. Louis, MO: Mosby.

Helikson, M., & Wolfson, P. (1993). Pediatric surgery: Surgical diseases of children. In P. Lawrence (Ed.), *Essentials of surgical specialties.* Baltimore: Williams & Wilkins.

Hellerstein, S. (1993). Fluid and electrolytes: Clinical aspects. *Pediatrics in Review, 14*(3), 103–115.

Horne, M., Heitz, U., & Swearingen, P. (1997). *Pocket guide to fluid, electrolyte, and acid-base balance* (3rd ed.). St. Louis, MO: Mosby.

Hunsberger, M. (1994). Principles of fluid and electrolyte maintenance. In C. Betz, M. Hunsberger, & S. Wright (Eds.), *Family-centered nursing care of children* (2nd ed.). Philadelphia: W.B. Saunders Company.

Klotz, R. (1998). The effects of intravenous solutions on fluid and electrolyte balance. *Journal of Intravenous Nursing, 21*(1), 20–26.

Letton, R., & Chwals, W. (1997). Homeostasis. In K. Oldham, P. Colombani, & R. Foglia (Eds.), *Surgery of infants and children.* Philadelphia: Lippincott-Raven Publishers.

Nachtsheim, B. (1999). Acute illness. In M. Broome & J. Rollins (Eds.), *Core curriculum for the nursing care of children and their families.* Pitman, NJ: Jannetti Publications, Inc.

O'Donnell, D., & Lathrop, J. (1993). *Pediatric fluids and electrolytes.* Milwaukee, WI: Maxishare.

Radhakrishnan, J., & Geissler, G. (1996). Pediatric surgery. In R. Condon & L. Nyhus (Eds.), *Manual of surgical therapeutics* (9th ed.). Boston: Little, Brown and Company.

Rice, H., Caty, M., & Glick, P. (1998). Fluid therapy for the pediatric surgical patient. *Pediatric Clinics of North America, 45*(4), 719–727.

Schwartz, S. (1999). *Principles of surgery companion handbook* (7th ed.). New York: McGraw-Hill.

Statter, M. (1992). Fluids and electrolytes in infants and children. *Seminars in Pediatric Surgery, 1*(3), 208–211.

CHAPTER 4

Nutrition in the Pediatric Surgical Patient

Annie McKenna and Jose M. Saavedra

Nutritional management of the pediatric surgical patient is both dynamic and challenging. The pediatric surgical patient carries the challenge of satisfying the increased nutritional and metabolic demands of surgical conditions in an individual who already bears the high energy requirements for growth. Recent advances in medical nutrition therapy have not only improved survival and decreased morbidity but have also minimized the impact on ultimate growth and development of children with adequate and safe provision of nutrients.

NUTRITION ASSESSMENT AND ESTIMATION OF NUTRITIONAL REQUIREMENTS

Nutritional assessment should be completed at the time of the initial visit and then continually during hospitalization and also when clinically indicated in the outpatient setting. Adequate assessment is necessary to identify patients in need of nutritional therapy or those at risk for malnutrition who may benefit from nutrition support in the preoperative or postoperative period.

Growth and Growth History

Infants and children should be weighed in kilograms (kg), measured for height or length in centimeters (cm), and head circumference should be measured in infants and children less than 2 years of age on admission to the hospital and during hospitalization. Children should be weighed with the appropriate size beam scale with minimal clothing and without shoes. Infants should be weighed naked. The length in children less than 2 years of age should be measured supine on a flat length board. Length and height should be obtained without shoes. These measurements should be plotted on age-specific and sex-specific growth curves; weight-age, height-age, weight-for-height using the National Center for Health Statistics (NCHS) growth curves. This is a simple and effective tool in identifying patients at nutritional risk. Individuals that are less than the 5th percentile for weight-age or height-age or those less than the 10th percentile for weight-for-height are at nutritional risk. A more detailed nutritional assessment and rehabilitation are warranted. If previous measurements are available, growth progress and deviations in growth rates can be followed. Growth rates that have dropped off (downward crossing of two major percentiles on NCHS curves) or sudden unexpected acceleration in growth should be investigated. Downward crossing of growth percentiles may be an indicator of failure to thrive as a result of medical, chromosomal, metabolic, nutritional, or environmental factors. Serial monitoring of arm anthropometrics (midarm circumference and triceps skinfold) is helpful when a child is either immobile for an extended time or for continued monitoring of fat and muscle deposition during nutritional rehabilitation (Chicago Dietetic Association and the South Suburban Dietetic Association, 1992).

Diet History

A detailed diet history documents current feeding practices and intake. A diet history, including a 24-hour recall, should be used to determine adequacy of intake and food preferences and to identify cultural or religious eating practices or food intolerances. Appetite, food allergies, gastrointestinal intolerance (diarrhea, constipation, vomiting, gastroesophageal reflux), and eating behaviors should be evaluated to help determine nutritional risk or previous intolerance. Estimation of dietary energy, protein, and micronutrient intake helps explain possible causes for failure to thrive, establish the nutritional risks of a surgical patient, and determine needs in the postoperative setting.

Estimating Energy and Protein Requirements

Measured energy expenditure (MEE) using indirect calorimetry is an accurate method of "estimating" energy needs. However, it is costly and time consuming and is not always available. Energy and protein requirements can be estimated using equations predicting resting energy expenditure (REE) on the basis of weight, sex, and age (Table 4–1) (National Research Council, 1989). These calculated values are not completely accurate for every individual but can be used as a guideline for initiating nutrition therapy or dietary planning. During hospitalization, infants' and children's energy and protein requirements change, depending on the injury (surgical, trauma, or burn) or infectious complications that may ensue. Metabolic requirements increase with a meal or with enteral feeding due to the thermic effect of food. The calculated REE must be increased an additional 5% to 10% if a patient is being enterally fed. Growth accounts for 1% to 2% of energy requirements beyond 2 years of age; infants require 5% to 30% additional calories for growth between birth and 1 year of age (Fomon, 1993). Energy requirements, therefore, can be divided into maintenance metabolic needs (REE, thermic effect of food, activity level, heat loss), growth, injury, and infection. Protein requirements generally correlate with energy needs based on REE. Protein delivery should constitute about 7% to 12% of total energy as calories.

The recommended dietary allowance (RDA) can be used as a guideline for determining initial requirements for energy and protein. Table 4–2 outlines the RDA for energy and protein on the basis of age. However, the RDA may overestimate energy needs initially, depending on the diagnosis and the time of injury or surgery.

The RDAs may need adjustment during illness or for children with a chronic disease. For example, children with neurologic injury may require less than the RDA for energy, protein, and micronutrients; whereas premature infants and infants and children with chronic lung disease, short bowel syndrome, immunodeficiency, cystic fibrosis, or congenital heart disease require additional energy, protein, and micronutrients to thrive and grow.

The addition of calories may be indicated depending on certain stress factors such as fever, minor surgery, major surgery, infection, or burns. Exhibit 4–1 (Wilmore, 1977) lists the recommended increases in energy on the basis of these specific stress factors. One should not consider the increases cumulatively; if a patient has more than one of the stressors, the largest percentage increase should be used to calculate caloric needs. For example, if a trauma patient with multiple fractures is septic, calories increase by 40% to 60% (moderate to severe infection).

Close nutritional monitoring and clinical assessment are necessary in the hospital setting, especially in the neonatal intensive care unit and the pediatric intensive care unit. The child's clinical course may change dramatically in a short period of time, and therefore energy and protein delivery will need to be continuously adjusted. Many problems are present with nutritional assessment and monitoring in the intensive care setting. Fluid status is extremely variable, and weight and visceral proteins are directly influenced by third spacing of fluid and diuresis. Therefore, subjective clinical assessment of the pediatric patient must be used in congruence with objective data.

Noncaloric Nutrients

Vitamins and minerals are essential micronutrients that serve as enzyme cofactors and structural components of the body. The micronutrient requirements of infants are derived from the nutrient content and volume of human milk consumed by a typical, healthy infant. For children and adolescents, the micronutrient requirements are based on the RDAs, which are derived from the average physiologic requirement for an absorbed nutrient (National Research Council, 1989).

Laboratory Data

A variety of laboratory tests are available to assess nutritional status. Vitamin (vitamins A, D, and E) and mineral (calcium, magnesium, phosphorus, copper, and zinc) serum levels may be useful in specific circumstances in individuals

Table 4–1 Predicting Resting Energy Expenditure from Body Weight (kg)

	Males		Females
Age Range (yr)	Equation To Derive Resting Energy Expenditure (kcal/day)	Age Range (yr)	Equation To Derive Resting Energy Expenditure (kcal/day)
0–3	$(60.9 \times wt) - 54$	0–3	$(61.0 \times wt) - 51$
3–10	$(22.7 \times wt) + 495$	3–10	$(22.5 \times wt) + 499$
10–18	$(17.5 \times wt) + 651$	10–18	$(12.2 \times wt) + 746$
18–30	$(15.3 \times wt) + 679$	18–30	$(14.7 \times wt) + 496$

Table 4–2 Recommended Dietary Allowance for Energy (kcal/kg) and Protein (gm/kg)

	kcal/kg/day	gm protein/kg/day
Infants		
0–6 mo	108	2.2
6–12 mo	98	1.6
Children		
1–3 yr	102	1.2
4–6 yr	90	1.1
7–10 yr	70	1.0
Males		
11–14 yr	55	1.0
15–18 yr	45	0.9
19–24 yr	38	0.8
Females		
11–14 yr	47	1.0
15–18 yr	40	0.8
19–24 yr	38	0.8

at risk or when supplementation to promote healing is necessary (see following). Laboratory assessment of renal and hepatic function (serum urea nitrogen, creatinine, liver enzymes, alkaline phosphatase, and bilirubins) helps in modifying requirements and delivery of nutrition according to the clinical situation. Evaluation of visceral protein status is particularly important. Hypoalbuminemia in the acute stressed state may indicate a faster catabolism or poor synthesis of proteins and protein loss. Postoperatively, persistent protein losses may be due to wounds, fistulas, or burns, dramatically increasing the need for energy and protein provision to maintain adequate synthesis and promote healing. Albumin and total protein have long half-lives (17–20 days) because of their large extravascular volume distribution and

Exhibit 4–1 Percentage Recommended Increase of Calorie Needs Based on Stress Factors

Fever—12% for every 1° >37°C
Minor surgery—10%
Major surgery—20%–30%
Long bone fractures—15%–30%
Infection—20% mild; 40% moderate; 60% severe
Multiple trauma with patient on ventilator—50%–70%
Long-term growth failure—35%–50%
Burns—25%–115% (depending on percent total body surface area burn)

also vary considerably depending on fluid status (Bernstein et al., 1995). Ongoing or acute protein evaluation can most effectively be assessed with prealbumin. Prealbumin is a rapid-turnover protein (half-life <48 hours) and is practical because it is the easiest of the rapid-turnover proteins to measure and the most free of interference compared with other acute-phase reactant proteins. Therefore, it is a good indicator of acute nutritional status and catabolic or anabolic state. Prealbumin declines to its lowest value in the postsurgical acute phase by the third to fifth postoperative day. Measurement should be initiated by that time to obtain a trend, and it can be used sequentially to evaluate the adequacy of nutritional support. Prealbumin should be measured biweekly in the early recuperative phase and more often in the critically ill patient with continued losses. Prealbumin concentrations of less than 11 mg/dl, assuming adequacy of liver synthetic capacity, indicate the need to initiate nutritional support (Bernstein et al., 1995).

METABOLIC CONSEQUENCES OF INJURY AND NUTRITIONAL REPLETION

The body's initial response to injury (e.g., surgery, sepsis, trauma, burns, acute inflammatory conditions) is the release of cytokines, which mediate the metabolic and immune response to injury. Counterregulatory hormones (e.g., catecholamines, glucagon, and cortisol) rapidly rise in response to cytokines. These counterregulatory hormones counteract the synthetic effects of insulin and insulin-like growth factor-1 (IGF-1) and cause a sequence of metabolic events that includes the catabolism of endogenous stores of protein, carbohydrate, and fat to fuel the body's ongoing metabolic response to stress. The loss of endogenous tissue because of a hypermetabolic and hypercatabolic state can lead to a poor clinical outcome in the absence of appropriate nutritional and metabolic support (Cerra, 1987; Frankenfield, Wiles, Bagley, & Siegel, 1994; Long, Schaffel, Geiger, Schiller, & Blakemore, 1979). As the body's acute metabolic response to injury resolves, anabolic metabolism adapts to restore catabolic losses. In children, the body now resumes growth. The goal then in the critically ill child is to initiate nutritional resuscitation early to promote growth recovery. The catabolic state also contributes to early nitrogen losses either caused by injury or starvation. The visceral protein (prealbumin, albumin, transferrin, and retinol-binding protein) stores are then depleted to provide energy for the body. Urinary nitrogen losses also increase as a result of protein and fat catabolism (gluconeogenesis in the liver and lipolysis). Not only are visceral proteins used for gluconeogenesis in the liver, but altered protein metabolism during acute metabolic stress also occurs. The liver preferentially synthesizes acute phase proteins (i.e., C-reactive protein), which start a cascade of events signaling an immune response and repair of the body (Pepys & Baltzs, 1983).

Nutritional Repletion during Metabolic Stress

Stress-related growth retardation results from cytokine-induced decreases in IGF-1 (Lazarus, Lowry, & Moldawer, 1992). Reductions in activity and insensible losses observed in sedated infants and children in the intensive care unit lead to reduced caloric requirements during the acute phase response to injury. Overfeeding then is a potential risk if caloric repletion is based on predicted requirements for healthy infants or children (Chwals, Lally, Woolley, & Mahour, 1988). As the acute phase response subsides and the body resumes anabolic metabolism (growth), usually within 5 days after injury or surgery, calorie administration should be progressively increased (Chwals, Letton, Jamie, & Charles, 1995). Close monitoring of prealbumin and C-reactive protein can assist in determining recovery from injury. Prealbumin levels will begin to rise and C-reactive protein levels should be less than 2 mg/dl.

Risks Associated with Overfeeding

Overfeeding the critically ill infant or child may lead to respiratory compromise or hepatic dysfunction. Overfeeding of carbohydrates, regardless of adequacy of energy, increases lipogenesis, which is an energy-requiring process characterized by an increase in carbon dioxide production (V_{CO_2}) relative to oxygen consumption (V_{O_2}). In infants, increased carbon dioxide production, resulting from excess carbohydrate administration, increases the respiratory rate that is necessary to remove excess CO_2. However, in the infant with chronic lung disease or acute pulmonary compromise, the body may be unable to compensate for the increased CO_2 production and, consequently, CO_2 retention may result. Substituting lipid for some of the carbohydrate administered may lead to reduced CO_2 production and lipogenesis (Delafosse et al., 1987; Piedboeuf, Chessex, Hazan, Pineault, & Lavoie, 1991). Hepatic cellular injury may also result in the face of overfeeding with excessive carbohydrate delivery because of increased insulin levels increasing glucose oxidation and lipogenesis. Hepatic cellular injury may therefore result from steatosis (deposition of fat in the liver) or intrahepatic cholestasis (Nussbaum & Fischer, 1991). Often during the initial hospitalization of a postsurgical or trauma patient, fluids are restricted and hyperglycemia is present. Therefore, the risk of overfeeding is minimal because of the inability to provide substrates (fluid, glucose) in excess amounts of need. However, it may be a risk in stable postoperative patients if substrate delivery is not limited and energy needs are overestimated.

ENTERAL NUTRITION SUPPORT

Enteral nutrition (EN) is the preferred method for meeting nutritional requirements of infants or children who have a functioning or partially functioning gastrointestinal tract but are unable or unwilling to safely and adequately achieve oral intake (Chicago Dietetic Association and the South Suburban Dietetic Association, 1992). EN is used in conjunction with an oral diet if intake is suboptimal or inadequate. EN may also be a transition method of weaning infants or children from parenteral nutrition to an oral diet. EN assists not only in nutrient delivery but is also critical in maintaining gastrointestinal mucosal integrity and immunologic function (Lo & Walter, 1993). This accelerates the time to full gut recovery, attenuates the hypermetabolic response to injury, is less costly than parenteral nutrition (Lipman, 1998), and may improve the outcome for critically ill or traumatized patients (Moore, Moore, Jones, McCroskey, & Peterson, 1989). EN support is a more efficient and physiologic use of nutrient substrates. In the critically ill surgical, trauma, or burn patient, enteral feedings may prevent the development of gastrointestinal bacterial translocation to the circulation and thus prevent the development of sepsis (Kudsk et al., 1992). EN decreases the risk of bacterial translocation and hepatobiliary complications often seen with parenteral nutrition support (Alverdy, Aoys, & Moss, 1988; Chellis, Price, & Dean, 1994; Deitch, Winterton, Li, & Berg, 1987; Moore et al., 1989; Ziegler, Smith, O'Dwyer, Demling, & Wilmore, 1988).

Enteral Access

Nutrient administration is primarily achieved by means of gastric or duodenal/jejunal feedings. Gastric feedings are the most practical and easiest route for short-term feedings; they are recommended when the risk of aspiration is minimal and tolerance is adequate. Duodenal/jejunal feedings are necessary when gastric feedings have failed because of upper gastrointestinal intolerance (poor gastric emptying, vomiting, aspiration) or if cardiopulmonary or neurologic status prevents placement or safe administration of gastric feedings. Jejunal access is typically obtained by several methods, including (1) passing a weighted feeding tube with or without a stylet into the stomach and relying on gastric motility for transpyloric migration (this can be done with varying success); (2) use of a weighted feeding tube, insufflation, and auscultation for postpyloric placement with confirmation from bile aspirate and alkaline pH (Ugo, Mohler, & Wilson, 1992); or (3) nonweighted silicone rubber nasoenteric tubes can be inserted using metoclopramide, air insufflation, and guide wire positioning (Chellis, Sanders, Dean, & Jackson, 1996) with or without endoscopic or fluoroscopic guidance (Oh, Mattox, Gelfand, Chen, & Wu, 1991).

Formula Selection

A primary consideration in choosing the appropriate formula includes identifying patient-specific nutrient requirements, including energy, protein, and fluid. Clinical status, disease state, gastrointestinal function, gastric or duodenal/jejunal administration, and length of nutrition support are also important factors to consider. The choice of formula is also age dependent and sometimes disease or injury specific (e.g., cystic fibrosis, necrotizing enterocolitis, short bowel syndrome, immunodeficiency, burn, or head trauma).

Breast milk is recommended for use in children less than 1 year old; if breast milk is not available, commercial infant formulas should be used. Standard infant formulas provide 20 kcal/oz and may be concentrated to increase caloric density while minimizing volume. Carbohydrate (Polycose, Moducal) or fat (MCT oil, Microlipid) modulars should be used to concentrate formulas greater than 24 kcal/oz. Some infants with cystic fibrosis or short bowel syndrome may have higher protein, vitamin, and mineral requirements because of increased losses; in that case infant formulas may be concentrated to 26 or 28 kcal/oz. In these situations, close monitoring is necessary to prevent electrolyte disturbances or dehydration. Powdered standard infant formula should be added to concentrate expressed breast milk to 30 kcal/oz. Table 4–3 outlines the indications for use and formula characteristics of the many specialized infant formulas available. Specific malabsorptive conditions (short bowel syndrome, intestinal resection, gastroschisis, intestinal atresia, biliary atresia) often require hydrolyzed protein or amino acid formulas with MCT oil to improve enteral absorption.

Prepared formulas for children greater than 1 year of age are available and convenient to use for enteral tube feedings. Fiber-supplemented formulas are now routinely used for long-term enteral support. Fiber may assist in increasing stool consistency with diarrhea and improve stool consistency and frequency in chronic constipation. Formula selection should once again be based on the child's clinical presentation (e.g., degree of malnutrition, presence of chronic disease, traumatic injury, or burns). Table 4–3 outlines a selection of current pediatric formulas available and a few adult formulas that may also be useful. For example, calorie-dense formulas (>1.5 kcal/ml) are adult product formulations that specifically meet the protein and micronutrient requirements of adult patients. However, some pediatric populations that have high energy demands (e.g., patients with burns, major surgery, or severe lung disease) or are severely fluid restricted (e.g., patients with closed-head injuries) may benefit from a concentrated formula, depending on fluid needs. The adequacy of micronutrient delivery should be evaluated to ensure appropriate delivery for a pediatric patient.

Types of Infusion

Intermittent (bolus) and continuous infusions, or a combination of both, are used for nutrient delivery. Intermittent gastric feedings can be administered over short periods of time (20 to 30 minutes) depending on tolerance. Intermittent or bolus feedings are practical for home enteral feedings because they allow ambulatory children to be more mobile between feedings. If continuous infusion is necessary because of poor nutrient absorption or feeding intolerance, portable feeding pumps are available. When feeding directly into the small bowel or if patients have delayed gastric emptying or gastroesophageal reflux, continuous infusion is recommended. Nocturnal continuous infusion is beneficial if the patient is receiving supplemental enteral nutritional support because it allows the patient to eat during the day.

Initiation and Advancement

Patients who have just received either a percutaneous endoscopic gastrostomy (PEG) or a surgical gastrostomy should initially receive an oral hydration solution (Pedialyte, Infalyte, etc.) to assess tolerance and adequacy of tube placement before initiating formula. If this is well tolerated, an isotonic formula can be administered at a rate of 1 to 2 ml/kg of body weight and advanced to the goal rate as tolerated over the next 24 to 48 hours. Guidelines for initiation and advancement of pediatric tube feedings are outlined in Exhibit 4–2.

PARENTERAL NUTRITION SUPPORT

Parenteral nutrition (PN) should be considered for infants and children in whom EN is either contraindicated or poorly tolerated. Congenital gastrointestinal malformations (gastroschisis, omphalocele, malrotation, intestinal atresias, meconium ileus requiring intestinal resection, Hirschsprung's disease), necrotizing enterocolitis, hypermetabolic states (burns, severe trauma, severe chronic lung disease, immunodeficiency), and organ failure are disease states in which PN support may be indicated. PN is often administered in conjunction with EN support, depending on the acuteness and severity of the injury or disease state. PN delivery should be considered in patients who are unable to tolerate adequate EN delivery for a significant period of time (>5 days) because of prolonged gastrointestinal dysfunction. The initiation of PN does not preclude the simultaneous administration of enteral feedings.

Table 4–3 Infant, Pediatric, and Disease-Specific Formulas

Formula Characteristics	*Indications for Use*	*Formulas*
Specialized infant formulas		
Premature infant formula, 12% protein, contains medium-chain triglyceride oil, additional calcium, phosphorus	Premature infants, infants with intrauterine growth retardation	Similac Special Care,[a] Enfamil Premature,[b] Enfamil 22,[b] Similac Neocare 22[a]
Protein hydrolysate infant formulas with medium-chain triglyceride oil	Malabsorption associated with bile acid deficiency, liver disease, short bowel syndrome, abnormal nutrient absorption	Pregestimil,[b] Alimentum[a]
Protein hydrolysate infant formulas without medium-chain triglyceride oil	Sensitive to soy or casein protein	Nutramigen[b]
Infant formula with medium-chain triglyceride oil	Severe steatorrhea, lymphatic anomalies	Portagen,[b] Tolerex[c] (for short periods of time, very low fat)
Elemental infant formulas	Severe malabsorption from short bowel syndrome, protein allergy	Neocate[d]
Pediatric formula selection		
Standard intact protein, lactose free, some medium-chain triglyceride oil, with and without fiber	Enteral tube feedings, 1 kcal/ml density, complete nutrition in 1,100 ml	Pediasure,[a] Pediasure with fiber,[a] Kindercal,[b] Resource for Kids[c]
Protein hydrolysate with maltodextrin and some medium-chain triglyceride oil	Gut atrophy or ischemic injury; malabsorption of fat, carbohydrate, or protein; poor tolerance to standard formulas	Peptamen Junior,[e] Propeptide for Kids,[f] Vital HN[a]
Elemental formulas with free amino acids	Severe gut injury leading to mucosal atrophy with poor tolerance of protein hydrolysate formula, food allergies, severe malabsorption, lymphatic anomalies	Vivonex Pediatric,[c] L-Emental Pediatric,[f] Vivonex Plus,[c] L-Emental Plus,[f] Tolerex,[c] Neocate One Plus,[d] Elecare[a]
Disease-specific formulas		
Calorie dense (>1.5 kcal/ml)	Fluid-restricted patients (head trauma, multiple traumas—fractures, wounds), patients with high energy demands (cystic fibrosis, pulmonary disease, immunodeficiency), renal patients	Nutren 1.5,[e] Nutren 2.0[e] (high medium-chain triglycerides), Pulmocare,[a] Deliver 2.0,[b] Ensure Plus,[a] Suplena,[a] Nepro[a]
High protein (>50 gm/L)	Patients with open wounds, burns, protein-losing enteropathy	Replete,[e] Promote,[a] Traumacal[b]
Glucose intolerance	Hyperglycemia associated with diabetes, chronic steroids, or immunodepressives	Glucerna,[a] Nutren 2.0[e]

[a] Ross Laboratories, Inc, Columbus, OH. [b] Mead Johnson Nutritionals, Evansville, IN. [c] Novartis, St. Louis Park, MN. [d] Scientific Hospitals Supplies, Gaithersburg, MD. [e] Nestle Clinical Nutrition, Deerfield, IL. [f] Nutrition Medicals, Inc, Minneapolis, MN.

Parenteral Access

Peripheral-vein parenteral nutrition (PPN) may be useful for 1 to 2 weeks of nutrition support, either to supplement enteral nutrition delivery or as the sole source of nutrition (Payne-James & Khawaja, 1993). The use of lipid emulsions in addition to protein and carbohydrate solutions enables safe nutrient delivery using a solution less than 900 mOsm/L (dextrose concentrations should not exceed 12.5 gm/dl). Highly concentrated dextrose solutions (>12.5 gm/dl) infused through a peripheral vein can quickly induce thrombophlebitis and therefore should only be infused in central venous catheters. PPN is indicated for patients when short-term need is anticipated and for whom PPN can complement

Exhibit 4–2 Guidelines for the Initiation and Advancement of Pediatric Tube Feedings

---

INTERMITTENT (BOLUS) FEEDINGS

1. Initiate at 2–5 ml/kg body weight per feeding every 3–4 hr and increase by 2–5 ml/kg body weight, every other feeding to goal rate, as tolerated.
2. Gastric residuals can be checked before each feeding. Common practice is to hold feedings if the volume is two times greater than the last feeding volume and recheck residuals in 1 hr and restart feedings at previous rate if residuals decreased.
3. Monitor for symptoms of upper gastrointestinal intolerance: gagging, retching, vomiting, regurgitation.

CONTINUOUS FEEDINGS

1. Initiate with 1–2 ml/kg/hr and advance every 4–8 hr by 1–2 ml/kg as tolerated until goal rate is reached. Initial volume should not exceed 55 ml/hr regardless of age or weight.
2. Adolescents can be started at 25–50 ml/hr, depending on clinical situation and expected tolerance. Advance to goal rate by increasing 25–50 ml/hr every 8–12 hr as tolerated.
3. Gastric residuals can be checked every 4 hr with nasogastric feedings in those at risk for aspiration. Common practice is to hold feedings for 1 hr if residual volume is greater than two times the volume previously infused, then recheck residuals. If residual decreased, resume feedings at previously tolerated rate.
4. Monitor for symptoms of upper gastrointestinal intolerance: gagging, retching, vomiting, regurgitation.
5. Do not check residuals on patients receiving transpyloric feedings because there is no reservoir in which formula can accumulate. Lower gastrointestinal intolerance such as abdominal distention or diarrhea may indicate feeding intolerance.

Note: Avoid advancing rate and formula strength simultaneously because if the patient becomes intolerant to the feedings, it will be unclear whether the intolerance is due to the increased rate or change in concentration.

---

early initiation of enteral feedings. PPN rarely provides more than 50% to 60% of energy needs. Central venous catheters are indicated in patients needing long-term (>2–4 weeks) partial PN or when all requirements need to be met parenterally. Peripherally inserted central catheters (PICCs) may be placed for long-term central PN if peripheral access is difficult to maintain during hospitalization and if the patient does not have a central catheter in place. The catheter tip is typically advanced to the junction of the superior vena cava with the right atrium to facilitate rapid dilution of the hyperosmolar solution with blood. Otherwise, if PICC access is not feasible, a long-term catheter (e.g., Hickman or Cook catheters) should be placed.

Parenteral Delivery and Monitoring

In infants and children requiring long-term PN, cyclic delivery (over 12–16 hours per day) has been shown to be safe and effective (Collier, Crough, Hendricks, & Caballero, 1994). Initially, close monitoring of blood sugar is necessary to evaluate tolerance of dextrose infusion. Hyperglycemia may occur during peak infusion times. Dextrose concentration or rate of infusion must be altered if this occurs. Tapering (over 1–2 hours) off the rate of infusion is important to slowly decrease the dextrose infusion and therefore prevent rebound hypoglycemia. PN infusion may also need to be al-

tered as a result of drug-nutrient incompatibilities. Specific antibiotics are not compatible with parenteral nutrition infusate or fat emulsions and should not be given simultaneously when contraindicated.

Parenteral Nutrient Delivery

Premature infants receiving PN support typically require 95 to 105 kcal/kg/day and 2.5 to 3 gm protein/kg/day to promote weight gain approximating the intrauterine growth rate (Putet, 1993). As a child grows, energy requirements generally decrease to 75 to 90 kcal/kg/day for 1- to 7-year-olds, 60 to 75 kcal/kg/day for children 7 to 12 years of age, and 30 to 60 kcal/kg/day for adolescents (Forlaw, Wong, & Little, 1995). Protein requirements vary, depending on the patient's surgical intervention, trauma, or presence of burns. Typically, critically ill or postsurgical infants and children require 2 to 3 gm protein/kg/day. Adolescents may require 0.8 to 2.5 gm protein/kg/day. Twenty to 60% of calories should come from carbohydrate (dextrose infusion), 7% to 20% from protein (depending on tolerance and protein losses), and 20% to 50% from fat. Micronutrient (vitamin and mineral) pediatric parenteral supplements are available and should be given on a daily basis for all patients receiving parenteral nutrition as their sole source of nutrition (Greene, Hambridge, Scanler, & Tsang, 1988).

Monitoring of Adequacy and Tolerance of Parenteral Nutrition

Monitoring parenteral nutrition is important to avoid complications. Baseline laboratory parameters, such as electrolytes and chemistries (calcium, phosphorus, liver function tests), and prealbumin and albumin should be obtained to evaluate renal function, glucose control, hydration, and baseline nutritional status before initiating PN. Monitoring for primary micronutrient deficiencies is important in patients receiving long-term PN in the hospital or home PN (see Table 4–4 for guidelines). Recommendations for monitoring of PN delivery in acute, hospitalized, and home PN support patients are outlined in Table 4–4.

Parenteral Nutrition Complications

The risks associated with PN complications can be reduced if a complete nutrition support team, including well-trained physicians, dietitians, nurses, and pharmacists, take part in the nutritional management of the patient. The most common problems associated with PN include glucose intolerance, hypertriglyceridemia, and electrolyte imbalances.

Hyperglycemia can typically be prevented with gradual advancement of dextrose solution by an increase of 5% per day. Electrolyte imbalances are typically associated with excessive losses as a result of diuresis, vomiting, and diarrhea or poor excretion caused by renal failure.

NUTRITIONAL MANAGEMENT OF THE BURN PATIENT

Nutrition management of the hypermetabolic burn patient is indisputably recognized as a crucial component of the overall treatment necessary to combat the deleterious effects of burn injury. Hypermetabolism associated with thermal injury is multifactorial. First, increased levels of circulating catecholamines, glucagon, and cortisol initiate the body's catabolism of endogenous stores of protein, carbohydrate, and fat. Second, increased body temperature caused by thermal injury increases metabolism. Evaporative losses from burn wounds and infectious complications are also known metabolic stressors in the face of tissue burns (Wallace, Caldwell, & Cone, 1994). Young pediatric burn patients (<3 years) are at significantly increased risk because they have higher maintenance fluids requirements to maintain ad-

Table 4–4 Recommended Schedule for Pediatric Parenteral Metabolic and Nutrition Monitoring

Parameter	Initial/Hospital Setting	Follow-up/Home
Metabolic (serum)[a]		
Electrolytes, glucose, BUN/creatinine	Daily/biweekly	Weekly to monthly
Ca, Phos, Mg, triglyceride	Biweekly/weekly	Weekly to monthly
Prealbumin/albumin	Biweekly/weekly	Weekly to monthly
Liver function tests, bilirubins	Biweekly/weekly	Weekly to monthly
Complete blood count/differential	Weekly	Weekly to monthly
Prothrombin time (PT/PTT)	Weekly	Weekly to monthly
Iron indices, trace elements	As indicated	Biannually to annually
Fat soluble vitamins, folate, B_{12}	As indicated	Biannually to annually
Carnitine, ammonia	As indicated	As indicated
Blood/catheter site cultures	As indicated	As indicated
Metabolic (urine)		
Glucose, ketones, specific gravity	As indicated	As indicated
Growth		
Weight	Daily	Biweekly to monthly
Height, head circumference	Weekly	Weekly to monthly
Body composition	Monthly	Monthly to biannually
Clinical parameters		
Vital signs[b]	Daily	Daily to as indicated
Intake and output	Daily	Daily to as indicated
Catheter site/dressing	2 to 4 times/day	2 times daily
Developmental milestones	As indicated	As indicated

Note: Frequency depends on clinical condition and tolerance.
[a] May need to check more frequently for metabolically unstable patients.
[b] Vital signs include respiratory rate, heart rate, temperature, and blood pressure.

equate hydration; they also have immature immune systems that do not respond to injury as well as their older counterparts (Durtschi, Kohler, Finley, & Heimbach, 1980). Infants and young children also have decreased endogenous energy reserves and, therefore, have rapid deterioration of fat and muscle mass (Harmel, Vane, & King, 1986). Although energy requirements are increased in infants and children with burns, the additional energy requirements necessary for growth and development may be depressed (Rutan & Herndon, 1990). Rutan and Herndon suggest that profound growth arrest or lack of growth occurs in the pediatric burn patient during the first year after the burn.

Estimating Energy and Protein Demands

Energy and protein requirements for the pediatric burn patient are typically estimated using one of the many predictive energy requirement calculations available. Recently, Mayes, Gottschlich, Khoury, and Warden (1996) compared some of the predictive equations commonly used, including (1) Long (Hunt & Groff, 1990), (2) revised Galveston (Hildreth, Herndon, Desai, & Broemeling, 1990), (3) Curreri Junior (Day et al., 1986), and (4) Davies and Liljedahl (Davies & Liljedahl, 1971), to measure energy expenditure (MEE) × 1.3, using indirect calorimetry, in thermally injured children less than 3 years of age. They found that the predictive equations overpredicted energy requirements of burned infants and toddlers by 13% to 80%. The discrepancy in predicting energy needs with the previously accepted predictive equations may in part be due to advancement in burn care and early closure of wounds, which would contribute to decreased energy requirements. The use of MEE × 1.3 in children less than 10 years of age resulted in preservation of at least 95% of preburn weight while ensuring adequate nutrition by maintaining respiratory quotient within the appropriate range.

If indirect calorimetry is not available to assess patient-specific energy needs, it is recommended that the revised Galveston formula (Exhibit 4–3) (Hildreth et al., 1990) be used to predict energy requirements of the pediatric burn patient because it only overestimated energy requirements by 13%, the least of all of the equations.

The pediatric burn patient has increased protein demands for replacement of nitrogen losses from wounds and urinary losses, as well as increased requirements for wound healing

and gluconeogenesis during the acute phase. Current recommendations are 1.5 to 3.0 gm protein/kg ideal body weight, depending on percent total body surface area (TBSA) burned (Rodriguez, 1995) or 20% of total kilocalories as protein (Waymack & Herndon, 1992).

Micronutrients

Thermal injury may result in increased losses of many micronutrients. Specific attention should be paid to phosphorus, magnesium, zinc, and water-soluble vitamins, which may become depleted because of wound or urinary losses. If severe hypophosphatemia results (<2 mg/dl), intravenous supplementation is recommended because of uncertain absorption of enteral phosphate administration. Additional vitamin and mineral supplements are recommended to promote wound healing, specifically, zinc, vitamin C, vitamin A, and the B vitamins as a result of increased energy metabolism. Table 4–5 lists the recommended vitamin and mineral supplements for patients with burns (Gottschlich & Warden, 1990).

Adequate Provision of Nutrients

Patients with less than 20% TBSA burns can typically achieve adequate oral intake if attention is given to adequacy of their food choices. When burn patients are unable to meet energy needs with oral intake alone, nutrition support is warranted. Nocturnal tube feedings may be adequate to supplement oral intake. EN support is the preferred route of nutrition delivery in the burn patient. Despite common concerns of postburn ileus, immediate intragastric feeding after burn injury (within 6 to 24 hours) is safe and effective (Hansbrough & Hansbrough, 1993; McDonald, Sharp, & Deitch, 1991). However, frequent NPO status caused by multiple surgical procedures may preclude adequate enteral provision of nutrients. In this situation, PN support should be initiated along with enteral support as feasible.

NUTRITIONAL MANAGEMENT: LIVER DISEASE AND LIVER TRANSPLANTATION

Liver disease presents many nutritional challenges, including hypermetabolism, enteropathy, and increased protein oxidation and poor protein synthesis. Patients with chronic liver disease and those patients awaiting liver trans-

---

Exhibit 4–3 Revised Galveston Formula for Predicting Energy Requirements in Pediatric (<12 yr) Burn Patients

$$1{,}800 \text{ kcal/m}^2 \text{ body surface area (BSA)} + 1{,}300 \text{ kcal/m}^2 \text{ body surface area burn (BSAB)}$$

Table 4–5 Recommendations for Vitamin and Trace Element Supplementation in Pediatric Burn Patients

%TBSA Burn	MVI/MIN	Vitamin C	Vitamin A	Zinc Sulfate
<10%–20% TBSA	1 QD	—	—	—
>10%–20% TBSA				
<3 years of age	1 QD	250 mg BID	5,000 IU QD	100 mg QD
>3 years of age	1 QD	500 mg BID	10,000 IU QD	220 mg QD

Note: MVI/MIN, Multivitamin with minerals; TBSA, total body surface area.

Table 4–6 Recommendations for Fat-Soluble Vitamin Supplementation in the Pediatric Patient with Cholestatic Liver Disease

Vitamin	Amount	Monitoring
Vitamin A (aqueous)	10,000–50,000 IU/day	Plasma retinol/retinol-binding protein
Vitamin E as TPGS[a]	25 IU/kg/day	Plasma vitamin E/total lipids
25-OH vitamin D[b]	2–4 µg/kg/day	Plasma 25-OH vitamin D
Vitamin K	2.5–5 mg/day	Prothrombin time

[a] TPGS, d-alpha tocopheryl polyethelen glycol-1000 succinate.
[b] 25-Hydroxycholecalciferol.

plantation have specific nutrient requirements and should be followed closely by a multidisciplinary liver/transplant team, including a gastroenterologist, surgeon, nurse, and dietitian. Patients with cholestasis typically require supplementation of fat-soluble vitamins (vitamin A, vitamin E, vitamin D, and vitamin K) (Table 4–6) (Novy & Schwarz, 1997). In addition, patients with cholestatic liver disease often benefit from specialized formulas that provide nutrients in a more absorbable form, including hydrolyzed protein, and a high percentage of kilocalories from fat, specifically medium-chain triglycerides. The hypermetabolic state and poor nutrient use often seen in patients with liver disease necessitates concentrating infant formulas, often to ≥32 kcal/oz to provide energy without excess fluid. The addition of medium-chain triglycerides (MCT oil) is necessary to provide absorbable energy. Close monitoring of growth is important in those patients awaiting liver transplantation. If growth failure is evident, the initiation of supplemental EN either at home or during hospitalization is necessary. Exhibit 4–4 outlines an algorithm for nutritional management of pediatric patients awaiting liver transplantation.

CONCLUSION

Nutritional monitoring with nutrition support using EN and PN when clinically indicated is a crucial component to the success of postsurgical pediatric patients and their ultimate well-being. Not only do minor and major surgeries place pediatric patients at risk for poor dietary intake postoperatively but recuperation and recovery may be stunted if adequate provision of nutrients is not maintained. Close monitoring of intake, laboratory data, growth, and clinical status allows for improved identification of nutrition risk and timely introduction of nutritional support.

Exhibit 4–4 Algorithim for Nutritional Management of Pediatric Patients before Liver Transplantation

> I. Provide oral nutrition in amounts estimated to meet needs for growth and development (~1.2–1.5 × recommended dietary allowance) and supplement fat-soluble vitamins in patients with cholestatic liver disease.
> II. Monitor weight, length, arm anthropometrics, and head circumference (<3 yr of age) frequently (every 2–3 mo).
> III. If growth failure occurs, initiate supplemental enteral tube feedings with a medium-chain triglycerides–containing formula.
> IV. Reserve parenteral nutrition for specific circumstances that limit enteral nutrition, such as recurrent variceal hemorrhage.
> V. Monitoring vitamin levels (adjust vitamin/mineral supplementation to prevent deficiency), intake, laboratory data, growth and clinical status allows for improved identification of nutrition risk and timely introduction of nutrition support.

REFERENCES

Alverdy, J.C., Aoys, E., & Moss, G. (1988). Total parenteral nutrition promotes bacterial translocation from the gut. *Surgery, 104*(2), 185–190.

Bernstein, L., Bachman, T.E., Meguid, M., Ament, M., Baumgartner, T., Kinosian, B., et al. (1995). Measurement of visceral protein status in assessing protein and energy malnutrition: Standard of care. *Nutrition, 11*(2), 169–171.

Cerra, R.B. (1987). Hypermetabolism, organ failure and metabolic support. *Surgery, 101*(1), 1–14.

Chellis, M.J., Price, M.B., & Dean, J.M. (1994). Cost effectiveness of early enteral feeding in critically ill children. *Critical Care Medicine, 22,* A156.

Chellis, M.J., Sanders, S., Dean, M., & Jackson, D. (1996). Bedside transpyloric tube placement in the pediatric intensive care unit. *Journal of Parenteral and Enteral Nutrition 20*(1), 88–90.

Chicago Dietetic Association and the South Suburban Dietetic Association. (1992). *Manual of clinical dietetics* (4th ed.). Chicago: The American Dietetic Association.

Chwals, W.J., Lally, K.P., Woolley, M.M., & Mahour, G.H. (1988). Measured energy expenditure in critically ill infants and children. *Journal of Surgical Research, 44*(5), 467–472.

Chwals, W.J., Letton, R.W., Jamie, A., & Charles, B. (1995). Stratification of injury severity using energy expenditure response in surgical infants. *Journal of Pediatric Surgery, 30*(8), 1161–1164.

Collier, S., Crough, J., Hendricks, K., & Caballero, B. (1994). Use of cyclic parenteral nutrition in infants less than 6 months of age. *Nutrition in Clinical Practice, 9*(2), 65–68.

Davies, J.W.L., & Liljedahl, S.L. (1971). Metabolic consequences of an extensive burn. In H.C. Polk & H.H. Stone (Eds.), *Contemporary burn management* (pp. 151–169). Boston: Little, Brown and Company.

Day, T., Dean, P., Adams, M.C., Luterman, A., Ramenofsky M.L., & Curreri, P.W. (1986). Nutritional requirements of the burned child: The Curreri junior formula. *Proceedings of the American Burn Association, 18,* 86.

Deitch, E.A. (1992). Multiple organ failure: Pathophysiology and future therapy. *American Surgery, 216,* 117–134.

Deitch, E.A., Winterton, J., Li, M., & Berg, R. (1987). The gut as a portal of entry for bacteremia: Role of protein malnutrition. *Annals of Surgery 205*(6), 681–691.

Delafosse, B., Bouffard, Y., Viale, J.P., Annat, G., Bertrand, O., & Motin, J. (1987). Respiratory changes induced by parenteral nutrition in postoperative patients undergoing inspiratory pressure support ventilation. *Anesthesiology, 66*(3), 393–396.

Durtschi, M.B., Kohler, T.R., Finley, A., & Heimbach, D.M. (1980). Burn injury in infants and young children. *Surgery Gynecology and Obstetrics, 150*(5), 651–656.

Fomon, S.J. (1993). *Nutrition of normal infants.* St. Louis, MO: Mosby.

Forlaw, L., Wong, M., & Little, C.A. (1995). Recommended daily allowances of maintenance parenteral nutrition in infants and children. *American Journal of Health-System Pharmacy, 52*(6), 651–653.

Frankenfield, D.C., Wiles, C.E., Bagley, S., & Siegel, J.H. (1994). Relationships between resting and total energy expenditure in injured and septic patients. *Critical Care Medicine, 22*(11), 1796–1804.

Gottschlich, M.M., & Warden, G.D. (1990). Vitamin supplementation in the patient with burns. *Journal of Burn Care and Rehabilitation, 11*(3), 275–279.

Greene, H.L., Hambridge, K.M., Scanler, R., & Tsang, R.C. (1988). Guidelines for the use of vitamins, trace elements, calcium, magnesium, and phosphorus in infants and children receiving total parenteral nutrition: Report of the subcommittee on pediatric parenteral nutrient requirements from the committee on clinical practice issues of the American Society for Clinical Nutrition. *American Journal Clinical Nutrition, 48*(5), 1324–1342.

Hansbrough, W.B., & Hansbrough, J.F. (1993). Success of immediate intragastric feeding of patients with burns. *Journal of Burn Care and Rehabilitation, 14,* 512–516.

Harmel, R.P., Vane, D.W., & King, D.R. (1986). Burn care in children: Special considerations. *Clinics in Plastic Surgery, 13*(1), 95–105.

Hildreth, M.A., Herndon, D.N., Desai, M.H., & Broemeling, L.D. (1990). Current treatment reduces calories required to maintain weight in pediatric patients with burns. *Journal Burn Care and Rehabilitation, 11,* 405–409.

Hunt, S.M., & Groff, J.L. (1990). Energy balance and weight control. In J Gomez (Ed.), *Advanced nutrition and human metabolism* (pp. 405–430). St. Paul, MN: West Publishing Co.

Kudsk, K.A., Croce, M.A., Fabian, T.C., Minard, G., Tolley, E.A., Poret, H.A., Kuhl, M.R., & Brown, R.O. (1992). Enteral versus parenteral feeding: Effects on septic morbidity after blunt and penetrating abdominal trauma. *Annals of Surgery, 215*(5), 503–513.

Lazarus, D.D., Lowry, S.F., & Moldawer, L.L. (1992). Cytokines acutely decrease circulating insulin-like growth factor-1 (IGF-1) and IGF binding protein-3 (IGFBP-3). *Surgical Forum, 43,* 92.

Lipman T.O. (1998). Grains or veins: Is enteral nutrition really better than parenteral nutrition? A look at the evidence. *Journal of Parenteral and Enteral Nutrition, 22*(3), 167–182.

Lo, C.W., & Walter, W.A. (1993). Changes in the gastrointestinal tract during enteral or parenteral feeding. *Nutrition Review, 47*(7), 193–198.

Long, C.L., Schaffel, N., Geiger, J.W., Schiller, W.R., & Blakemore, W.S. (1979). Metabolic response to injury and illness: Estimation of energy and protein needs from indirect calorimetry and nitrogen balance. *Journal of Parenteral and Enteral Nutrition, 3*(6), 452–456.

Mayes, T., Gottschlich M.M., Khoury, J., & Warden, G.D. (1996). Evaluation of predicted and measured energy requirements in burned children. *Journal of the American Dietetics Association, 96,* 24–29.

McDonald, W.S., Sharp, C.W., & Deitch, E.A. (1991). Immediate enteral feeding in burn patients is safe and effective. *Annals of Surgery, 213*(2), 177–183.

Moore, F.A., Moore, E.E., Jones, T.N., McCroskey, B.L., & Peterson, V.M. (1989). TEN versus TPN following major abdominal trauma-reduced septic morbidity. *The Journal of Trauma, 29*(7), 916–923.

National Research Council. (1989). *Recommended dietary allowances* (10th ed.). Washington, DC: National Academy Press.

Novy, M.N., & Schwarz, K.B. (1997). Nutritional considerations and management of the child with liver disease. *Nutrition, 13*(3), 177–184.

Nussbaum, M.S., & Fischer, J.E. (1991). Pathogenesis of hepatic steatosis during total parenteral nutrition. In L.M. Nyhus (Ed.), *Surgery annual.* Norwalk, CT: Appleton & Lange.

Oh, D.J., Mattox, H.E., Gelfand, D.W., Chen, M.Y., & Wu, W.C. (1991). Enteral feeding tubes: Placement by using fluoroscopy and endoscopy. *American Journal of Radiology, 157,* 769–771.

Payne-James, J.J., & Khawaja, H.T. (1993). First choice for parenteral nutrition: the peripheral route. *Journal of Parenteral and Enteral Nutrition, 17*(5), 468–478.

Pepys, M.D., & Baltzs, M.L. (1983). Acute phase proteins with special reference to c-reactive protein and related proteins (Pentaxins) and serum amyloid A protein. *Advances in Immunology, 34,* 141–211.

Piedboeuf, B., Chessex, P., Hazan, J., Pineault, M., & Lavoie, J. (1991). Total parenteral nutrition in the newborn infant: Energy substrates and respiratory gas exchange. *Journal of Pediatrics, 118*(1), 97–102.

Putet, G. (1993). Energy. In R.C. Tsang, A. Lucas, R. Uauy, & S. Zlotkins (Eds.), *Nutritional needs of the preterm infant* (pp. 15–28). Baltimore: Williams & Wilkins.

Rodriquez, D.J. (1995). Nutrition in major burn patients: State of the art. *Support Line, 17*(4), 1–8.

Rutan, R.L., & Herndon, D.N. (1990). Growth delay in postburn pediatric patients. *Archives Surgery, 125*(3), 392–395.

Ugo, P., Mohler, P., & Wilson, G. (1992). Bedside postpyloric placement of weighted feeding tubes. *Nutrition in Clinical Practice, 7,* 284–287.

Wallace, B.H., Caldwell, F.T., & Cone, J.B. (1994). The interrelationship between wound management, thermal stress, energy metabolism, and temperature profiles of patients. *Journal of Burn Care and Rehabilitation, 15,* 499–508.

Waymack, J.P., & Herndon, D.N. (1992). Nutritional support of the burned patient. *World Journal of Surgery, 16*(1), 80–86.

Wilmore, D.W. (1977). *The metabolic management of the critically ill.* New York: Plenum Publishing.

Ziegler, T.R., Smith, R.J., O'Dwyer, S.T., Demling, R.H., & Wilmore, D.W. (1988). Increased intestinal permeability associated with infection in burn patients. *Archives of Surgery, 123*(11), 1313–1319.

SUGGESTED READINGS

Bresson, J.L., Bader, B., Rocchiccioli, F., Mariotti, A., Ricour, C., Sachs, C., & Rey, J. (1991). Protein-metabolism kinetics and energy-substrate utilization in infants fed parenteral solutions with different glucose-fat ratios. *The American Journal of Clinical Nutrition, 54,* 370–376.

Davis, A. (1994). Indications and techniques for enteral feedings. In S.B. Baker, R.D. Baker, & A. Davia (Eds.), *Pediatric enteral nutrition* (pp. 67–93). New York: Chapman & Hall.

Hofmann, A.F. (1995). Defective biliary secretion during total parenteral nutrition: Probable mechanisms and possible solutions. *Journal Pediatric Gastroenterology and Nutrition, 20,* 376–390.

Marian, M. (1993). Pediatric nutrition support. *Nutrition in Clinical Practice, 8*(5), 199–209.

Moss, R.L., Das, J.B., Ansari, G., & Raffensperger, J.G. (1993). Hepatobiliary dysfunction during total parenteral nutrition is caused by infusate, not the route of administration. *Journal of Pediatric Surgery, 28*(3), 391–396.

Page, C.P. (1989). The surgeon and gut maintenance. *American Journal Surgery, 158*(6), 485–490.

Shattuck, K.E., Grinnell, C.D., & Rassin, D.K. (1993). Amino acid infusions induce reversible, dose related decreases in bile flow in the isolated rat liver. *Journal Parenteral and Enteral Nutrition, 17,* 171–176.

Wilmore, D.W., Smith, R.J., O'Dwyer, S.T., Jacobs, D., Zeigler, T., & Wang, Y. (1988). The gut: A central organ after surgical stress. *Surgery, 104,* 917–923.

CHAPTER 5

Vascular Access

Melanie A. Kenney

INTRODUCTION

Central venous catheters have advanced greatly during the last 30 years. Early animal studies demonstrated the safety and efficiency of administering hyperosmolar solutions through a central venous catheter (Dudrick, Wilmore, Vars, & Rhoads, 1968). The animals demonstrated adequate growth and development and a decreased incidence of thrombosis when the catheter tip was threaded into the superior vena cava. In a case study Wilmore and Dudrick (1968) provided an infant with fluids and nutrition by means of a central venous catheter. After 44 days of intravenous nutrition, the infant's growth was appropriate for a 2-month-old child. Today central venous catheters are used to provide parenteral nutrition solutions, access for blood sampling, medications, and fluids or to monitor a patient's hemodynamic stability. This chapter describes the various types of vascular access devices available, the care and maintenance of these devices, and the complications associated with their use.

CATHETER TYPES

Two general types of central venous catheters exist: long term (partially implanted and totally implanted) and short term. Each catheter type has different features consistent with the anticipated duration of pediatric venous access required. Long-term central venous catheters provide vascular access for prolonged or lifelong therapies (e.g., chemotherapy, hemophilia therapy, parenteral nutrition, or other extended intravenous therapies). Short-term catheters function similarly to long-term catheters, but the duration of therapy is expected to be more limited.

Long-Term Partially Implanted Devices (Hickman, Broviac, Groshong, Cook)

The first category, partially implanted venous access devices, are those commonly referred to by the name of the manufacturer or inventor, Hickman, Broviac, Groshong, and Cook. These are single-lumen or multiple-lumen catheters that are surgically placed in subcutaneous tunnels. The distal portion of the catheter exits the skin at what is referred to as the "exit site."

These catheters also feature a Dacron cuff that remains in the subcutaneous tunnel and promotes the surrounding tissue to adhere to the cuff. This anchoring process requires several days to weeks. Theoretically, the cuff prevents the inadvertent removal or dislodgment of the catheter. The cuff also provides a mechanical barrier that inhibits the migration of organisms from the exit site along the catheter in the subcutaneous tunnel (Figure 5–1). These features, the subcutaneous tunnel and the Dacron cuff, have been theorized as reasons for the lower infection rates of these catheters compared with short-term catheters (Baranowski, 1993; Rostad, 1992). In addition, some catheters have two cuffs. One is the Dacron cuff and the other is an antimicrobial cuff that is located closer to the exit site to discourage bacterial migration in the initial postplacement period.

The Groshong catheter developed in 1978 has an additional unique feature to its design. The catheter tip is closed and has a pressure-sensitive valve inside it. The pressure of introducing infusions or medications creates positive pressure and opens the valve outward. When negative pressure or suction is applied, the valve opens inward and allows blood sampling from the catheter (Figure 5–2). When the catheter is not in use, the valve is closed, which prevents blood backflow into the catheter. Therefore, this catheter does not require heparin as a flush solution or the use of a clamp when changing the cap or intravenous tubing (Baranowski, 1993; Thomason, 1991).

Long-Term Totally Implanted Devices

The second category of long-term venous catheters is the totally implanted vascular devices (TIDs). These catheters

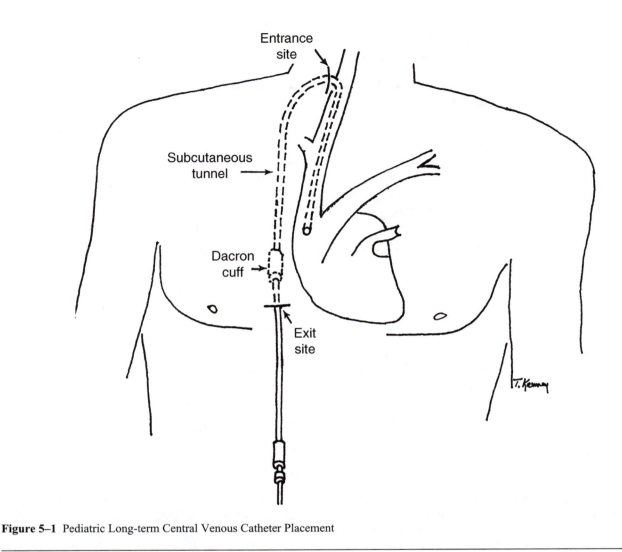

Entrance site

Subcutaneous tunnel

Dacron cuff

Exit site

T. Kenney

Figure 5–1 Pediatric Long-term Central Venous Catheter Placement

are also surgically tunneled under the skin but possess a subcutaneous port or reservoir, with a self-sealing septum that is implanted in the body. The septum is accessed by means of a noncoring or Huber needle through the skin (Figure 5–3). The ports require less frequent maintenance, are much less noticeable, and facilitate optimal body image. Because the port is completely covered by the skin, the patient is able to more freely participate in activities such as swimming and contact sports (Camp-Sorrell, 1992; Gullo, 1993).

Theoretically, patients with TIDs experience fewer infectious complications. However, variable infection rates have been reported when comparing totally implanted to partially implanted catheters. The results range from significantly lower infectious complications for totally implanted devices to comparable rates between the two catheter types (Groeger et al., 1993; LaQuaglia et al., 1992; Wiener et al., 1992). See Table 5–1 for a summary of the advantages and disadvantages of the types of long-term devices.

Short-Term Central Venous Catheters

Short-term central venous catheters provide central access but they lack the features of a Dacron cuff and extensive subcutaneous tunnel. The traditional short-term central venous catheters are those inserted into the subclavian, jugular, or femoral veins and then sutured to the skin (Figure 5–4). These catheters are available in single-lumen or multi-lumen capabilities.

A second type of short-term central venous catheter is the peripherally inserted central catheters (PICC). These catheters are placed in a variety of veins and threaded to either a peripheral or central tip location (Figure 5–5). Total parenteral nutrition can be administered only after the central tip location is verified by radiographic films. Peripheral parenteral nutrition is given through a line that does not have the tip centrally placed. Kearns, Coleman, and Wehner (1996) found that for PICCs placed in the upper extremity,

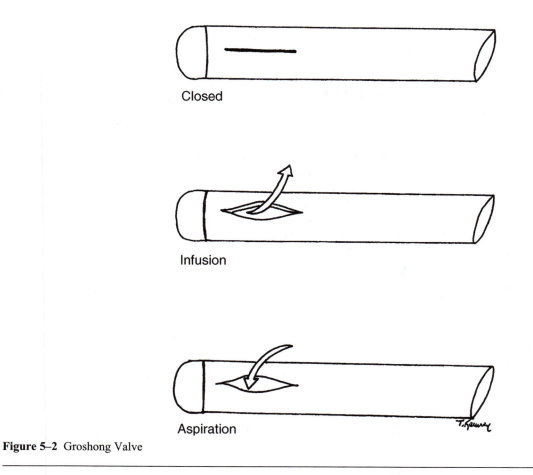

Figure 5–2 Groshong Valve

advancing the catheter tip in a central vein reduced the occurrence of thrombosis. The PICCs do not require surgical insertion and have been placed in interventional radiology suites and by registered nurses in home, hospital, or clinic settings. PICCs are available in a variety of lumen sizes ranging from 2F to 5F, with single-lumen or double-lumen styles. The 2F catheter is not suitable for administration or aspiration of blood samples (BeVier & Rice, 1994; East, 1994; Frey, 1995; LaRue, 1995; Miller & Dietrick, 1997). Bahruth (1996) was the first to report the vasoconstriction or vasos-

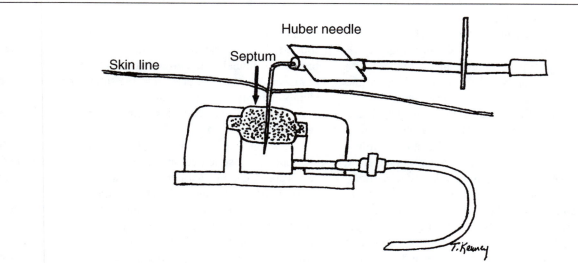

Figure 5–3 Totally Implanted Device (Port)

Table 5–1 Comparisons of Long-term Devices

Partially Implanted Devices	*Totally Implanted Devices*
Advantages	Advantages
No needle sticks	Few activity/clothing restrictions
Easy to initiate intravenous access	Less obvious to casual observer
Technically simple to place and remove	Improved body image
Device less expensive	Minimal care required
Can be removed at bedside/office setting with sedation	Fewer complications
Disadvantages	Disadvantages
Frequent flushing	Needle stick for each access
Dressing to maintain	Greater expense associated with placement
Cost and time required to care for line	Waiting time required when EMLA used
Catheter can be pulled on/broken	Requires a second operation for removal
Dressing change may be uncomfortable	Requires specific equipment (Huber needle) for access

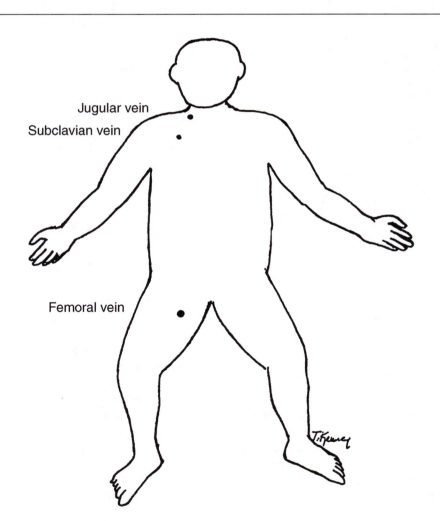

Jugular vein

Subclavian vein

Femoral vein

Figure 5–4 Traditional Short-term Placement Sites

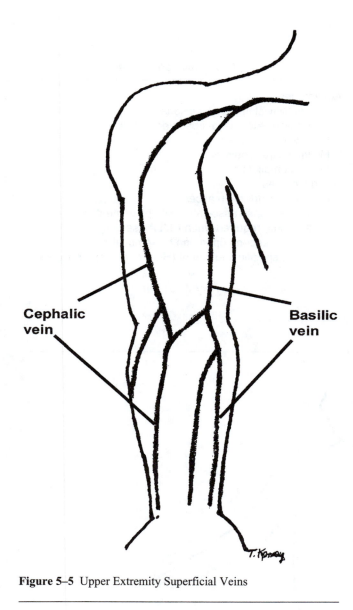

Figure 5–5 Upper Extremity Superficial Veins

pasm that resulted from the application of topical anesthetic cream before placement of a PICC.

CARE AND MAINTENANCE OF CENTRAL VENOUS CATHETERS

Specific policies and procedures are required for the care and maintenance of vascular access devices. Controversy exists about the use of sterile technique versus clean procedures to change dressings and access TIDs. Discussion follows about the care and maintenance of central venous catheters. Appendix 5–A provides a caremap for the patient with a vascular access device.

Antiseptic Agents

The principles of the various antiseptic agents used for dressing change had traditionally been extrapolated from research that studied hand washing of hospital personnel using 70% alcohol and 10% povidone-iodine (Ayliffe, Babb, & Davies, 1988; Rotter, Koller, & Wewalka, 1980). Other trials compared 2% chlorhexidine with these agents when used for catheter dressing changes (Larsen & Thurston, 1997; Maki, Ringer, & Alvarado, 1991; Shapiro, Bond, & Garman, 1990). The 2% chlorhexidine has shown greater antiseptic efficacy; however, as Freiberger (1994) reported, 2% chlorhexidine is not a commercially available product in the United States. The antiseptic agent should be applied using a circular motion, moving from the inside outward. The solution should be applied using a scrubbing technique and allowed to dry (Hadaway, 1998).

Topical Ointment

The use of topical antimicrobial ointment such as 10% povidone-iodine or polyantibiotic ointment is controversial. Some studies have reported that the ointment contributes to decreased infection (Moran, Atwood, & Rowe, 1965; Norden, 1969), whereas other studies have not yielded these same conclusions (Jones, 1998; Maki & Band, 1981; Zinner et al., 1969). Polyantibiotic ointments that are not fungicidal have been shown to contribute to an increased risk of *Candida* colonization of central catheters (Adal & Farr, 1996; Maki & Band, 1981; Zinner et al., 1969). Topical mupirocin or Bactroban applied to the exit site is an effective antimicrobial against staphylococcal species. However, Bactroban does not provide antimicrobial coverage against other organisms (*Physicians Desk Reference*, 1996). Therefore, ointments are rarely routinely used at the catheter exit site today. Their use should be reserved for treatment of organism-specific exit site infections.

Dressing Material

The use of transparent semipermeable dressings instead of the traditional dressing of gauze and tape is a growing trend. The transparent dressings (Tegaderm, Op-Site, Op-Site IV 3000) facilitate securing the central venous catheter, which is a priority for pediatric patients. These dressings also allow for the visual observation of the exit site, less frequent dressing changes, and a greater ability for the patient to bathe or shower without saturating the exit site. The type of dressing material recommended has an impact on the desired frequency of dressing changes. The traditional dressing requires more frequent changes than the transparent dressing. Some researchers report that transparent dressings contribute to increased microbial colonization of the exit site and result in increased infection rates (Conly, Grieves, & Peters, 1989; Dickerson, Horton, Smith, & Rose, 1989), whereas others have reported no difference in catheter colonization and infection rates between the dressing type used (Maki & Ringer, 1987; Young, Alexeyeff, Russell, & Thomas, 1988). Two studies with pediatric subjects compared gauze dressings with transparent dressings and found no significant differences in the incidence of bacterial growth or positive skin cultures (Freiberger, Bryant, & Marino, 1992; Shivnan et al., 1991). The use of a highly permeable transparent dressing resulted in fewer catheter-related infections compared with traditional gauze and transparent dressing groups (Treston-Aurand, Olmsted, Allen-Bridson, & Craig, 1997). Taylor et al. (1996) found a significant increase in microbial growth for the transparent dressing group in their neonatal intensive care patients. However, because this microbial growth did not correlate with an increased sepsis rate, this study recommended the use of transparent dressings for the pediatric population.

Flush Maintenance

The flush solution is yet another issue of controversy for central catheter care. The recommended concentration, amount, and frequency of heparin used to maintain the patency of the central catheter and prevent thrombosis vary. Fry (1992) compiled a survey regarding flushing protocols for all intravenous catheters. This survey revealed a great variation in protocols ranging from a frequency of every 2 hours to every week, with the heparin concentration ranging from 10 units/ml to 1,000 units/ml. This survey provided minimal or no outcome evidence to support specific clinical practices. The use of the lowest possible concentration of heparin is recommended, and it is acceptable that the amount of flush should fill the volume of the catheter and add-on tubing times two (Intravenous Nursing Standards of Practice, 1998). Mechanical measures that use positive pressure flushing techniques or closing the catheter clamp while maintaining pressure on the syringe plunger should be incorporated into the flushing maintenance regimen (Hadaway, 1998).

Heparin is not used with Groshong catheters because the pressure-sensitive valve eliminates the need for heparinization. Research has been conducted to suggest that 0.9% saline is as effective as heparin for peripheral catheters (Epperson, 1984; Goode et al., 1991). A study of obstetric patients found that heparin was needed to maintain peripheral catheter patency because normal saline was not as effective (Meyer, Little, Thorp, Cohen, & Yeast, 1995). The practice of maintaining central venous catheters with saline has not been tested. Future research will determine whether saline is an effective flush for central venous catheters.

Cleansing Catheter Junction/Cap

Sitges-Serra et al. (1984) documented that catheter sepsis does originate from infected central venous catheter hubs, thus emphasizing the need for junctional care. The protocol for cleaning the catheter connection or infusion cap varies using sterile versus aseptic procedures. Seventy percent alcohol and/or povidone-iodine may be used as antiseptic agents (Ruschman & Fulton, 1993). Mechanical barriers such as sterile 2 × 2s may be used when opening the catheter connection to decrease the potential for contamination. The Intravenous Nursing Standards of Practice (1998) report that the optimal time for changing the infusion cap is unknown. Their recommendation is to change the cap at least every 7 days and immediately if residual blood is observed in the cap or if the integrity of the cap may have been compromised.

In 1992, needleless systems were introduced to help make the environment safer for health care providers (Horner, 1998). Danzig et al. (1995) studied the occurrence of bloodstream infections of home intravenous infusion patients using one type of needleless system. The parenteral nutrition patients were found to have a higher rate of infections than patients receiving other therapies. The authors believed that the nutrient-rich parenteral nutrition solutions remained in the infusion cap and became contaminated with subsequent cap manipulations. Different product lines of needleless systems are available. The selection of a particular system should include consideration of the number of pieces required. This will have a direct impact on the time and ease of assembly when using the system.

Accessing an Implanted Port

The patient's skin over and surrounding the port must be prepared before the insertion of the noncoring or Huber needle. This is referred to as "accessing" the implanted port. The Huber needle, which has a noncoring point, must be used because it slices the port septum, thus preserving its integrity. An issue of controversy is whether sterile or clean gloves are necessary when accessing a port. Long and Ovaska (1992) and Schulmeister (1987) found no febrile episodes or septicemia occurred with either method.

After the needle placement is confirmed by blood aspiration and normal saline flush, the needle must be secured and stabilized to prevent needle dislodgment during use. Strips of tape may be used or a formal dressing applied (see "Dressing Material" discussion above). For continued intravenous access, the dressing and Huber needle must be changed. A weekly change is the most commonly reported frequency. To maintain catheter patency, it is recommended that an implanted port be flushed with 5 ml of 100 units/ml heparin after each use. The heparin flush can be effective for up to 1 month when the port is not accessed (Baranowski, 1993; Camp-Sorrell, 1992; Gullo, 1993).

The psychological consequences and pain associated with the use of a needle to obtain vascular access is a definite disadvantage of the implanted port type of central venous catheter. The use of a topical anesthetic, such as eutectic mixture of local anesthetics (EMLA) helps minimize the pain or discomfort reported by patients (Koren, 1993). The EMLA cream should be applied and covered with a transparent dressing at least 1 hour before accessing the port.

POTENTIAL COMPLICATIONS

Potential complications occurring with central catheters can be categorized into two groups: infectious or mechanical. Infections with central venous catheters occur as a localized infection or a systemic infection.

Infectious Complications

Localized Infections

A localized infection occurs at the exit site of short-term or long-term central venous catheters. The signs and symptoms include erythema, edema, drainage, and tenderness at the exit site. Fever may be present. The most common organism involved is *Staphylococcus epidermidis. Staphylococcus aureus, Pseudomonas* species, and *Mycobacterium* species may also be involved (Jones, 1998). Topical and/or systemic antibiotic therapy is needed. Clinicians may also determine that catheter removal or replacement is warranted for tunnel track infections or for exit site infections that recur when antibiotic therapy is concluded (Jones, 1998).

Systemic Infections

Historically, a positive blood culture meant immediate removal of the central venous catheter. More recently, depending on the type of organism isolated and the child's particular infectious history, systemic infections have been successfully treated with appropriate antibiotics and without requiring catheter removal. Many authors report the occurrences and circumstances regarding infectious complications in their patients. Wiener et al. (1992) analyzed the insertion and reason for removal of venous access devices for children with cancer. Infection was the most frequent complication reason for removal of a device. This study did not identify a difference between the number of partially implanted catheters and totally implanted devices removed because of infection. However, a large number of partially implanted catheters were inadvertently removed because of dislodgment and, therefore, could not acquire an infection. A weakness of this study was the inability to collect data on complications that occurred during the life of the catheter. The

authors could not determine infection rates because they were only aware of infections that were the reason for the catheters to be removed. Jones, Konsler, Dunaway, Lacey, and Azizkhan (1993) also investigated pediatric hematology-oncology patients with central venous catheters. They found a greater rate of catheter infection within the first 3 months after the device was placed. They also noted that children younger that 2 years of age had an increased incidence of catheter infection. Kurkchubasche, Smith, and Rowe (1992) discovered that children with short bowel syndrome had a higher incidence of catheter sepsis (7.8/1,000 catheter days) compared with non–short bowel syndrome children (1.3/1,000 catheter days). The non–short bowel syndrome children had *Staphylococcus* species isolated most (88%) of the time from their blood cultures. The short bowel syndrome group showed *Staphylococcus* 38%, yeast 23%, and gram-negative rods 27% of the time. Buchman et al. (1994) reviewed the catheter-related infections of home parenteral nutrition patients discharged from their institution. This included both adult and pediatric patients. Their findings revealed that although the incidence of catheter infection was low for home parenteral nutrition patients, there was a significantly greater occurrence of catheter sepsis and exit site infections in children compared with adults.

Another consideration in the event of infection is the documented relationship between catheter-related sepsis and the presence of vascular thrombosis (Raad et al., 1994). Jones, Konsler, and Dunaway (1996) instilled the amount of 5,000 IU/ml of urokinase needed to fill the catheter lumen and let it dwell for 1 hour before the urokinase was removed. This procedure was repeated the following day, then an antibiotic course was given. This protocol was used when positive blood cultures persisted or the same organism reoccurred.

Mechanical Complications

Occlusion

Resistance of flow when flushing or attempting to administer intravenous fluid is characteristic of an occluded central venous catheter. It is imperative to determine the history and characteristics of this malfunction to decide whether the occlusion is from a clot or thrombus versus a precipitation of intravenous medication or fluid. A perceived occlusion may be investigated radiographically. Stephens, Haire, and Kotulak (1995) radiographically examined 200 dysfunctional central venous catheters. They found 58% of the catheters were occluded as a result of thrombus. Before any treatment, mechanical maneuvers should be tried, such as repositioning the patient, coughing, deep breathing, and having the patient raise his or her arms above the head. The dressing should be removed to determine whether the catheter is kinked by the dressing or sutures, if present (Bagnall-Reed, 1998).

A clotted catheter usually has a history of slight resistance over the past few days, with increasing difficulty in flushing. The history may also reveal difficulty or inability to obtain blood samples from the catheter. Urokinase is a thrombolytic agent that is effective in clearing catheters occluded by clot or thrombosis. Urokinase (5,000 IU/ml) can first be administered by bolus in a syringe, and then the patency of the catheter is checked over time (Cunningham & Bonam-Crawford, 1993; Holcombe, Forloines-Lynn, & Garmhausen, 1992; Wachs, 1990). A second bolus of urokinase may be recommended if the return of patency is not achieved from the first dose of urokinase and left to dwell for 12 hours (Wiener & Albanese, 1998) or overnight (Hadaway, 1998). Continuous infusion of low-dose urokinase (200 units/kg/hr) over 12 to 24 or more hours has been used to clear catheters that remain occluded after urokinase is administered by the bolus method (Bagnall, Gomperts, & Atkinson, 1989; Bagnall-Reed, 1998).

However, the U.S. Food and Drug Administration issued a drug warning on January 25, 1999 (U.S. FDA, 1999a) and an update on March 16, 1999 (U.S. FDA, 1999b) regarding urokinase use. The FDA advised that urokinase be reserved for use only after other alternatives have been considered and urokinase is determined by the physician to be critical to the care for that patient. Other thrombolytic agents to consider for use include streptokinase and tissue plasminogen activator (t-pa).

In contrast, a precipitated catheter is seen with a sudden, complete inability to flush or infuse through the catheter. Drug or solution incompatibilities occur by inappropriate drug preparation or the mixing of incompatible medications or solutions (Hadaway, 1998). Evaluating the intermittent intravenous medications and the components of the intravenous solution should reveal the cause of the precipitated catheter. The clinician must know the chemicals involved in the precipitate when attempting to clear the catheter. Various precipitates and their treatments have been reported. Calcium phosphorus precipitates have been treated with 0.1 N hydrochloric acid (Hashimoto, Morgan, Kenney, Pringle, & Alcorn, 1986; Holcombe et al., 1992; Kupensky, 1995). Shulman, Barrish, and Hicks (1995) used a model to demonstrate that even a daily infusion of hydrochloric acid over an 8-week interval did not cause visible damage to central catheters. Pennington and Pithie (1987) reported experience using an ethanol solution to clear catheters occluded with lipid material associated with "three-in-one" (dextrose, amino acid, and lipid emulsion in same solution) parenteral nutrition. Werlin et al. (1995) and Borg, Timmer, and Kam (1992) also reported the efficacy of ethanol and hydrochloric acid to clear partially and totally implanted catheters.

Emergency Care of Broken/Damaged Central Catheters

The patient or caregiver must be prepared to clamp the catheter between the child and damaged or broken area of the catheter should the central venous catheter become damaged or broken. The patient or caregiver should be educated in performing a temporary repair by inserting the appropriate-sized blunt needle into the catheter lumen. A temporary repair kit can easily be assembled for the family/caregiver, which includes flushing supplies, sterile scissors, alcohol swabs, appropriate-sized blunt needle, and tongue depressor. The corresponding permanent repair kit is obtained from the manufacturer of the particular PICC or partially implanted catheter. This permanent repair is performed by a member of the health care team.

Implanted Port-Specific Complications

Twiddler's Syndrome

Patients with the nervous habit of "twiddling" their implanted ports could actually displace, curl, or kink the catheters. Twiddler's syndrome was originally associated with patients after pacemaker insertion, but it has also been reported in patients with implanted ports (Gebarski & Gebarski, 1984). Servetar (1992) reported the first incidence of twiddler's syndrome in a pediatric patient. The patient's port site was edematous and tender on one occasion but was resolving. Before administering a vesicant solution, a chest radiograph film revealed the catheter had migrated out of the vein and the catheter had multiple revolutions in the subcutaneous tunnel. On questioning, the mother recalled noticing the patient playing with his port. This episode illustrates the need to observe for itching, scrubbing, or excess touching of the port and the need to obtain a history from the caregiver when the port area appears tender, to have changed location, or has signs of infection present.

Needle Dislodgment/Extravasation

The anatomic placement of the implanted port may be a factor in the incidence of needle dislodgment. A port placed in excessive adipose tissue, near breast tissue, and over the pectoral muscle near the axilla not only makes accessing the port more difficult, but the movement of the arms and shoulders could also potentially cause accidental needle dislodgment (Camp-Sorrell, 1998). Other causes of extravasation include migration of the catheter into a smaller vein (Ingle, 1995). Conditions that change intrathoracic pressure such as coughing, sneezing, heavy lifting, or forceful flushing of the catheter could result in catheter tip migration (Hadaway, 1998). The presence of thrombus or fibrin sheath formation at the catheter tip is also associated with extravasation. The flow of infusate is obstructed at the catheter tip, which causes the infusate to flow back along the catheter into the subcutaneous tissue (Mayo & Pearson, 1995). The presence or absence of a blood return and patient discomfort should be assessed with each accessing. The port should flush easily without erythema or edema observed at the Huber needle site. If the device has a history of no blood return, a dye study should be obtained to evaluate the needle placement and catheter position before it is used to infuse a vesicant (Chrystal, 1997). If it is uncertain whether needle dislodgment/extravasation occurred, a physician should be consulted. Appropriate treatment of the suspected or known ex-travasation is determined by the type of infusate that was administered.

CONCLUSION

The use and maintenance of vascular access catheters is a rapidly growing and evolving area of health care. Many issues relevant to the care and maintenance of these catheters remain controversial. With continued research and outcome reporting, children requiring central venous access can safely receive a variety of medications and fluids through these devices.

REFERENCES

Adal, K., & Farr, B. (1996). Central venous catheter-related infections: A review. *Nutrition, 12,* 208–213.

Ayliffe, G., Babb, J., & Davies, J. (1988). Hand disinfection: A comparison of various agents in laboratory and ward studies. *Journal Hospital Infection, 11,* 226–243.

Bagnall, H., Gomperts, E., & Atkinson, J. (1989). Continuous infusion of low-dose urokinase in the treatment of central venous catheter thrombosis in infants and children. *Pediatrics, 83,* 963–966.

Bagnall-Reed, H. (1998). Diagnosis of central venous access device occlusion. *Journal of Intravenous Nursing, 21,* 115–121.

Bahruth, A. (1996). Peripherally inserted central catheter insertion problems associated with topical anesthesia. *Journal of Intravenous Nursing, 19,* 32–34.

Baranowski, L. (1993). Central venous access devices: Current technologies, use, and management strategies. *Journal of Intravenous Nursing, 16,* 167–194.

BeVier, P., & Rice, C. (1994). Initiating a pediatric peripherally inserted central catheter and midline catheter program. *Journal of Intravenous Nursing, 17,* 201–205.

Borg, F., Timmer, J., & Kam, S. (1992). Use of sodium hydroxide solution to clear partially occluded vascular access ports. *Journal of Parenteral and Enteral Nutrition, 17,* 289–291.

Buchman, A., Moukarzel, A., Goodson, B., Herzog, F., Pollack, P., Reyen, L., Alvarez, M., Ament, M., & Gornbein, J. (1994). *Journal of Parenteral and Enteral Nutrition, 18,* 297–302.

Camp-Sorrell, D. (1992). Implantable ports: Everything you always wanted to know. *Journal of Intravenous Nursing, 15,* 262–273.

Camp-Sorrell, D. (1998). Developing extravasation protocols and monitoring outcomes. *Journal of Intravenous Nursing, 21,* 232–239.

Chrystal, C. (1997). Administering continuous vesicant chemotherapy in the ambulatory setting. *Journal of Intravenous Nursing, 20,* 78–88.

Conly, J., Grieves, K., & Peters, B. (1989). A prospective, randomized study comparing transparent and dry gauze dressings for central venous catheters. *Journal of Infectious Diseases, 159,* 310–319.

Cunningham, R., & Bonam-Crawford, D. (1993). The roles of fibrinolytic agents in the management of thrombotic complications associated with vascular access devices. *Nursing Clinics of North America, 28,* 899–900.

Danzig, L., Short, L., Collins, K., Mahoney, M., Sepe, S., Bland, L., & Jarvis, W. (1995). Blood stream infections associated with a needleless intravenous infusion system in patients receiving home infusion therapy. *JAMA, 273,* 1862–1865.

Dickerson, N., Horton, P., Smith, S., & Rose, R. (1989). Clinically significant central venous catheter infections in a community hospital: Association with type of dressing. *Journal of Infectious Diseases, 160,* 720–721.

Dudrick, S., Wilmore, D., Vars, H., & Rhoads, J. (1968). Long-term total parenteral nutrition with growth, development, and positive nitrogen balance. *Surgery, 64,* 134–140.

East, S. (1994). Planning, implementation, and evaluation of a successful hospital-based peripherally inserted central catheter program. *Journal of Intravenous Nursing, 17,* 189–192.

Epperson, E. (1984). Efficacy of 0.9% sodium chloride injection with and without heparin for maintaining indwelling intermittent injection sites. *Clinical Pharmacy, 3,* 626–629.

Freiberger, D. (1994). The use of Hibiclens™ in pediatric central venous line skin care. *Journal of Pediatric Nursing, 9,* 126–127.

Freiberger, D., Bryant, J., & Marino, B. (1992). The effects of different central venous line dressing changes on bacterial growth in a pediatric oncology population. *Journal of Pediatric Oncology Nursing, 9,* 3–7.

Frey, A. (1995). Pediatric peripherally inserted central catheter program report. *Journal of Intravenous Nursing, 18,* 280–291.

Fry, B. (1992). Intermittent heparin flushing protocols. *Journal of Intravenous Nursing, 15,* 160–163.

Gebarski, S., & Gebarski, K. (1984). Chemotherapy port "twiddler's syndrome": A need for preinjection radiography. *Cancer, 54,* 38–39.

Goode, C., Titler, M., Rakel, B., Ones, D.S., Kleiber, C., Small, S., & Triolo, P.K. (1991). A meta-analysis of effects of heparin flush and saline flush: Quality and cost implications. *Nursing Research, 40,* 324–329.

Groeger, J., Lucas, A., Thaler, H., et al. (1993). Infectious morbidity associated with long-term use of venous access devices in patients with cancer. *Annals Internal Medicine, 119,* 1168–1174.

Gullo, S. (1993). Implanted ports technologic advances and nursing care issues. *Nursing Clinics of North America, 28,* 859–871.

Hadaway, L. (1998). Major thrombotic and nonthrombotic complications. *Journal of Intravenous Nursing, 21,* 143–160.

Hashimoto, E., Morgan, D., Kenney, M., Pringle, K., & Alcorn, A. (1986). Blocked TPN catheters: Clots aren't the only culprit. *Journal of Parenteral and Enteral Nutrition, 10,* 17S.

Holcombe, B., Forloines-Lynn, S., & Garmhausen, L. (1992). Restoring patency of long-term central venous access devices. *Journal of Intravenous Nursing, 15,* 36–41.

Horner, K. (1998). Technology assessment of two needleless systems. *Journal of Intravenous Nursing, 21,* 203–208.

Ingle, R. (1995). Rare complications of vascular access devices. *Seminars in Oncology Nursing, 11,* 184–193.

Intravenous Nursing Standards of Practice. (1998). *Journal of Intravenous Nursing, 21* (suppl).

Jones, G. (1998). A practical guide to evaluation and treatment of infections in patients with central venous catheters. *Journal of Intravenous Nursing, 21,* 134–142.

Jones, G., Konsler, G., & Dunaway, R. (1996). Urokinase in the treatment of bacteremia and candidemia in patients with right atrial catheters. *American Journal Infection Control, 24,* 160–166.

Jones, G., Konsler, G., Dunaway, R., Lacey, S., & Azizkhan, R. (1993). Prospective analysis of urokinase in the treatment of catheter sepsis in pediatric hematology-oncology patients. *Journal of Pediatric Surgery, 28,* 350–357.

Kearns, P., Coleman, S., & Wehner, J. (1996). Complications of long arm-catheters: A randomized trial of central vs peripheral tip location. *Journal of Parenteral and Enteral Nutrition, 20,* 20–24.

Koren, G. (1993). Use of the eutectic mixture of local anesthetic in young children for procedure-related pain. *Journal of Pediatrics, 122,* S30–S35.

Kupensky, D. (1995). Use of hydrochloric acid to restore patency in a occluded implantable port. *Journal of Intravenous Nursing, 18,* 198–201.

Kurkchubasche, A., Smith, S., & Rowe, M. (1992). Catheter sepsis in short-bowel syndrome. *Archives of Surgery, 127,* 21–25.

LaQuaglia, M., Lucas, A., Thaler, H., Friedlander-Klar, H., Exelby, P., & Groeger, J. (1992). A prospective analysis of vascular access device-related infections in children. *Journal of Pediatric Surgery, 27,* 840–842.

Larsen, L., & Thurston, N. (1997). Research utilization: Development of a central venous catheter procedure. *Applied Nursing Research, 10,* 44–51.

LaRue, G. (1995). Improving central placement rates of peripherally inserted catheters. *Journal of Intravenous Nursing, 18,* 24–27.

Long, M., & Ovaska, M. (1992). Comparative study of nursing protocols for venous access ports. *Cancer Nursing, 15,* 18–21.

Maki, D., & Band, J. (1981). A comparative study of polyantibiotic and iodophor ointment in prevention of vascular catheter-related infection. *American Journal of Medicine, 70,* 739–744.

Maki, D., Ringer, A., & Alvarado, C. (1991). Prospective randomized trial of povidone-iodine, alcohol, and chlorhexidine for prevention of infection associated with central venous and arterial catheters. *Lancet, 338,* 339–343.

Maki, D., & Ringer, M. (1987). Evaluation of dressing regimens for prevention of infection with peripheral intravenous catheters: Gauze, a transparent polyurethane dressing, and an iodophor-transparent dressing. *JAMA, 258,* 2396–2403.

Mayo, D., & Pearson, D. (1995). Chemotherapy extravasation: A consequence of fibrin sheath formation around venous access devices. *Oncology Nursing Forum, 22,* 675–680.

Meyer, B., Little, C., Thorp, J., Cohen, G., & Yeast, J. (1995). Heparin versus normal saline as a peripheral line flush in maintenance of intermittent intravenous lines in obstetric patients. *Obstetrics and Gynecology, 85,* 433–436.

Miller, K., & Dietrick, C. (1997). Experience with PICC at a university medical center. *Journal of Intravenous Nursing, 20,* 141–147.

Moran, J., Atwood, R., & Rowe, M. (1965). A clinical and bacteriologic study of infections associated with venous cutdowns. *New England Journal of Medicine, 272,* 554–560.

Norden, C. (1969). Application of antibiotic ointment to the site of venous catheterization: A controlled trial. *Journal Infectious Diseases, 120,* 611–615.

Pennington, C., & Pithie, A. (1987). Ethanol lock in the management of catheter occlusion. *Journal of Parenteral and Enteral Nutrition, 11,* 507–508.

Physicians Desk Reference. (1996). Montvale, NJ: Medical Economics Co.

Raad, I., Luna, M., Khalil, S., Costerton, J., Lam, C., & Bodey, G. (1994). The relationship between the thrombotic and infectious complications of central venous catheters. *JAMA, 271,* 1014–1016.

Rostad, M. (1992). Intravenous access part 3. Venous access devices. *Urologic Nursing, 12,* 130–135.

Rotter, M., Koller, W., & Wewalka, G. (1980). Povidone-iodine and chlorhexidine gluconate containing detergents for disinfection of hands. *Journal of Hospital Infection, 1,* 149–158.

Ruschman, K., & Fulton, J. (1993). Effectiveness of disinfected techniques on intravenous tubing latex infection ports. *Journal of Intravenous Nursing, 16,* 304–308.

Schulmeister, L. (1987). A comparison of skin preparation procedures for accessing implanted ports. *National Intravenous Therapy Association, 10,* 45–47.

Servetar, E. (1992). A case of twiddler's syndrome in a pediatric patient. *Journal of Oncology Nursing, 9,* 25–28.

Shapiro, J., Bond, E., & Garman, J. (1990). Use of a chlorhexidine dressing to reduce microbial colonization of epidural catheters. *Anesthesiology, 73,* 625–631.

Shivnan, J., McGuire, D., Freedman, S., Sharkazy, E., Bosserman, G., Larson, E., & Grouleff, P. (1991). A comparison of transparent adherent and dry sterile gauze dressings for long-term central catheters in patients undergoing bone marrow transplant. *Oncology Nursing Forum, 18,* 1349–1356.

Shulman, R., Barrish, J., & Hicks, J. (1995). Does the use of hydrochloric acid damage silicone rubber central venous catheters? *Journal of Parenteral and Enteral Nutrition, 19,* 407–409.

Sitges-Serra, A., Puig, P., Linares, J., Perez, J., Farrero, N., Jaurrieta, E., & Garau, J. (1984). Hub colonization as the initial step in an outbreak of catheter-related sepsis due to coagulase negative staphylococci during parenteral nutrition. *Journal of Parenteral and Enteral Nutrition, 8,* 668–672.

Stephens, L., Haire, W., & Kotulak, G. (1995). Are clinical signs accurate indicators of the cause of central venous catheter occlusion? *Journal of Parenteral and Enteral Nutrition, 19,* 75–79.

Taylor, D., Myers, S., Monarch, K., Leon, C., Hall, J., & Sibley, Y. (1996). Use of occlusive dressings on central venous catheter sites in hospitalized children. *Journal of Pediatric Nursing, 11,* 169–173.

Thomason, S. (1991, October). Using a Groshong central venous catheter. *Nursing 91,* 58–60.

Treston-Aurand, J., Olmsted, R., Allen-Bridson, K., & Craig, C. (1997). Impact of dressing materials on central venous catheter infection rates. *Journal of Intravenous Nursing, 20,* 201–206.

U.S. Food and Drug Administration (FDA). (1999a). "Important Drug Warning." http://www.fda.gov/cber/ltr/abb012599.htm. Accessed 17 June 1999.

U.S. Food and Drug Administration (FDA). (1999b). "Update on Abbokinase (Urokinase)." http://www.fda.gov/cber/infosheets/abb031699.htm. Accessed 17 June 1999.

Wachs, T. (1990). Urokinase administration in pediatric patients with occluded central venous catheters. *Journal of Intravenous Nursing, 13,* 100–102.

Werlin, S., Lausten, T., Jessen, S., Toy, L., Norton, A., Dallman, L., Bender, J., Sabilan, L., & Rutkowski, D. (1995). Treatment of central venous catheter occlusions with ethanol and hydrochloric acid. *Journal of Parenteral and Enteral Nutrition, 19,* 416–418.

Wiener, E., & Albanese, C. (1998). Venous access in pediatric patients. *Journal of Intravenous Nursing, 21,* 122–133.

Wiener, E., McGuire, P., Stolar, C., Rich, R., Albo, V., Ablin, A., Betcher, D., Sitarz, A., Buckley, J., Krailo, M., Versteeg, C., & Hammond, G. (1992). The CCSG prospective study of venous access devices: An analysis of insertions and causes for removal. *Journal of Pediatric Surgery, 27,* 155–164.

Wilmore, D., & Dudrick, S. (1968). Growth and development of an infant receiving all nutrients exclusively by vein. *JAMA, 203,* 860–864.

Young, G., Alexeyeff, M., Russell, D., & Thomas, R. (1988). Catheter sepsis during parenteral nutrition: The safety of long-term OpSite dressings. *Journal of Parenteral and Enteral Nutrition, 12,* 365–370.

Zinner, S., Denny-Brown, B., Braun, P., Burke, J., Toala, P., & Kass, E. (1969). Risk of infection with indwelling intravenous catheters: Effects of application of antibiotic ointment. *Journal of Infectious Diseases, 120,* 616–619.

Appendix 5–A

Caremap for Vascular Access

	Preplacement/Day of Placement	*Postplacement*
Treatment		Begin and advance feedings as bowel sounds return Resume normal nonstrenuous activity
Medications	Give perioperative antibiotics as indicated, i.e., ___ (drug name) @ ___ mg/kg/day q___h Pain medications per institution protocol, i.e., ___ (drug name) @ ___ mg/kg/day	Heparin ___ units/ml ___ ml as needed Postprocedure antibiotics as ordered Pain medication as ordered
Assessment and monitoring	Weight QD Intake and output Vital signs q1h x 2, then q4h Assess dressing dry and intact	Vital signs q8h Assess dressings Assess incisions/exit site/port site
Consults	Anesthesia Social service as necessary Translator as needed Child life	Home nursing agency as needed Vendor for discharge vascular access supplies
Tests	CBC Doppler ultrasonography to assess vein patency as indicated	

Education	Preprocedure teaching as appropriate for infant/child developmental stage	Begin vascular access teaching and return demonstrations with patient/caregiver:
		    Dressing change
		    Flush maintenance
		    Emergency care of damaged catheter
		    Accessing implanted port
		    Monitoring for systemic/localized infection

Discharge planning	Discuss type of vascular access with patient/family Involve patient/family in selection of type of access as indicated Assess caregiver's ability to learn home vascular access care	Recommend to caregiver that any individual supervising child (teacher, child care provider) be prepared to clamp broken catheter Coordinate additional intravenous therapies Correlate home nursing visits as needed Arrange for delivery of vascular access supplies Arrange for follow-up appointments

CHAPTER 6

Pain Management and Sedation in Children

Wendy Lord Mackey

PAIN IN CHILDREN: AN OVERVIEW

Definition of Pain

The International Association for the Study of Pain Subcommittee on Taxonomy (1979) defines pain as "an unpleasant sensory and emotional experience connected with actual or potential tissue damage, or described in terms of such damage." According to McCaffery (1979), pain defies definition. However, she does offer a more liberal and operational definition by stating pain is "whatever the experiencing person says it is, existing whenever he says it does" (p. 11). McGrath supports McCaffery's definition of pain and further specializes it to the pediatric population by stating, "the answer to understanding a child's pain comes from the children themselves, not from us (medical and nursing professionals) blindly applying adult perceptions to their world" (Helwig, 1990, p. 130). Further, children are not small adults and may not demonstrate or even verbalize their pain in the way adults do. This makes the job of pain control in the child very difficult.

Many factors may determine how a child responds to pain, such as developmental age, cognitive and developmental level, procedure or condition causing pain, coping style, advance preparation for the procedure or condition, sex, birth order, culture, personality, temperament, past experiences, parental response to pain, and type of pain (acute or chronic) (Eland & Anderson, 1977; McCrory, 1991; Ross & Ross, 1988). Several factors that increase the experience of pain are fear, anxiety, and depression (Berde, 1989). Further, Anna Freud speculated that the meaning of a painful experience may be influenced by the child's type and depth of fantasy aroused by it (Eland & Anderson, 1977). Therefore, it is imperative that clinicians consider the procedure, treatment, and actual pain experience for each child.

Pathophysiology of Pain

Physiologic pain is the result of stimulation of nociceptors. Nociceptors (or pain sensors) are free nerve endings located throughout the body in the skin, muscle, blood vessels, and organs. The transmission of the pain impulses occurs by way of two different types of afferent fibers, thereby creating two types of pain sensation. These fibers ascend to the brain and are called A-delta fibers and C-delta fibers (Sinatra, 1992). A-delta fibers are myelinated, thereby transmitting pain impulses very rapidly, resulting in sharp, pricking, localized sensations. These fibers are responsible for the withdrawal response from a painful stimuli. C-delta fibers are unmyelinated, smaller fibers. These fibers conduct impulses more slowly and are responsible for dull, persistent, diffuse pain or chronic, burning, aching pain. The afferent fibers transmit the nociceptive signals to the dorsal horn of the spinal cord. Cell bodies and dendrites from within the dorsal horn relay the sensory messages to higher neurocenters, including the thalamus, cerebral cortex, limbic system, hypothalamus, areas of the frontal lobe, and cingulate gyrus (Fitzgerald & Anand, 1993).

The psychobiological aspect is an integral part of the pathophysiology of pain, with the affective and cognitive mechanisms of the experience often as important as the actual tissue damage (McGrath & Craig, 1989). A common misconception is that neonates do not feel pain as a result of an immature nervous system. Neonates do feel pain. Anand and Hickey have concluded that "pain pathways, as well as cortical and subcortical centers necessary for pain perception, are well developed late in gestation, and neurological systems well known to be associated with pain transmission and modulation are also intact and functional" (Schechter, 1989, p. 786).

DEVELOPMENTAL CONSIDERATIONS IN PEDIATRIC PAIN CONTROL

Developmental level is an important factor to consider when managing children in pain. Throughout the childhood years, they are continually expanding their individual capacities physically, cognitively, emotionally, socially, and psychologically. Further, children often regress cognitively and emotionally under the stress of pain, illness, and hospitalization (Ross & Ross, 1988). Table 6–1 explores the developmental influences on pain behavior and expression.

Cognitive development has an impact on a child's communication about pain. Infants are behaviorally disorganized when agitated and distressed. The influence of cognitive development on pain in infants is poorly understood at this time. Older infants and toddlers have greater communication skills to let others know when it hurts. They often know some words that denote pain, such as owie, boo-boo, or hurt. Children older than 3 years of age have the ability to identify the intensity of pain when provided with the appropriate measurement device (Beyer & Wells, 1989). Pain scales give children permission to express their pain while following the rules of appropriate behavior (Broome, Bates, Lillis, & McGahee, 1990). Adolescents have the abstract ability to easily quantify and qualify their pain experiences. However, according to Favaloro (1988), adolescents have difficulty expressing their true feelings regarding pain. Some adolescents will deny having any pain because of their fear of addiction, the treatment, or being thought of as a baby. Adolescents are also developmentally egocentric in their thinking. They may not verbalize their pain, assuming that the clinician is aware of their pain and has done everything possible to alleviate it (McCaffery & Beebe, 1990). Consequently, it is equally important to assess for nonverbal indications of pain (behavioral and physiologic) even when the adolescent (and child) denies having pain. Common behavioral changes include irritability, restlessness, depression, agitation, and refusal to cooperate (Wong & Baker, 1988).

Fear is an important emotional response when focusing on pain in children. The fear of what is happening, strange surroundings, people, sounds, smells, and a lack of control may be overwhelming for any child, which in turn may exacerbate the perception of pain (Broome et al., 1990; McGrath, Thurston, Wright, Preshaw, & Fermin, 1995; McGrath & Craig, 1989). This fear may be lessened or controlled with developmentally appropriate explanations and preparation. Often, children refuse to report pain because they fear the treatment (Eland & Anderson, 1977; McGrath & Craig, 1989; Wong & Baker, 1988). The child may deny the pain until it is out of control, at which time a much larger dose of analgesia may be indicated to make the child comfortable (Rauen & Ho, 1989).

PAIN ASSESSMENT AND MEASUREMENT

Pain assessment requires a multidimensional approach, accumulating information from a variety of sources including the pain history, pain interview, a variety of measurement tools and thorough, ongoing evaluations and reassessments. A pain history is an interview between a health care provider and the child and family to learn about the child's experience with pain, acute and chronic, including the child's reporting style, coping mechanisms, and pain language. Ideally, the interview takes place preoperatively or before the pain event. The interview is an ideal time to provide information regarding the general pain management plan, answer questions, and correct misconceptions. The pain interview pertains to the communication between the child and/or family and the health care provider when the child is experiencing pain. Information regarding the nature of the pain, intensity, duration, sensation, and what makes it feel better or worse must be gathered. Follow-up and continued assessment is imperative. It is important to remind the child and family at regular intervals to report any pain when it occurs or changes (McCaffery, 1979).

The presence of pain, the intensity of that pain, and the impact of the pain on the individual should be accurately identified when making a pain assessment (Slack & Faut-Callahan, 1991). All individuals have their own beliefs, attitudes, and experiences regarding pain, all of which have an impact on their perception of another individual's pain (Colwell, Clark, & Perkins, 1996; French, Painter, & Coury, 1994; Mackey, 1993). Imposing beliefs and attitudes about pain on the patient should be avoided.

Self-Reporting Measures

Self-reporting measures rely on the individual experiencing pain to elicit a score that represents the pain experienced. This method of measurement is the best indicator of the intensity of an individual's pain. Numerous research studies have found that children as young as 3 years of age are able to indicate the intensity and location of their pain when provided with an appropriate tool (Abu-Saad, 1984; Aradine, Beyer, & Tompkins, 1987; Beyer & Wells, 1989; Eland & Anderson, 1977; Hester, 1979). These tools allow the child to discriminate the intensity of the pain. Scales range from "no pain" to "the worst pain imaginable." It is important to remember that a child's rating is personal and unique and should not be compared with another child's pain rating. The ratings are only valid and meaningful when compared with the same child's pain rating at different times and occasions (Kuttner, 1997). These tools are practical for clinical use and relatively easy to administer.

However, many difficulties remain in using these tools in children. All tools rely on a certain developmental, verbal, and cognitive level on the part of the child to communicate an

Table 6–1 Pain Behaviors, Expressions, Fears, and Sources of Comfort during the Various Stages of Growth and Development

Development Stage	Potential Pain Behaviors	Potential Modes of Expression	Predominant Fears	Potential Sources of Comfort
Infant (0–12 months): Dependent on others for all needs. Forms meaningful relationship with primary caregiver. Develops best when needs are consistently and effectively met and anxiety and mistrust when they are not. "Stranger" anxiety develops at about 8 months. Receives stimulation and gratification through mouth.	Total body movements Lack of responsiveness to feeding Changes in alertness Lack of contentment Sleep disturbances Poor responsiveness to caregivers Withdrawal, unusual stillness	Crying (quality) Whimpering Facial expression	Separation from parents Fear of strangers	Presence of primary caregiver or consistent nurses Sucking, self-comforting (soother, blanket, etc.) Holding, rocking Favorite toy, object, photograph Medication
Toddler (1–3 years): Develops autonomy through exploration. Shame and doubt if assertiveness nonacceptable or actions ineffective. Egocentric. Tolerates minimal separation from primary caregiver only. Opposes everything— "no." "Separation anxiety" 8–24 months. Gratification from control of muscles. Thought derives from sensation and movement.	Clinging to primary caregiver Rejection of all others Refusing food/toileting; regression to infant behaviors Decreased exploration of the environment Flailing arms and legs, holding body rigid Touching hurting body part	Crying (varies from whimpering to outright scream) Refusal of everything Withdrawal Anxious facial expression or hiding face Describing pain as "hurt" or "owie" (location not specific)	Separation from parents or primary caregivers Fear of immobility and restraint	Presence of primary caregiver or consistent nurses Special toys or objects Rocking, holding Distraction activities—stories, television, music Self-comforting—sucking, holding on to special blanket Medication
Preschooler (3–5 years): Becoming more of an individual and tolerating longer separation. Mastering of play and movement, control of bowel and bladder functions, ability to initiate interactions. Magical thinking—some difficulty distinguishing fantasy and reality. Develops conscience and learns to share.	Immobility, rigidity Clinging to anyone Crying, kicking Regression to previous stages (e.g., loss of bowel and bladder control) Disinterest in normal play and tasks Anxiety	Crying (screaming) Shrieking (without tears) Withdrawal Concerned only with how pain affects him or her Able to describe pain's location and intensity; "bad tummy ache" or "legs hurt" Fearful of pain-relieving interventions and incessantly asking questions, "What are you doing?" "Why?"	Separation from parents, siblings, home environment Fear that pain is punishment Fear of body mutilation	Presence of family, consistent staff Familiar toys, books, etc. Games and play activities (distraction techniques) Regular caregivers performing painful procedures Fantasy Increased mobility (e.g., going to the playroom) Asking child what has helped relieve pain in the past and using child's suggestions and simple participation Simple routines and explanations Medication

continues

Table 6-1 continued

Development Stage	Potential Pain Behaviors	Potential Modes of Expression	Predominant Fears	Potential Sources of Comfort
School-age Child (6–12 years): Develops industry through mastery of new skills and rewards for them or inferiority if not. Enjoys structure and rules. Becomes competitive. Values peers. Bases conclusions on perceptions—beginning of logical thought.	Wide variance in behavior from hyperactivity to extreme passivity Unstable moods and temperament Demanding Overt aggression, anger Not caring for self Temper outbursts Withdrawal, extreme quietness, lying with eyes closed, "tuning out" Regression to earlier behaviors—e.g., panic attacks, bedwetting, impulsiveness Anxious facial expressions and poor eye contact	Able to more accurately describe location and intensity of pain May groan, wince, scream, but try to hold back tears and "be brave" May deny any pain in presence of peers Demand scientific explanations of how pain treatments and procedures affect body functioning May ask for pain medications providing they are *not* injections	Fear of feeling inferior Separation from peers Fear of mutilation Fear of rejection Fear of loss of self-control	Relationship with peers Ability to engage in tasks Presence of supportive, understanding adult Explanations at a level the child can understand Encourage participation in care Hypnosis and biofeedback Medication
Adolescent (13+ years): Vacillates between dependence and independence. Logical thought and deductive reasoning. Peer acceptance crucial. Self-control, body image, body changes, sexuality, and role development are very prominent concerns.	As above, there may be a wide range of behaviors and regression to previous stages Withdrawal, depression Aggressiveness, teasing Manipulation Poor eating and hygiene Refusal of care	Able to describe pain—location, intensity, and duration May verbalize desire for pain medications May refuse pain interventions in presence of peers	Fear of losing control Fear of changes in self-concept and body image Fear of loss of independence Separation from peers Concerns regarding future (e.g., relationships, sexual competency, fertility, etc.)	Relationships with peers and friends Consistency of roommates Consistency of caregivers Interests; hobbies Family members—may prefer siblings to parents at times Self-hypnosis, self-relaxation Control over the situation Solitude Medication

accurate score. Second, many children may communicate invalid information and scores. Numerous factors may affect a child's pain score such as nausea, constipation or gas, position, fear or anxiety, and the presence or absence of parents or significant others (Beyer & Wells, 1989). It is important to evaluate all these factors to elicit a valid and reliable subjective pain score.

Observer Report Measures

Often, observer reporting measures are used by individuals to quantify the child's pain in an objective way. This method is indicated and useful for children who are unable to communicate (preverbal, unconscious, language barrier, and developmental delay).

Behavioral Observations

Another valuable method of measuring pain is through the observation of behaviors. This method is based on the assumption that certain behaviors correlate with certain types and degrees of pain. Behaviors that are commonly used to identify the presence of pain are facial expressions, vocalization, and posture/movement. Several scales and tools have been developed that focus on this type of pain information. Most behavioral scales are based on the summation of scores of various behaviors.

Behavioral observations are sometimes difficult to interpret. Behavior that indicates pain often mimics other stressors experienced by children, such as hunger, separation, or the discomfort of a wet diaper (Hester & Barcus, 1986). These types of tools are useful in the assessment of preverbal or unconscious children when used in correlation with other assessments. Their independent use may be insufficient or misleading (Colwell et al., 1996).

Physiologic Measurements

Pain can have an impact on a variety of physiologic measures, such as respiratory rate, heart rate, blood pressure, perspiration, and a variety of biologic and hormonal measures. However, these measures do not exclusively indicate pain. Pain perception initiates a stress response and may cause a person to be tachycardic, tachypneic, and hypertensive. Yet, absence of these physiologic phenomenon does not necessarily mean lack of pain. The body is often quick to adapt to these physiologic changes and to establish a new equilibrium. This is especially true for patients who have long-term or chronic pain (Fitzgerald & Anand, 1993).

NONPHARMACOLOGIC METHODS OF PAIN MANAGEMENT IN CHILDREN

Nonpharmacologic methods of pain control are an integral part of the care of all children experiencing pain. By defini-

tion, nonpharmacologic pain management is an extremely general and broad topic, including all interventions used to control pain, except pharmacologic ones. Children are filled with fantasy and magical thinking and desire coping mechanisms to guide them away from a frightening, unfamiliar, or painful situation. This section describes a variety of general topics, all of which contribute to the nonpharmacologic milieu of pain management.

Separation from parents can be stressful for the hospitalized child and contribute to pain sensation. Most hospitals have adopted liberal policies concerning parental presence, including 24-hour rooming in capabilities. Empowering the parents to care for and comfort their child is important.

Control and predictability are vitally important to a child. The very nature of the hospital is one of little control. The child is submerged in an environment with different people, smells, noises, sounds, food, and activity. Creating an institutional philosophy incorporating the concepts and interventions identified in Exhibit 6–1 will help to comfort the child and family and offer more predictability (Schechter, Blankson, Pachter, Sullivan, & Costa, 1997).

Preparation enables a child to become acquainted with a situation or procedure before the event. Fear of the unknown is an anxiety-provoking experience for a child. Individuals under stress experience difficulty processing and coping with new experiences. Allowing a child to visualize the environment or play with some of the equipment that will be used before the actual event increases coping at the time of the painful procedure or event (Broome, 1990; Heiney, 1991; Mansson, Fredrikzon, & Rosberg, 1992). It also provides the child and family time to plan coping strategies for a difficult situation. Exhibit 6–2 offers some guidelines for preparation of children and families for health care experiences.

Mind-Body Techniques

Mind-body methods are active treatments that use both mental and physical functions to modify, modulate, or relieve pain (Kuttner, 1997). They engage and promote an individual's personal coping abilities, enabling success and mastery over a situation.

Anyone who has a relationship with the child is qualified to implement the interventions. Health care professionals have an obligation to assist their patients and families in learning methods to minimize pain and facilitate coping during painful situations. Although practice does enhance the success of these interventions, they can be used during the painful event with minimal preparation (Kuttner, 1997). The key is to experiment and practice them on a colleague, friend, or family member and use them yourself. Feeling comfortable with these techniques helps the child, family, and other members of the health care team use them. A summary of the most common mind body techniques follows.

Exhibit 6–1 Increasing Control and Predictability in the Hospital Setting

- Comfort items: Allowing the child to have comfort items, such as favorite toys or security items, pictures of family, friends, or pets, musical tapes, or videos, all may help to make the environment more familiar and personal and less threatening. Allowing children to wear their own clothes and have their own bed linens may also help.
- Comfort measures: This includes providing a comfortable environment for the child. Ensure the appropriate lighting, room temperature, and noise control. Make provisions for being held or rocked. Positioning is an important aspect of comfort measures. A new theory is emerging called "positioning for comfort." This involves using various patient positions during procedures that promote the comfort of the child.
- The treatment room: The treatment room is a place where any invasive procedure should take place. The child's bed, on the other hand, should remain a safe place. Routine, noninvasive examinations, assessments, and vital signs will occur there, but nothing invasive or painful. Some children will voice a preference to have certain things done in their bed, and these requests for the most part should be honored. For example, one child may prefer to have their central line dressing change done in bed versus going to the treatment room. The following passage basically summarizes a child-safe environment.

  "There is a room where you have your IV done, the treatment room. Having your own room with friends, it's the thing in the hospital that's like your own home. It's a place for you to lie and stay and sleep. It can be nice and comfy. If you have an IV there, or even a finger stick, it doesn't feel like you're even at home! Only getting your IV out in your room is really okay" (Alex [age 7], personal interview).

  Ensuring compliance with this concept and philosophy is important. Although it does take a little more time to move the child from his or her room into the treatment room, it will benefit the child and health care team.
- The playroom: The playroom should be a child's safe haven. The playroom belongs to the children. It is filled with fun things. Absolutely no procedures or examinations occur in the playroom. If it is necessary for a child to be examined or have vital signs while in the playroom, they leave and return once the intervention is completed. The only medical thing that occurs in the playroom is medical play and preparation. It is not uncommon to see children in the playroom giving a needle or intravenous to their doll or playing with casting material or bandages.

Exhibit 6–2 Preparing Children and Families for Health Care Experiences: Guidelines from the ACCH Child Life Research Project

- Give priority to children and families who are assessed at high risk for vulnerability to stress.
- Assess each child's present knowledge, understanding, and appraisal of the situation before deciding what information to share with the child.
- Select materials and style of presentation to match the child's cognitive level, experience, and interest.
- Use minimally threatening, age-appropriate language.
- Provide accurate information about what the child will actually experience. Avoid providing irrelevant details.
- Describe the procedure in terms of the child's sensory experiences (including all five senses), the sequence of events, and the anticipated duration.
- Describe the steps involved in the procedure, demonstrating with actual medical equipment when possible.
- Encourage the child to handle and explore the actual medical equipment that he or she will see during the procedure.
- Describe, draw, or demonstrate with dolls behaviors that are expected of the child during each step of the procedure (such as a position).
- Discuss different options of how the child might effectively cope during the procedure.
- Provide the child with opportunities to rehearse effective coping behaviors (directly or with a doll).
- Discuss with parents ways they can support their child during and after procedures.
- Encourage the child (and family members) to ask questions and express feelings.
- Assess the child's understanding and assimilation of the information (through verbal feedback or by observing the child's play or demonstration of the procedure).
- Explore parents' understanding of their child's concerns and fears and assess family responses to the preparation.
- Do not force information on children if they clearly indicate that they do not want to hear or experience it.

Breathing/Blowing Techniques

Breathing and blowing techniques are powerful distraction tools with the added benefit of slowing down respirations and promoting relaxation. Implementing this technique avoids the first response most children have to pain, breath holding, which in fact heightens pain sensation. The breathing essentially consists of taking in a long, deep breath through the nose and slowly blowing it out through the mouth. Fantasy elements can be added to assist the child such as blowing out pretend candles or the light of a flashlight, blowing up a pretend balloon, or taking in big breaths to help them float. Suggestive language, such as, "blow away the owie" may also enhance effectiveness. This technique can be used successfully even in the toddler years with the assistance of bubbles or other blow toys and activities. Being creative is the key.

Initially, most children do better if their coach breathes with them and encourages them. This offers a twofold advantage to the coach (often the parent), whose tension and stress is controlled by the effects of the breathing, as well as providing them with a tool effective in contributing to the management of the child's stress and pain (McDonnell & Bowden, 1989). When proficient, many children implement this technique independently. Breathing techniques assist in the management of acute and chronic episodes of pain and other discomforts such as nausea. Some children use this technique in combination with other strategies such as imagery.

Hypnosis

Hypnosis is the ability to focus attention and become absorbed in an altered state of consciousness whereby perceptions and sensations can be enhanced, modified, or changed (Kuttner, 1997). It is an internal imaginative mind-body process. The goal of hypnosis in pain management is to empower the child to take control of the pain versus the usual passive role and state of helplessness. The key is to enable the child to focus attention on the task of undoing the pain versus focusing on the pain itself. For example, empower the child to untie the pain knot or change the sensation of the pain from a burning to a tingling sensation (Kuttner, 1997).

Relaxation

Relaxation involves the voluntary relaxation of muscles in the body, thereby decreasing stress and anxiety and increasing coping abilities. It strives to clear the mind and body of all internal and external influences. Numerous methods induce relaxation, including successive tension-relaxation methods and yoga-style breathing with suggestions for calmness and guided release of tension from head to toe (Durham & Frost-Hartzer, 1994; Kuttner, 1997).

Guided Imagery

Imagery is a cognitive-behavioral technique that requires the child to create an image of something that is not actually present while in a relaxed state. It draws on the child's active imagination, allowing the coach to guide the child through the painful, often frightening, event that leaves the child with feelings of security, control, and success (Yaster, Krane, Kaplan, Cote, & Lappe, 1997). The child's attention is refocused away from the problem toward a new image. The image can be one that the child creates, an actual event (such as a birthday party or baseball game), or a story portrayed and delivered by the coach. The incorporation of senses, including sound, vision, taste, smell, movement, position, and touch, brings the image to life. Some children want to vocally participate in the imagery, and others prefer to just listen. The child needs support and coaching at least initially to participate in this method, especially when pain intensity increases. This method may be effective for children with chronic pain or children who undergo repeated painful events.

Distraction Methods

Distraction methods are reality-based, cognitive-behavioral techniques whereby the child focuses attention on an external object, separate from the pain, to maximize coping. This method can implement one or a number of senses, including visual, auditory, tactile, and taste and may be used with any age group. Other techniques such as breathing or relaxation are often used in conjunction with distraction. Table 6–2 offers a variety of distraction tools with the corresponding age group for which they are most useful.

PHARMACOLOGIC MANAGEMENT OF PAIN

Pharmacologic management of pain in children involves numerous drugs and routes. The following is a summary of nonopioid analgesics, opioid analgesics, antagonists, local anesthetics, and sedatives. Table 6–3 describes the most commonly used medications.

Nonopioid Analgesia

Nonopioid analgesics act at the level of the peripheral nervous system by inhibiting the production of prostaglandin (Yaster et al., 1997). They are effective in increasing pain relief when used in combination with other types of analgesics without increasing the risk of dose-related side effects such as respiratory depression. Nonopioid analgesics all have a ceiling therapeutic dose, where increasing the dose above the recommended therapeutic dosing range does not increase the analgesic effect.

Table 6–2 Developmental Approaches with Distraction Resources

Distraction Resource	Newborn	Infant	Toddler	Preschool	School Age	Adolescent
Music	X	X	X	X	X	X
Rattle, sound toys		X	X	X		
Bubbles		X	X	X	X	X
Magic wands			X	X	X	X
Videos		X	X	X	X	X
Walkman				X	X	X
Party blowers			X	X	X	X
Stickers			X	X	X	X
Baby toys		X	X	X		
I spy books				X	X	X
Guided imagery				X	X	X
Travel games				X	X	X
Gameboy/Sega					X	X
Massage	X	X	X	X	X	X
Magazine/book				X	X	X
Pinwheels			X	X	X	X
Musical/popup books			X	X	X	
View master			X	X	X	
Kaleidoscope			X	X	X	X
Stress balls					X	X
Talking	X	X	X	X	X	X
Singing	X	X	X	X	X	X

Corticosteroids

Corticosteroids are used in combination with other analgesics in the critically ill patient. Corticosteroids (most commonly prednisone and dexamethasone) are therapeutic in the management of pain associated with swelling such as joint pain from rheumatologic disorders, nerve pressure pain, and pain from bone metastases and brain tumors (Shannon & Berde, 1989).

Opioid Analgesia

An opioid can be defined as a medication that has a morphine-like effect (Leith & Weisman, 1997b). Opioids are the mainstay for the treatment of acute and chronic severe pain, including postoperative pain, post-traumatic pain, sickle-cell pain, and chronic cancer pain. They are not optimally therapeutic in the treatment of neuropathic pain (Shannon & Berde, 1989). Opioids do not have a ceiling effect. Analgesic effect increases with increased dosing, as do the risk of respiratory depression and other side effects. The most effective analgesic program using opioids is one that is titrated to optimal analgesic effect and minimal side effects.

The pharmacokinetics of how opioids work in treating and preventing pain is complex. Most opioids are agonists (neurotransmitters) and occupy pain receptor sites in the central nervous system that initiate a pharmacologic effect. The most common opioid receptors include mu, kappa, delta, and sigma receptors. Each of these receptors has prototype agonists causing various clinical effects. The medications most commonly used to treat pain are mu agonists, responding to morphine, methadone, fentanyl, meperidine, and codeine, among others. The agonists reach the receptor sites in the central nervous system in one of two ways: systemic circulation across the blood-brain barrier (intravenous, intramuscular, transdermal, transmucosal administration) or direct placement or diffusion into the cerebrospinal fluid (intrathecal or epidural administration) (Yaster & Maxwell, 1993).

Route of Administration

Opioids can be administered by a multitude of routes, including oral, rectal, buccal, nasal, transdermal, subcutaneous, intramuscular, intravenous, and epidural. The goal in administering safe and therapeutic opioids is to maintain a plasma level that lies above the effective analgesic threshold and below the level of respiratory depression or coma. The patient's clinical status and pain level determine the most appropriate route.

Table 6–3 Medication Used in Pediatric Pain Management

Classification	Medication (administration routes and dosing guidelines)	Comments
Nonopioids	Acetaminophen (PO/PR) 10–15 mg/kg q4h orally or rectally	• Therapeutic in the management of pain and fever. • Safe and effective for use in all children including newborns and premature infants.[a,b] The hepatic metabolic systems in the newborn are immature, which in fact is protective because it results in decreased production of the toxic metabolites of acetaminophen.[c] • Little anti-inflammatory effect. • Do not divide suppositories, medication not evenly dispersed.
	Aspirin (PO) 10–15 mg/kg q4h orally	• Use with caution: Associated with Reye's syndrome. • Used primarily in children with rheumatic disorders. • Very effective analgesic with anti-inflammatory properties.
Nonsteroidal anti-inflammatory drugs (NSAIDs)	Ibuprofen (PO) 3–10 mg/kg q6h orally	• Superior anti-inflammatory effects along with analgesia. • Side effects include gastrointestinal bleeding, gastric upset, hematologic disturbances (primarily related to platelet function and prolongation of bleeding times) and alteration in renal function.[d] • Food may decrease the incidence of gastric upset and ulceration. • NSAIDs primarily bind with protein and may interfere with the absorption of other medications.[d]
	Ketorolac (PO/IV) Loading dose: 1 mg/kg IV x1, then 0.5 mg/kg q6h IV 10 mg orally/dose for adolescents	• Currently the only NSAID approved for IV use. • Not recommended for use >3 days. • Loading dose should be given when initiating therapy. • IV dose may be given IM.
Opioids	Morphine (IV/PO) 0.05–0.1 mg/kg 2–3 hr IV 0.03–0.06 mg/kg/hr cont IV infusion 0.3 mg/kg q3–4h orally Neonates and infants <4 mo 0.02–0.05 mg/kg IV q3–4h 0.01–0.02 mg/hr, cont infusion	• Morphine is the standard against which all other opioids are compared. • Inexpensive and easily administered. • Note dosing differences in neonates.
	MS Contin (PO) 0.3 mg/kg q8–12h orally	• Slow release form of morphine. • Do not crush tablets.
	Fentanyl (IV, transdermal, epidural, transbuccal) 0.01 mg/kg q1–2h IV Neonates and infants <4 mo 0.0001–0.002 IV bolus	• Fentanyl has a rapid onset (1 minute) and short duration (30–45 minutes), making it an ideal medication for use with short painful procedures.[e] • It is extremely lipophilic, readily penetrating all membranes, including the blood-brain barrier. • Sufentanyl and alfentanyl, the more potent relatives of fentanyl, are extremely therapeutic drugs; however, they should be reserved for use by anesthesiologists only.

continues

Table 6–3 continued

Classification	Medication (administration routes and dosing guidelines)	Comments
	0.001–0.02 hourly infusion	• Fentanyl is 100 times more potent than morphine. • It has less of a histamine release, resulting in less pruritus and vasodilation.[f] • Chest wall rigidity is a serious side effect that can occur with rapid infusion, making ventilation impossible at times. It can be treated with muscle relaxants such as succinylcholine or pancuronium, or with naloxone.[g] • Fentanyl Oralet is a transbuccal preparation of fentanyl and has been quite successful when taken as a premedication before a painful procedure or surgery.[h–j] • A transdermal fentanyl patch is available. Fentanyl is bound to a patch that is placed on the skin. Therapeutic levels are reached approximately 12 hours after patch placement and reported to be fairly consistently maintained.
	Codeine (PO) 1 mg/kg q4–6h orally	• Codeine is the most commonly prescribed oral opioid analgesia for children. It is most commonly prescribed in combination with acetaminophen, also referred to as Tylenol #3. • Codeine is often the drug of choice when a child is able to take food/drink orally and can safely and easily be used in the outpatient setting.
	Demerol (IV) 1 mg/kg	• Although pharmacokinetically similar to morphine at equianalgesic doses (morphine is 10 times more potent); the clinical use of meperidine is limited. After repeated doses of meperidine, there is an accumulation of its metabolite, normeperidine, which may produce tremors, muscle twitching, hyperactive reflexes, and convulsions.[a] • The use of meperidine causes hyperpyrexia, delirium, seizures, and death when administered to patients taking monoamine oxidase inhibitors.[k] • There is no clear clinical advantage to using meperidine over morphine, although some clinicians maintain that it is more effective for smooth muscle pain, as with gynecologic procedures and biliary colic.[g]
	Methadone (IV, PO) 0.1–0.2 mg/kg q4h IV (initially) x2 then 0.05 mg/kg IV q4–6h 0.2–0.4 mg/kg q8–12h orally	• Absorbed extremely slowly and has a long duration of action (12–36 hr). • Often used in the treatment of long-term or chronic pain. With routine scheduled dosing, plasma levels can be maintained similar to a continuous intravenous infusion of morphine.[k] • Very therapeutic when prescribed using a sliding scale, where the dose is dependent on the pain the patient has at the time of the dose. • It can also be used in combination with other drugs to tackle any breakthrough pain. • Produces less sedation, euphoria/dysphoria, and constipation than morphine.[l]
	Hydromorphone (PO, IV, epidural)	• Similar to morphine except that it is 8 to 10 times more potent. • The incidence of central nervous system depression, nausea, and pruritus may be less than morphine in some patients.[k]
Sedatives— benzodiazepines		• Benzodiazepines are clinically useful as premedications for surgery and procedures and as general sedatives in the intensive care unit setting. They are powerful anxiolytics and amnesic agents.[f] • No analgesic properties. • Sedative and respiratory depressant effects are increased with concomitant opioid administration.

continues

Table 6–3 continued

Classification	Medication (administration routes and dosing guidelines)	Comments
	Midazolam (PO, PR, IV) 0.05–0.1 mg/kg IV q2–4h 0.5 mg/kg orally	• Clinically versatile, well-tolerated drug with profound amnesic effect. • It provides rapid sedation and is very short acting, making it especially useful for short procedures. Many studies report the safe and therapeutic effects of midazolam administered by way of numerous routes, when used for sedation in pediatric patients.[m–o]
	Diazepam (PO, PR) 0.2–0.3 mg/kg orally 0.02–0.1 mg/kg q6–8h IV	• Numerous disadvantages including a contraindication in the neonatal period and in patients with hepatic dysfunction. Incompatible with many intravenous solutions and long duration of action.[p]
	Chloral hydrate (PO, PR) 50–100 mg/kg orally	• Most commonly used as a sedative in young children before nonpainful procedures such as diagnostic imaging or ophthalmic examinations. • There has been controversy regarding the safe and effective use of chloral hydrate.[q–s] • Should always be administered in a safely monitored environment because deaths from respiratory arrest have been reported.[p] There is no antagonist for chloral hydrate at this time.
Antagonist	Naloxone (IV) 0.01 mg/kg	• A complete opioid antagonist. It is powerful in reversing the effects of agonist-opioids. Naloxone is nonselective, reversing all aspects of the agonist, side effects, and analgesia. • The most effective dosing of naloxone involves the titration by small increments to reverse the unwanted effects without completely reversing all aspects of the opioid.[f] • Naloxone overdose is a potential complication and results in tachycardia, tachypnea, hypertension, nausea, vomiting, and possible sudden death from cardiac fibrillation.[e] • The effect of naloxone is short acting (30–45 min). Careful monitoring is warranted to observe for the return of the unwanted side effects.[p] • Often, repeated doses are needed in narcotized patients with respiratory suppression. Naloxone drips are helpful in controlling various uncomfortable side effects such as puritus and urinary retention when other measures have been unsuccessful. When dosed appropriately, the naloxone infusions do not seem to interfere with the analgesic effects of the opioids.
	Flumazenil (IV) 0.003–0.005 mg/kg	• A benzodiazipine antagonist. • Very short-acting agent and therefore will often require repeated doses when used to reverse long-acting benzodiazepines such as diazepam. • A very specific inhibitor that focuses on reversing the convulsant and anxiolytic properties of the benzodiazepines and, to a lesser extent, it reverses the sedative and motor incoordination properties.[r]
Local anesthetics (topical preparation)	EMLA (eutectic mixture of local anesthetics)	• Contains a combination of lidocaine and prilocaine. • It is a white cream that is applied topically and is covered with an occlusive dressing. • Also available in a ready to use anesthetic disk. • After being left in place for longer than 1 hr, the surface beneath the cream is anesthetized for up to 4 hr. Its application is useful and indicated whenever there is an invasive penetration of intact skin on an awake child.[t–v]

continues

Table 6–3 continued

Classification	Medication (administration routes and dosing guidelines)	Comments
		• It is ideal for procedures such as venipunctures, accessing ports, circumcisions, draining abscess, and immunizations. • Its limiting factor is the 1-hr delay after application, although with thoughtful planning, this does not have to be an issue.

TAC		• TAC is a combination of local anesthetic solutions (tetracaine, 0.5%; adrenaline [epinephrine, 1:2,000], and cocaine, 11.8%) used topically for laceration repairs.[w] The prepared solution is placed into the wound, and covered with a TAC-saturated gauze for 10 to 15 min.
		• The use of TAC is contraindicated in the following clinical situations:
		  – Lacerations on areas supplied by end arteries, such as the digits, penis, and nose, because of the vasoconstricting properties of both epinephrine and cocaine.
		  – Lacerations on or close to any mucous membranes because of the cocaine content. Ingestion can be life threatening.
		  – Children with an allergy to PABA-containing lotions or local anesthetics.[w]

Nummy Stuff		• Topical application of a local anesthetic by iontophoresis (the administration of drugs, whereby an external electric field propels the ionizable drug molecules transdermally).[x] • Procedure takes 10–30 min based on the power level of electrophoresis used. • This is a new product and little clinical research is available on its efficacy and safety at this time.[x]

[a] Forest, Clements, & Prescott, 1982. [b] Berde, 1989. [c] Berde, 1991. [d] Tyler, 1994. [e] Yaster & Maxwell, 1993. [f] Shannon & Berde, 1989. [g] Yaster & Deshpande, 1988. [h] Weisman, 1995. [i] Schecter, Weisman, Rosenblum, Bernstein, & Conrad, 1995. [j] Epstein et al., 1996. [k] Leith & Weisman, 1997a. [l] Vetter, 1989. [m] Sievers, Yee, Foley, Blanding, & Berde, 1991. [n] Theroux et al., 1993. [o] Tolksdorf, Elick, & Amberger, 1991. [p] Cote, 1994. [q] Lipshitz, Marino, & Sanders, 1993. [r] Anderson, Zeltzer, & Fanurik, 1993. [s] Steinberg, 1993. [t] Koren, 1993. [u] Benini, Johnston, Faucher, & Aranda, 1993. [v] Weatherstone et al., 1993. [w] Yaster, Tobin, & Maxwell, 1993. [x] Ashburn et al., 1997.

Intravenous administration of opioids is the most reliable method of delivery. When plasma-opioids are in the therapeutic range, they provide the patient with prompt pain control. Continuous infusions are a practical and therapeutic method of intravenous delivery (Berde, 1991; Leith & Weisman, 1997a; Vetter, 1989). Intermittent administration of intravenous opioids commonly produces fluctuating plasma drug levels, which results in cycles of pain, comfort, and sedation (Bender, Weaver, & Edwards, 1990). This cycle exposes the patient to unnecessary opioid toxicities while only providing intermittent pain control.

The use of patient-controlled analgesia (PCA) and epidural analgesia are other effective methods of pain control. They are discussed in detail later in this chapter. There is absolutely no physiologic or emotional advantage to the administration of any analgesic by injection (Hendrickson et al., 1990; Liu & Northrop, 1990). Oral administration of opioids is the route of choice in most situations when a child is able to tolerate oral intake. It is often not an option for children in the initial postoperative period because of an ileus or when children have nausea and vomiting or severe mucositis.

Dose Scheduling

For most analgesics to be effective in controlling severe pain, adequate blood levels must be maintained by around-the-clock administration. Most analgesics in pediatrics are ordered on an as-needed (PRN) basis. PRN was thought to be the appropriate approach to pain control before there was sufficient knowledge regarding analgesic plasma levels

(Eland, 1988). Unfortunately, PRN is often interpreted as meaning "as little as possible" as opposed to "as needed." For many clinicians, this requires the child to feel severe pain before another dose of analgesia may be administered and only if the allotted time has passed since the last dose (Berde, 1989).

Side Effects of Opioids

Opioids produce a host of side effects, including respiratory depression, pruritus, nausea/vomiting, urinary retention, urticaria, decreased gastrointestinal motility or ileus, and sedation. These side effects can often add to the discomfort of the patient. Careful monitoring and anticipation of these effects avoid untoward complications. The side effects are primarily dose related and can be easily controlled with dose adjustments and various clinical antidotes. Table 6–4 provides a summary of some of the most common side effects and complications. Tolerance, dependence, and addiction are all phenomena associated with the use of opioids. Clearly defining these three phenomena increases understanding in the clinical setting (Exhibit 6–3).

Sedatives

Because of the emotional, psychological, and behavioral components of pain, sedation is often an important component in pain management. Sedatives are effective when used in conjunction with an opioid. However, they should not be used in place of opioids when analgesia is needed. The goal of pain management is to provide analgesia, not to render the child too sleepy to complain or resist. Refer to Table 6–3 for specific drug information.

Antagonists

Antagonists are drugs that occupy specific receptor sites and block the activity of neurotransmitters (or agonists). Table 6–3 provides information on the two most commonly used antagonists: naloxone and flumazenil.

Local Anesthetics

Local anesthetics are drugs that block the neural impulses along both central and peripheral nerve pathways (Yaster, Tobin, & Maxwell, 1993). Unlike most other medications, they must be deposited directly into the area at which an effect is desired. Local anesthetics are extremely effective in obliterating pain sensation with minimal physiologic effects. They are primarily used to treat pain as part of a regional anesthetic technique, including topical application (Table 6–3), local infiltration, peripheral nerve blocks, intravenous regional anesthesia (Bier Blocks), and epidural or spinal anesthesia.

Buffering the local anesthetic decreases the acidity of the solution and thereby decreases the burning sensation commonly described with its infiltration (McKay, Morris, & Mushlin, 1987). Buffering is accomplished by mixing 1 part 8.4% sodium bicarbonate (1 mEq/ml) with 10 parts lidocaine (1% to 2%; ± epinephrine) (Wong, 1996). A small-gauge needle (30-gauge) is used when injecting the local anesthetic to decrease the discomfort from the needle stick. Wound infiltration with local anesthetic is commonly practiced by some surgeons before wound closure in the operating room. This technique has been successful in decreasing the incidence of postoperative pain and decreasing the amount of postoperative analgesia required (Yaster et al., 1997).

Epinephrine, a vasoconstrictor, is often added to local anesthetics. It decreases the vascular absorption of the local anesthetic. This lengthens the time of the sensory block by almost 50% and decreases peak plasma levels by up to a third. Solutions containing epinephrine should *never* be used in areas supplied by end arterials, such as the digits and penis (Yaster et al., 1993). Its addition may cause necrosis or ischemia to the injected area (Yaster et al., 1993).

Toxicity

The most significant concern related to the use of local anesthetics is the risk of toxicity. Local anesthetics can have an impact on the function of any excitable membrane, including the heart or brain, and at the neuromuscular junction, when toxic levels are reached systemically (Denson & Mazoit, 1992). Although routine clinical use of these agents at accepted dosages does not result in toxic systemic and tissue concentrations, the accidental intravascular or excessive extravascular administration can have catastrophic consequences on the cardiovascular and central nervous systems (Denson & Mazoit, 1992).

Whenever local anesthetics are used in combination with each other, the toxicities of the agents are cumulative and should not be considered individually (Broadman & Rice, 1988). The addition of epinephrine decreases systemic absorption. Mild side effects representing increasing plasma levels include tinnitus, light-headedness, visual and auditory disturbances, restlessness, and muscular twitching. These can progress into severe side effects as the plasma levels rise, including seizures, arrhythmias, coma, cardiovascular collapse, and respiratory arrest (Yaster et al., 1993). Fortunately, toxic reactions have rarely been reported in children (Broadman & Rice, 1988; Yaster et al., 1993).

PATIENT-CONTROLLED ANALGESIA

Definition

Liu and Northrop (1990) describe patient-controlled analgesia (PCA) as a "human-operated, closed loop, analgesic

Table 6–4 Side Effects of Opioids

Side Effect	Cause and Effect	Care and Nursing Interventions
Respiratory depression (most serious side effect)	• Too much opioid. • Accumulation of the opioid over a period of time. • Concurrent administration of other opioids or sedatives. • Progression of respiratory depression commences with a decreased respiratory rate, followed by a decrease in tidal volume, and eventually apnea. • Opioids also diminish the body's protective response to hypoxia and hypercarbia.[a]	• Careful and astute monitoring and assessment of a patient's respiratory function is essential. • Frequent and consistent assessment of the patient's respiratory rate, rhythm, depth, and level of consciousness are indicated. • Monitoring will depend on the age of the child, his or her medical condition and history, and the medications that are being administered. Children at high risk for respiratory compromise include premature infants, infants less than 3 months of age, patients with an altered mental status or fixed neurologic impairments, airway compromise (including tracheomalasia and snoring), and respiratory insufficiency including a history of apnea or asthma.[a,b] • Electronic monitoring including pulse oximetry and apnea monitors should be considered, especially in the younger age groups and high-risk patients. • When respiratory depression or distress occurs, support respirations, notify the physician, and administer an appropriate dose of naloxone. • Naloxone will often wear off before the return of regular respiratory status. More than one dose or a continuous infusion may be indicated. • Management of the child's pain is still essential. Discontinuation of all pharmacologic interventions is not an appropriate clinical option.
Pruritus (most common side effect)	• The opioid triggers a histamine release that causes the itchiness. • May be experienced anywhere on the body, most prevalent on the forehead and nasal region in children.	• Often controlled by the administration of an antipruretic such as diphenhydramine. • If unsuccessful, change opioids. • Continuous low-dose infusion of naloxone in the maintenance fluids often works well in the case of intravenous and epidural opioid infusions.
Nausea and vomiting		• Administer antiemetics. • Sometimes the infusion drugs or rate can be changed to alleviate the problem. • Rule out other potential reasons for the nausea and vomiting (i.e., blocked or malpositioned nasogastric sump tube, bowel obstruction, concomitant medical therapy).
Urinary retention	• Retention occurs because of relaxation of the detrussor muscle in the floor of the bladder.[c]	• Examine the abdomen carefully assessing for bladder distention. • Monitor the patient's intake and output. • If the patient is unable to void, urinary catheterization is indicated. Often the child will regain normal voiding patterns after a single catheterization.
Decreased gastrointestinal motility	• Opioids inhibit smooth muscle motility, causing a decrease in small and large intestine peristalsis along with an increase in the tone of the pyloric sphincter, ileocecal valve, and the anal sphincter.[d]	• Encourage ambulation. • Ensure adequate fluids and high-fiber diets. • Stool softeners or laxatives are sometimes prescribed for patients taking opioids for more than 3 or 4 days.

[a] Leith & Weisman, 1997a. [b] Shannon & Berde, 1989. [c] Naber, Jones, & Halm, 1994. [d] Yaster & Maxwell, 1993.

Exhibit 6–3 Tolerance, Dependence, and Addiction

- Tolerance refers to the altered effect of a drug, in which an increasing amount of a drug is needed to produce the same therapeutic effect.[a] Some drugs are more apt to produce tolerance (i.e., fentanyl); however, tolerance does not commonly occur until 1 or 2 weeks after therapy is initiated. Treatment involves titrating the opioid to an appropriate therapeutic range.
- Dependence can be defined as a physiologic state produced by the discontinuation of an agent that has been administered for an extended period of time and results in an abstinence syndrome.[a] Treatment of the dependence can be achieved by using a tapering cycle over a period of time. Commonly, tapering cycles involve decreasing the amount of drug by 10% every day or every other day. The key is to identify patients at risk for this syndrome before drug withdrawal and to carefully monitor for signs of withdrawal while titrating their drugs. Signs of opioid abstinence syndrome (a.k.a., withdrawal syndrome) include tachycardia, hypertension, insomnia, sweating, yawning, agitation, restlessness, vomiting, diarrhea, and abdominal cramping.[b]
- Addiction refers to the psychological need for a drug and is characterized by drug-seeking behavior.[a] Individuals who need medications for reasons of pain control do not take them for the "high feeling" but for relief from pain. Although dependence on opioids is relatively common in the setting of long-term medically indicated opioid use, true addiction is extremely rare. This is a major fear of many children and their parents and sometimes causes a great deal of reluctance in taking a prescribed opioid.

[a] Tyler, 1994. [b] Yaster & Maxwell, 1993.

drug injection system . . . designed to alleviate pain" (p. 1147). The basic PCA system provides the patient with a hand-held button that the patient is instructed to press whenever in need of pain relief. A preset opioid dose is administered intravenously each time the button is pressed. Each pump is equipped with a lockout interval, which is a preset inactivation time interval, and is controlled by the computerized timing device within the pump, between patient-initiated doses. The pump may also be set for a maximum dose per hour(s). This lockout feature helps to prevent overdoses. The benefits of PCA are numerous as outlined in Exhibit 6–4.

Delivery Methods

PCA is delivered by interval dosing or continuous basal infusion with interval dosing. Continuous infusions are also possible using the PCA pump. The goal of the continuous infusion method is to maintain constant therapeutic levels of opioid in the blood; however, the patient has no way of instilling extra doses. Interval dosing allows for small, predetermined amounts of opioid to be given intravenously at frequent intervals to keep the blood levels within a therapeutic and safe range. This avoids inadequate or excessive blood levels of opioid.

Continuous basal infusion with intermittent dosing involves both functions. The continuous basal infusion helps to maintain a constant baseline level of comfort. When the patient begins to feel pain or is preparing for a painful event (ambulation, dressing change, etc.), the basal infusion can be supplemented with periodic, patient-controlled, small additional doses of analgesia (Bender et al., 1990; Berde, Beate, Yee, Sethna, & Russo, 1991; Gureno & Reisinger, 1991).

This method is effective in providing more consistent therapeutic opioid levels during sleep (Berde et al., 1991).

Patient Selection

PCA is a safe and effective mode of analgesia delivery in children, when it is used on the appropriate patient (see Exhibit 6–5). For PCA to work effectively, the child must be

Exhibit 6–4 Benefits of Patient-Controlled Analgesia

- Adequate and therapeutic pain control
- Less sedation
- Patient satisfaction
- Smaller overall use of narcotics
- More consistent analgesia blood levels
- Minimal side effects
- Feelings of self-control
- No delay between perception of pain and administration of analgesia
- Less respiratory depression and increased pulmonary function
- Earlier ambulation and resumption of activities of daily living
- Lack of injections
- Improvement of the quality of the nurse-patient relationship
- Reduces nursing staff work load
- Allows for wide variability between patients
- Suitable for all types of acute and chronic pain

Exhibit 6–5 Patient Understanding of Patient-Controlled Analgesia before Initiation

- PCA will help control the pain but not completely obliterate it.
- PCA can be used prophylactically to avoid pain associated with pain-inducing events (i.e., ambulation, procedures).
- Truthfully communicate any adverse effects or pain when they occur.
- Not to expect others to push the button, he or she should be in complete control of the device.
- There are numerous safety features programmed into the device to prevent overdosing.

physically able to activate the pump and understand the basic concept of PCA and causal relationships (usually attained between the ages of 6 and 9 years). If this is not present, the child is at risk for overuse or underuse of PCA. Adequate patient and family instruction regarding PCA is necessary along with ongoing support and encouragement for the patient from nursing staff and parents. Numerous reports have demonstrated the safe and effective use of parent-controlled or nurse-controlled analgesia used in children developmentally inappropriate for conventional PCA (Fulton, 1996; Gureno & Reisinger, 1991; Kanagasundaram, Cooper, & Lane, 1997; O'Halloran & Brown, 1997).

The most ideal opioid to use with PCA is one that has rapid onset of analgesic action, effectiveness in controlling the pain, intermediate duration of action, minimal tolerance or dependency effects, and minimal side effects (White, 1988). Although no perfect opioid exists, morphine tends to be the opioid used most frequently with PCA both clinically and in research (White, 1988).

Side Effects and Complications with PCA

Common side effects experienced by patients receiving pain control by means of PCA are related to the opioids. Therefore, the side effects are not specific to the PCA but to the medications themselves. The clear advantage to the use of PCA is that the patient not only has control over the pain or lack of pain but also has control over the side effects. Serious complications can occur from malprogramming or malfunction of the infusion device.

EPIDURAL PAIN CONTROL

Definition

Regional analgesia refers to the delivery of pain-relieving drugs, including opioids and local anesthetics, into the epi-

dural, caudal epidural, and intrathecal (spinal) routes. The drugs are administered by means of a small flexible catheter for intermittent or continuous infusions or by way of a small needle for a single bolus administration.

Spinal Anatomy and Pain Physiology

The spinal column and brain are covered by three membranes including, from the outermost layer in, the dura mater, the arachnoid, and the pia mater. Cerebrospinal fluid is contained in the subarachnoid space between the pia mater and the arachnoid membrane. The epidural space is a potential space located between the spinal dura mater and the vertebral canal. It extends from the cranium to the sacrum and is composed of loose connective tissue, fat, and blood vessels. It functions as a cushion or shock absorber around the spinal cord (Yaster et al., 1997).

Pain impulses are transmitted from the site of pain to the dorsal horn of the spinal column by way of sensory nerve fibers. Substance P is a neurotransmitter that resides in the dorsal horn. It transmits pain impulses by way of the lateral spinothalamic tract to the thalamus, where the impulses are transmitted to the cerebral cortex. When opioids are administered into the epidural space, they slowly diffuse into the cerebrospinal fluid, bind to the opioid receptors in the dorsal horn, thereby blocking substance P, and block the transmission of the pain impulse (Fitzgerald & Anand, 1993).

Catheter Placement

Epidural catheters are usually placed in children in the operating room. The desired location of the catheter tip is at the level of the surgical site or the dermatome level of the source of pain. Catheter placement is verified by the anesthesiologist. The catheter is covered with a sterile occlusive dressing at the exit site. It is preferable not to cover the site with any gauze so that it may be easily visualized without dressing removal. The catheter is often taped up the patient's back to the shoulder or upper chest area for easy access and to avoid pressure areas at the hub site. Nursing care of the epidural catheter focuses on careful assessment of the patient's vital signs and oxygenation, respiratory status, pain assessment, level of sedation, catheter site, and presence of side effects. Table 6–5 outlines the numerous nursing considerations in relation to common side effects.

Agents and Administration Techniques

All drugs administered into the epidural region must be preservative free because preservatives may cause neurotoxicity and severe spinal cord injury (Naber, Jones, & Halm, 1994). Local anesthetics administered in the epidural space cut off pain signals in the dorsal root ganglion, whereas opio-

Table 6–5 Side Effects of Epidural Analgesia with Nursing Considerations

Side Effect	Cause and Effect	Care and Nursing Interventions
Respiratory depression	• Too much opioid or local anesthetic (wrong dose, wrong concentration, or pump malfunction). • Accumulation of the opioid over a period of time. • Rostral spread of the opioid. • Misplacement of the catheter in the intrathecal space or vasculature. • Concurrent administration of other opioids systemically. • There are two key times when the patient is at the greatest risk for this complication. The first is within the first hour of the injection or infusion, caused by systemic absorption of the opioid. The second is 6 to 12 hours after initiation of the infusion secondary to cerebral migration of the drug.[a]	• Hourly assessment of the patient's respiratory rate, rhythm, depth, and level of consciousness are indicated for the first 24 hr. • Electronic monitoring such as pulse oximetry and apnea monitors, especially in the younger age groups and high-risk patients. • Head of the bed should be maintained in at least a 30-degree head-up position. • Verify the drugs and doses and the infusion pump to identify any potential problems or issues. • If respiratory depression or distress occurs, it is essential to support respiration, notify the physician, and administer an appropriate dose of naloxone. • Naloxone will often wear off before the return of regular respiratory status. Multiple doses or a continuous infusion may be indicated. • Ensure pain control. Management of the child's pain may continue with an epidural infusion once the respiratory crisis is resolved and the appropriate changes are made to the child's infusion or pump. • If the respiratory depression is the result of a misplaced catheter, catheter removal by anesthesia is indicated. • Intubation is indicated when respiratory paralysis occurs.
Urinary retention	• May be caused by both local and opioid analgesia. • Patient may not feel the urge to void with bladder distention because of the sensory or motor block produced by the local anesthetic. • Opioids cause a relaxation of the detrussor muscle in the floor of the bladder that may result in retention.[b]	• Careful abdominal examinations assessing for bladder distention and monitor the patient's intake and output. • Urinary catheterization is indicated when patient is unable to void. • Often the child will regain normal voiding patterns after a single catheterization. • Some clinicians advocate for indwelling bladder catheterization while the patient has an epidural catheter in place.
Sensory and motor deficits	• Changes in sensation to the lower extremities, including motor weakness, motor blocks, tingling, and numbness may occur as a result of the effects of the local anesthetic.	• Safety is of vital importance to ensure that a child does not fall because of the alteration in sensation. • Careful explanations are essential to help children cope with this side effect and to help them understand that they will regain full feeling and movement of their extremities. • Concentration of the local anesthetic may be decreased or eliminated from the infusion to reverse this side effect.
Infection	• Fortunately very rare.[c]	• Meticulous aseptic technique is required during epidural placement and all subsequent care. • Nursing assessment should include a careful evaluation for infection (fever, drainage, redness, or tenderness at the exit site, nuccal rigidity) on a routine basis.[d] • The dressing should be occlusive, but clear, allowing for frequent observation of the catheter exit site.

continues

Table 6–5 continued

Side Effect	Cause and Effect	Care and Nursing Interventions
		• The frequency of dressing changes and tubing changes is controversial and depends on the institution's policy. However, all soiled or disrupted dressings should be changed. • All epidural solutions are changed on a 24–hr basis. • Only preservative-free solutions should be used for cleansing at the hub (i.e., alcohol). • When infection is suspected, the epidural catheter is pulled by anesthesia and cultured. Antibiotics are prescribed as needed.
Spinal headache	• The result of a dural penetration or leak. Cerebral spinal fluid leaks from the intrathecal space into the dura. • Symptoms include extreme headache, photophobia, tinnitus, diplopia, and increased discomfort in an upright position.[b]	• Bedrest, hydration, and analgesia. • In some patients an autologous blood patch is applied. Blood is injected through the catheter to seal the dural puncture and prevent further cerebral spinal fluid leak.
Pruritus and nausea or vomiting		• Often remedied by the administration of antipruritics or antiemetics. • Sometimes the infusion drugs or rate is changed to alleviate the problem. • If unsuccessful, a continuous low-dose infusion of naloxone in the maintenance fluids is administered with excellent results.

[a] Weisman, 1996. [b] Naber et al., 1994. [c] Sethna, Berde, Wilder, & Strafford, 1992. [d] Dunajcik, 1988.

ids occupy opiate receptors in the dorsal horn, thereby blocking pain pathways inside the spinal cord (Dunajcik, 1988). The analgesic effects of local anesthetics and opioids are synergistic when administered epidurally and offer a higher therapeutic ratio when administered together versus independently (Berde, 1989). Table 6–3 offers information regarding commonly used epidural medications.

The two most commonly used local anesthetics for epidural analgesia include lidocaine and bupivacaine. Bupivacaine offers the advantage of a prolonged duration of action and decreased incidence of motor block over lidocaine (Berde, 1989). The higher the concentration of the drug, the greater the sensory block and potential for motor block. Regardless of the agent and concentration used, careful attention must be given to the overall dose of the local analgesic administered.

A number of safe and therapeutic choices exists for epidural opioids, the most common being morphine, hydromorphone, and fentanyl. The choice of drug depends on the patient's age and history, the procedure, the location of the catheter tip, the dermatomal level or levels of the pain, and the preference of the physician and institution. Rostral spread refers to the cephalic migration of a drug. Drugs that are more hydrophilic, such as morphine and hydromorphone, have an increased affinity to water and therefore a greater rostral spread. These agents are useful when the catheter tip lies well below the surgical site or when many dermatomal levels are involved by the pain or surgical site (Weisman, 1996). However, the risk of respiratory depression is greater when using hydrophilic opioids as opposed to lipophilic opioids. Lipophilic agents, such as fentanyl, are indicated when the catheter tip is at the dermatomal level of the pain and for patients who are at high risk for respiratory depression.

The preferred method of epidural administration is by continuous infusion. Patient-controlled epidural analgesia may be added to the continuous infusion. Single-shot caudal epidurals or "kiddie caudals" are another method of epidural analgesia. This technique can provide postoperative analgesia for a range in time (6 to 18 hours), depending on the medications administered. One-day surgery patients may also benefit from this technique if only a local anesthetic is administered. Any child who receives epidural opioids must be closely monitored within the hospital for 24 hours after the caudal administration due to the risk of respiratory depression. There are two key times when the patient is at the greatest risk for this complication. The first is within the first hour of the injection because of systemic absorption of the opioid. The second is 6 to 12 hours after the injection secondary to cerebral migration of the drug (Weisman, 1996). An overview of the nursing considerations can be found in Table 6–5.

SEDATION

Children may require sedation to help them hold still for a procedure, which may or may not be painful. Some procedures require a combination of analgesic or amnesic effects and sedation. In 1985, the American Academy of Pediatrics developed guidelines for the use of depressant pharmacologic agents in children as a result of the increasing use of these agents in nontraditional clinical settings (American Academy of Pediatrics, 1985). The guidelines were revised in 1992 to reflect an increased understanding of monitoring needs for children receiving sedation (American Academy of Pediatrics, 1992).

Definitions

Sedation is a physical state that is on a continuum that ranges from the awake state to general anesthesia. One must be prepared to deal with situations when a child passes from one stage on the continuum into another. The American Academy of Pediatrics (1992) has defined the various states of sedation as follows: Conscious sedation is a medically controlled, depressed level of consciousness that allows the patient to maintain protective reflexes, independently maintain a patent airway, and the ability to respond to verbal or tactile stimuli. Deep sedation and general anesthesia refer to a medically controlled, depressed level of consciousness (or unconsciousness) from which the patient is not easily aroused (or unarousable). The patient may have partial or complete loss of protective reflexes, including airway maintenance, and is unable to respond purposefully to physical stimulation or verbal command.

Equipment, Facilities, and Personnel

The practitioner and facility must be capable of safely treating any of the complications of conscious sedation, including vomiting, seizures, anaphylaxis, and cardiopulmonary arrest (American Academy of Pediatrics, 1992).

Minimal requirements include the availability of (1) monitoring equipment (pulse oximetry and blood pressure monitoring), (2) emergency equipment (emergency code cart including age-appropriate drugs and equipment to resuscitate a nonbreathing patient, defibrillator, positive pressure oxygen delivery system, suction equipment with appropriate catheters, supplies to initiate and maintain vascular access), (3) backup emergency services with a protocol for implementation and use, and (4) qualified practitioners and personnel who are competent in providing pediatric life support and establishing intravenous access.

Patient Screening

The patient must have a responsible and competent person accompany them home after the procedure. (Often two people are recommended, especially if one individual must drive or if the child is very young or developmentally delayed). What is the child's medical condition? The American Society of Anesthesiologists physical status classification system (ASA classification) is used to identify appropriate candidates for sedation. Patients with a classification of I or II are often considered appropriate candidates (American Academy of Pediatrics, 1992). A health history and physical examination must be completed, including documentation of age and weight, allergies, drug use, relevant medical history and family history, review of systems, and vital signs. All pertinent laboratory results must be reviewed. An evaluation of the child's oral intake must be completed. It is also important to consider medications the child may be taking and identify their potential impact on the procedure or drug interactions.

Perisedation Period

The practitioner(s) responsibilities include (1) the administration of the pharmacologic agents inducing sedation and (2) the treatment of the patient undergoing the procedure. (The practitioner must have a clear understanding of the pharmacokinetics of the drugs being administered, including onset time, duration, principal effect, side effects and their treatment, routes of administration, and dosing [Cote, 1994].)

The support personnel responsibilities include (1) ongoing monitoring of appropriate physiologic parameters and (2) assisting in any supportive or resuscitative procedures required. The number of support personnel needed to be available depends on the procedure. It is always imperative to have the resources available to deal with an emergency situation. If the child should become deeply sedated, the level of vigilance must be increased to provide one-on-one observation, monitoring, and documentation of the patient's condition. Backup personnel who are expert in airway management, emergency intubation, and advanced cardiopulmonary resuscitation must be available should complications arise (American Nurses Association, 1992). It is not feasible to appropriately monitor a patient who is deeply sedated while assisting with a procedure (American Nurses Association, 1992; Cote, 1994).

The Prescription of Sedation

Whenever sedation is required for patient care, one must consider a number of factors pertaining to the patient and procedure to choose an appropriate cocktail. An overview of the pharmacologic agents used for sedation can be found in Table 6–3.

The Procedure

What is the procedure being performed? Is it painful or nonpainful? This information is important to determine the need for analgesia. Does the procedure require the child to be motionless? The answer to this question is important in determining the level of sedation required and the appropriate drugs to use. How long will the procedure take? This information is helpful to determine the appropriate pharmacologic agent. If the anticipated procedure time is short, then short-acting agents, such as fentanyl and midazolam, may be used.

The Patient

What are the child's past experiences with sedation and which agents were used? Data from patient screening (noted previously) should be taken into account, as well as the level of anxiety and agitation. This information will help determine whether an anxiolytic or amnesic agent is needed. One must consider the access routes that a patient has available for use. For example, if a child is NPO, oral administration may not be feasible. If a child has no vascular access, certain drugs will be ruled out.

Postprocedure Care

It is imperative to continue diligent monitoring of the patient's status after the procedure until the child returns to a preprocedural level of functioning. If a discrepancy exists between prelevel and postlevel functioning at the time of discharge, it must be carefully documented and justified. The child needs to be monitored in an environment where the appropriate medical personnel and equipment are readily available. This does not include the back corridor of the emergency department or a waiting area where the appropriate staff is not closely monitoring the patient. It is not uncommon for a child to pass into a deep sedation after the procedure. This results from a lack of external stimulation (completion of the procedure), continued drug uptake, delayed excretion, and pharmacodynamics (Cote, 1994). Pulse oximetry monitoring until the child is fully awake is a sensitive and practical method of monitoring patients for adverse physiologic effects.

The American Academy of Pediatrics (1992) has outlined a number of recommended discharge criteria, which are as follows: (1) the patient has satisfactory and stable cardiovascular function and airway patency, (2) the patient can be aroused easily and has intact protective reflexes, (3) the patient can talk if developmentally appropriate, (4) the patient can sit up unassisted if developmentally appropriate, (5) a child who is very young or developmentally compromised should return to his or her normal level of responsiveness, and (6) an adequate state of hydration exists.

Once the patient is considered medically safe for discharge, written instructions should be given to the accompanying adult. The instructions should outline information about who and when to call in an emergency, routine follow-up care, and diet. Ideally, two responsible adults should accompany the child on discharge.

CONCLUSION

Many advances have been made in the past 15 years in the area of understanding the mechanisms of pain and its management. These advances have significantly improved pain control for children. This chapter provided an overview of pain assessment, management, and sedation with a focus on the pediatric surgical patient. Nurses caring for pediatric surgical patients use a variety of pain management methods and techniques to achieve effective pain control and sedation.

REFERENCES

Abu-Saad, H. (1984). Assessing children's responses to pain. *Pain, 19,* 163–171.

American Academy of Pediatrics, Committee on Drugs. (1992). Guidelines for monitoring and management of pediatric patients during and after sedation for diagnostic and therapeutic procedures. *Pediatrics, 89*(6), 1110–1115.

American Academy of Pediatrics, Committee on Drugs, Section on Anesthesiology. (1985). Guidelines for the elective use of conscious sedation, deep sedation and general anesthesia in pediatric patients. *Pediatrics, 76,* 317–321.

American Nurses Association. (1992). Position statement on the role of the registered nurse in the management of patients receiving IV conscious sedation for short-term therapeutic, diagnostic, or surgical procedures. *The American Nurse, February,* 7–8.

Anderson, C., Zeltzer, L., & Fanurik, D. (1993). Procedural pain. In N. Schechter, C. Berde, & M. Yaster (Eds.), *Pain in infants, children and adolescents.* Baltimore: Williams & Wilkins.

Aradine, C., Beyer, J., & Tompkins, J. (1987). Children's pain perceptions before and after analgesia: A study of instrument construct validity. *Journal of Pediatric Nursing, 3,* 11–23.

Ashburn, M., Gauthier, M., Love, G., Basta, S., Gaylord, B., & Kessler, K. (1997). Iontophoretic administration of 2% lidocaine HCl and 1:100,000 epinephrine in humans. *The Clinical Journal of Pain, 13,* 22–26.

Bender, L., Weaver, K., & Edwards, K. (1990). Postoperative patient-controlled analgesia in children. *Pediatric Nursing, 16*(6), 549–554.

Benini, F., Johnston, C., Faucher, D., & Aranda, J. (1993). Topical anesthesia during circumcision in newborn infants. *JAMA, 270,* 850–853.

Berde, C. (1989). Pediatric postoperative pain management. *Pediatric Clinics of North America, 36*(4), 921–937.

Berde, C. (1991). The treatment of pain in children. In M. Bond, J. Charlton, & C. Woolf (Eds.), *Proceedings of the VIth World Congress on Pain*. New York: Elsevier Science.

Berde, C., Beate, L., Yee, J., Sethna, N., & Russo, D. (1991). Patient-controlled analgesia in children and adolescents: A randomized, prospective comparison with intramuscular administration of morphine for postoperative analgesia. *Journal of Pediatrics, 118*(3), 460–466.

Beyer, J., & Wells, N. (1989). The assessment of pain in children. *Pediatric Clinics of North America, 36*(4), 837–851.

Broadman, L., & Rice, L. (1988). Pediatric regional anesthesia and perioperative analgesia. *Perioperative Pediatric Analgesia, 2*(3), 386–407.

Broome, M. (1990). Preparation of children for painful procedures. *Pediatric Nursing, 16*(6), 537–541.

Broome, M., Bates, T., Lillis, P., & McGahee, T. (1990). Children's medical fears, coping behaviors, and pain perceptions during a lumbar puncture. *Oncology Nursing Forum, 17*(3), 361–366.

Colwell, C., Clark, L., & Perkins, R. (1996). Postoperative use of pediatric pain scales: Children's self-report versus nurse assessment of pain intensity and affect. *Journal of Pediatric Nursing, 11*(6), 375–382.

Cote, C. (1994). Sedation for the pediatric patient. *Pediatric Clinics of North America, 41*(1), 31–52.

Denson, D., & Mazoit, J. (1992). Physiology and pharmacology of local anesthetics. In R. Sinatra, A. Hord, B. Ginsberg, & L. Preble (Eds.), *Acute pain: Mechanisms & management*. St. Louis, MO: Mosby.

Dunajcik, L. (1988). Controlling the dangers of epidural analgesia. *RN, 10*, 40–45.

Durham, E., & Frost-Hartzer, P. (1994). Relaxation therapy for children and families. *Maternal Child Nurse, 19*, 222–225.

Eland, J. (1988). Pharmacologic management of acute and chronic pain. *Comprehensive Pediatric Nursing, 11*, 93–111.

Eland, J., & Anderson, J. (1977). The experience of pain in children. In A. Jacox (Ed.), *Pain: A source book for nurses and other health professionals*. Boston: Little, Brown and Company.

Epstein, R., Mendel, H., Witkowski, T., Waters, R., Guarniari, K., Marr, A., & Lessin, J. (1996). The safety and efficacy of oral transmucosal fentanyl citrate for preoperative sedation in young children. *Anesthesia and Analgesia, 83*, 1200–1205.

Favaloro, R. (1988). Adolescent development and implications for pain management. *Pediatric Nursing, 14*(1), 27–29.

Fitzgerald, M., & Anand, K. (1993). Developmental neuroanatomy and neurophysiology of pain. In N. Schechter, C. Berde, & M. Yaster (Eds.), *Pain in infants, children and adolescents*. Baltimore: Williams & Wilkins.

Forest, J., Clements, J., & Prescott, L. (1982). Clinical pharmacokinetics of paracetamol. *Clinical Pharmacokinetics, 7*, 93–107.

French, G., Painter, E., & Coury, D. (1994). Blowing away shot pain: A technique for pain management during immunization. *Pediatrics, 93*(3), 384–388.

Fulton, T. (1996). Nurses' adoption of a patient-controlled analgesia approach. *Western Journal of Nursing Research, 18*(4), 383–396.

Gaines, L. (1998). *Developmental approaches with distraction resources*. Unpublished work.

Gaynard, L., Wolfer, J., Goldberger, J., Thompson, R., Redburn, L., & Laidley, L. (1990). Preparing children and families for health care experiences: Guidelines from the ACCH Child Life research project. *Psychosocial care of children in hospitals: A clinical practice manual from the ACCH Child Life Research Project*. Bethesda, MD: The Association for the Care of Children's Health.

Gureno, M., & Reisinger, C. (1991). Patient controlled analgesia for the young pediatric patient. *Pediatric Nursing, 17*(3), 251–254.

Heiney, S. (1991). Helping children through painful procedures. *American Journal of Nursing, November*, 20–25.

Helwig, D. (1990). Pediatric pain and polar bears. *Canadian Medical Association Journal, 143*(2), 130–131.

Hendrickson, M., Myre, L., Johnson, D., Matlak, M., Black, R., & Sullivan, J. (1990). Postoperative analgesia in children: A prospective study of intermittent intramuscular injection versus continuous intravenous infusion of morphine. *Journal of Pediatric Surgery, 25*(2), 185–191.

Hester, N. (1979). The preoperational child's reaction to immunization. *Nursing Research, 28*, 250–254.

Hester, N., & Barcus, C. (1986). Assessment and management of pain in children. *Pediatrics: Nursing Update: Continuing Professional Education Center, Inc., 1*(14), 1–7.

International Association for the Study of Pain, Subcommittee on Taxonomy. (1979). Pain terms: A list with definitions and notes on usage. *Pain, 6*, 249–252.

Joyce, T. (1993). Topical anesthesia and pain management before venipuncture. *Journal of Pediatrics, 122*(5), S24–S29.

Kanagasundaram, S., Cooper, M., & Lane, L. (1997). Nurse-controlled analgesia using a patient-controlled analgesia device: An alternative strategy in the management of severe cancer pain in children. *Journal of Paediatric Child Health, 33*, 352–355.

Koren, G. (1993). Use of the eutectic mixture of local anesthetics in young children for procedure-related pain. *Journal of Pediatrics, 122*(5), S30–S35.

Kuttner, L. (1997). Mind-body methods of pain management. *Child and Adolescent Psychiatric Clinics of North America, 6*(4), 8–10.

Leith, P., & Weisman, S. (1997a). Pharmacologic interventions for pain management in children. *Child and Adolescent Psychiatric Clinics of North America, 6*(4), 12–21.

Leith, P., & Weisman, S. (1997b). The management of painful procedures in children. *Child and Adolescent Psychiatric Clinics of North America, 6*(4), 11–21.

Lipshitz, M., Marino, B., & Sanders, S. (1993). Chloral hydrate side effects in young children: Causes and management. *Heart & Lung, September/October*, 408–414.

Liu, F., & Northrop, R. (1990). A new approach to the modeling and control of postoperative pain. *IEEE Transactions on Biomedical Engineering, 37*(12), 1147–1157.

Mackey, W. (1993). *An analysis of numerous factors affecting patient-controlled analgesia efficacy in children*. Unpublished thesis, Yale University.

Mansson, M., Fredrikzon, B., & Rosberg, B. (1992). Comparison of preparation and opioid-sedative premedication in children undergoing surgery. *Pediatric Nursing, 18*(4), 337–342.

McCaffery, M. (1979). *Nursing management of the patient with pain* (2nd ed.). Philadelphia: J.B. Lippincott.

McCaffery, M., & Beebe, A. (1990). Myths and facts . . . about pain in children. *Nursing, 20*(7), 81.

McCrory, L. (1991). A review of the second international symposium on pediatric pain. *Pediatric Nursing, 17*(4), 366–369.

McDonnell, L., & Bowden, M. (1989). Breathing management: A simple stress and pain reduction strategy for use on a pediatric service. *Issues in Comprehensive Pediatric Nursing, 12,* 339–344.

McGrath, D., Thurston, N., Wright, D., Preshaw, R., & Fermin, P. (1995). Comparison of one technique of patient controlled postoperative analgesia with intramuscular meperidine. *Pain, 37,* 265–270.

McGrath, P., & Craig, K. (1989). Developmental and psychological factors in children's pain. *Pediatric Clinics of North America, 36*(4), 823–835.

McKay, W., Morris, R., & Mushlin, P. (1987). Sodium bicarbonate attenuates pain on skin infiltration with lidocaine, with or without epinephrine. *Anesthesia and Analgesia, 66,* 572–574.

Naber, L., Jones, G., & Halm, M. (1994). Epidural analgesia for effective pain control. *Critical Care Nurse, October,* 69–85.

O'Halloran, P., & Brown, R. (1997). Patient-controlled analgesia compared with nurse-controlled infusion analgesia after heart surgery. *Intensive and Critical Care Nursing, 13,* 126–129.

Rauen, K., & Ho, M. (1989). Children's use of patient-controlled analgesia after spine surgery. *Pediatric Nursing, 15*(6), 589–593.

Ross, D., & Ross, S. (1988). Assessment of pediatric pain: An overview. *Comprehensive Pediatric Nursing, 11,* 73–91.

Schechter, N. (1989). The undertreatment of pain in children: An overview. *Pediatric Clinics of North America, 36*(4), 781–793.

Schechter, N., Blankson, V., Pachter, L., Sullivan, C., & Costa, L. (1997). The ouchless place: No pain, children's gain. *Pediatrics, 99*(6), 890–893.

Schechter, N., Weisman, S., Rosenblum, M., Bernstein, B., & Conrad, P. (1995). The use of oral transmucosal fentanyl citrate for painful procedures in children. *Pediatrics, 95*(3), 335–339.

Sethna, N., Berde, C., Wilder, R., & Strafford, M. (1992). The risk of infection from pediatric epidural analgesia is low. Unpublished abstract.

Shannon, M., & Berde, C. (1989). Pharmacologic management of pain in children and adolescents. *Pediatric Clinics of North America, 36*(4), 855–871.

Sievers, T., Yee, J., Foley, M., Blanding, P., & Berde, C. (1991). Midazolam for conscious sedation during pediatric oncology procedures: Safety and recovery parameters. *Pediatrics, 88*(6), 1172–1179.

Sinatra, R. (1992). Pathophysiology of acute pain. In R. Sinatra, A. Hord, B. Ginsberg, & L. Preble (Eds.). *Acute pain: Mechanisms & management.* St. Louis, MO: Mosby.

Slack, J., & Faut-Callahan, M. (1991). Pain management. *Nursing Clinics of North America, 26*(2), 463–473.

Steinberg, A. (1993). Should chloral hydrate be banned? *Pediatrics, 92*(3), 442–446.

Stevens, B. (1989). Nursing management of pain in children. In R. Foster, M. Hunsberger, & J. Anderson (Eds.), *Family-centered nursing care of children.* Philadelphia: W.B. Saunders Company.

Theroux, M., West, D., Corddry, D., Hyde, P., Bachrach, S., Cronan, K., & Kettrick, R. (1993). Efficacy of intranasal midazolam in facilitating suturing of lacerations in preschool children in the emergency department. *Pediatrics, 91*(3), 624–627.

Tolksdorf, W., Elick, C., & Amberger, M. (1991). Premedication in preschool children with oral, rectal and nasal midazolam. *Anesthesia and Analgesia, 72,* 297.

Tyler, D. (1994). Pharmacology of pain management. *Pediatric Clinics of North America, 41*(1), 59–69.

Vetter, T. (1989). Postoperative analgesia for the pediatric patient. *Wellcome Trends in Anesthesiology, 7*(3), 3–9.

Weatherstone, K., Rasmussen, L., Erenberg, A., Jackson, E., Claflin, K., & Leff, R. (1993). Safety and efficacy of a topical anesthetic for neonatal circumcision. *Pediatrics, 92,* 710–714.

Weisman, S. (1995). Fentanyl Oralet for bone marrow aspiration/lumbar puncture. Abbott Park, IL: Abbott Laboratories.

Weisman, S. (1996). *Epidural anesthesia in pediatrics.* Unpublished work; Yale University School of Medicine, Department of Anesthesiology.

White, P. (1988). Use of patient-controlled analgesia for management of acute pain. *JAMA, 259*(2), 243–245.

Wong, D. (1996). *Wong and Whaley's clinical manual of pediatric nursing* (4th ed.). St. Louis, MO: Mosby.

Wong, D., & Baker, C. (1988). Pain in children: Comparison of assessment scales. *Pediatric Nursing, 14(*1), 9–17.

Yaster, M., & Deshpande, J. (1988). Management of pediatric pain with opioid analgesics. *Journal of Pediatrics, 113,* 421–429.

Yaster, M., Krane, E., Kaplan, R., Cote, C., & Lappe, D. (1997). *Pediatric pain management and sedation handbook.* New York: Mosby Year-Book.

Yaster, M., & Maxwell, L. (1993). Opioid agonists and antagonists. In N. Schechter, C. Berde, & M. Yaster (Eds.), *Pain in infants, children and adolescents.* Baltimore: Williams & Wilkins.

Yaster, M., Tobin, J., & Maxwell, L. (1993). Local anesthetics. In N. Schechter, C. Berde, & M. Yaster (Eds.), *Pain in infants, children and adolescents.* Baltimore: Williams & Wilkins.

CHAPTER 7

Caring for the Child with Technology Needs in the Home

Kimberly Haus McIltrot and Laura Phearman

INTRODUCTION

The discharge of children with complex health needs from the hospital to the home setting requires a collaborative relationship between the health care team, home care agencies, educational system, payers (insurance companies), and the family. A recent survey revealed that approximately 30% of children less than 18 years of age have a chronic illness or disability, and many of these children require technologic support (Patterson & Blum, 1996). Apnea monitors, dialysis, infusion therapies, and ventilators are a few examples of technologic support being used in the home setting (Smith, 1995). The increased use of technology in the home requires an appropriate plan of care and knowledgeable caregivers. Experienced pediatric home care nurses are essential to provide education, assessment, and nursing care (Petit de Mange, 1998). Hospital costs are rising, health care benefits are changing, and home care is a viable alternative for families of children with complex needs (Schuman, 1997). This chapter discusses planning, funding, specific technologic services, educational issues, and family coping strategies related to providing care for the technology-dependent child in the home.

DEVELOPING A PLAN OF CARE FOR HOME

The goal of home care is to provide safe and effective medically necessary care in the home. This alternative to inpatient medical and nursing care includes nursing services, durable medical equipment (DME), rehabilitation services, social services, and educational support in the home. Discharge planning requires care coordination and anticipation of future needs. The health care team assists the family in accessing community supports and services needed to care for the child with technology needs at home (Goldberg, 1993). The role of the home care nurse is to educate and encourage independent caregiving by the parents and to provide a range of services, such as simple dressing changes, ostomy care, or the infusion of intravenous antibiotics. Case managers are also responsible for ordering DME, such as wheelchairs and hospital beds, that facilitate the transition home.

Coordination of effective care for high-risk children involves case management and must use individualized care plans. Case managers assess progress toward stated goals, authorize and monitor referrals for related services, and provide family support and caregiver training. It is important to involve the family in development of the plan of care to ensure success. The family provides valuable feedback regarding the overall quality of the services and effectiveness of the plan.

Not all situations are amenable to home care; guidance from health care professionals helps the family determine whether the technology regimens are realistic. Home care for young children has value because it allows the child to be in a "normal" environment. However, this can only happen if resources provided in the home lead to some semblance of normal life (Lindsay, 1999). Jennett's (1986) framework is a useful tool for determining whether technology in the home setting is appropriate. This tool evaluates the use of technology in the home by asking the questions: (1) Is it likely to be unsuccessful in achieving therapeutic purpose, given the child's condition? (2) Is it unnecessary? Could the therapeutic objective be met with simpler means? (3) Is it unsafe in that complications of the technology outweigh benefits? (4) Is it unkind in that the resulting quality of life for patient and family is poor? (5) Is it unwise? Does applying the technology deliver community resources that could better be used elsewhere?

After establishing that home care is a reasonable option for a child with complex health care needs, the health care team conducts a needs assessment and devises a discharge plan with the family. A complete needs assessment for children with complex health problems includes personal, physical, family, school, and community assessments (Guillett, 1998).

The discharge assessment should include the child's current level of function and a review of systems. The physical assessment should be focused on the systems affected by the illness, disability, or chronic condition (Guillett, 1998). Functional health patterns should be assessed, including cognitive-perceptual, activity-exercise, nutritional-metabolic, elimination, and sleep. Cognitive-perceptual patterns include language, visual acuity, hearing, fears and sensitivities, grade in school, and the parents' perception of the child's abilities. It is also important to note the therapies provided at school or in outpatient settings.

Home care providers assess the environment before discharging children with complex needs (Guillett, 1998). Evaluation of the environment includes consideration of the home, family, school, neighborhood, and community. The home environment assessment includes safety, accessibility of the equipment, appropriate electrical hook-ups, and access to generators and telephone service. Structural changes, including larger doorways, ramps, and electrical rewiring, may be necessary to accommodate the needs of the child.

Assessment of the family as part of the home environment includes family members, folk health practices, values, knowledge level, health of the family members, coping skills, and support systems (Guillett, 1998). Nursing visits or shifts of nursing care may be needed to supplement the care family members provide. Social work consults facilitate the family's coping with the stress of providing complex care in the home on a long-term basis.

Discharge information is often overwhelming for families. Before discharge, an educational and skills checklist should be completed. Refer to Exhibit 7–1 for an example of necessary discharge information.

An educational or developmental assessment is essential in considering the whole child. Health care providers should encourage and facilitate regular school attendance to normalize the tasks of children. Success in school is essential to the development of positive self-esteem. The health care provider needs to complete home tutoring forms for children who are absent for longer than 30 days or if a chronically ill child is expected to have intermittent absences related to hospitalization or medical visits. Referrals to local infant and toddler programs for chronically ill toddlers and preschoolers is essential to identify delays in fine or gross motor skills, poor oral motor skills, or cognitive deficits.

Community resources vary greatly; therefore, an assessment of the availability of emergency services, transportation, neighborhood resources for respite care, support groups, and church supports is essential. Many times the ser-

Exhibit 7–1 Necessary Discharge Information

- Medical summary
- Medical discharge orders
- Nursing discharge orders
- Outline of child's typical day
- Medications, including action and use, dosage and frequency, route, side effects, and storage instructions
- Special treatment instructions
- Nutritional needs
- Instruction on use and maintenance of equipment
- When to call the doctor
- Phone numbers of physicians, utility companies (phone, gas, and electric), fire department, paramedics, nursing agencies, equipment companies, and pharmacy
- Home equipment and supply list
- Names and phone numbers of contact people at school
- Learning needs
- Rehabilitation needs (physical, occupational, and speech therapy)

vices exist but the health care providers and families must be creative in mobilizing the resources. For example, the fire department or first responder teams may help in transporting or lifting individuals in and out of apartments or housing.

FUNDING AND SERVICES

Reimbursement issues often affect decisions regarding home care. Insurance companies contract with specific home care agencies to provide DME and nursing services. Funding for portable equipment, formula, and enteral feeding supplies may be denied or severely limited. Specific equipment may be chosen because the insurance company will reimburse for it, but it may not be optimal; nursing services may be limited to visits only, not shifts of care (Zerwekh, 1995). Case managers identify resources available from the primary insurance company, and if resources are limited, alternative payment mechanisms are pursued, such as blending state resources with commercial insurance or referrals to Medicaid Waiver programs. All children are not covered by medical insurance, and, in fact, children are the largest group of uninsured or underinsured individuals in the United States (Mauldon, Leibowitz, Buchanan, Damberg, & McGuigan, 1994). These children rely on public support, but state laws governing social programs are not standard between states. In addition, qualifications for federal programs are changing and becoming more restrictive in nature, resulting in inconsistent funding of home care services. Case managers and social workers collaborate in discharge planning to identify financial resources that facilitate discharge to home and to assist with the complicated process of obtaining funding for services in the home setting. Exhibit 7–2 reviews funding options for children without commercial insurance or as a supplement for an existing policy.

In the past, fee-for-service insurance programs allowed children with chronic or disabling conditions to receive care from tertiary care centers, specialty clinics, and specialists who were experienced in dealing with complex care issues. At present, commercial insurance plans, along with Medicaid, are shifting toward fully capitated arrangements with health maintenance organizations (HMOs). With capitation, each diagnosis is assigned a dollar amount for reimbursement, and the institution must then provide care within that assigned dollar amount unless there is an appeal for additional resources. Many children with chronic or disabling conditions are now receiving care in an HMO system designed to decrease the use of specialists (Mauldon et al., 1994).

The chronically ill child requires a health care network that includes primary care pediatricians, pediatric specialists, mental health care providers, hospitals, home agencies, and ancillary therapists. A mechanism to assess quality assurance or utilization review is an essential component of monitoring cost and quality outcomes for chronically ill children. To date, no outcome differences have been found between the HMO and fee-for-service groups in their efforts to reduce hospitalization rates and control hospital costs (Szilagyi, 1998). Refer to Exhibit 7–3 for suggested questions for families to discuss with the plan provider about the network and care options when evaluating various plans.

Exhibit 7–2 Funding Options

1. Medicare: usually for the elderly but also includes children with renal failure
2. Medicaid: provides access to health care for families below the poverty level, which is determined by each state
3. Medicaid waiver: established for children with many needs; does not consider family income
4. Supplement Social Security: established by the states for children with long-term disabilities
5. Women, Infants and Children (WIC): federal nutrition program that provides assistance with formula and food
6. Privately funded grants and special interest groups, for example, the Lion's Club, Shriner's, Make a Wish Foundation
7. Nonprofit organizations, for example, the American Heart Association, the American Cancer Society, the Muscular Dystrophy Association
8. Community funding, for example, local churches and service organizations

Exhibit 7–3 Evaluating the Plan Provider

- What are the primary care provider's knowledge, expertise, and training to care for my child?
- What is the primary care provider's willingness to listen and learn from me the parent?
- What is my child's access to pediatric specialists? Is there an option for second opinions?
- What is the length of time that we have to wait for plan approval of a recommended service and how long does it take to get appointments for the service?
- What level of communication can I expect between the health care providers and myself regarding my child's condition?
- Is adequate information about the coverage and grievance procedures available?

TECHNOLOGY SERVICES IN THE HOME

Respiratory Support

Concomitant respiratory problems may be found in neonates or children with a surgical problem. Oxygen is provided in the home in liquid cylinders by way of nasal cannula, face mask, or ventilator. A portable oxygen tank is provided for clinic appointments or time away from home. Periodic monitoring of oxygen saturations with a pulse oximeter may be required.

A respiratory therapist or nurse employed by the DME company instructs parents and caregivers on the correct operation of equipment and how to troubleshoot potential false alarm situations and equipment malfunctions. Before discharge, families are instructed in basic cardiopulmonary resuscitation for infants and children and the fire department is contacted to monitor the home for any gas leaks. Safety procedures, such as the safe storage of oxygen and no smoking, need to be observed in the home. The health care provider should ensure that DME companies and supply vendors provide 24-hour service to manage potential equipment failures. Discharge instructions include emergency phone numbers with providers familiar with the child and his or her specific needs.

Children with tracheostomies are another group of children requiring respiratory services at home. Refer to Chapter 12 for further information. Stable ventilator-dependent children are also managed at home. Families and care providers undergo intensive training learning how to assemble ventilator circuits, operate controls, change settings, determine the correct source of alarms, clean and maintain equipment, set up and deliver breathing treatments, and perform emergency measures (Hilton & Gold, 1989). Home ventilator patients often have shift nursing care, and the family must adjust to the stress of having health care providers in their home environment for prolonged periods of time.

Nutritional Therapy

Children with congenital or acquired surgical problems, such as gastroschisis, necrotizing enterocolitis, or gastroesophageal reflux, may require supplemental nutritional therapy in the home. The child whose oral intake does not provide adequate calories for growth and development is an appropriate candidate for home parenteral or enteral nutrition therapy. The caregivers involved must learn to perform all the procedures for the administration of parenteral or enteral nutrition, in addition to the maintenance of a central venous catheter and gastrostomy, jejunostomy, or nasogastric tube.

Some children are unable to consume an adequate diet through the oral route because of problems with absorption or the inability to protect their airway. In this group of children, nutrition is provided by means of an enteral or parenteral route. The enteral route is preferred because it aids in adaptation of the gut to maximize absorption capability. Enteral feedings may be administered through nasogastric or gastrostomy tubes. Silicone elastomer (Silastic) and polyurethane nasogastric tubes are flexible and have a longer indwelling life than polyvinyl chloride tubes. The tubes need to be changed by a trained individual every 30 days (Young & White, 1992). Most parents prefer skin level gastrostomy tubes that are more comfortable for the child and difficult to dislodge. Skin level devices, known as buttons, interfere less than traditional gastrostomy tubes with the activities of daily living (Huth & O'Brien, 1987). Refer to Chapter 16 for further discussion of gastrostomy tubes.

Parenteral feeding is administered through a variety of devices that provide access to the central venous system. These devices require more meticulous care than enteral feeding tubes and can result in serious complications. Refer to Chapter 5 for further discussion of these devices and Chapter 4 for further information on parenteral and enteral feedings.

Several practical concerns exist regarding the physical environment of the home to consider before discharge. A telephone is necessary so that the family has the ability to contact and follow the instructions of the health care providers if problems arise, especially during a nighttime infusion. A discussion of the layout of the home is required, in particular the location of steps, the location of the bathroom in relation to the living and sleeping areas, and carpeting. Infants in an infant carrier can be placed in a small wagon with enteral pumps for easier movement throughout the home. Coat hangers can be used as portable infusion bag holders, which are convenient for cars and strollers. A baby monitor can be used to hear pump alarms when the child is sleeping and the parents are in another area of the home. A child on home total parenteral nutrition (TPN) requires a separate refrigerator or space in the existing refrigerator for supplies, pumps with battery backup for power outages, and a suitable area to store intravenous tubing. The family should notify the local electric company to put the household on a priority list to resume power in the event of an outage. Refer to Exhibit 7–4 for home requirements for technology-assisted children.

The home equipment may differ from the hospital equipment, requiring more nursing support for the first few days of therapy. The home care nurse instructs and supervises the family in independent administration of infusions such as intravenous antibiotics or fluid replacements. Infants require pumps that are not capable of free flow to prevent accidental overadministration. The connections should be taped along the enteral or parenteral line to prevent accidental dislodgment.

The time and attention required for complex medical therapies strain family relationships. The health care provider and family need to encourage sibling involvement by asking for their help in bringing diapers or playing with the ill child. The family needs to make adjustments that result when one member has dietary restrictions. Compressing the infusion time of nutritional solutions, known as creating a window or cycling, helps to normalize family activities. The window period, when infusions are off, allows the child to be free from equipment. The health care provider must assess the family schedule or routines to determine the optimal time for the window period. Many families prefer to infuse during the evening and night so that the window is during the daytime hours. Daytime windows facilitate the child's return to school or finding suitable child care providers for younger children (Loan, Kearney, Magnuson, & Williams, 1997).

Attending youth camps or family vacations can be less stressful with nutritional coordination provided by regional and national vendors. Many families choose to travel with a 1-day supply of formula or TPN and rely on the delivery of

---

Exhibit 7–4 Home Requirements

- Smoke detector
- Fire extinguisher
- Electrical service and outlets adequate to handle equipment
- Backup power source (generator or batteries)
- Telephone
- Heat
- Refrigeration for some medications and TPN
- Water
- Space for equipment and supplies
- Accessible entry and exit

additional equipment and solutions to the camp or vacation destination. This is convenient for the family and ensures safe storage of solutions and enables the family to plan outings with ease.

EDUCATION

The technology-dependent child presents special challenges in educational planning and service provision in order to address his or her health care needs at school (Goldberg, 1993). The Individuals with Disabilities Education Act (IDEA) of 1990 mandates that state and local educational agencies serve all children with disabilities. Services included in these regulations are as follows: Early identification and assessment of developmental delays, medical services, occupational therapy, parent counseling and training, physical therapy, school health services, and transportation (IDEA of 1990 Regulations 300.16). Congress also amended the IDEA to include assistive technology services and devices that are used to increase or improve the students' functional capabilities (IDEA of 1990 Regulations 300.5 and 300.6). The related services may only be available for students who have an individualized educational program (IEP) that documents the need for special services. Students qualify for an IEP only if they are placed in special education. However, technology-dependent children with special health care needs may not require specially designed instructions (Palfrey, Singer, Raphael, & Walder, 1990; Walker, 1987). These children can be protected under the Americans with Disabilities Act (ADA) of 1990. This law prevents discrimination against an individual because of their disability. The central component of this law requires that states provide education at the public expense. The education plan must meet the standards of the state educational agency, and related services must be provided in the least restrictive environment (Hamilton & Vessey, 1992). Often, the educational programs for students with complex health care needs are planned and implemented at the local level. Geiger and Schilit (1988) suggest the appointment of an individual to plan, administer, and coordinate integrated programming that increases communication and ensures the success of these programs.

Educators formally evaluate the abilities of the child with complex health care needs. Alternative response methods may be required in children with physical or cognitive deficits to obtain an accurate measure of their abilities. For example, a child with a tracheostomy or on a ventilator may have difficulty communicating verbally with the evaluator. The educational program developed should be accompanied by backup strategies to deal with long absences from school caused by illness. The plan needs to be flexible and dynamic to encompass changes in the child's medical condition.

Health care instructions with emergency plans are also developed individually for the child and school. A successful program requires collaboration and communication between the family, medical personnel, and policy makers (Clatterbuck, Jones, Turnbull, & Moberly, 1998).

The role of the nurse or health care provider is one of educating families and school personnel about the child's condition and providing appropriate anticipatory guidance. Topics to address include clinical condition, medication and treatments, school readiness, lifestyle choices, promotion of self-esteem and coping strategies, and transition to adulthood (Vessey, 1997). The nurse can advocate for the family directly with the educational system or recommend local or state advocacy groups for additional assistance.

FAMILY COPING STRATEGIES

Parents of children with complex health care needs require knowledge and skill in normal parenting issues and information specific to their situation. Parents must gain expertise in technologies while grieving for the "perfect" child of their dreams (Jenkins, 1996). The health care provider needs to support the parent through the grieving process. Moses (1993) described the five grieving stages as denial, anxiety, depression, anger, and guilt. Each of these stages has behaviors that can serve useful purposes for limited periods but are not helpful for extended periods. Denial of the child's handicap or illness can allow time for the parents to discover personal strengths that they can use to understand information and help offered by others. Anxiety can be used to mobilize and focus the parents' energies to cope with current demands. Depression is the most frequently identified behavior. It can provide a defining competence, values, capabilities, and potency. Anger can enable a parent to reassess and reconstruct beliefs concerning fairness and justice. Guilt may be the mechanism that enables the parents to reexamine and redefine their sense of meaning, importance, and responsibility within the context of the loss.

A supportive environment is necessary for parents to work through the grieving process. A nonjudgmental climate gives the parents permission to express emotions, to think, and to move through the stages of grief. The health care provider assists parents in using their existing support system and helps them inventory their resources so they do not feel alone. The provider arranges follow-up communication and uses anticipatory guidance that builds on the parents' existing knowledge base, validates concerns, focuses on the future, and encourages developmental progress. The positive interactions between the child and parents should be reinforced and the parents' ability to identify and respond to the child's special needs should be complimented (Jenkins, 1996). Parents who focus exclusively on the needs of the child with complex health care needs lose sight of their own needs or the needs of their other family members. Additional parental concerns include finances, altered career goals, and job sacrifices.

A source of support for families with medically complex children is the parents of other ill children. Networking often occurs informally during the child's hospitalization. Families exchange telephone numbers, addresses, or attend parent support groups. Diagnosis-related support groups are a valuable source of information and support for newly diagnosed families. Family Voices is a national grassroots clearinghouse for information and education regarding the health care needs of children with special needs. The purpose of this group is to give families a voice in the national health care reform debate. The group is also involved in managed care; Medicaid; access to specialty care; hospital policies; welfare reform; and corporate health policies at local, state, and federal levels (Arango, 1997). Many other information and support networks are available for families with access to the Internet and electronic mail to obtain information about their child's diagnosis and treatment (Yerks, 1996). Appendix A found at the end of this text includes a list of family resources.

Caring for a technology-dependent child in the home stresses the parental relationship. Often the parental relationship suffers because attention is focused on the technology-assisted child. Areas of difficulty include communication and information sharing, defining roles and responsibilities, and intimacy (Kahn, 1997). It is important for couples to communicate well, listen to each other, and learn to compromise. Home care may affect responsibilities if one spouse has to stop working. Frequently, one spouse has the primary responsibility of caring for the technology-assisted child. Both partners need to be valued for their roles. Companionship and sexuality is also important in the marital relationship, and time needs to be set aside to enjoy each other (Kahn, 1997).

Siblings act as support for each other in ordinary times and during crisis. Healthy siblings have both negative and positive perceptions of the impact of chronic illness on the family. They may feel loving, protective, jealous, angry, or a combination of feelings. Siblings need a safe environment to express these feelings. The parents need to reassure them that these feelings are normal and expected and that they are loved and are important members of the family (Kahn, 1997). Peer support groups can serve as a forum for discussion of many issues. Older siblings who have learned positive coping strategies serve as resources for children who have recently learned that their sibling has a chronic illness. Health professionals help siblings deal with misconceptions about the illness causes and consequences that may lead to a closer sibling relationship (Desiree & Jessee, 1996). Siblings need to be included in the family decision making when appropriate. Parents should schedule special events and outings for the siblings to spend special time together. Also support groups or camps for the siblings, such as Siblings of Cancer Patients, help them adjust to the situation.

Having health care professionals in the home can cause tension. The home is a private domain and is now open for public view. It is important for the health care provider and family to keep relationships on a professional basis. The health care provider should respect the family's cultural heritage, customs, religious beliefs, and health care practices (McNeal, 1998). Together, the health care provider and family should establish roles, rules, and responsibilities. Families must plan for the care of other children in the home because the health care provider is legally only responsible for the technology-dependent child. With good communication and planning, the family and health care provider can become a "team" and provide optimal care (Kahn, 1997).

Respite care or child care that is provided by someone other than the parents may be difficult for the family to identify. Resources that some families have used as supports include schools, extended family members, community groups such as church volunteers and hospice, and volunteer health care providers (Youngblood, 1994). Parents of technology-dependent children cope with the economic hardship of providing for their child's needs. Often, both parents must work outside of the home to meet their financial responsibilities. This necessitates pursuing day care services (Stutts, 1994). Finding acceptable day care services may be difficult when the child has special needs (Delaney & Zolondick, 1991). Medically fragile day care centers are lacking, and if available, the services may not be covered by insurance. These day care centers provide an alternative to home care or prolonged hospitalization. Parents who use these prescribed child care centers report fewer communicable diseases, lower monthly nursing costs, and improved coping levels (Stutts, 1994).

It is not always possible to care for the technology-dependent child in the home. Transfer to a long-term care facility, local hospital, or hospice program may be the best choice. It is important that the family does not feel like they have failed the child if an alternate site to home is selected. The needs and well-being of the child and family unit are the first priority.

CONCLUSION

When the child with complex health care needs is able to be cared for at home, the child and family can concentrate on being a unit and integrating back into the community. Home health teams are an integral part of making home care of the technology-dependent child a safe and effective environment for meeting health care needs.

REFERENCES

Arango, P. (1997). Family voices: Building voices for our children with special health care needs. *Pediatric Nursing, 23*(4), 400–402.

Burns, M., & Thornam, C. (1993). Broadening the scope of nursing practice: Federal programs for children. *Pediatric Nursing, 19*(6), 546–553.

Clatterbuck, C., Jones, D., Turnbull, H., & Moberly, R. (1998). Planning educational services for children who are ventilator assisted. *Children's Health Care, 27*(3), 185–204.

Delaney, N., & Zolondick, K. (1991). Day care for technology-dependent infants and children: A new alternative. *Journal of Perinatal and Neonatal Nursing, 5*, 80–85.

Desiree, D., & Jessee, P. (1996). Impact of a chronic illness in childhood: Siblings' preconceptions. *Issues in Comprehensive Pediatrics Nursing, 19*, 135–147.

Geiger, W., & Schilit, J. (1988). Providing appropriate education environments. In L. Sternberg (Ed.), *Educating students with severe or profound handicaps* (2nd ed., pp. 17–51). Rockville, MD: Aspen Publishers.

Goldberg, E. (1993). Getting off to a good start: Transition planning for children with chronic health conditions. *Network*, Summer, 9–10.

Guillett, S. (1998). Assessing the child with disabilities. *Home Healthcare Nurse, 16*(6), 403–407.

Hamilton, B., & Vessey, J. (1992). Pediatric discharge planning. *Pediatric Nursing, 18*(5), 475–478.

Hilton, T., & Gold, P. (1989). Hospital to home for the ventilator-assisted patient: The future is now! *Homecare Connection, 2*, 1–5.

Huth, M., & O'Brien, M. (1987). The gastrostomy feeding button. *Pediatric Nursing, 13*, 241–245.

Jenkins, R.L. (1996). Grieving the loss of the fantasy child. *Home Healthcare Nurse, 14*(9), 691–696.

Jennett, B. (1986). *Technology medicine: Benefits and burdens.* New York: Oxford University Press.

Kahn, P. (1997). *When your child is technology assisted: A home care guide for families.* Wolfeboro, NH: L & A Publishing/Training.

Lindsay, K. (1999). Challenges in pediatric home care. *Canadian Nurse, 95*(3), 61–2.

Loan, T., Kearney, P., Magnuson, B., & Williams, S. (1997). Enteral feeding in the home environment. *Home Healthcare Nurse, 15*(8), 531–536.

Mauldon, J., Leibowitz, A., Buchanan, J.L., Damberg, C., & McGuigan, K.A. (1994). Rationing or rationalizing children's medical care: Comparison of a medicaid HMO with fee-for-service care. *American Journal of Public Health, 84*, 899–904.

McNeal, G. (1998). Diversity issues in the homecare setting. *Critical Care Nursing Clinics of North America, 10*(3), 357–368.

Moses, K. (1993). *Resource networks, crisis, trauma, and loss.* Evanston, IL: Consultation and Training Services.

Palfrey, J., Singer, J., Raphael, E., & Walder, D. (1990). Providing therapeutic services to children in special educational placements: An analysis of the related service provisions of Public Law 94–142 in five urban school districts. *Pediatrics, 85*(4), 518–524.

Patterson, J., & Blum, R. (1996). Risk and resilience among children and youth with disabilities. *Archives of Pediatric and Adolescent Medicine, 150*, 692–698.

Petit de Mange, E. (1998). Pediatric considerations in homecare. *Critical Care Nursing Clinics of North America, 10*(3), 339–346.

Schuman, A. (1997). Home sweet home: The best place for pediatric care. *Issues in Contemporary Pediatrics, 14*(3), 91–95.

Smith, C.E. (1995). Technology and home care. *Annual Review of Nursing Research, 13*, 137–167.

Stutts, A. (1994). Selected outcomes of technology dependent children receiving home care and prescribed child care services. *Pediatric Nursing, 20*(5), 501–507.

Szilagyi, P. (1998). Managed care for children: Effect on access to care and utilization of health services. *The Future of Children, 8*(2), 39–59.

Vessey, J. (1997). School services for children with chronic conditions. *Pediatric Nursing, 23*(5), 507–510.

Walker, D. (1987). Chronically ill children in schools: Programmatic and policy directions for the future. *Rheumatic Diseases of Childhood, 13*, 113–121.

Wells, N., & O'Neil, M. (1996). *Family perspective on managed care. Family Voices Pilot Survey Report.* Boston: Federation for Children with Special Needs.

Yerks, A. (1996). The internet and pediatric nursing: Guide to the information superhighway. *Pediatric Nursing, 22*, 11–14.

Young, C., & White, S. (1992). Tube feeding at home. *American Journal of Nursing*, April, 45–53.

Youngblood, A. (1994). Families with medically fragile children: An exploratory study. *Pediatric Nursing, 20*(5), 463–467.

Zerwekh, J. (1995). High-tech home care for nurses. *Home Healthcare Nurse, 13*(1), 9–15.

CHAPTER 8

The Death of a Child

Kelly A. Jedlicki

The death of a child alters the expected sequence of life events (Milo, 1997; Murphy, 1996). In pediatric surgery, death can be anticipated, as in a child with end-stage liver disease or neuroblastoma, or unexpected, as in trauma. It is imperative that the care delivered surrounding the death of the pediatric surgical patient meets the needs of the dying child and the child's family. Regardless of the family composition, all members require support during this stressful event. This chapter discusses the care of the dying child, the child's family, and others involved in the child's life, including the nursing staff. The chapter also includes suggested interventions for the period of time after the death of the child.

UNEXPECTED LOSS

The death of a child is often considered worse than the death of an adult, perhaps because the child has not experienced a long chronological life. Parents describe the death of a child as one of the most painful and stressful experiences endured (Milo, 1997; Nesbit, Hill, & Peterson, 1997). Families view the death of a family member as one of the most severe stressors a family may experience (Moriarty, Carroll, & Cotroneo, 1996). Sudden or unanticipated death can be even more stressful because there was not time to prepare for the death psychologically (Barakat, Sills, & LaBagnara, 1995). Sudden death is often a result of trauma. The death of a previously healthy child may be overwhelming. Parents may experience feelings of guilt, especially if the death was potentially preventable. Provide the family with immediate factual information to help them deal with feelings of responsibility and guilt (Barakat et al., 1995).

ANTICIPATED LOSS

The death of a child who has been chronically ill is also devastating to a family. Unlike families who lose a healthy child suddenly, families of chronically ill children often face two losses (Milo, 1997). First, parents suffer from the loss of the dream of a "normal" healthy infant or child; then they confront the loss of their child (Milo, 1997). Many times the family's entire life and schedule are centered around caring for the chronically ill child. The death is not only a loss of the child but also a loss of the routine, schedule, and relationships with the medical professionals surrounding the child. Grief is not lessened for families who lose a chronically ill child. Parents of chronically ill children disagree with the statement that "it was for the best," and most would willingly have continued to parent and care for the child for many more years if given the option (Milo, 1997). Parents of children with a genetic illness, such as cystic fibrosis, or a congenital defect, such as tracheoesophageal fistula, feel responsible for the child's illness and death. The family of a child with a chronic illness has an opportunity to experience anticipatory loss and grief so that they can gradually prepare themselves for the death of the child. However, these families are going through this process suffering from the prolonged stress of a terminal illness (Barakat et al., 1995). Nurses may find it difficult to deal with the death of a chronically ill child, particularly if strong relationships have formed between the nurse and the child and family. Remaining objective and maintaining a professional relationship are essential when caring for the chronically ill child and family.

CARING FOR THE PEDIATRIC SURGICAL PATIENT

The Dying Child

"A dying child is a living child we care for until death" (Dawson, 1995, p. 1534). Honesty is essential when establishing a relationship with the dying child and family (Olson,

1997). Information concerning the child's care and prognosis should be shared with the child and family as appropriate. The developmental level of the child should be considered to give information effectively. For example, descriptions such as "death is like falling asleep" should be avoided with the preschooler because this can lead to nightmares or fear of sleeping (Aldrich, 1996). Hiding facts or avoiding questions leads to mistrust and affects the nurse-patient relationship.

A child's question of whether he or she is going to die requires an age-appropriate answer. Negotiate with the family in advance as to what information should be shared with the child. Dying children sense that talk about death upsets their parents so children often avoid the topic with their parents. Children may approach the nurse with their concerns. The nurse can then facilitate communication between the child and family. Dying children may also be concerned that their parents will not answer their questions about death honestly (Olson, 1997). Children involved in the decision-making process surrounding their own death are less likely to experience anxiety, withdrawal, and isolation than those children "protected" from knowledge about their impending death (Faulkner, 1997). Caring for the child and the family who refuses to share information about death with the child can be a dilemma for the health care team. Social workers, chaplains, and child life specialists may be of assistance to the child and family, as well as the staff. It may be useful to share factual information or research with the family about children's knowledge of their own dying and to convene a patient care conference.

Palliative Care

When a child is terminally ill, the focus of care shifts from cure to symptom control. At this time, the goals of the health care team should be the most effective use of pain medication for the child and physical, psychological, and spiritual support for the child and family. The child should be helped to function at the maximum level of his or her ability, so that the child and family can spend time doing those things most meaningful to them. Comprehensive and successful pain management requires around-the-clock medication with additional administration of medication as needed. Adequate pain control is integral to ensuring quality of life for the dying child. There may be times when members of the health care team or the family disagree among themselves regarding the amount of pain medication necessary and the effects it may have on the child's physiologic status. No evidence exists that adequate pain control hastens a child's death (Martinson, 1995). When controversy exists as to how to manage the child's pain, a team meeting should be considered to re-examine the goals of treatment and to formulate a formal plan.

The Role of Hospice

During the last three decades, many hospice programs specifically designed for children and their families have developed (Martinson, 1993). These programs allow for dying children to be cared for in their homes instead of in the hospital. Many families choose this option with the provision that there is adequate support available from the health care team. See Exhibit 8–1 for key components of a pediatric hospice program. The main principle of hospice care is to "offer developmentally appropriate palliative and supportive care to any child with a life-threatening condition in any appropriate setting" (Children's Hospice International, 1993). Families who care for the dying child at home need specific information about the expected course of the disease and what signs and symptoms suggest impending death. It is also helpful to discuss a plan of action for when death does occur (Goldman, 1996).

Care of the Body

After the death of a child, the nurse must continue to render care to both the child and the family. Respect and dignity should be maintained for the deceased's body. To avoid causing additional pain to the family, continue to keep the child covered and move the child's body gently as needed (Olson, 1997). Privately clean and prepare the body for the family to view. Apply baby lotion to the child's skin or petroleum jelly to the child's cracked lips as needed. The family may wish to participate in the final bath (Parkman, 1992; Wong, 1997). Many parents cherish this last bath. If possible, remove all tubes and equipment. This may be prohibited if an autopsy will be performed or if the death is rendered a coroner's case. Place a favorite toy, blanket, or outfit at the child's side or on the bed while the family is viewing the child. The toy or blanket can accompany the body to the funeral home, which can alleviate the parents' feelings that the child is all alone.

Exhibit 8–1 Key Components of a Pediatric Hospice Program

1. 24-hr availability of experts in pediatric and family care
2. 24-hr availability of experts in pediatric palliative care
3. An identified professional to coordinate care and communicate among the family, caregivers, the local hospital, and the specialty clinic or hospital
4. Respite care facilities
5. Immediate access to hospital care as needed

CARING FOR THE ENTIRE FAMILY

Informing the parents or legal guardian of the death is difficult. The nurse should make every effort to be present when the physician is telling the family about the child's death to help the family to understand what is being told to them and to answer any questions. The family may need guidance in contacting other family members and clergy and in choosing a funeral home. Oftentimes, a social worker or chaplain is available to assist in the process. Occasionally, the nurse must inform family members by telephone of the recent death of the patient. Be concise and factual with the information. For example, say, "your child has sustained a serious injury that caused his death" or "he quit breathing and his heart stopped permanently." Avoid phrases such as "we lost her" or "she is gone" that may have an unclear meaning to the family.

People grieve differently. Societal values and culture affect the grieving process. Kubler-Ross (1969) described six stages of parental reactions to the loss of a child's health. The six stages are shock, denial, guilt, anger, sadness, and resolution and reorganization. Miles (1985) developed a parental grief model that divides the grief process into three phases: (1) a period of shock and numbness, (2) a period of intense grief, and (3) a period of recovery with reorganization. Immediately after the death of a child, the primary focus of the health care team is to assist the family through the shock phase. Parents describe this phase as a "feeling of unreality or being outside of themselves and watching things happen" (Wells, 1996, p. 59). Although the nurse cannot take away the terrible pain of the child's death, helpful interventions can be initiated. This may require colleagues relieving the nurse of other responsibilities. These activities include being a presence to the family, listening, calling the child by name and touching the child, encouraging the family to talk about the child by asking them questions, and expressing personal sadness about the child's death (Wells, 1996).

Removal of Life Support

In some instances there comes a time in the child's course of care when the family must make a decision whether to withdraw extraordinary medical interventions. The nurse should be honest and direct with the family. They may have unrealistic expectations or be hoping for a miracle. Emotions affect the family's ability to concentrate and make rational decisions (Kruger, 1992). Often, information will need to be repeated (Parkman, 1992). Kirschbaum (1996) studied 20 families involved in the decision to authorize, withdraw, or forgo authorization of life-sustaining treatment of a child. Several factors had an impact on the parents' decision making, including (1) their desire for their child to experience

life, (2) their wish to limit their child's suffering, (3) their desire to protect their child's quality of life, (4) their belief that their child's illness affected the child so much that the child no longer seemed like himself or herself, (5) their desire to do what was in the best interest of their child, (6) the importance of the nuclear and extended family, (7) the role of faith and prayer, and (8) their respect for technology. In this study, parents appreciated the opportunity to participate in the challenging decisions regarding life support with their seriously ill children. Chaplains and social workers can reinforce information and offer support to the family. Offer baptism or last rites to the parents as appropriate. When the decision to withdraw life support is made, first turn off the alarms and monitors. This allows the family to focus on the child.

Organ Donation

Most states have a Required Request law that mandates that hospitals approach families of eligible donors to give them the opportunity to donate organs and tissue (Siminoff & Saunders Sturm, 1998). The Joint Commission of Accreditation of Health Care Organizations (Joint Commission) mandates Required Request policies as part of its accreditation requirements for hospitals (Siminoff & Saunders Sturm, 1998). The state's organ procurement organization has transplant coordinators available to help staff determine eligibility to donate.

The transplant coordinators may initiate and discuss the option of donation with families or they may guide the staff on how to approach the family (Siminoff, Arnold, & Caplan, 1995). In some states, only representatives of the organ procurement agency or identified designated requesters may broach the subject of organ donation with the family. The transplant coordinators can address family concerns such as financial costs and disfigurement of the child. Reassure the family that the organ procurement agency provides for all expenses incurred by the decision to donate organs and that if the family desires, an open casket for viewing is still possible.

If the child's death is due to severe head injury, organ donation may be a real option for the family. For many families, organ donation offers a positive note to a tragic and horrible event (Nesbit et al., 1997). The appropriate timing, positive attitude, and manner are essential when approaching the family to request organ donation (Parkman, 1992; Siminoff et al., 1995). Information about the death and organ donation should not be presented at the same time. The family is less likely to agree to donation at that time and later may regret not donating (Siminoff & Saunders Sturm, 1998). There needs to be an interim after explaining the concept of brain death to the family and informing the family of the child's death that allows them time to comprehend and accept that death has occurred (Olasky & Gerdes, 1996). When the family has accepted the reality of the child's death, they can be informed of the option for organ or tissue donation (Coolican, 1987; Nesbit et al., 1997). To not offer the family the opportunity to donate organs is equivalent to making the decision not to donate for them (Olasky & Gerdes, 1996).

Autopsy

Autopsies are required by law in many states when the cause of death is traumatic, perioperative, or unknown. The physician should discuss the need for or the possibility of an autopsy after the family has had time to assimilate the news of the death. Carefully seek permission when an autopsy is requested for medical study or research. Families may hesitate to give permission if they believe their child is going to be "cut up" for research. Families should be reassured that autopsy will not prohibit an open casket for viewing or delay the burial. A plan should be established with the family to help them obtain and review the results of the autopsy with a physician if they desire (Ahrens, Hart, & Maruyama, 1997).

Final Viewing

The family should be prepared for what to expect before they view the child. Discuss the medical equipment that remains in the child. If the death was related to trauma, describe any injuries the child may have sustained. Do not restrict the family's last visit with the child (Parkman, 1992; Wong, 1997). Allow them to have anyone they choose in the room with them (Parkman, 1992). Ideally, someone should be holding or rocking the child when the family enters the room. The family should not be led into the room to view the child and immediately be left alone. A member of the health care team must be present initially to answer questions and demonstrate concern and support. Then, the family should be offered time alone with the child, with the assurance that the staff is readily available and information on how to obtain assistance during their viewing (Parkman, 1992).

Offer families a rocking chair so that they may sit to hold and rock the child (Wong, 1997). Families often cherish the final time spent rocking the child. This time should not be limited and may last from a few minutes to several hours (Parkman, 1992; Wong, 1997). Flexibility in meeting each family's needs provides for a caring and supportive environment to the family.

If possible, offer the family a photograph, lock of hair, ink handprint, or cast molds of the child's hands (Nesbit et al., 1997; Olson, 1997; Parkman, 1992). In one retrospective study (Ahrens et al., 1997), 92% of parents indicated they would have wanted a physical memento of their child. In this study, parents were clear, however, that the memento should not be given at the time they are told of the child's death.

Rather, they would prefer to receive it after they had spent some time with the child's body or even a few weeks after the child's death. Many neonatal and pediatric units have instant cameras and ink pads. Emergency departments and units that apply casts have plaster that can be used for creating hand molds. Ask the parent's permission before cutting a lock of hair. Parents may choose to cut the lock of hair, obtain the handprint, make the hand mold, or take the photograph themselves.

Families often feel awkward, empty, or lost when it is time to leave the hospital. Transportation issues should be discussed to ensure the family's safety (Olson, 1997). The family should be sent home with written information about grief and loss and support groups that they can refer to at a later date. The nurse should offer a good-bye handshake, hug, or pat on the back to show concern and sympathy as appropriate.

Care of the Siblings

Death is difficult for everyone involved. Some believe that it is extremely difficult for children and adolescents to deal with because they may not fully comprehend what has occurred and the ramifications (Aldrich, 1996). Children have limited experience with death to help them comprehend and cope with the death of a loved one (Robinson & Mahon, 1997). Children and adults grieve differently (Aldrich, 1996). The family may choose to inform the siblings of the child's death, or the family may request that a member of the health care team do so. Often child life specialists, social workers, and chaplains help families tell siblings.

The sibling's developmental level should be considered when helping the family to determine what information to share and to anticipate how the child may respond. The concept of death closely follows Piaget's cognitive stages. Infants and toddlers have no concept of death but respond to parental emotions (Barakat et al., 1995). Toddlers are egocentric and cannot separate fact from fantasy, so they are unable to comprehend death. They may persist in wanting to visit the deceased and talk as if the child was still living (Whaley & Wong, 1991). Routines and rituals are important to toddlers, so changes can produce anxiety and behavioral changes such as regression or anger.

Preschool children, ages 3 to 5 years, view death as a temporary or reversible condition. They are egocentric and, therefore, may think that their own thoughts or actions caused the death (Barakat et al., 1995; Faulkner, 1997). They have an immature concept of time, so they do not understand the universality of death. Because preschoolers accept the literal meaning of words, phrases such as "we lost him," "she has gone to sleep forever," or "he has gone away" should not be used (Aldrich, 1996). These phrases can cause anxiety and a possible fear of sleeping or the dark. Some preschoolers respond to death by regressing to earlier developmental skills or behaviors such as thumbsucking and bedwetting. Others may respond by complaining of somatic illnesses or physical symptoms such as headaches or stomach aches (Aldrich, 1996; Dixon & Stein, 1992; Olson, 1997; Whaley & Wong, 1991).

School-age children, ages 6 to 12 years, view death as irreversible or permanent. However, they are unable to comprehend their own mortality (Barakat et al., 1995; Whaley & Wong, 1991). They may personify death as the "grim reaper" or the "bogeyman" (Behrman, 1992; Whaley & Wong, 1991). School-age children are interested in the details of death such as coffins, postmortem care, and body decomposition (Faulkner, 1997; Whaley & Wong, 1991). They may associate bad thoughts or actions as the causative factor of the death (Faulkner, 1997). Siblings may have fears or feelings that they caused the death (Parkman, 1992). They may have feelings of guilt if the death was related to an accident.

Adolescents also view death as irreversible. They have a mature understanding of death but may deny their own mortality through risk-taking behaviors (Barakat et al., 1995; Faulkner, 1997). They also may experience feelings of guilt. They have an idealistic view of the world that may hinder their understanding and acceptance of rituals, customs, funeral rites, and ceremonies. Adolescence is a transition phase from childhood to adulthood, so reactions to death can vary greatly (Whaley & Wong, 1991). When told of the death, the adolescent may have no reaction, experience physical symptoms, or express emotions associated with grief.

Siblings should be allowed to view the deceased (Parkman, 1992; Whaley & Wong, 1991). The siblings should be prepared for what to expect before the viewing to avoid fear and emotional trauma. Before the sibling is brought in, the child should be covered to keep any tubes and wires from view (Parkman, 1992). Families should be encouraged to allow siblings to attend memorial services or funerals (Barakat et al., 1995; Behrman, 1992). Preconceived ideas are often worse than the actual experience. Siblings' questions should be answered honestly. All members of the health care team can assist siblings with their overwhelming feelings about death by listening and answering questions. Often parents are unable to provide adequate support to siblings because they are confronting their own grief. Some hospitals, hospices, and community agencies now offer support groups to meet the needs of grieving children (McGlauflin, 1994).

Care of Families on the Hospital Unit where Death Has Occurred

Many times, a child may die in an intensive care unit or on a medical-surgical unit. While the child was on the unit, the family may have developed relationships or friendships with other families experiencing the same stress and fears of having a hospitalized child. After the death of a child, the "other" families are often left to deal with the death alone. The death of another child can augment the stress of having a sick child (Johnson, 1997). The "other" families may have a child with a condition similar to the one that led to the death of the child. These parents may fear that their child might also die. The "other" families may experience guilt that their child lived while another died. These families must confront their fears of death and their inability to protect their child from death (Johnson, 1997; Kruger, 1992). Witnessing a child's death, especially more than one death, may cause families to question the quality of care their child is receiving (Johnson, 1997).

The health care team is often so focused on caring for the family of the dying or deceased child that the "other" families' fears and feelings may go unnoticed. Avoiding communication with the "other" families can have a negative impact on the grieving experience (Miles, 1985). The coping skills of the "other" families may be compromised if they believe their needs are minor or insignificant compared with those of the family that just suffered the death of a child (Johnson, 1997). Not addressing the "other" families' needs can ultimately affect the health care team's relationships with those families. Without breaching patient confidentiality, these families need reassurance that the staff is affected by the death (Johnson, 1997). Acknowledging the "other" families' concerns and feelings is essential. The "other" families should be allowed to vent their sadness and grief (Johnson, 1997). Unit-based family support groups, led by a social worker and staff nurse, can help these families cope with their fears and feelings and clarify misconceptions (Ladebauche, 1992). Chaplains can also assist with meeting the needs of the "other" families when the health care team is focusing on the care of the dying patient and his or her family (Johnson, 1997).

NURSES WHO CARE FOR DYING CHILDREN

Nurses require support when dealing with the death of a pediatric surgical patient. Nurses must be aware of the stress a death can create for them, as well as for the rest of the health care team (Davies et al., 1996). Open discussion about feelings and expressing emotions helps professionals come to terms with loss. Showing feelings of loss and sadness, such as crying, is therapeutic and should not be viewed negatively (Aldrich, 1996; Davies et al., 1996; Wong, 1997). Nurses who express their feelings can also act as a role model for children, as well as for other adults, and give others permission to grieve (Aldrich, 1996). To effectively continue to care for children, nurses need to cope through maintaining self-awareness and general good health and by making use of available support systems. Professional support groups tend to be more therapeutic and supportive than social groups (Davies et al., 1996; Olson, 1997). Professional groups offer nurses an opportunity to share experiences and coping skills (Davies et al., 1996; Olson, 1997). Other helpful activities include attending ethics rounds, exercise, and maintaining a balance between work and home (Olson, 1997).

AFTER THE DEATH

The health care team must be available to the family even after the death. After the initial shock, the family may want to discuss and review details, events, or circumstances around the death. Reassure parents and guardians that everything possible was done for the child and that the child did not suffer. Families may request guidance regarding the effects of any genetic cause of the child's death on future children or how to cope with their grief. Provide information regarding genetic counselors and support groups such as Compassionate Friends (Moriarty et al., 1996; Parkman, 1992). Oliver and Fallat (1995) researched the effects of a child's traumatic death on the parents. The results indicated that the parents' grief response was considered therapeutic in 7 of 29 parents and pathologic in the other 22. The parents whose grief was therapeutic, although profoundly affected by the pain of the child's death, were able to work through the grief and integrate the child's life and death with their own ongoing life. In contrast, the parents whose grief was pathologic could not get past the death of the child, even years later. These authors challenge the health care team to "take initiative to involve parents in available care systems" (p. 306) such as organized support and self-help groups.

Attendance by members of the health care team at memorial services or funerals is an individual decision (Barakat et al., 1995; Wong, 1997). Some professionals find closure in attending memorial services, and some believe that it is an extension of caring. Families should be supported as they move through the grief process by the nurse making follow-up calls or sending correspondence such as a sympathy card, photographs, a lock of hair, or handprints (Parkman, 1992; Wong, 1997). This continued contact with the family is often therapeutic and appreciated because other support may be

Exhibit 8–2 Example of Key Elements of One Bereavement Program

1. Within 48 hours: phone call to the family by the attending physician to express condolences and answer questions
2. Within one week: sympathy card sent to the family signed by the health care team and phone call to the family by a representative of the bereavement program
3. At 2 weeks and 2, 3, 4, 5, 6, 9, and 12 months after the child's death: individualized letters sent to the family containing information about grief education and support materials
4. Within 3 months: invitation to the parents to meet with the attending physician and bereavement program staff to discuss any concerns, questions, guilty feelings, or other issues
5. Throughout the year: periodic phone calls from nurses and bereavement program staff
6. Annually: Day of Remembrance
7. At 13 months after the death: evaluation of the bereavement program

transient or diminished as family and friends may have begun to withdraw after the funeral (Barakat et al., 1995). Many hospitals have formal bereavement programs to provide continued contact with the family when other support has decreased. Bereavement programs often acknowledge the child's birthday and the anniversary of the death (Nesbit et al., 1997; Ruden, 1996). See Exhibit 8–2 for key elements of one bereavement program.

CONCLUSION

The death of a child, whether anticipated or unexpected, presents many challenges to the nurses involved. Nurses must care for the dying child, the child's family, other patients' families, and each other. There are special considerations regarding palliative care, hospice, removal of life support, organ donation, and autopsy. Finally, long-term support to the family after the child's death is of paramount importance.

REFERENCES

Ahrens, W., Hart, R., & Maruyama, N. (1997). Pediatric death: Managing the aftermath in the emergency department. *The Journal of Emergency Medicine, 15*(5), 601–603.

Aldrich, L. (1996). Helping children cope with the death of someone close. *CARING Magazine, 15*(12), 64–66.

Barakat, L., Sills, R., & LaBagnara, S. (1995). Management of fatal illness and death in children or their parents. *Pediatrics in Review, 16*(11), 419–423.

Behrman, R. (1992). *Nelson textbook of pediatrics* (14th ed.). Philadelphia: W.B. Saunders Company.

Children's Hospice International. (1993). Standards of hospice care for children. *Pediatric Nursing, 19*(3), 242–243.

Coolican, M. (1987). Katie's legacy. *American Journal of Nursing 87*(4), 483–485.

Davies, B., Cook, K., O'Loane, M., Clarke, D., MacKenzie, B., Stutzer, C., Connaughty, S., & McCormick, J. (1996). Caring for dying children: Nurses' experiences. *Pediatric Nursing, 22*(6), 500–507.

Dawson, S. (1995). A dying child. *Canadian Family Physician, 41,* 1534–1540.

Dixon, S., & Stein, M. (1992). *Encounters with children: Pediatric behavior and development* (2nd ed.). St. Louis, MO: Mosby.

Faulkner, K. (1997). Talking about death with a dying child. *American Journal of Nursing, 97*(6), 64–69.

Goldman, A. (1996). Home care of the dying child. *Journal of Palliative Care, 12*(3), 16–19.

Johnson, A. (1997). Death in the PICU: Caring for the "other" families. *Journal of Pediatric Nursing, 12*(5), 273–277.

Kirschbaum, M. (1996). Life support decisions for children: What do parents value? *Advances in Nursing Science, 19*(1), 51–71.

Kruger, A. (1992). Parents in crisis: Helping them cope with a seriously ill child. *Journal of Pediatric Nursing, 17*(2), 133–140.

Kubler-Ross, E. (1969). *On death and dying.* Indianapolis, IN: Macmillan Publishing USA.

Ladebauche, P. (1992). Unit based family-support groups: A reminder. *MCN, 17,* 18–21.

Martinson, I. (1993). Hospice care for children: Past, present and future. *Journal of Pediatric Oncology Nursing, 10*(3), 93–98.

Martinson, I. (1995). Improving care of dying children. In Caring for patients at the end of life [special issue]. *Western Journal of Medicine, 163,* 258–262.

McGlauflin, H. (1994). What one small hospice learned from its grieving children's program. *The American Journal of Hospice & Palliative Care, 11*(2), 36–39.

Miles, M. (1985). Helping adults mourn the death of a child. *Issues in Comprehensive Pediatric Nursing, 8,* 219–241.

Milo, E. (1997). Maternal responses to the life and death of a child with a developmental disability: A story of hope. *Death Studies, 21,* 443–476.

Moriarty, H., Carroll, R., & Cotroneo, M. (1996). Differences in bereavement reactions within couples following death of a child. *Research in Nursing & Health, 19,* 461–469.

Murphy, S. (1996). Parent bereavement stress and preventive intervention following the violent deaths of adolescent or young adult children. *Death Studies, 20,* 441–452.

Nesbit, M.J., Hill, M., & Peterson, N. (1997). A comprehensive pediatric bereavement program: The patterns of your life. *Critical Care Nurse Quarterly, 20*(2), 48–62.

Olasky, K., & Gerdes, K. (1996). Management of the pediatric organ donor: Psychological factors, understanding of brain death important. *Nephrology News & Issues, 10*(8), 22–23, 30.

Oliver, R., & Fallat, M. (1995). Traumatic childhood death: How well do parents cope? *The Journal of Trauma, Injury, Infection, and Critical Care, 39*(2), 303–308.

Olson, M. (1997). *Healing the dying.* Albany, NY: Delmar Publishers.

Parkman, S. (1992). Helping families say good-bye. *MCN, 17,* 14–17.

Robinson, L., & Mahon, M. (1997). Sibling bereavement: A concept analysis. *Death Studies, 21,* 477–499.

Ruden B. (1996). Bereavement follow-up: An opportunity to extend nursing care. *Journal of Pediatric Oncology Nursing, 13*(4), 219–225.

Siminoff, L., Arnold, R., & Caplan, A. (1995). Health care professional attitudes toward donation: Effect on practice and procurement. *The Journal of Trauma, Injury, Infection, and Critical Care, 39*(3), 553–559.

Siminoff, L., & Saunders Sturm, C. (1998). Nursing and the procurement of organs and tissues in the acute care hospital setting. *Nursing Clinics of North America, 33*(2): 239–251.

Stewart, E. (1995). Family-centered care for the bereaved. *Pediatric Nursing, 21*(2), 181–184, 187.

Wells, E. (1996). Assisting parents when a child dies in the ICU. *Critical Care Nurse, 16*(1), 58–62.

Whaley, L., & Wong, D. 1991. *Nursing care of infants and children.* St. Louis, MO: Mosby.

Wong, D. (1997). *Whaley & Wong's essentials of pediatric nursing.* St. Louis, MO: Mosby.

PART II

Surgical Procedures Using Innovative Technology

CHAPTER 9

Fetal Surgery

Lori J. Howell, Susan K. Von Nessen, and Kelli M. Burns

INTRODUCTION

The focus of this chapter is to describe those fetal diagnoses that may be considered for prenatal surgery. For most, detection of a fetal anomaly leads to a change in the timing, mode, or location of delivery to improve the maternal-infant outcome. For a few severely affected fetuses, fetal surgery may be the best option. Each of these anatomic malformations presents with a spectrum of severity, and only those fetuses with life-threatening or severely debilitating anomalies are considered candidates for fetal surgery (Table 9–1).

The incidence, embryology, prenatal diagnosis, and in utero repair of anatomic malformations are described. Postnatal repair is detailed elsewhere in the appropriate chapters in this text. In addition, the role of the surgical nurse using a critical pathway in providing preoperative, intraoperative, and postoperative nursing care is presented. Finally, the role of a center for fetal diagnosis and treatment is discussed.

FETAL CONGENITAL DIAPHRAGMATIC HERNIA

Congenital diaphragmatic hernia (CDH) occurs in approximately 1 in 2,400 live births, with left-sided hernias occurring about seven times more frequently than right-sided hernias. CDH occurs when the pleuroperitoneal canal fails to close and the abdominal viscera migrate into the thoracic cavity, compressing the existing fetal lung and preventing normal pulmonary development (Figure 9–1). Many recent advances have been made in the care of these challenging infants including extracorporeal membrane oxygenation (ECMO) (Bartlett, Gazzaniga, & Toomasian, 1986; Stolar, Dillon, & Reyes, 1988), high-frequency oscillatory ventilation (Tamura et al., 1988), and nitric oxide. In one prospective study, despite optimal postnatal care, fetuses with isolated CDH diagnosed before 25 weeks' gestation had

a mortality rate of 58% (Harrison, Adzick, Estes, & Howell, 1994), and most data support that early prenatal diagnosis is associated with a poor prognosis (Flake, 1997).

Prenatal Diagnosis and Indication for Fetal Surgery

Because the prognosis of CDH is not universally fatal, selecting the most severely affected fetuses with CDH is critical. It now appears liver herniation into the chest is a predictor of poor outcome in fetal CDH (Albanese et al., 1998). Liver herniation is detected by following the umbilical vein and ductus venous above the level of the diaphragm with color flow Doppler ultrasonography. More recently, the use of ultrafast fetal magnetic resonance imaging (MRI) has become an even better technique to detect liver position and does not require maternal sedation or fetal paralysis to prevent motion artifact (Hubbard, Adzick, Crombleholme, & Haselgrove, 1997). The use of sonographic determination of the lung/head ratio (LHR) is also used as a predictor of survival in fetal CDH (Metkus, Filly, Stringer, Harrison, & Adzick, 1996). The LHR is a measurement of the right lung at the level of the atria expressed as a ratio to the head circumference, where an LHR less than 1 is associated with 90% mortality. Careful sonographic evaluation is also important to rule out syndromes such as Fryn's syndrome. This syndrome is an autosomal recessive condition with multiple defects, including CDH, and is associated with mental retardation in those who survive but is generally lethal because of the severe pulmonary hypoplasia associated with CDH (McPherson, Ketterer, & Salsburey, 1993). A chromosome analysis is completed by amniocentesis, chorionic villus sampling, or percutaneous umbilical blood sampling to rule out abnormalities such as trisomy 13, 18, mosaic tetrasomy 12 p (Bergoffen, Prunett, & Campbell, 1993), and others. Fetal surgery is not offered when a chromosomal abnormality

95

Table 9–1 Conditions Amenable to Fetal Surgery

Congenital Anomaly	Prenatal Effects	Postnatal Outcome	Fetal Surgical Procedure	Postnatal Surgical Procedure
Congenital diaphragmatic hernia	Lung hypoplasia	Pulmonary failure	Tracheal occlusion	CDH repair
Congenital cystic adenomatoid malformation	Lung hypoplasia Hydrops > death	Pulmonary failure Death	Open fetal lobectomy —	—
Sacrococcygeal teratoma	Hydrops > death Maternal mirror syndrome		Tumor debulking	Complete resection
Urinary tract obstruction	Hydronephrosis Oligohydramnios Pulmonary hypoplasia	Renal and pulmonary failure	Vesicoamniotic shunt; fetoscopic laser ablation of valves	± Urethral valve ablation
Neck masses	Airway obstruction Polyhydramnios	Asphyxia Prematurity	EXIT procedure	± Tumor resection

is detected. A fetal echocardiogram is performed to rule out structural heart disease. Thus, a mother is considered a candidate for fetal surgery for CDH when her fetus has an isolated CDH with liver herniation into the chest, an LHR less than 1, and is less than 26 weeks' gestation. In addition, the fetus must have a structurally normal heart by fetal

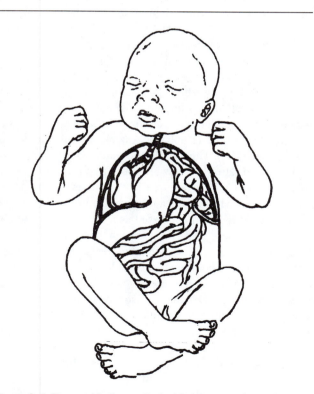

Figure 9–1 Fetus with Severe Left-sided CDH Showing Herniation of Liver, Bowel, and Stomach Causing Mediastinal Shift and Bilateral Lung Compression

echocardiogram and no chromosomal abnormality. Only the most severely affected fetuses are considered candidates for prenatal surgery because of additional risk to the mother as an innocent bystander trying to help her fetus.

Fetal Surgery Technique for CDH

The therapeutic strategy for fetal CDH is to promote lung growth by impeding the normal egress of lung fluid by tracheal occlusion. The lungs enlarge and push the viscera back into the abdomen (Hedrick, Estes, Sullivan, Adzick, & Harrison, 1994a; Wilson, DiFiore, & Peters, 1993). Fetal surgery involves a general anesthesia for the mother and fetus; a maternal laparotomy, hysterotomy, or fetoscopic trocar placement through the uterus; exposure of the fetal neck; and dissection to the fetal trachea where clips are applied. At delivery, the mother undergoes general anesthesia, laparotomy, hysterotomy, and exposure of the fetal head and neck, where clip removal is performed while the fetus is on placental bypass. This procedure is called the ex-utero intrapartum treatment (EXIT). A bronchoscopy of the fetal airway is performed, exogenous surfactant is instilled if the fetus is premature, and the airway is intubated. Umbilical lines are placed, the cord is clamped and cut, and the neonate is taken to the adjacent operating room for the remainder of the resuscitation. Once stabilized, a standard repair of the CDH is performed usually several weeks later, often with a synthetic patch because these diaphragmatic defects are typically quite large. Thus, the goal of fetal surgery in the fetus with a severe CDH is to decrease the severity of pulmonary hypoplasia.

FETAL LUNG LESIONS

There are two types of thoracic masses, congenital cystic adenomatoid malformation of the lung (CCAM) and bronchopulmonary sequestration (BPS), that are sometimes amenable to prenatal resection. CCAM is a benign pulmonary lung mass characterized by an overgrowth of the terminal bronchioles that form various-sized cysts (Adzick, Harrison, Crombleholme, Flake, & Howell, 1998). CCAMs develop during the first 6 weeks of gestation and generally arise from one lobe. CCAMs are classified into three types on the basis of the size and distribution of the cysts. Type I CCAMs contain macrocysts; type II CCAMs are both cystic and solid, whereas type III CCAMs are microcystic or solid in appearance. Bronchopulmonary sequestration (BPS) is a mass of abnormal lung tissue that receives an anomalous blood supply from a feeding vessel off the aorta and does not communicate with the tracheobronchial tree by normally related bronchi. BPSs may be intralobar (90%) or extralobar (10%) (Rowe, O'Neill, & Grosfeld, 1995). A recent report describes a "hybrid" mass that has histologic findings similar to a CCAM, with an anomalous blood supply (Cass et al., 1997). Both types of masses may compromise lung growth and thus lead to lung hypoplasia.

Prenatal Diagnosis of a Thoracic Mass and Indication for Fetal Surgery

The diagnosis of a fetal thoracic mass is made by ultrasonography. The differential diagnoses include CDH, bronchogenic/neuroenteric cysts, bronchial atresia, pleural effusions (usually of infectious origin), and congenital high airway obstruction (CHAOS) (Hedrick et al., 1994b). Prenatally detected CCAM and BPS have a much higher mortality than those diagnosed after birth. The mortality underestimation occurs because some fetuses die in utero, whereas others with large masses resulting in pulmonary hypoplasia require urgent removal in the delivery room and do not survive resuscitation and transfer to a tertiary center. Those fetuses with fetal hydrops caused by large mass compression have a dismal prognosis without prenatal intervention (Adzick et al., 1998).

Once a diagnosis of a fetal CCAM is made, ultrasonographic surveillance to detect tumor growth leading to hydrops is critical. Serial sonography is often performed several times per week for large masses. If the mass appears to regress in size or stabilize, the frequency of the ultrasonography is decreased. However, for those masses that increase in size the heart may become displaced, impede venous return, and result in fetal hydrops. Fetal hydrops is a precursor of fetal death and is the only indication for fetal surgery (Adzick et al., 1998). Typically, fetal hydrops is demonstrated by the following progression of findings: fetal ascites, placentomegaly, and skin and scalp edema. Chromosome analysis is not necessary to proceed with fetal surgery because there appears to be no abnormal chromosomal association with CCAM. A large CCAM also can have health

implications for the mother known as the "maternal mirror syndrome." This pre-eclamptic state can be life threatening to the mother as she mirrors the condition of the sick fetus. Fetal surgery will not cure this maternal hyperdynamic state, and if the mother chooses to continue the pregnancy without fetal surgery in the face of a hydropic fetus, she must be closely monitored for hypertension, proteinuria, and edema (Adzick et al., 1993).

Fetal Surgery Technique for CCAM

For the hydropic fetus with a CCAM diagnosed before 32 weeks of gestation, fetal surgery can be considered (Figure 9–2). Fetal surgery involves maternal-fetal general anesthesia, laparotomy, hysterotomy, and fetal exposure of the presenting side of the CCAM. A fetal thoracotomy and lobectomy are then performed. Operative time is usually quite short, and blood loss is typically minimal. The fetus is then returned to the womb to await delivery. Unlike fetal surgery for CDH, the Caesarean delivery is performed by the obstetricians with neonatal resuscitation immediately available. Prenatal surgery has dramatically improved the outcome for fetuses with hydrops associated with CCAM. In one reported series 13 hydropic CCAM fetuses underwent fetal surgery and 8 survived with an excellent quality of life (Adzick et al. 1998; Flake & Howell, 1998).

FETAL SACROCOCCYGEAL TERATOMA

Sacrococcygeal teratoma (SCT) is the most common tumor found in the newborn, with a reported incidence of 1 in 35,000 to 40,000 live births (Pantoja, Llobet, & Gonzalez-Flores, 1976). Fetal SCT is a tumor arising from the presacral space that may grow to massive proportions. Teratomas are embryonal neoplasms derived from totipotential cells that contain tissue from two or three germ cell layers (ectoderm, endoderm, and mesoderm) (Flake, 1993). SCTs arise from the coccyx bone.

The American Academy of Pediatrics Surgical Section suggests four classifications according to location (Altman, Randolph, & Lilly, 1974). Type I tumors are external with little presacral component (Figure 9–3). Type II tumors have more external than intrapelvic components, whereas type III tumors, although obvious externally, have more internal components. A type IV tumor is located entirely within the pelvis and may go unrecognized until symptomatic. These tumors are classified according to histologic findings. Type I histologic findings are mature and well differentiated and may contain endodermal, mesodermal, or ectodermal tissue. These tumors are usually benign. Type II histologic findings are immature and contain embryonal elements and may become malignant. Type III histologic findings are malignant and contain elements of the yolk sac (Altman et al., 1974).

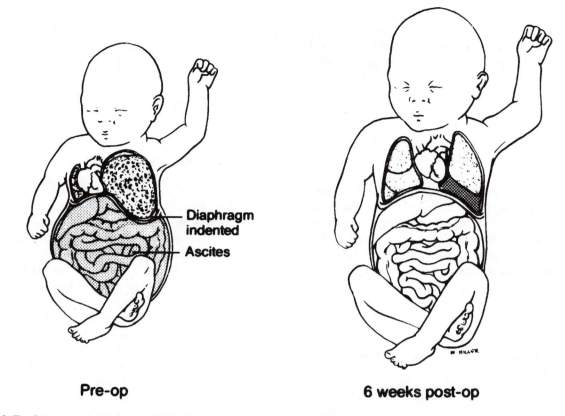

Figure 9–2 Fetal Anatomy in Hydropic CCAM Preoperatively and 6 Weeks after Fetal Surgery

Prenatal Diagnosis of SCT and Indication for Fetal Surgery

Fetal SCT is diagnosed by prenatal ultrasonography. As with other fetal diagnoses, most fetal SCTs can be managed with routine prenatal care. For those fetuses with large SCTs, who show no signs of hydrops, a Caesarean section is recommended to prevent dystocia, tumor rupture, and exsanguination (Flake, 1993). Preterm delivery caused by polyhydramnios may affect morbidity and mortality. The mechanism of polyhydramnios in SCT is not completely understood but seems to accompany the development of placentomegaly and may be the first sign that the tumor is affecting the fetus (Holzgreve, Flake, & Langer, 1990). Fetal SCTs are followed with serial ultrasonographic studies using color and power Doppler ultrasonography to identify those fetuses with large, vascular lesions who are at risk for fetal death as a result of high output cardiac failure. Ultrasonography is useful to determine fetal hemodynamics such as inferior vena caval dilation and increased cardiac output, as well as placental thickness, as a predictor for fetal hydrops. As with other fetal conditions that result in poor placental perfusion and endothelial cell injury, maternal mirror syndrome

may be seen (Flake, 1993). The indication for fetal SCT resection is a type I SCT with hydrops evidenced by placentomegaly and increased combined ventricular output.

Fetal Surgery Technique for SCT

The presumed cause of fetal hydrops is a vascular steal by the teratoma, placing an increased work load on the fetal heart (Flake, 1993). Emergency debulking of the tumor is done as a palliative measure to reduce the cardiac work load. The mother and fetus receive a deep inhalation anesthetic. A maternal laparotomy and hysterotomy are performed, allowing exposure of the fetal buttocks with the attached tumor. Because the tumor can be larger than the fetus, uterine relaxation is critical. The anus is identified and the fetal skin is incised posterior to the anorectal sphincter to avoid injury to the continence mechanism. A tourniquet is then applied to the base of the tumor and cinched down gradually to the vascular pedicle. Tumor debulking is then performed with a stapler. Care is taken to avoid tumor rupture. The entire fetal procedure typically is performed in less than 15 minutes with minimal blood loss (Flake, 1993). Delivery is performed by obstetricians in the high-risk setting with neonatal resuscitation immediately available. Once the neonate is stabilized, a complete resection of the mass including the coccyx is performed. Of the four fetal SCT resections performed, one has survived (Adzick, Crombleholme, Morgan, & Quinn, 1997). Three earlier losses occurred as the result of maternal mirror syndrome, uncontrolled preterm labor, and an intraoperative complication during the postnatal coccyxgectomy (Flake & Howell, 1998).

OBSTRUCTIVE UROPATHY

Obstructive uropathy refers to multiple conditions that may cause an obstruction in the urinary system, such as ureteropelvic junction obstruction, posterior urethral valves, ureterocele, megaureter, multicystic kidney, duplex collecting system, and prune belly syndrome (Figure 9–4). Most of these anomalies require surgery after birth. Most fetuses with obstructive uropathy are male, but obstructions do occur in females and are usually associated with ureteropelvic junction obstruction, ectopic ureterocele, and cloacal abnormalities (Lebowitz & Griscom, 1997). The most common cause of obstruction in the male is posterior urethral valves, which has a reported incidence of 1 in 5,000 to 8,000 (Casale, 1990). Obstruction of the fetal urinary tract may result in renal damage, which ranges from hydronephrosis to renal dysplasia. The obstruction leads to a decrease or absence of amniotic fluid, resulting in fatal pulmonary hypo-

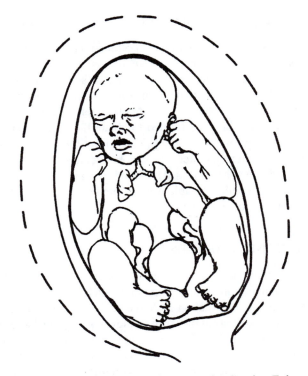

Figure 9–4 Fetus with Obstructive Uropathy Causing Enlarged Bladder, Dilated Ureters and Kidneys, and Oligohydramnios Causing Pulmonary Hypoplasia and Club Feet

plasia, Potter's facies, and contractures (Harrison, Ross, Noall, & de Lorimier, 1983).

Prenatal Diagnosis of Obstructive Uropathy and Indication for Fetal Surgery

Ultrasonographic evaluation and urine sampling of fetuses with obstructive uropathy have helped to explain the natural history of this process and formulate selection criteria for intervention. Ultrasonographic examination indicating poor renal function is evidenced by the development of cortical cysts and renal echogenicity indicating renal dysplasia. Poor renal function is likely when elevated fetal urinary electrolytes (sodium and chloride) and beta-2 microglobulin are noted (Freedman et al., 1997).

Fetal urine sampling techniques involve three percutaneous aspirations of the fetal bladder usually several days apart. The first and second urine samples can be stale and results unreliable. The third aspiration provides the most reliable indicator of kidney function (Johnson et al., 1994). The indications for fetal intervention include bilateral obstructive uropathy, known onset of oligohydramnios, normal chromosomes, favorable urine electrolytes and beta-2 microglobulins, and the absence of renal echogenicity and cortical cysts.

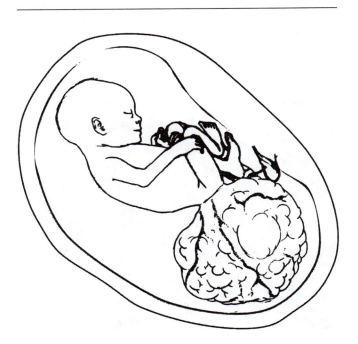

Figure 9–3 Fetus with Huge Type I Sacrococcygeal Teratoma Tumor

Fetal Surgery Technique for Obstructive Uropathy

At present, the most widely accepted method for decompressing the fetal urinary tract is the use of a double pigtailed catheter placed percutaneously with sonographic guidance. However, the catheter lumen can become occluded, migrate, or injure the fetus during placement. Most recently, fetoscopy has been performed to ablate the valves using a Yanitrium Aluminum Garnet (YAG) laser through an antegrade approach (Quintero, Reich, & Puder, 1994). Despite the treatment techniques developed and available for obstructive uropathy, reliable ways of predicting long-term renal function are still needed.

GIANT NECK MASSES

Giant fetal neck masses such as cervical teratomas, hygromas, hemangiomas, and anomalies such as CHAOS can cause airway obstruction at delivery. CHAOS is characterized by a blockage at the laryngeal level or laryngeal atresia. Fetal neck mass disorders can result in profound hypoxia and even death as a result of the inability to obtain an airway after birth. Although fetuses with these conditions do not undergo fetal surgery in the classic sense (i.e., the fetus is not returned to the womb after the operation), they can undergo multiple procedures for up to an hour while still attached to the placental circulation (Leichty et al., 1997; Skarsgard et al., 1996).

Prenatal Diagnosis of Giant Neck Masses and Indication for Fetal Surgery

Accurate diagnosis of these anomalies with prenatal ultrasonography (Figure 9–5A) and ultrafast fetal MRI (Figure 9–

5B) (Hubbard, Crombleholme, & Adzick, 1998) ensures appropriate preparation for a planned delivery to rule out anomalies, establish fetal growth, and detail characteristics of the fetal airway anatomy. A complete obstetric history and physical and genetic evaluation is also performed. For example, polyhydramnios caused by esophageal compression of the neck mass causes distention of the uterus and may lead to preterm labor. Genetic abnormalities such as 69XXX or syndromes such as Fraser's syndrome can be associated with CHAOS (Hedrick et al., 1994b). A triploidy chromosomal abnormality, 69XXX is characterized by marked lateral physical asymmetry, syndactly, and often associated with a myelomeningocele. Fraser's syndrome is an autosomal recessive disorder in which laryngeal atresia and renal agenesis are common findings. These conditions are usually fatal in pregnancies that reach full term. A fetal echocardiogram is performed to rule out structural abnormalities and to identify impending hydrops.

Fetal Surgery Technique for Giant Neck Mass

The EXIT procedure is a technique first described for delivery of a fetus in which tracheal occlusion had been performed in cases of severe CDH (Bealer et al., 1995; Skarsgard et al., 1996). This technique was modified to allow time to obtain an airway in a near-term fetus with a giant neck mass (Leichty et al., 1997). Maternal-fetal anesthesia is provided to enhance uterine relaxation, a crucial point to preserve uteroplacental circulation. A maternal laparotomy and an amniotic fluid reduction is performed through a uterine trocar for patients with severe polyhydramnios. When possible, a lower uterine segment hysterotomy is performed to expose the fetal head, neck, and thorax. A classical Caesar-

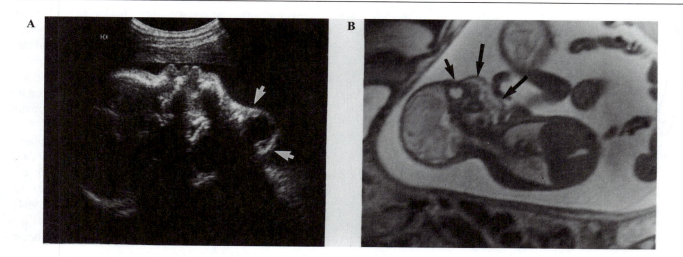

Figure 9–5 A, Conventional Ultrasound Image. B, High-speed Magnetic Resonance Image of Same Fetus with a Giant Neck Mass. Arrows indicate neck mass.

ean delivery is necessary when extension of the head and neck cannot be done because of tumor size. The head, neck, thorax, and one arm are then delivered. Fetal pulse oximetry is applied to monitor the fetal heart rate and hemoglobin saturation continuously. Multiple procedures can be performed for up to an hour before clamping the cord and subsequent delivery. These procedures may include laryngoscopy, bronchoscopy, intubation, exogenous surfactant instillation, placement of umbilical lines, and in rare instances, tumor resection. The advantage of this technique is that multiple procedures may be performed without anoxic insult because of maternal-placental "bypass" before delivery (Leichty et al., 1997).

Patient Selection Process

When a fetal abnormality amenable to fetal intervention is diagnosed, the prospective parents have three choices. If the gestation is before 24 weeks, termination of the pregnancy may be an option. After 24 weeks, continuation of the pregnancy and providing for the best postnatal care may be the parents' decision. For some, intervening before birth may be the option selected. Parents need to be supported regardless of their decision to minimize feelings of guilt later.

An evaluation for fetal surgery consists of outpatient diagnostic tests and a review of the results by a multidisciplinary team (Figure 9–6). The detailed sonographic survey is performed to confirm the diagnosis, detect any additional fetal abnormalities, and assess the presence and severity of hydrops. A fetal echocardiogram is performed to assess any structural abnormalities of the heart and in certain diagnoses such as cervical teratomas to assess subtle hemodynamic changes. Ultrafast fetal MRI is a newer modality that provides striking anatomic detail and is particularly useful for diagnostic dilemmas, confirmation of liver position in CDH fetuses, and obtaining lung volumes as a predictor of pulmonary hypoplasia. If genetic karyotyping is not done at the referring institution, an amniocentesis, chorionic villus sampling, or percutaneous blood sampling is obtained to rule out chromosomal abnormalities associated with certain fetal diseases. Rapid karyotyping can be performed for emergency problems by fluorescent in situ hybridization (FISH). This diagnostic procedure provides information about chromosomes 13, 18, and 21 and sex. Finally, an informed consent conference is held with the family, fetal/pediatric surgeon, obstetric specialists, fetal and obstetric anesthesiologists, the social worker, and nurse coordinator to review the test results and explain the available options for the pregnancy. All

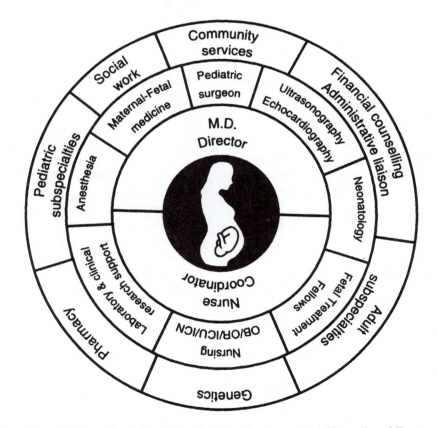

Figure 9–6 The Expertise of Many Different Specialists Is Required by a Center for Fetal Diagnosis and Treatment

these services should be coordinated so that the family can learn of the fetus' anomaly and options in an unhurried, comprehensive manner.

The informed consent conference provides an in-depth description of the fetal surgery procedure, results from the procedure, maternal risks, potential benefits, and alternatives. If the family opts for planned delivery and postnatal surgery, the surgeon counsels the parents regarding the anomaly, the surgical repair, and the anticipated neonatal course. Arrangements are then made for maternal transport and planned delivery at the tertiary center. If the fetus has a fatal defect not amenable to fetal or postnatal surgery or if the parents opt to terminate the pregnancy, the parents receive counseling from the reproductive geneticist. Follow-up telephone and written consultation are provided immediately to the referring physician.

MATERNAL-FETAL MANAGEMENT

The management of the mother from admission to discharge is detailed in the critical pathway for fetal surgery (Appendix 9–A).

Preoperative

Once the complete evaluation indicates that the mother and fetus are candidates for fetal surgery and the parents choose to proceed, the preoperative admission is arranged. The mother undergoes further preoperative teaching and preparation with the nurse coordinator and obstetric nurse specialist, including a tour of the obstetric and neonatal units. The mother has a preoperative history and physical examination completed by the obstetrician and the anesthesiologist, and any additional questions and concerns are answered. The mother is admitted the night before surgery to the labor and delivery unit, where the mother and fetus are monitored, an intravenous line is started, and an indomethacin suppository is administered to promote uterine relaxation.

Perioperative

The morning of surgery, uterine contractions and fetal well-being are assessed by the tocodynamometer. Support stockings are placed to prevent an embolic event. An epidural catheter is placed for postoperative pain management for the mother and the fetus. The mother receives a second indomethacin suppository. She is then brought to the operating room for anesthetic induction and intubation (Figure 9–7). Once the mother is asleep, an arterial line and an additional intravenous line are placed. A Foley catheter is inserted into the bladder, and the sequential compression device to prevent embolic events is activated. The mother is then prepped

and draped in preparation for the fetal surgery. After sonography confirms no change from the preoperative evaluation, a low transverse maternal laparotomy is made. Sterile sonography is then used to mark the placental edges. If the placenta is anterior, the uterus must be lifted up so that the hysterotomy can be made on the posterior aspect of the uterus. If the placenta is posterior, the hysterotomy is made on the anterior side of the uterus. The hysterotomy is performed with a specially devised stapler, being careful to avoid the placenta (Harrison & Adzick, 1993). The arm of the fetus is brought out and a miniaturized fetal pulse oximeter is applied and secured with a transparent dressing and foil. The affected portion of the fetus is then exteriorized and the fetal surgery as described in the preceding sections is performed. The pulse oximetry is removed and the hysterotomy is closed with reinfusion of warmed normal saline with an antibiotic substituted for the previously removed amniotic fluid. The maternal abdomen is then closed, and a transparent dressing is applied to allow for the postoperative sonographic evaluations.

Postoperative

The mother is awakened and extubated in the operating room and then transported to the maternal-fetal intensive care unit (FICU) where intensive monitoring is provided for 48 to 72 hours. The FICU is a devoted area where maternal-fetal intensive care is provided, including arterial access, hemodynamic monitoring and special fetal monitoring, and tocolysis and vasoactive drug administration. Careful fluid management is critical to avoid hypovolemia, which leads to poor uterine perfusion, or hypervolemia, which can induce pulmonary edema when magnesium sulfate and beta-mimetics are used for tocolysis. Daily ultrasonographic surveillance for fetal well-being and amniotic fluid levels is done. A daily echocardiogram is also performed while the mother is receiving indomethacin to assess ductal constriction and tricuspid regurgitation of the fetal heart. Once the preterm labor is controlled, the monitoring lines are removed and tocolysis is weaned to subcutaneous terbutaline. The epidural catheter and the Foley catheter are then removed. The mother typically remains in the hospital for 5 to 7 days and remains on modified bedrest for the duration of her pregnancy on subcutaneous tocolysis.

Discharge Planning and Follow-up

Plans are made for discharge to the nearby Ronald McDonald House by the nurse coordinator. This planning requires preauthorization for home monitoring and tocolytic administration. The Ronald McDonald House has wheelchair accessibility and provides a pager for immediate patient access. In most surgery cases, the family remains near

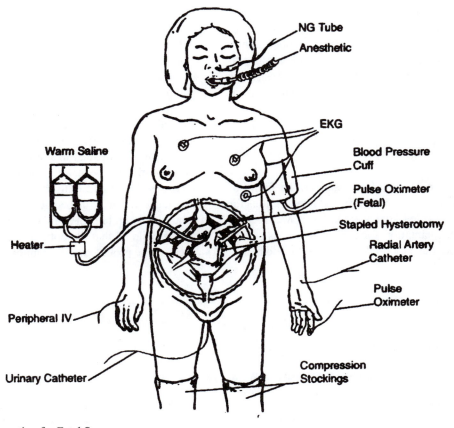

Figure 9–7 Maternal Preparation for Fetal Surgery

the hospital for frequent sonographic evaluations and obstetric care for the duration of the pregnancy.

THE FETAL DIAGNOSIS AND TREATMENT CENTER

A center for fetal diagnosis and treatment provides a coordinated approach to the care of the mother and fetus with an anomaly using the many necessary specialists and state-of-the-art facilities required (Howell, Adzick, & Harrison, 1993). Because the center focuses on maternal-fetal problems, this model offers a systematic approach for diagnosing and providing treatment options; thus expert, coordinated, efficient, and compassionate care is offered to parents facing a decision about their unborn child.

The institutional setting for a center must be able to provide a combination of clinical and basic science research with complex antepartum, intrapartum, and postpartum clinical care for the maternal-fetal patient. An active maternal transport system, and high-risk obstetric and neonatal units are essential. A neonatal resuscitation room adjacent to the operating suite must be available to provide immediate neonatal care and surgical intervention to critically ill newborns as necessary. In addition to the setting, numerous items have required miniaturization, adaptation, and sterilization, including special surgical instruments, specially devised staplers, atraumatic retractors, the level I intrauterine warming device, fetal medications, and fetal intravenous access equipment (Harrison & Adzick, 1993).

In addition to the necessary medical specialists, nurses trained in the management of high-risk obstetric patients are crucial, and education about fetal surgery is provided on an ongoing basis to nursing staff. A center should provide community education regarding the most current information related to prenatal diagnosis and treatment and immediate phone consultation and review of sonographic materials. A toll-free number such as 1-800-IN-UTERO at the Children's Hospital of Philadelphia should be established for consultations for families seeking information about their unborn child. A patient education video and web page detailing fetal anomalies and supporting literature, such as www.fetal-surgery.chop.edu, is available to provide further education.

Many additional resources are required by a center for fetal diagnosis and treatment. For example, The Ronald McDonald House or guesthouse catering to pregnant women on bedrest is crucial to provide a "home away from home."

Staff education regarding pregnant patients may be necessary. The "Adopt a Mommy to Be" program to provide support for fetal surgery mothers on bedrest was subsequently developed and implemented. Also, travel funds are necessary to provide immediate transportation needs. Assistance must be sought from numerous committees and family agencies to provide additional needs.

FUTURE DIRECTIONS

Although beyond the scope of this chapter, the future of fetal therapy is evolving to include prenatal interventions for severe myelomeningocele (Adzick et al., 1998; Meuli et al., 1995), cellular transplantation for such diseases as severe combined immunodeficiency (Flake et al., 1996), and hemo-globinopathies and gene therapy for metabolic diseases such as cystic fibrosis (Sylvester, Yang, Cass, Crombleholme, & Adzick, 1997). Further evolutions in fetal treatment will include minimally invasive approaches to reduce the risk to the mother and fetus and broaden the applications for fetal surgery (Yang & Adzick, 1998).

Ongoing assessment, evaluation, and outcome (Flake & Howell, 1998) of all clinical experience must be reviewed, analyzed, and reported in the literature. Only then will the natural history of fetal anatomic abnormalities be clarified for obstetricians, neonatologists, pediatricians, and pediatric surgeons. The mandate to the surgical nurse providing care to a fetal, neonatal, or pediatric surgery patient is to understand the natural history of the disease and the future effects on the child so that the optimal care and anticipatory guidance can be provided to the family.

REFERENCES

Adzick, N.S., Crombleholme, T.M., Morgan, M.A., & Quinn, T.M. (1997). A rapidly growing fetal teratoma. *Lancet, 349,* 538.

Adzick, N.S., Harrison, M.R., Crombleholme, T.M., Flake, A.W., & Howell, L.J. (1998). Fetal lung lesions: management and outcome. *American Journal of Obstetrics & Gynecology, 128,* 884–889.

Adzick, N.S., Harrison, M.R., Flake, A.W., Howell, L.J., Golbus, M.S., & Filly, R.A. (1993). Fetal surgery for congenital cystic adenomatoid malformation. *Journal of Pediatric Surgery, 28,* 806–812.

Albanese, C.T., Lopoo, J., Goldstein, R.B., Filly, R.A., Feldstein, V.A., Calen, P.W., Jennings, R.W., Farrell, J.A., & Harrison, M.R. (1998). Fetal liver position and perinatal outcome for congenital diaphragmatic hernia. *Prenatal Diagnosis, 18,* 1138–1142.

Altman, R.P., Randolph, J.G., & Lilly, J.R. (1974). Sacrococcygeal teratoma: American Academy of Pediatrics Surgical Section Survey 1973. *Journal of Pediatric Surgery, 9,* 389.

Bartlett, R.H., Gazzaniga, A.B., & Toomasian, J. (1986). Extracorporeal membrane oxygenation (ECMO) in neonatal respiratory failure, 100 cases. *Annals of Surgery, 204,* 236–242.

Bealer, J.F., Skarsgard, E.D., Hedrick, M.H., Meuli, M., Vanderwall, K.J., Flake, A.W., Adzick, N.S., & Harrison, M.R. (1995). The PLUG odyssey: Adventures in experimental fetal tracheal occlusion. *Journal of Pediatric Surgery, 30,* 361–365.

Bergoffen, J.A., Prunett, H., & Campbell, T.J. (1993). Diaphragmatic hernia in tetrasomy 12 p Mosaicism. *The Journal of Pediatrics, 122,* 603–606.

Casale, D. (1990). Early urethral surgery for posterior urethral valves. *Urologic Clinics of North America, 17*(2), 361–371.

Cass, D.L., Crombleholme, T.M., Howell, L.J., Stafford, P.W., Ruchelli, E.D., & Adzick, N.S. (1997). Cystic lung lesions with systemic arterial blood supply: A hybrid of congenital cystic adenomatoid malformation and bronchopulmonary sequestration. *Journal of Pediatric Surgery, 32,* 986–990.

Flake, A.W. (1993). Fetal sacrococcygeal teratoma. *Seminars in Pediatric Surgery, 2,* 113.

Flake, A.W. (1997). Fetal surgery for congenital diaphragmatic hernia. *Seminars in Pediatric Surgery, 5,* 266–274.

Flake, A.W., & Howell, L.J. (1998). *Pediatric surgery and urology: Long term outcomes.* Philadelphia: W.B. Saunders Company.

Flake, A.W., Roncarolo, M.G., Puck, J.M., Ameida-Proada, G., Evans, M.I., Johnson, M.P., Abella, E.M., Harrison, D.D., & Zanjani, E.D. (1996). Treatment of X-linked severe combined immunodeficiency (X-SCID) by the in utero transplantation of paternal bone marrow. *New England Journal of Medicine, 335,* 1806–1810.

Freedman, A.L., Bukowski, T.P., Smith, C.A., Evans, M.I., Berry, S.M., Gonzalez, R., & Johnson, M.P. (1997). Use of urinary Beta 2 microglobulin to predict severe renal damage in fetal obstructive uropathy. *Fetal Diagnosis & Therapy, 12,* 1–6.

Harrison, M.R., & Adzick, N.S. (1993). Fetal surgical techniques. *Seminars in Pediatric Surgery, 2,* 136–142.

Harrison, M.R., Adzick, N.S., Estes, J.M., & Howell, L.J. (1994). A prospective study of the outcome for fetuses with diaphragmatic hernia. *JAMA, 271,* 382–384.

Harrison, M.R., Ross, N.A., Noall, R.A., & de Lorimier, A.A. (1983). Correction of hydronephrosis: I. The model: Fetal urethral obstruction produces hydronephrosis and pulmonary hypoplasia. *Journal of Pediatric Surgery, 8,* 247–256.

Hedrick, M.H., Estes, J.M., Sullivan, K.M., Adzick, N.S., & Harrison, M.R. (1994a). Plug the lung until it grows (PLUG): A new method to treat congenital diaphragmatic hernia in utero. *Journal of Pediatric Surgery, 29,* 612–617.

Hedrick, M.H., Ferro, M.M., Filly, R.A., Flake, A.W., Harrison, M.R., & Adzick, N.S. (1994b). Congenital high airway obstruction syndrome (CHAOS): A potential for perinatal intervention. *Journal of Pediatric Surgery, 29,* 271–274.

Howell, L.J., Adzick, N.S., & Harrison, M.R. (1993). The fetal treatment center. *Seminars in Pediatric Surgery, 2,* 143–146.

Holzgreve, W., Flake, A.W., & Langer, J. (1990). A fetal sacrococcygeal teratoma. In M.R. Harrison, M.S. Golbus, & R.A. Filly (Eds.), *The unborn patient: Prenatal diagnosis and treatment* (2nd ed.) (pp. 460–469). Philadelphia: W.B. Saunders Company.

Hubbard, A.M., Adzick, N.S., Crombleholme, T.M., & Haselgrove, J.C. (1997). Left-sided congenital diaphragmatic hernia: Value of prenatal MR imaging in preparation for fetal surgery. *Radiology, 203,* 636–640.

Hubbard, A.M., Crombleholme, T.M., & Adzick, N.S. (1998). Prenatal MRI evaluation of giant neck masses in preparation for the fetal exit procedure. *American Journal of Perinatology, 15,* 253–257.

Johnson, M.P., Bukowski, T.P., Reitleman, C., Isada, N.B., Pryde, P.G., & Evans, M.I. (1994). In utero surgical treatment of fetal obstructive uropathy: A new comprehensive approach to identify appropriate candidates for vesicoamniotic shunt therapy. *American Journal of Obstetrics & Gynecology, 170,* 1770–1779.

Lebowitz, R.L., & Griscom, N.T. (1997). Neonatal hydronephrosis—146 cases. *Radiology Clinics of North America, 15,* 49–59.

Leichty, K.W., Crombleholme, T.M., Flake, A.W., Morgan, M.A., Kurth, D.C., Hubbard, A.M., & Adzick, N.S. (1997). Intrapartum airway management for giant fetal neck masses: The EXIT procedure (ex utero intrapartum treatment). *American Journal of Obstetrics & Gynecology, 177*(4), 870–874.

McPherson, E.W., Ketterer, D.M., & Salsburey, D.J. (1993). Pallister Killian and Fryn's syndrome: Nosology. *American Journal of Medical Genetics, 47,* 241–245.

Metkus, A.P., Filly, R.A., Stringer, M.D., Harrison, M.R., & Adzick, N.S. (1996). Sonographic predictors of survival in fetal diaphragmatic hernia. *Journal of Pediatric Surgery, 31,* 148–152.

Meuli, M., Meuli-Simmen, C., Hutchins, G.M., Yingling, C.D., McBiles-Hoffman, K., Harrison, M.R., & Adzick, N.S. (1995). In utero surgery rescues neurologic function at birth in sheep with spina bifida. *Nature Medicine, 1,* 342–347.

Pantoja, E., Llobet, R., & Gonzalez-Flores, B. (1976). Retroperitoneal teratoma: Historical review. *Journal of Urology, 115,* 52.

Quintero, R., Reich, H., & Puder, K. (1994). Umbilical cord ligation of an acardiac twin by fetoscopy at 19 weeks gestation. *New England Journal of Medicine, 330,* 469–470.

Rowe, M.I., O'Neill, J.A., & Grosfeld, F. (1995). *Essentials of pediatric surgery* (pp. 366–372). St. Louis, MO: Mosby.

Skarsgard, E.D., Chitkara, L.L., Krane, A.J., Riley, E.T., Halamek, L.P., & Dedo, H.H. (1996). The OOPS procedure (operation on placental support): In-utero airway management. *Journal of Pediatric Surgery, 31*(6), 826–828.

Stolar, C., Dillon, P., & Reyes, C. (1988). Selective use of extracorporeal membrane oxygenation in the management of congenital diaphragmatic hernia. *Journal of Pediatric Surgery, 23,* 207–211.

Sylvester, K.G., Yang, E.Y., Cass, D.L., Crombleholme, T.M., & Adzick, N.S. (1997). Fetoscopic gene therapy for congenital lung disease. *Journal of Pediatric Surgery, 32,* 964–969.

Tamura, M., Tsuchida, Y., Kawano, T., Honna, T., Ishibashi, R., Iwanaka, T., Morita, Y., Hashimoto, H., Tada, H., & Miyasaka, K. (1988). Piston-pump-type high frequency oscillatory ventilation for neonates with congenital diaphragmatic hernia: A new protocol. *Journal of Pediatric Surgery, 23,* 478–482.

Wilson, J.M., DiFiore, J.W., & Peters, C.A. (1993). Experimental fetal tracheal ligation prevents the pulmonary hypoplasia associated with fetal nephrectomy: Possible application for congenital diaphragmatic hernia. *Journal of Pediatric Surgery, 28,* 1433–1439.

Yang, E.Y., & Adzick, N.S. (1998). Fetoscopy. *Seminars in Laparoscopic Surgery, 5,* 31–39.

Appendix 9–A

Critical Pathway for Fetal Surgery

	Outpatient		Obstetric Services	Maternal-Fetal ICU — — — — — — — — — — →		
Date	/ /	/ /	/ /	/ /	/ /	/ /
	Pre Adm	Pre Adm	Day 1 Day of Adm	Day 2 DOS	Day 3 POD 1	Day 4 POD 2
Admission and discharge planning	Preauthorization for fetal surgery Travel/lodging arrangements		Lodging arrangements for post hosp initiated	UR updates		Preauthorization for outpatient services/ home care
Consults	Pedi Surgeon Perinatologist Neonatalogist Anesthesiologist Sonographer Social worker Other	Informed Consent Conference	Pedi Surgeon Perinatologist Anesthesiologist	Social worker	Social worker	Social worker
Labs	Chromosomes AFP		CBC PLTS TXC unit glucose AST, Lytes, Cr, BUN, UA	CBC glucose BUN/CR Lytes/Mg/Phos/Ca ABG	CBC glucose BUN/CR Lytes/Mg/Phos/Ca ABG	CBC glucose BUN/CR Lytes/Mg/Phos/CA ABG
Diagnostic tests	Level II SONO ECHO ultrafast fetal MRI		EKG	SONO ECHO Chest X-ray	SONO ECHO Chest X-ray	SONO ECHO
Activity			Ad Lib	Lateral bedrest Modified Trendelenberg turn q2h	Modified Trendelenberg turn q2h	Modified Trendelenberg turn q2h
Diet/nutrition			Reg NPO after MN	NPO/NG	NPO/NG	NG dc'd NPO
Routine medications						
Pain management				Epidural	Epidural	Epidural
Antibiotics				1g q12h	1g q12h	1g q12h
Tocolytics			Indocin MgSO4	Indocin MgSO4	Indocin MgSO4	Indocin MgSO4
Treatment/ interventions			Compression stockings ordered Weight	Hibiclens shower Compression stockings Weight I&O q1h Foley	Compression stockings Weight I&O q1h Foley	Compression stockings Weight I&O q1h Foley
Fluids			PIV	PIV	PIV	PIV
Respiratory therapy			Teach ICS	Postop: O2 per face mask or NP pulse ox ICS q1h W/A	Postop: O2 per face mask pulse ox ICS q1h W/A	SaO2 >95 + PRN

Courtesy of The Children's Hospital of Philadelphia, Philadelphia, Pennsylvania.

		Obstetric Services				Ronald McDonald House
/ /	/ /	/ /	/ /	/ /		
Day 5 POD 3	Day 6 POD 4	Day 7 POD 5	Day 8 POD 6	Day 9 POD 7	Discharge Outcomes	
	Arrange home monitoring		Arrange f/u appointments	Arrange f/u appointments	Lodging arranged near CHOP. Authorization for home monitoring secured	
Social worker	Social worker	Social worker Neonatologist	Social worker	Social worker	Oriented to OB/ICN for delivery. Emergency/OB f/u	
CBC Glucose BUN/CR Lytes/Mg/Phos/Ca ABG					Normal labs	
SONO ECHO	SONO	SONO	SONO	SONO	AFI > 5 good fetal movement	
Modified Trendelenberg Dangle	Dangle BRP	BRP/shower	BRP/shower Ambulate room	BRP/shower Ambulate hall	Shower/BRP Amb short distances	
Clear liquids	Clear liquids	Reg	Reg	Reg	Bedrest Diet	
		FeSO4, Prenatal vitamins, Colace	FeSO4, Prenatal vitamins, Colace	FeSO4, Prenatal vitamins, Colace	Taking prenatal vitamins Fe + Colace	
Epidural	PO Narcotic Tylenol	PO Narcotic Tylenol	PO Narcotic Tylenol	Tylenol	Pain score <3	
1g q12h					No antibiotics, afebrile	
D/C Indocin Terb pump basal + bolus	Terb pump	Terb pump	Terb pump	Terb pump	Terb pump uterine activity <5/hr	
Compression stockings D/C Foley Weight I&O q1h	Weight Bedpan I&O q shift	Weight I&O q shift	D/C I&O		No emboli Voids q shift	
PIV	TKO	Saline lock	Saline lock	D/C PIV		
SaO2 >95 + PRN	Postop: D/C ICS D/C O2 sats				Lungs clear	

continues

Appendix 9–A continued

Date	Outpatient		Obstetric Services	Maternal-Fetal ICU — — — — — — — — — — — — →		
/ /	Pre Adm	Pre Adm	Day 1 Day of Adm	Day 2 DOS	Day 3 POD 1	Day 4 POD 2
Assessment		Nsg hx OB hx	H&P baseline Tocodynamometer baseline	Tocodynamometer baseline & continuous VS PE incision	Tocodynamometer continuous VS PE incision	Tocodynamometer continuous VS PE incision
Patient teaching	Video Booklet	Tour OBI/ICU/ICN	Preop teaching checklist	Family support & updates	Family support & updates	Family support & updates
Alt in comfort				Verbalizes acceptable level of pain Able to cooperate with activities	Verbalizes acceptable level of pain	Verbalizes acceptable level of pain
Alt in skin integrity				Incision intact Transparent dressing intact	Incision intact Transparent dressing intact	Incision intact without redness or drainage Transparent dressing intact
Anxiety/coping	Asks appropriate questions. Verbalizes concerns regarding self and fetus. Identifies coping style.	Asks appropriate questions. Verbalizes concerns regarding self and fetus. Identifies coping style.	Exhibits mild to severe anxiety. Able to cooperate with care.	Able to cooperate with care. Able to be calmed. Begins to use functional coping mechanisms.	Verbalizes fears and concerns. Receives info. Participates in care.	Receives and retains info. Participates in care. Uses coping mechanisms effectively.
Alt in elimination			Urine output >30 cc/ hr. Bowel sounds min or abs. Abd soft, nondistend.	Urine output >30 cc/ hr. Bowel sounds min or abs. Abd soft, nondistend.		Voiding q4h
Fetal well-being			Baseline FHR >120, <160	Baseline FHR >120, <160		
Uterine activity a) average UC's/hr b) cervical status			No cervical change <6 UC's/hr	No cervical change <6 UC's/hr	No cervical change <6 UC's/hr	

— — →	Obstetric Services	— — — — — — — — — — — — — — →			Ronald McDonald House
/ /	/ /	/ /	/ /	/ /	
Day 5 POD 3	Day 6 POD 4	Day 7 POD 5	Day 8 POD 6	Day 9 POD 7	Discharge Outcomes
Tocodynamometer continuous VS	VS q2–4 h PE incision continuous tocodynamometer	VS q4–6h PE incision continuous tocodynamometer	VS q6h PE incision continuous tocodynamometer	VS q sh Tocodynamometer PE incision	Afebrile VSS No adverse periodic changes No cervical changes contractions <6/hr on terbutaline pump
Bedrest Terb pump Overview	Initiate PTL checklist Terb pump	PTL checklist Incisional care Demand bolus and basal rate	PTL checklist Terb pump syringe	Complete PTL checklist Terb pump checklist Changes Terb pump syringe	Teaching checklist complete Terb pump Resource—who & when to call
Verbalizes acceptable level of pain	Verbalizes acceptable level of pain Takes PO pain med	Verbalizes acceptable level of pain PO pain med	Verbalizes acceptable level of pain Takes pain med pm	Verbalizes acceptable level of pain	Pain at acceptable level with PO meds
Incision intact without redness or drainage Transparent dressing intact	Incision intact without redness or drainage Transparent dressing intact	Incision intact without redness or drainage Transparent dressing intact	Incision intact without redness or drainage Transparent dressing intact	Incision intact without redness or drainage Transparent dressing removed	Incision intact without redness or drainage
Receives and retains info. Participates in care. Uses coping mechanisms effectively.	Receives and retains info. Participates in care. Groups requests. Able to make decisions.	Retains info.	Retains info. Participates in care. Discusses plan for home care. Makes decisions.	Retains info. Verbalizes ability to manage at home. Support systems adequate. Makes decisions.	Verbalizes ability to manage at home with continuing care arrangements.
Voiding q2–4h	Voiding q2–4h	Voiding q2–4h	Voiding q2–4h	Voiding q2–4h	Voiding q2–4h Bowel pattern established
					No cervical change <6 UC's/hr

CHAPTER 10

Minimally Invasive Surgery in Infants and Children

Allen F. Browne and Nancy J. Tkacz

Minimally invasive surgery (MIS) is a general term that describes diagnostic and therapeutic surgical procedures performed with instruments placed through cannulas. MIS is known as minimal access surgery and video-assisted surgery. Laparoscopy (or peritoneoscopy) is the term used for MIS performed in the abdominal cavity (Figure 10–1); thoracoscopy is the term used for MIS performed in the thoracic cavity.

The past several years have witnessed a tremendous growth in MIS in the pediatric population. The development of improved technology enables pediatric surgeons to perform an increasing number of laparoscopic and thoracoscopic procedures previously performed by means of laparotomy or thoracotomy (Gans, 1994; Schropp, 1994b). Each specific procedure (e.g., cholecystectomy or Nissen fundoplication) is performed in MIS with the same series of steps as in the open approach. Differences between the two techniques include the size of wounds, the amount of tissue exposed, and the degree of tissue manipulation that occurs when gaining access to the operative field.

Advantages of MIS can include shorter hospitalizations, decreased costs, less postoperative pain, an earlier return to normal activity, and improved cosmetic results (Holcomb, 1994). Disadvantages may include intraabdominal injury, hemorrhage, or gas embolism with trocar insertion; expensive operative equipment; increased intraoperative time; and the inability to perform the specific procedure as effectively with the MIS technique as opposed to the open technique (Lobe, 1994).

This chapter reviews the historical development of MIS in children and describes the instrumentation used for these

procedures. Specific pediatric anesthetic considerations are discussed. A general overview of laparoscopy and thoracoscopy is presented. The chapter concludes with a discussion of nursing implications and future research considerations.

HISTORICAL DEVELOPMENT

The evolution of minimally invasive surgery parallels technological advances in lighting, imaging, and video monitors. The initial problem with MIS was the lack of an adequate light source. Desormeaux in 1867 is credited with inventing the first functional endoscope that used a kerosene lamp for light (Gans, 1994). Electric light as a source of endoscopic illumination followed in 1868. In 1911, Ott, Kelling, and Jacobeus performed the first light source–illuminated laparoscopy in humans (Schropp, 1994b). Imaging was immensely improved in 1948 by the development of the Hopkins rod-lens system. This system enlarged the endoscope's viewing angle and increased light transmission, thereby producing a brighter, more useful image. The cold, fiberoptic light source was introduced in 1966 and refinements of this system are in use today.

Laparoscopy remained primarily a gynecologic tool until 1987 when Mauriat performed the first laparoscopic cholecystectomy (Schropp, 1994b). The adaptation of laparoscopy as a tool for general surgeons was facilitated and stimulated by the development of cameras that transfer the image of the operative field to one or more monitors. With this "video assistance," multiple surgeons and instruments are involved in the operative procedure. As general surgeons developed their laparoscopic skills, the scope of adult laparoscopic surgery expanded to include appendectomies, bowel resections, splenectomies, herniorrhaphies, and Nissen fundoplications.

Few surgeons performed pediatric laparoscopic procedures before 1970 because instrumentation was too large for the

Acknowledgments: We thank Albert W. Dibbins, MD, and Michael R. Curci, MD, for their assistance and support in the preparation of this chapter.

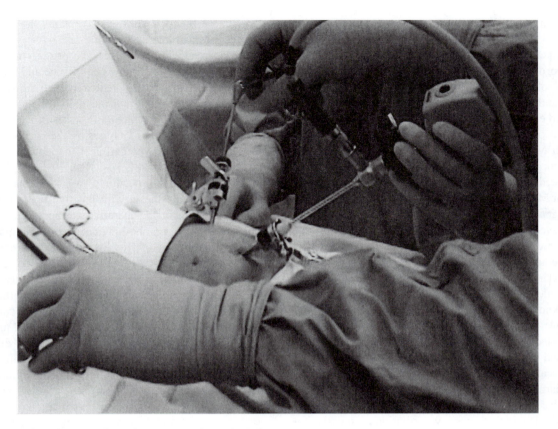

Figure 10–1 Trochar Placement for Pyloromyotomy in a 4-kg Infant

small body cavities of children. In 1969, Gans introduced improved, smaller instruments with superior fiberoptic light sources developed in Germany (Gans, 1994). With the introduction of video assistance in the late 1980s, pediatric surgeons developed their laparoscopic skills and MIS equipment improved. Now a wide range of operations is performed in children of all sizes and ages.

Jacobeus first performed thoracoscopy in 1910. He described introducing a cystoscope into the pleural space to dissect adhesions in patients with pulmonary tuberculosis (Schropp, 1994a). Rodgers and Talbert introduced modern pediatric thoracoscopy in 1976. They performed biopsies of pulmonary and pleural lesions in children ranging in age from 17 months to 16 years (Rodgers, 1994). Video assistance and recent improvements in thoracoscopic instrumentation allow pediatric surgeons to apply thoracoscopy to many diagnostic and therapeutic problems ranging from decortication for empyema to ligation of patent ductus arteriosus.

INSTRUMENTATION

Most MIS instruments did not exist more than 30 years ago. The development of the Hopkins rod-lens system al-

lowed transmission of a bright light and a high-quality image through a small tube. This light is termed a "cold light" because the light source is remote from the body cavity. Although small endoscopes provide excellent images, the limiting factor continues to be the brightness of the light. The larger the endoscope diameter, the more light that can be transmitted (Moir, 1993). Telescopes offer different degrees of field of view, magnification, and angle. Thus, options for various operative procedures and surgeon preferences are provided.

The video camera converts the image into an electronic signal that is transmitted to the video monitor. The most common type of video camera attaches to the outer end of the telescope and captures the image coming through the telescope. Newer systems involve a "chip camera" placed on the inner end of the telescope. Chip cameras are cooler, require less light, and produce a better picture (Kimber, Spitz, & Cuschieri, 1997; Rothenberg, 1994). However, size and expense limit their use.

Video cameras can auto-adjust the brightness of the light source to compensate for reflection off peritoneal surfaces or surgical instruments. Video cameras can be connected to a VCR or a still image printer for documentation of the procedure (Hertzmann, 1994). Recent improvements in video cameras and monitors allow the entire operating team to view the operative field image simultaneously, which improves coordination of the team's efforts. With all team members looking at the same picture, the manipulation of retractors and instruments by multiple personnel becomes a coordinated effort (Holcomb, 1994).

The goal of MIS is to perform standard surgical procedures with MIS techniques rather than open techniques. Standard surgical instruments such as forceps, dissectors, scissors, needle drivers, clip appliers, and staplers have been adapted for MIS (Holcomb, 1994). Endoscopic surgeons use scissors that are straight-edged, curved, or hooked. Hemostasis is achieved with endoscopic clips, staplers, sutures, and cautery. Needle drivers with tips identical to those used in open procedures are passed through the laparoscopic port. Suturing is then performed as in a standard open case. Knot tying is achieved by using a standard instrument-tie technique, preknotted suture, or by extracorporeal knots (Hertzmann, 1994).

Lasers, electrocautery, and harmonic scalpels are energy sources used for coagulation and transection of tissue. The harmonic scalpel facilitates tissue transection and coagulation. The harmonic scalpel uses a rapidly oscillating blunt tip that transects the tissue and provides hemostasis (Rogers & Lobe, 1995). The high-frequency oscillation is an easier energy source to control than laser or electrocautery. Harmonic scalpel instruments can be used to grasp and retract, as well as transect and coagulate, thereby shortening operative times. Cost, safety, surgical skill level, and personal preference are factors a surgeon considers when choosing a method of tissue dissection, transection, and coagulation.

Laparoscopic specimen removal is sometimes possible through the largest cannula. Tissue can be placed in a plastic bag before removal to avoid spillage into the operative field. Occasionally, the specimen is too large to pass through a cannula. Options then include morcellation (fragmenting) of the specimen in the bag, enlarging one of the incisions, making a new incision, or using a natural orifice such as the anus.

ANESTHETIC MANAGEMENT

MIS spans a spectrum ranging from elective, outpatient procedures to emergency laparoscopy/thoracoscopy on a critically ill child. As in all surgery, anesthetic technique is tailored to the child's specific clinical condition. However, unique considerations exist for the anesthesia and analgesia needs of children undergoing MIS.

Anesthetic options for MIS include local anesthetic infiltration, regional anesthesia, and general anesthesia (McGahren, Kern, & Rodgers, 1995). Although all three of these options are currently used in the adult and adolescent population, general anesthesia remains the only practical choice for most infants and children.

In laparoscopic procedures, the primary anesthetic concern is the reduction in lung compliance and functional pulmonary residual capacity created by both the Trendelenburg position and insufflation of the abdomen with carbon dioxide gas (CO_2). These factors may result in hypoxemia. In addition, absorption of CO_2 gas by the peritoneum may result in significant hypercarbia if inadequate ventilation is provided (Tobias, 1998).

In thoracoscopic procedures, the use of standard general endotracheal anesthesia with positive pressure ventilation inflates the lung on the operative side and obscures the surgical field. Therefore, one-lung anesthesia with positive pressure ventilation is preferred for thoracoscopic cases. In older children (more than 40 kg), a double-lumen endotracheal tube provides effective one-lung ventilation. By use of this technique, either lung can be ventilated in isolation. Also, the anesthesiologist can change from one-lung to two-lung ventilation without repositioning the endotracheal tube (Tobias, 1994). However, double-lumen endotracheal tubes are too large for the airways of infants and smaller children. Therefore, selective endobronchial intubation of either the right or left mainstem bronchus is performed. Selective endobronchial intubation allows one-lung ventilation of the contralateral lung, allows collapse of the lung on the operative side, and provides optimal visualization of the operative field (Tobias, 1994). Another alternative is to use the laparoscopic CO_2 insufflator to create a low-pressure (5 mm Hg) tension pneumothorax in the pleural space on the operative side.

After anesthesia induction, an incision is made into the pleural space. The cannula and telescope are placed through this incision and a pneumothorax is created. Subsequent cannulas are inserted under thoracoscopic visualization. Positioning of subsequent cannulas depends on the procedure and size of the patient. Potential risks of this procedure include hypotension related to decreased venous return from excessive intrathoracic pressure and the inadvertent injection of air into the pulmonary vasculature (Tobias, 1994). Although these events are possible, most children tolerate the pneumothorax without difficulty. At the end of the procedure, the pneumothorax is evacuated and two-lung ventilation is resumed. Reversal of anesthesia and extubation proceed routinely.

Postoperative analgesia is achieved by wound infiltration with a local anesthetic, intravenous or oral narcotics, nonsteroidal anti-inflammatory agents, and/or acetaminophen. Pain control is tailored to the individual needs of the child. In general, children undergoing MIS report less postoperative pain compared with children who experience the same procedure performed by the standard open method (Austin, 1994; Nymberg & Crawford, 1996; Valdes & Boudreau, 1996).

BASIC LAPAROSCOPY

Before beginning a laparoscopic procedure, video monitors should be positioned to provide the surgeon and assistants with an unobstructed view of the "operating field." The patient is positioned, prepped, and draped so that the operation can be converted to an open procedure if necessary (Holcomb, 1994). To decompress both the stomach and the bladder, a nasogastric tube and Foley catheter are inserted after anesthesia induction, minimizing possible injury to these organs.

Abdominal access is achieved by either a Hasson approach or by Veress needle puncture. In the Hasson approach, the peritoneum is opened and a cannula is inserted under direct vision. When using the Veress needle, the peritoneum is punctured followed by insufflation of the peritoneal cavity and the blind insertion of a trocar and cannula (Lobe, 1994).

Insufflation of the peritoneum is most commonly achieved with CO_2 gas. The intraabdominal pressure is monitored to prevent high abdominal pressures (greater than 15 mm Hg) that can adversely affect the child's hemodynamic status. Gasless laparoscopy using metal or wire struts as abdominal wall lifters is evolving in pediatric MIS. The potential advantages of these lifting devices include simplification of trocars, decreased cost, and no loss of pressure in the abdomen (and no visual loss of the operative field) when CO_2 gas is suctioned or inadvertently interrupted (Georgeson, 1998a).

After a cannula has been inserted and the abdomen insufflated, the lens with the camera is introduced and a general inspection of the abdominal cavity is performed. The remaining trocars are then placed under laparoscopic visualization to minimize the chance of inadvertent injury. The specific procedure is then performed. After the procedure has been completed, the surgeon makes a final inspection of the abdominal cavity and the CO_2 used for insufflation is allowed to escape. The trocars are removed under laparoscopic visualization and the final cannula is removed. The trocar wounds are closed and dressed.

Potential complications specific to laparoscopy include puncture of intestine or blood vessels by either the Veress needle or the trocars, insufflation of CO_2 into a large vessel (gas embolism), abdominal wall hematomas, and incisional hernias (Chen, Schropp, & Lobe, 1996; Lobe, 1994). Although the incidence of these events is small, early recognition can prevent further complications.

Several considerations specific to pediatric laparoscopy exist because of the child's small intraabdominal space. Decompression of the stomach (nasogastric tube) and bladder (Foley catheter) is particularly important to both protect these organs and to expand the intraabdominal workspace.

Also, wide placement of the trocars on the abdomen is often necessary to maximize the working angle of the instruments. Some surgeons believe that the routine use of the Hasson technique for abdominal access, which allows for direct visualization during insertion of the umbilical cannula, minimizes the chance of injury to abdominal structures (Holcomb, 1994), but this is controversial. Many surgeons use the Veress needle technique in selected patients with good results.

BASIC THORACOSCOPY

Thoracoscopy was initially used in the 1920s to dissect pulmonary adhesions resulting from tuberculosis. Poor exposure of the operative field because of inadequate equipment resulted in the abandonment of thoracoscopy for thoracotomy. Thoracoscopy enjoyed resurgence in the 1980s as visualization improved with the advent of superior equipment and advances in pediatric anesthesiology (Rogers & Lobe, 1995). Indications for thoracoscopy presently include evaluation of trauma, recurrent pneumothoraces, resection and/or biopsy of tumors, removal of cysts, and evacuation of fluid and decortication for empyema (Rothenberg & Chang, 1997b; Schropp, 1994a).

Several advantages of thoracoscopy over thoracotomy exist. The three to four trocar punctures of thoracoscopy in contrast to the rib spreading, muscle cutting incision of a thoracotomy decrease postoperative pain and promote a rapid return to preoperative activity level. Children requiring chemotherapy or radiation treatments are able to resume their treatment protocols sooner (Pesetski, 1995). Postoperative chest tubes are often unnecessary. A decrease in morbidity results in shorter hospitalizations and therefore lower costs. Finally, thoracoscopy is easily converted to an open procedure if necessary (Schropp, 1994a).

The major contraindication to thoracoscopy is the inability to establish and maintain adequate access to the operative field. Other clinical situations precluding the use of this procedure include coagulopathy or deep pulmonary parenchymal lesions. In the past, the patient's size was a limiting factor but now 2-mm sheaths and shorter, small-diameter instruments are making thoracoscopy possible on infants less than 6 months of age (Burke, 1997; Kimber et al., 1997).

Because trocar placement is critical to the success of thoracoscopy, accurate preoperative evaluation by magnetic resonance imaging, computed tomography scan, fluoroscopy, and radiographs becomes essential (Rodgers, 1994). The thoracoscopic patient is positioned specific to the surgical approach chosen by the preoperative evaluation. As with laparoscopy, the patient is widely prepped and draped in the event that the procedure is converted to open thoracotomy.

After anesthesia induction, the initial trocar is placed and a pneumothorax is created for visualization of the operative field (Rothenberg, 1994). Further trocars are placed under camera visualization. After the specific procedure is completed, trocars are removed and the field is inspected before camera removal. One trocar site is used for a chest tube if needed. The remaining wounds are closed and dressed.

Potential complications include tension pneumothorax, hemorrhage, or gas embolism created by trocar introduction into the thoracic cavity (Schropp, 1994a). It is also possible to injure subdiaphragmatic organs such as the liver or spleen with secondary trocar insertions. Trocar insertion under camera visualization can prevent this complication.

SPECIFIC PROCEDURES

A wide variety of MIS operative procedures are reported in the pediatric literature. Table 10–1 includes procedures currently reported as being performed with the use of laparoscopic and thoracoscopic techniques.

The most common laparoscopic procedures currently include (1) cholecystectomy (Holcomb, 1998b), (2) appendectomy (Blakely et al., 1998), (3) management of nonpalpable testis (Brock, Holcomb, & Morgan, 1996; Koo & Bloom, 1998), (4) evaluation for inguinal hernia (Holcomb, 1998a), (5) fundoplication for gastroesophageal reflux (Georgeson, 1998b; Rothenberg, 1998a), (6) splenectomy (Farah et al., 1997; Rothenberg, 1998b), (7) resection and pull-through for Hirschsprung's disease (Rothenberg & Chang, 1997a; Wulkan & Georgeson, 1998), (8) pyloromyotomy (Bufo et al., 1998; Rothenberg, 1997), and (9) evaluation of acute conditions of the abdomen (Lobe, 1997).

Thoracoscopy is currently used for (1) tumor biopsy (Rothenberg, Wagner, Chang, & Fan, 1996); (2) patent ductus arteriosus ligation, vascular ring division, and cardioscopy (Burke, 1997); and (3) management of pleural effusions,

empyemas, and recurrent pneumothoraces (Rothenberg & Chang, 1997b). The reader is referred to the reference list for more detailed discussions of specific MIS procedures.

NURSING CONSIDERATIONS

Clinical Implications

MIS procedures are changing the traditional pathways of patients in the health care system. Health care practitioners need to make adjustments in existing practice to respond to the shift from inpatient to ambulatory care and shorter hospitalizations. Optimal collaboration and cooperation is needed between community, ambulatory, and inpatient caregivers. A critical pathway for laparoscopic fundoplication is provided in Appendix 10–A.

Preoperative/Ambulatory Setting

Children undergoing MIS receive a thorough preoperative assessment. The child's preoperative physical status is established and the advantages, disadvantages, and potential complications of the procedure are discussed with the patient and family. Families are reminded that conversion from an MIS approach to an open approach may be necessary in the event that the operation cannot be performed satisfactorily with MIS techniques or if complications occur. Complications such as excessive bleeding, bowel perforation, an inability to accurately define the anatomy, or an inability to perform the procedure result in conversion to an open technique (Holcomb, 1994; Lobe, 1994).

The child and family often spend less time in the traditional inpatient setting when undergoing an MIS procedure. Therefore, preoperative assessment and education are shifting to the community setting (Nymberg & Crawford, 1996). Family preparation and education for laparoscopic procedures need to be very focused. Expanding preoperative edu-

Table 10–1 Reported Pediatric Laparoscopic and Thoracoscopic Procedures

Laparoscopic Procedures	*Thoracoscopic Procedures*
Adrenalectomy	Blebectomy
Bowel resection	Collateral vessel division
Excision of Meckel's diverticulum	Diaphragm plication
Excision of ovarian cyst	Evacuation of bronchogenic cyst
Ladd's procedure (malrotation)	Lobectomy
Ligation of veins for varicocele	Lung biopsy
Nephrectomy	Pericardiectomy
Oophorectomy	Release of scoliotic anterior spine
Trauma exploration	
Ventriculoperitoneal shunt	
Vagotomy	

cation into the initial office evaluation or preoperative visit can facilitate this goal (Bozzette, 1998).

Preoperative instructions specific to MIS include the following. Multiple small incisions are made rather than one larger incision. Drains such as nasogastric tubes and Foley catheters are routinely placed during the operation and removed at the end of the case. Postoperative pain may include areas remote from the incisions. For example, shoulder pain may develop because of diaphragmatic irritation from the CO_2 gas used for abdominal insufflation.

Families often require assistance in making the transition from a traditional to an MIS approach. Some families may interpret the child's early discharge home to the parent's care as an overwhelming responsibility. Preoperative and postoperative involvement of community nursing resources becomes increasingly important as families are required to view surgical procedures from a wellness perspective rather than the traditional dependent role (Tkacz, 1994).

Perioperative Setting

MIS and its technology have had a profound impact on the role of the perioperative nurse. In addition to traditional operative skills, perioperative nurses are now responsible for the operation and troubleshooting of video cameras, monitors, recorders, fiberoptic light sources, printers, endoscopes, and instruments with multiple, fragile parts (Mailhot, 1996). Equipment is often awkward and space consuming. Visibility is frequently limited because MIS is performed in a darkened room to enhance the video monitor picture.

The establishment of an MIS coordinator and core team is necessary for an effective MIS program (Charney, 1996; Kenyon, Lenker, Bax, & Swanstrom, 1997). The MIS team coordinator oversees all endoscopic equipment, ensures that all nurses performing MIS are knowledgeable and proficient, schedules to ensure 24-hour coverage of MIS-experienced staff, and serves as a contact for vendors and service personnel (Austin, 1994; Valdes & Boudreau, 1996). In addition, coordinators function as liaisons between surgeons, operating room personnel, and management. The coordinator remains current on operative and technical aspects of MIS and serves as an advisor for MIS-related issues such as staff education, equipment purchases, and budgetary concerns.

The establishment of an MIS core team increases the skillful management of the operation and decreases operative time (Kenyon et al., 1997). MIS requires the use of highly technical equipment such as video cameras, monitors, insufflators, and VCRs. Perioperative nurses knowledgeable in the use, care, and placement of this equipment contribute to smoother transition between cases, longevity of expensive instruments, and minimal conversions to open procedures related to equipment failure or personnel inexperience.

The MIS circulating nurse understands the operative procedure from both MIS and open approach perspectives. The circulator is responsible for minimizing intraoperative problems and facilitating the procedure (Valdes & Boudreau, 1996). Minimally invasive procedures require the presence of specialized, space-occupying equipment in addition to standard instruments, which must be on standby in the room. The circulating nurse must pay specific attention to personnel traffic patterns, location of electrical outlets and cords, and the potential for sterile field contamination. Careful orchestration of personnel and equipment by the circulator ensures patient and staff safety. The circulator is also responsible for all documentation, which includes videotaping the procedure in addition to completing standard written forms.

Patient preparation consists of prepping and draping for the MIS procedure with the possibility of conversion to an open procedure. The scrub nurse inspects all MIS equipment preoperatively to ensure its proper functioning. MIS instruments have many small, moveable parts, which can be broken during sterilization or storage between cases (Valdes & Boudreau, 1996). Ongoing assessment of equipment avoids prolonged anesthesia and operating time caused by intraoperative equipment or instrument failure.

Postanesthesia nurses also have made adjustments in postoperative assessment and patient education (Forrest, 1993). The body often responds to MIS with less of a stress response than with traditional open procedures. This physiologic change has implications for postoperative fluid, pain, pulmonary, and activity management. Postoperative medical and nursing care is adjusted to the child's specific response to the perceived surgical stress. Postoperative management is also influenced by the child's rapid return to the community, which again necessitates adjustments in traditional approaches to fluid, pain, and activity.

Discharge teaching by postanesthesia and ambulatory nurses becomes critically important as families are asked to learn important information at a time of increased personal stress. Written information, visual aids, and follow-up phone calls are useful techniques for many families. Reinforcement of the surgeon's specific postoperative instructions offers the family further opportunities to seek information and guidance (Valdes & Boudreau, 1996).

Community Setting

Follow-up by nurses in community, primary care, and surgical office settings allows for reinforcement of postoperative education in addition to assessing for complications and ongoing educational needs. Community health agencies are experiencing a shift from clients who require surgical wound care to those whose major needs are education and support of their self-care (Tkacz, 1994). MIS incisions/scars are placed differently than those used with the traditional approach. Also, smaller scars tend to be less obvious over time. Families should be encouraged to remind future health care professionals of the MIS approach used with the child's surgery because some of the "usual" clues (e.g., right lower quadrant scar of open appendectomy) will be absent.

Educational Implications

The ongoing development of MIS presents implications for nursing education. Nursing curriculums must provide students with exposure to endoscopic procedures throughout the entire continuum of care (Nymberg & Crawford, 1996). A tremendous need also exists to include endoscopic nursing education by staff development programs in both community and inpatient settings (Charney, 1996). As medical and nursing practitioners become more comfortable with MIS, the technique will be used for a wider spectrum of diagnostic and therapeutic procedures. Expanded nursing roles such as the laparoscopic nurse practitioner are being developed to address the needs created by MIS (Williams, 1996).

Research Implications

The implications for nursing research in pediatric endoscopic surgery are vast. Little research exists to address these emerging clinical and educational questions. The efficiency and success of patient and family education techniques must be evaluated. Studies are needed to determine the most effective way for nurses in all health care settings to communicate in a concise, expedient manner.

Evaluation of the care, maintenance, and cost of minimally invasive technology and equipment is needed. Cost/benefit analyses offer timely information in determining the most practical and efficient use of available technology (Reichert, 1993). Nursing can provide ongoing research into the cost-effectiveness of disposable versus reusable equipment. To be accurate, cost/benefit analyses should evaluate the entire period of time that the child is in the medical system rather than simply operative or hospitalization costs. A more rapid return to home decreases hospital costs, but costs relating to lost wages by caregivers (parents) who remain out of work during their child's recuperative period need to be considered.

Prospective, randomized comparisons of MIS versus an open technique for specific procedures will objectively provide rationale for the type of approach best suited for each specific procedure. Factors to be analyzed include, but are not limited to, morbidity, mortality, complications, comfort, length of hospital stay, cost, and patient satisfaction. Accurate outcome and cost analysis research will guide practitioners to choose the most effective and beneficial method (Mellinger & Ponsky, 1996).

FUTURE CONSIDERATIONS

The ongoing development of technology combined with the expertise and imagination of clinicians continues to cre-

ate realities from possibilities. The concept of collaboration has expanded beyond medical and nursing professionals to include scientists, bioengineers, and computer programming specialists. Ongoing development is occurring simultaneously in both the clinical and technological arenas.

Clinical

Fetoscopic Surgery

Fetoscopy now offers the promise of intervention for congenital anomalies in utero through the ongoing development of instrumentation, technology, and access systems (Kimber et al., 1997). Fetoscopy is the application of microlaparoscopic technology to fetal diagnosis and therapeutic intervention. Fetoscopic procedures currently in development are focusing on congenital anomalies such as hydronephrosis, congenital diaphragmatic hernia, and myelomeningocele. Minimally invasive fetal surgery may reduce the risks seen in open in-utero surgery. These risks include uterine irritation, fetal stress, and preterm delivery (Yang & Adzick, 1998).

Neuroendoscopic Surgery

Advances in illumination, miniaturization, and optics now enable pediatric neurosurgeons to address distal intracranial pathologic conditions with MIS under the guidance of direct visualization. MIS, combined with stereotactic or image-guided localization, has become a viable combination of technologies, extending the boundaries of modern pediatric neurosurgery (Wilson & Drake, 1998). Neuroendoscopic surgery allows access to deep intracranial structures by way of small incisions with decreased trauma to nearby neural tissue in select patient groups (Gerzeny & Cohen, 1998).

Technology

Despite the advances in MIS, many technical limitations remain. Operating suites are far from "user friendly" as bulky equipment encroaches on the operative field. Loss of depth perception from the human eye to the video monitor and the inability to palpate body tissue directly can be problematic. Inaccessibility to the operative field in small infants caused by a restriction on the angles of MIS instruments continues to challenge bioengineers, the endoscopic surgeon, and the MIS team (Mailhot, 1996). Redesigning the operating room workspace, improving the surgeon's ability to manipulate tissue, reducing the effects caused by long instruments, and improving the team's limited field of vision will continue to advance the field of MIS.

The operating room is being redefined through various technologies. Remote-controlled video monitors and printers allow the circulating nurse to turn on the monitor, record the procedure, and print still pictures while remaining remote from the sterile field and drapes. Operating rooms are being redesigned to accommodate video equipment. Accessory equipment is being ceiling mounted with suspended electrical cords. Equipment is becoming smaller, computer controlled, simpler to use, and easier to store (Mailhot, 1996).

However, difficulties remain. The cost of new technology limits centers where MIS is not the primary recipient of surgical resources. And although suspending video monitors from the ceiling may allow for better "traffic control," the more ergonomic position for practitioners is currently an image projected to a podium placed at the level of the operative field. This allows the team to look "down" at the same angle as the operative instruments and prevents back and neck strain.

The most promising MIS technologies are a part of a greater scheme known as the Information Age of the twenty-first century. A fundamental change has occurred in the realization and implementation of digital information. Medical images, patient records, laboratory tests, vital signs, and physiologic data are now capable of being converted to a digital format and displayed to medical professionals on monitors rather than paper charts, radiographic films, or pathology slides. Three technologies hold particular promise for MIS: robotics, telepresence, and virtual reality (Satava, 1996).

Robotics

Robotics is an intelligent machine that manipulates real objects under the supervisory control of a human (Satava, 1996). Several types of robotic systems are being developed.

The automatic robotic system offers the promise of high precision that can be programmed to complete specific tasks. This system is particularly suited to the fields of orthopaedics, neurosurgery, and ophthalmology, which require a higher degree of accuracy than is capable by the human hand (Eckberg, 1998; Goh, Krishnan, & Seah, 1996).

The remote-controlled robotic system is being developed to allow a surgeon dexterity, tactile sensation, and feedback from a remote workstation. The surgeon "performs" the surgical maneuvers that, by means of satellite, are executed by the robotic manipulator at the surgical site. This technology could enhance the ability of the surgeon to perform a difficult procedure with the assistance of robotic control. Or the robot could perform a procedure in a place too dangerous or distant for the surgeon to realistically operate in person (Satava, 1996).

The manually controlled (voice activated) robotic system has become a realization. This robot is being used to control the video camera during MIS. The robot obeys voice commands and moves the video camera as directed by the surgeon's voice (Goh et al., 1996). The robot is programmed to recognize only the voice of the operator and follows simple commands such as "left" and "right."

Telepresence

Telepresence is defined as human control over a remote manipulator of objects at a distant site in the real world (Satava, 1996). This remote-controlled system addresses the three main deficiencies of MIS: (1) absence of three-dimensional vision; (2) poor dexterity; and (3) lack of sensory feedback. Telepresence surgery is performed at a remote operative site with a robotic dexterous manipulator and a stereoscopic camera. The surgeon operates at a workstation with a 3-dimensional monitor and instrument handle controllers that have dexterity and sensory feedback similar to instruments in open procedures (Satava, 1996). This prototype is currently undergoing military field training evaluation.

Virtual Reality

In contrast to telepresence, virtual reality is an imaginary world created by computer graphic programs where imaginary objects can be manipulated (Satava, 1996). These sophisticated programs "allow" a person to enter the created world and explore its contents. The educational possibilities of this technology appear limitless. The "Visible Human Project" is the recreation of a virtual cadaver, which promises the capability of "exploring" the inner workings of this "human's" anatomy. Use of virtual reality technology will permit members of the MIS operative team to practice their technique on a surgical simulator just as pilots currently practice take-offs and landings using flight simulators.

CONCLUSION

Although applications of MIS to the pediatric population appear limitless, it is important to continually assess which surgical approach is in the best interest of the individual child. The pediatric expertise of the surgeon, anesthesiologist, and nursing staff, along with their comfort with MIS, should be thoroughly considered. The management of available resources is also important.

The experimental techniques of today are rapidly becoming tomorrow's established standard of care. All health professionals should take the responsibility to develop expertise with these new techniques. The challenge of the future is appropriate application of these procedures while maintaining the child's safety as the foremost concern.

REFERENCES

Austin, B.A. (1994). Perioperative nursing considerations for minimally invasive surgical procedures. In T.E. Lobe & K.P. Schropp (Eds.), *Pediatric laparoscopy and thoracoscopy* (pp. 67–80). Philadelphia: W.B. Saunders Company.

Blakely, M.L., Spurbeck, W.W., Laksman, S., Hanna, K., Schropp, K.P., & Lobe, T.E. (1998). Laparoscopic appendectomy in children. *Seminars in Laparoscopic Surgery, 5*(1), 14–18.

Bozzette, M. (1998). Endoscopic surgery in infants and children: New approaches for surgical problems. *Journal of Pediatric Nursing, 13*(4), 252–261.

Brock, J.W., Holcomb, G.W., & Morgan, W.M. (1996). The use of laparoscopy in the management of the nonpalpable testis. *Journal of Laparoendoscopic Surgery, 6*(Suppl. 1), S35–S39.

Bufo, A.J., Merry, C., Shah, R., Cyr, N., Schropp, K.P., & Lobe, T.E. (1998). Laparoscopic pyloromyotomy: A safer technique. *Pediatric Surgery International, 13*(4), 240–242.

Burke, R.P. (1997). Minimally invasive techniques for congenital heart surgery. *Seminars in Thoracic and Cardiovascular Surgery, 9*(4), 337–344.

Charney, F. (1996). Minimally invasive surgery equals maximum education. *Minimally Invasive Surgical Nursing, 10*(2), 69–71.

Chen, M.K., Schropp, K.P., & Lobe, T.E. (1996). Complications of minimal-access surgery in children. *Journal of Pediatric Surgery, 31*(8), 1161–1165.

Eckberg, R. (1998). The future of robotics can be ours. *AORN Journal, 67*(5), 1018–1023.

Farah, R.A., Rogers, Z.R., Thompson, W.R., Hicks, B.A., Guzzetta, P.C., & Buchanan, G.R. (1997). Comparison of laparoscopic and open splenectomy in children with hematologic disorders. *Journal of Pediatrics, 131*(1), 42–45.

Forrest, D.M. (1993). Practical points in the postoperative management of a laparoscopic inguinal herniorrhaphy patient. *Journal of Post Anesthesia Nursing, 8*(4), 280–285.

Gans, S.L. (1994). Historical development of pediatric endoscopic surgery. In G.W. Holcomb (Ed.), *Pediatric endoscopic surgery* (pp. 1–8). Norwalk, CT: Appleton & Lange.

Georgeson, K.E. (1998a, May). Instrumentation. In K.E. Georgeson & E.P. Tagge (Course Directors), *Advanced minimal access pediatric surgery workshop.* Workshop conducted by American Pediatric Surgical Association, Charleston, South Carolina.

Georgeson, K.E. (1998b). Laparoscopic fundoplication and gastrostomy. *Seminars in Laparoscopic Surgery, 5*(1), 25–30.

Gerzeny, M., & Cohen, A.R. (1998). Advances in endoscopic neurosurgery. *AORN Journal, 67*(5), 957–965.

Goh, P., Krishnan, S.M., & Seah, J. (1996). Robotics. In R. Savalgi & H. Ellis (Eds.), *Clinical anatomy for laparoscopic and thoracoscopic surgery* (pp. 281–301). New York: Radcliffe Medical Press.

Hertzmann, P. (1994). Instrumentation for endoscopic surgery. In T.E. Lobe & K.P. Schropp (Eds.), *Pediatric laparoscopy and thoracoscopy* (pp. 6–24). Philadelphia: W.B. Saunders Company.

Holcomb, G.W. (1994). Diagnostic laparoscopy: Equipment, technique, and special concerns in children. In G.W. Holcomb (Ed.), *Pediatric endoscopic surgery* (pp. 9–20). Norwalk, CT: Appleton & Lange.

Holcomb, G.W. (1998a). Diagnostic laparoscopy for congenital inguinal hernia. *Seminars in Laparoscopic Surgery, 5*(1), 55–59.

Holcomb, G.W. (1998b). Laparoscopic cholecystectomy. *Seminars in Laparoscopic Surgery, 5*(1), 2–8.

Kenyon, T.A., Lenker, M.P., Bax, T.W., & Swanstrom, L.L. (1997). Cost and benefit of the trained laparoscopic team: A comparative study of a designated nursing team vs. a nontrained team. *Surgical Endoscopy, 11*(8), 812–814.

Kimber, C., Spitz, L., & Cuschieri, A. (1997). Current state of antenatal in utero surgical interventions. *Archives of Disease in Childhood, 76,* F134–F139.

Koo, H.P., & Bloom, D.A. (1998). Laparoscopy for the nonpalpable testis. *Seminars in Laparoscopic Surgery, 5*(1), 40–46.

Lobe, T.E. (1994). Basic laparoscopy. In T.E. Lobe & K.P. Schropp (Eds.), *Pediatric laparoscopy and thoracoscopy* (pp. 81–93). Philadelphia: W.B. Saunders Company.

Lobe, T.E. (1997). Acute abdomen: The role of laparoscopy. *Seminars in Pediatric Surgery, 6*(2), 81–87.

Mailhot, C.B. (1996). The future of minimally invasive surgery. *Nursing Management, 27*(10), 32Y, 32AA.

McGahren, E.D., Kern, J.A., & Rodgers, B.M. (1995). Anesthetic techniques for pediatric thoracoscopy. *Annals of Thoracic Surgery, 60*(4), 927–930.

Mellinger, J.D., & Ponsky, J.L. (1996). Recent publications in laparoscopic surgery: An overview. *Endoscopy, 28,* 441–451.

Moir, C.R. (1993). Diagnostic laparoscopy and laparoscopic equipment. *Seminars in Pediatric Surgery, 2*(3), 148–158.

Nymberg, S.M., & Crawford, A.H. (1996). Video-assisted thoracoscopic releases of scoliotic anterior spines. *AORN Journal, 63*(3), 561–575.

Pesetski, J.R. (1995). Laparoscopy and thoracoscopy in infants and children. *Seminars in Perioperative Nursing, 4*(2), 146–150.

Reichert, M. (1993). Laparoscopic instruments. *AORN Journal, 57*(3), 637–655.

Rodgers, B.M. (1994). Thoracoscopy. In G.W. Holcomb (Ed.), *Pediatric endoscopic surgery* (pp. 103–118). Norwalk, CT: Appleton & Lange.

Rogers, D.A., & Lobe, T.E. (1995). Thoracoscopic surgery in children. In R.A. Dieter (Ed.), *Thoracoscopy for surgeons: Diagnostic and therapeutic* (pp. 185–191). New York: Igaku-Shoin.

Rothenberg, S.S. (1994). Thoracoscopy in infants and children. *Seminars in Pediatric Surgery, 3*(4), 277–282.

Rothenberg, S.S. (1997). Laparoscopic pyloromyotomy: The slice and pull technique. *Pediatric Endosurgery & Innovative Techniques, 1*(1), 39–41.

Rothenberg, S.S. (1998a). Experience with 220 consecutive laparoscopic Nissen fundoplications in infants and children. *Journal of Pediatric Surgery, 33*(2), 274–278.

Rothenberg, S.S. (1998b). Laparoscopic splenectomy in children. *Seminars in Laparoscopic Surgery, 5*(1), 19–24.

Rothenberg, S.S., & Chang, J.H. (1997a). Laparoscopic pull-through procedures using the harmonic scalpel in infants and children with Hirschsprung's disease. *Journal of Pediatric Surgery, 32*(6), 894–896.

Rothenberg, S.S., & Chang, J.H. (1997b). Thoracoscopic decortication in infants and children. *Surgical Endoscopy, 11,* 93–94.

Rothenberg, S.S., Wagner, J.S., Chang, J.H., & Fan, L.L. (1996). The safety and efficacy of thoracoscopic lung biopsy for diagnosis and treatment in infants and children. *Journal of Pediatric Surgery, 311*(1), 100–104.

Satava, R.M. (1996). Future directions. In B.V. MacFadyen Jr. & J.L. Ponsky (Eds.), *Operative laparoscopy and thoracoscopy* (pp. 929–939). Philadelphia: Lippincott-Raven Publishers.

Schropp, K.P. (1994a). Basic thoracoscopy in children. In T.E. Lobe & K.P. Schropp (Eds.), *Pediatric laparoscopy and thoracoscopy* (pp. 94–104). Philadelphia: W.B. Saunders Company.

Schropp, K.P. (1994b). History of pediatric laparoscopy and thoracoscopy. In T.E. Lobe & K.P. Schropp (Eds.), *Pediatric laparoscopy and thoracoscopy* (pp. 1–5). Philadelphia: W.B. Saunders Company.

Tkacz, N.J. (1994). Pediatric laparoscopy and thoracoscopy. *Nursing Clinics of North America, 29*(4), 671–680.

Tobias, J.D. (1994). Anesthetic management for endoscopic procedures. In G.W. Holcomb (Ed.), *Pediatric endoscopic surgery* (pp. 163–172). Norwalk, CT: Appleton & Lange.

Tobias, J.D. (1998). Anesthetic considerations for laparoscopy in children. *Seminars in Laparoscopic Surgery, 5*(1), 60–66.

Valdes, M.P., & Boudreau, S.A. (1996). Video-assisted thoracoscopic ligation of patent ductus arteriosus in children. *AORN Journal, 64*(4), 526–535.

Williams, M. (1996). The expanding role of the nurse in laparoscopic surgery. *British Journal of Theatre Nursing, 6*(4), 34–35.

Wilson, J.T., & Drake, J.M. (1998). Technical aspects of endoscopy. In R. Tasker & P. Gildenberg (Eds.), *Stereotactic and functional neurosurgery* (pp. 373–377). New York: McGraw-Hill.

Wulkan, M.L., & Georgeson, K.E. (1998). Primary laparoscopic endorectal pull-through for Hirschsprung's disease in infants and children. *Seminars in Laparoscopic Surgery, 5*(1), 9–13.

Yang, E.Y., & Adzick, N.S. (1998). Fetoscopy. *Seminars in Laparoscopic Surgery, 5*(1), 31–39.

Appendix 10–A

Critical Pathway for Laparoscopic Nissen Fundoplication

	ASU/PACU	POD #1	POD #2	POD #3
Assessment	Vital signs q1h PACU Vital signs q4h per pediatric routines I + O Dressings dry Incisions intact UO—1–2ml/kg/hr Transfer to pediatric unit	Vital signs q4h I + O Dressings dry Incisions intact Abdomen soft Bowel movement/flatus	Vital signs q4h I + O Dressings dry Incisions intact Abdomen soft Bowel movement/flatus	DC vital signs DC I + O Dressings dry Incisions intact Abdomen soft Bowel movement/flatus
Treatments	CPT q2h Pulse oximetry	CPT q4h Pulse oximetry	DC CPT DC oximetry	
Lines	PIV—maintenance + ½ volume	PIV—maintenance volume	Heparin lock PIV	DC PIV
Medications	Ketorolac IV q6h X 8 doses MS PRN	Ketorolac IV q6h (complete dosing) Tylenol PRN	Tylenol PRN	Tylenol PRN
Activity	OOB to chair in evening	Ambulate TID and PRN	Ambulate TID and PRN	Ambulate ad lib
Diet	NPO	Clear liquids	Blenderized foods—no solids allowed	Blenderized foods
Referrals	Dietary Child life Social work screen	Follow-up with referrals	Follow-up with referrals	Finalize discharge instructions suggested by consults Follow-up with primary care MD
Patient teaching	Orientation to perioperative experience Assess discharge needs	Begin diet teaching— will be on blenderized foods for 4–6 weeks; PO supplements as needed; stress importance of no solid food	Reinforce dietary teaching: discuss how to transition to solids after 4–6 wk of blenderized foods Ensure that family owns or has access to blender	Finalize dietary education Written instructions to family as appropriate Dressing removal POD #7 Bath POD #7 Activity as tolerated without restrictions
Discharge planning	Notify home care services (if existing) of admission	Follow-up with home services PRN	Follow-up with home services PRN	Discharge Follow-up with surgeon 2 wk

PART III

Nursing Care of Children with Surgical Lesions of the Head, Neck, and Thoracic Cavity

CHAPTER 11

Common Cysts

M. Elizabeth Foster

Discovery of a lump or bump on a child initiates a cascade of parental anxiety and action that prompts a visit to the pediatrician. Despite parental fears, most unexplained superficial lumps carry a low risk of malignancy in the pediatric population. Many lumps and bumps are seen and carefully observed or treated by primary care physicians. Those that classically present as specific lesions or fail to respond to various salts and salves, antibiotics, steroids, and reassurance are often referred to a pediatric surgeon. Embryologic accidents result in numerous reparable conditions that may present as lumps or bumps. This chapter focuses on the more common cysts and superficial lumps and includes branchial cleft remnants, thyroglossal duct cyst, lymphangioma, vascular anomalies, lymphadenitis, dermoid cyst, and ganglion cyst. Excluded are torticollis, teratomas, dermatologic lesions, tumors, and cystic lesions of internal organs. Table 11–1 summarizes the standard surgical approach to common cysts in childhood, and Appendix 11–A is a generic critical pathway for ambulatory surgery. Information specific to the surgical excision of the cyst is discussed in each section.

BRANCHIAL CLEFT REMNANTS

During the fifth week of embryologic development, major head and neck structures are formed from a series of four internal pharyngeal pouches and external clefts separated by five pharyngeal arches. The external and middle ear, mandible, larynx, laryngeal muscles, nerves and vessels, thyroid gland, parathyroid glands, and thymus gland are among these structures. Pharyngeal arches contain mesenchymal tissue that becomes cartilage, bone, muscle, and blood vessels. Arches are covered externally with squamous epithelium (ectoderm) and internally with cuboidal epithelium (endoderm). Ectodermal tissues become skin over the lower face and neck, ear, thyroid, and cricoid cartilages and bone.

Endoderm forms blood vessels and mucous membranes of the pharynx. Mesoderm forms facial and laryngeal muscle and cranial nerves V, VII, IX, and X (trigeminal, facial, glossopharyngeal, and vagus, respectively). The pharyngeal arches, pouches, and clefts are known as branchial (gill-like) arches, pouches, and clefts, although human embryos do not develop gills (Skandalakis, Gray, & Todd, 1994b; Soper & Pringle, 1986).

Incomplete, failed, or persistent embryologic development of the branchial arches results in several anomalies or defects in the neck. Two common branchial cleft remnants are branchial cleft sinuses and cysts. As the arch structures finish forming, the branchial pouches and clefts obliterate; if obliteration is incomplete, a sinus tract, fistula, or cyst is the result. Sinuses and cysts are more common than true fistulas. Branchial cleft remnants originating from the second arch are the most common, followed by those of the first arch. Third and fourth arch anomalies are rare (Friedberg, 1989; Roback & Telander, 1994; Soper & Pringle, 1986).

Preauricular sinuses are tracts that remain after formation of the external ear from the first and second arches. It is believed these are not true branchial cleft remnants but are the result of abnormal infolding and entrapment of epithelium during the external ear formation. These sinuses are autosomal dominant with incomplete penetrance and usually present as a preauricular or helical pit. Bilateral presentation occurs in 25% of affected individuals (Friedberg, 1989). The pits may fill with debris and become infected; surgical excision is indicated for cosmetic reasons or to prevent recurrent infections in those previously infected.

True first branchial cleft anomalies are rare but do occur as cysts that lie in front, behind, or below the earlobe or in the submandibular area (see Figure 11–1). A first branchial sinus has an external opening below the mandible and above the hyoid bone. Some sinus tracts have internal openings to

Table 11–1 Summary of Common Cysts and the Straightforward Surgical Approaches (complexity, clinical data, cyst physiology, and complications potentially alter the surgical approach and outcome and are excluded from this listing.)

Cyst	Location	Surgical Indications	Incision	Wound Closure	Complications
First branchial cleft	In front, behind, or below earlobe	Risk of infection	Curved, vertical incision in front of ear down to jaw	Subcutaneous with topical collodion or wound closure strips	Facial nerve paralysis, damage to parotid gland, infection, recurrence
Second branchial cleft	Lower third and anterior border of sternocleido-mastoid	Risk of infection	Elliptical around opening of sinus or cyst; second stepladder (occasional)	Subcutaneous with topical collodion or wound closure strips	Hypoglossal and glossopharyngeal nerve damage, bleeding, infection, recurrence
Thyroglossal duct cyst	Midline over or above hyoid bone; moves up with swallowing or tongue thrust	Risk of infection	Transverse just above cyst	Subcutaneous with topical collodion or wound closure strips	Respiratory distress, dysphagia, infection, bleeding, recurrence
Cystic hygroma	Posterior triangle of neck, axilla	Risk of infection, airway obstruction	Transverse to accommodate removal	Subcutaneous or sutured with drain(s)	Airway obstruction, edema, bleeding, infection, facial nerve damage, recurrence
Hemangioma	Anywhere	Rare; threat to facial or vital structures; extreme size; cosmetic	Transverse to accommodate removal	Subcutaneous or sutured with or without drain(s)	Bleeding, infection, recurrence
Capillary malformation	Anywhere	Cosmetic	None; laser	None	Failure, bleeding, infection
Arteriovenous malformation	Anywhere	Severe bleeding	Depends on location	Subcutaneous with nonabsorbable skin sutures	Bleeding, pain, infection, recurrence
Venous malformation	Anywhere	Decrease bulk of lesion; cosmetic	Depends on location	Subcutaneous with nonabsorbable skin sutures	Bleeding, pain, infection, recurrence
Dermoid cyst	Palpebral ridge of eye	Risk of infection; cosmetic	Transverse to accommodate removal	Subcutaneous with topical collodion or wound closure strips	Infection
Ganglion cyst	Dorsal or palmar surface of wrist, foot	Risk of infection; pain; interference with joint function	Transverse to accommodate removal	Subcutaneous with nonabsorbable skin sutures	Recurrence, infection

the external ear canal and are true fistulas (Soper & Pringle, 1986). In close proximity to these tracts are the facial nerve (cranial nerve VII) and the parotid gland, which increases the risk and difficulty of surgical excision. Lymphadenitis is the differential diagnosis with first branchial remnants. Complete surgical excision of first branchial remnants is indicated to prevent infection and should be performed in the absence of inflammation and infection. The operation requires general anesthesia, nerve stimulators and probes, and

adequate exposure of the facial nerve and parotid gland by means of a curved, vertical incision in front of the ear carried down to just below the jaw. A drain may be placed if fluid or pus is encountered during excision. Wound closure is performed in layers with absorbable sutures, and the skin closed subcutaneously. Topical collodion or wound closure strips may be applied. Mild paresis of the facial nerve frequently occurs and should resolve within 6 weeks of the procedure. Complications include persistent facial nerve paralysis, wound infection, or recurrence caused by incomplete excision (Soper & Pringle, 1986).

Second branchial cleft remnants present as sinus tracts during the first decade of life and as cysts during the second decade. A skin tag or ectopic cartilage (see Figure 11–2) is often present at the opening, and occasionally the tract may be palpated deep in the neck. The sinus or cyst is usually located on the lower third and anterior border of the sternocleidomastoid muscle. Differential diagnoses include cystic hygroma and lymphadenitis. Complete surgical excision is indicated for second branchial sinuses and cysts to prevent infection and should be performed in the absence of inflammation and infection. General anesthesia, good airway control, and slight hyperextension of the neck are required throughout the procedure. An external sinus is approached by means of an elliptical incision around the opening, preferably in a skin crease (see Figure 11–3); cysts are approached similarly and the incision is made around the cyst. If bilateral cysts are present, both may be removed during the same operation. A second (stepladder) incision may be required in an older child when the sinus is low on the sternocleidomastoid to facilitate complete removal of the tract. This allows adequate exposure of the carotid artery branches and the hypoglossal and glossopharyngeal nerves (cranial nerves XII and IX, respectively). Wound closure is done in layers, without a drain, and the skin is closed with subcutaneous sutures. Complications include infection, recurrence because of in-

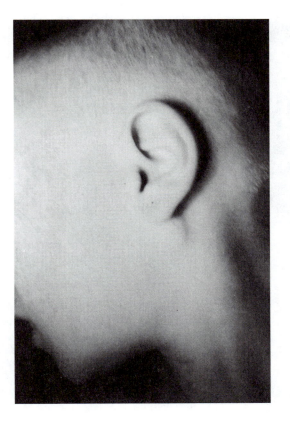

Figure 11–1 First Branchial Cleft Cyst Located below the Earlobe

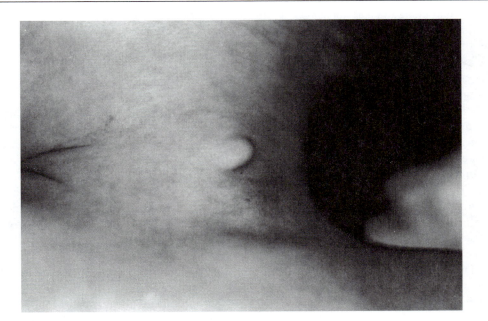

Figure 11–2 Second Branchial Cleft Remnant with Skin Tag Marking the Site of the Lesion

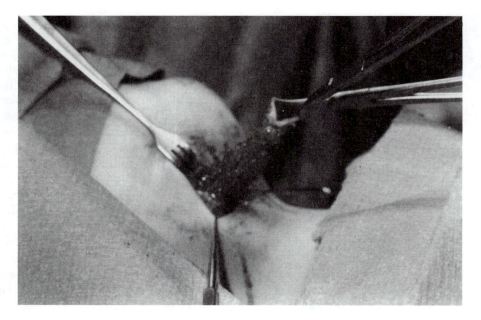

Figure 11–3 Excision of a Second Branchial Cyst and Sinus Tract

complete excision, bleeding, and damage to cranial nerves IX and XII (Friedberg, 1989; Roback & Telander, 1994; Soper & Pringle, 1986). First and second branchial sinuses and cysts are lined with stratified squamous epithelium and may contain skin appendages such as sweat glands, hair follicles, and sebaceous glands. Cartilage and muscle tissue have also been identified in the histologic study of these lesions (Bill & Vadheim, 1955).

Third branchial cleft remnants are rare and are often located near the thyroid and along the anterior border of the sternocleidomastoid muscle at the clavicular insertion. Differential diagnoses of third branchial cleft remnants include thymic cyst, cystic hygroma, and ectopic bronchogenic cyst. Fourth branchial cleft remnants are also rare and are located low in the neck similar to third cleft remnants (Soper & Pringle, 1986).

Infection and drainage are common presenting signs of branchial cleft remnants. Preoperative nursing care of children with branchial cleft cysts includes monitoring compliance of medical regimen and education related to hospital-specific ambulatory surgery procedures and process. Most children are discharged several hours after the procedure with the exception of those with respiratory or anesthesia complications. Nursing care includes instructions to the parent(s) about wound care, activity, pain control, bathing, diet, and complications. Discharge instructions for parents should include information about complications such as late stridor, dysphagia, and cranial nerve injury. Table 11–2 may be used as a guide for cranial nerve function assessment. Regular diet is resumed when the child is fully alert and able to swallow

liquids without aspiration. Normal activity is resumed on postoperative day (POD) 2, with instruction to avoid strenuous activity for 5 to 7 days and trauma to the operative area. Sponge bathing is recommended until POD 3. A follow-up visit is planned to assess wound healing, nerve damage, and any signs of recurrence. Topical antibiotic ointments and creams are not recommended for incision care, but oral antibiotics may be prescribed for several days for patients with a previous infection. Pain control is achieved with narcotic agents on POD 1 and 2 and nonnarcotic agents thereafter as needed. Collodion or wound closure strips applied to the incision are left to peel off spontaneously, usually by POD 5 to 7.

THYROGLOSSAL DUCT CYST

Development of the thyroid gland occurs between the third and tenth week of embryologic development, with the beginning marked by an endodermal thickening in the primitive pharynx. The thickening becomes a diverticulum at the posterior third of the tongue (foramen caecum) and then develops a bilobed shape as it projects downward on its tract. By the tenth week, the thyroid is in its normal adult position and the tract remains connected to the tongue, but the tract's channel obliterates. The tract is behind, in front of, or, rarely, through the hyoid bone. Persistence of the tract permits the accumulation of a colloidlike material secreted by the epithelial lining of the tract. A thyroglossal duct cyst is the result of this accumulation and usually appears between the second and tenth year of life (Skandalakis et al., 1994b; Solomon & Rangecroft, 1984). Distribution between sexes is equal, and

Table 11–2 Cranial Nerve Assessment Guidelines for Postoperative Care of the Child Undergoing Excision of a Cystic Lesion of the Head or Neck

Cranial Nerve	Name	Function	Assessment
5	Trigeminal	Motor—jaw movement Sensory—sensation on face	Clench teeth Sharp or dull pain sensation on face Hot or cold sensation on face Corneal reflex Infants <4 mo: rooting reflex
7	Facial	Motor—facial muscle movement Sensory—taste on anterior two thirds of tongue	Facial symmetry Raise eyebrows Frown Close eyes tight Show teeth Smile Puff out cheeks Infants: observe facial symmetry while crying
9	Glossopharyngeal	Motor—swallowing Sensory—sensation on tongue, pharynx, and eardrum; taste	Listen for hoarseness or speech changes Watch movement of uvula when patient says "ah" Gag reflex
10	Vagus	Motor—movement of palate, pharynx, larynx Sensory—sensation in pharynx and larynx	Same as for glossopharyngeal
12	Hypoglossal	Motor—tongue movement	Stick out tongue Look for asymmetry or deviation from midline Tongue strength Infants: pinch nostrils and look for baby to open mouth and raise the tip of the tongue

the cyst is seen as an asymptomatic midline neck mass over the hyoid bone (see Figure 11–4). Classically, the cyst is round and firm with no external opening and moves up with tongue thrust or swallowing. The cyst may be seen just lateral to the midline, usually to the left, and is rarely seen in the foramen caecum or suprasternally. Differential diagnoses include ectopic thyroid, thyroid nodule, cervical lymphadenopathy, hemangioma, lipoma, and midline dermoid cyst. Oral flora may infect the thyroglossal duct cyst through the thyroglossal duct, causing an eruption through the skin, erythema, and tenderness over the cyst (Solomon & Rangecroft, 1984; Soper & Pringle, 1986).

Surgical excision is indicated at diagnosis unless infection is present. The Sistrunk procedure (Sistrunk, 1928) involves excising the cyst and its tract upward to the base of the tongue, including dividing and removing part of the hyoid bone adjacent to the tract (see Figure 11–5). General anes-thesia, good airway control, and midline positioning of the head are required, and the cyst is approached through a transverse incision at or just above the cyst. The cyst and tract are dissected, and the tract is ligated at the foramen caecum. Wound closure is done in layers and the skin is closed subcutaneously. Collodion and/or wound closure strips are placed over the incision, and a drain is not necessary unless fluid or pus is encountered during excision (Soper & Pringle, 1986). Histologic examination reveals the cyst is usually lined with ciliated columnar respiratory epithelium or stratified squamous epithelium (Sade & Rosen, 1968). Complications include infection, recurrence as a result of incomplete excision, bleeding, and airway obstruction resulting from edema or bleeding. Perioperative nursing care of children with thyroglossal duct cysts is similar to that of children with bronchial cleft cysts. Uncomplicated excisions and postoperative courses permit discharging the child several hours after the

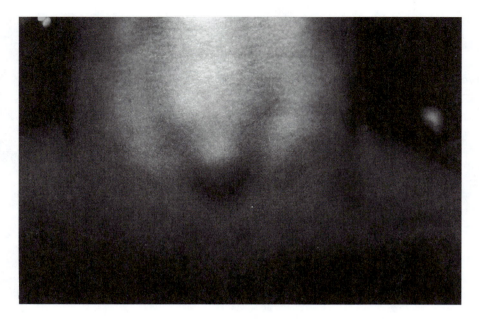

Figure 11–4 Thyroglossal Duct Cyst Presents as a Midline Mass over the Hyoid Bone

procedure. A 23-hour observance is indicated after excision of a thyroglossal duct cyst if any hint of airway problems is suspected or noted postoperatively or if a drain is in place.

LYMPHANGIOMA (CYSTIC HYGROMA)

Lymphangiomas are characterized by the presence of fluid-filled, endothelium-lined spaces derived from lymphatic vessels. Three types of lymphangiomas are described as: (1) simple—capillary-sized, thin-walled lymph channels, (2) cavernous—dilated lymph channels, and (3) cystic—cysts of varying sizes with thick fibrous walls. When the cystic type of lymphangioma is located in the primitive jugular lymph sac, it is called a cystic hygroma. Lymphatic tissue and fluid are unable to drain in normal channels and become sequestered in a loculated mass (Skandalakis, Gray, &

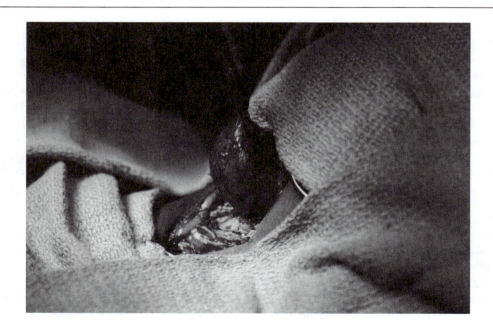

Figure 11–5 Excision of Thyroglossal Duct Cyst. The tract is excised up to the foramen caecum of the tongue.

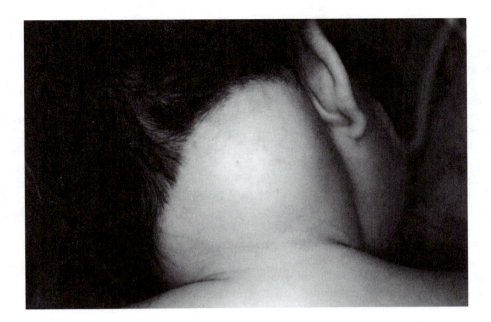

Figure 11–6 Cystic Hygroma in the Posterior Neck

Ricketts, 1994a). Although most cystic hygromas are located in the neck and axilla, some call cystic lymphangiomas anywhere on the body cystic hygromas (see Figures 11–6 and 11–7). Ninety percent of cystic hygromas are seen before 2 years of age. Diagnosis of fetal cystic hygroma by sonography before 30 weeks gestation is strongly associated with chromosome and structural anomalies that often result in fetal death. Chromosome anomalies include Turner's syn-

drome (45X) and Down syndrome (trisomy 21). Structural defects are cardiac, renal, neural tube, eye, skeletal, anorectal, or genital in origin (Chervenak et al., 1983; Langer et al., 1990).

Enlargement of the cystic hygroma progresses with the child's growth and is hastened by bacterial or viral infection. Spontaneous regression is rare; surgical excision offers the best hope of a cure. The common presentation is a soft, pain-

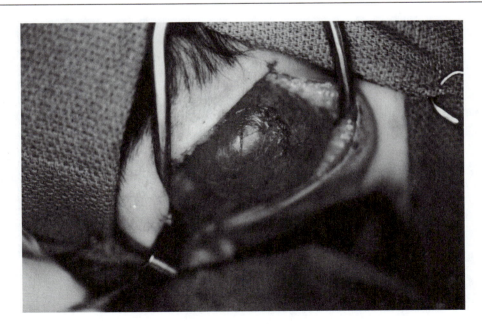

Figure 11–7 Operative View of Cystic Hygroma in Figure 11–6. The mass is clear and loculated.

less mass in the posterior triangle of the neck. The mass is loculated, fluctuant, not attached to skin, not movable on deep palpation, and transilluminates. Cystic hygromas are benign and have no symptoms of their own, but their growth may cause dysphagia and dyspnea because of airway obstruction. Extensive radiologic studies are not necessary to diagnose cystic hygroma because of its uniqueness; however, a computed tomographic scan is helpful in defining the boundaries of the lesion and its invasion of surrounding structures. Differential diagnoses include branchial cleft cyst, hemangioma, dermoid cyst, and lipoma (Filston, 1994; Ravitch & Rush, 1986).

Surgical excision is indicated at diagnosis unless inflammation or infection is present. The cystic hygroma is approached through a transverse cervical incision large enough to accommodate removal (see Figure 11–8). General anesthesia, good airway control, and positioning of the head away from the affected side are required for the procedure. Some lesions are excised simply, others require extensive dissection, and a few are unresectable. Sclerotherapy has been shown to aid with regression for cystic hygromas that are unresectable. Axillary hygromas are approached by means of incision in an axillary skin crease with the arm raised during the procedure. Mediastinal extension is approached from the cervical incision alone or by extending the incision down the anterior midline. Splitting the sternum may be necessary to remove the cyst wholly. A drain(s) is (are) placed to capture any residual lymph fluid or blood after extensive resection (Filston, 1994; Ravitch & Rush,

1986). Complications include recurrence requiring reoperation, injury to the mandibular branch of the facial nerve, lingual edema, bleeding, infection, and airway obstruction (Filston, 1994; Ninh & Ninh, 1974).

Nursing care of the child undergoing resection of a cystic hygroma includes airway management and monitoring, fluid balance, cranial nerve function assessment (see Table 11–2), pain control, and nutrition for wound healing. Supporting the family's adjustment to a potentially disfiguring lesion and/or scar on the child is important. Intensive care monitoring is required after an extensive resection, and nurses must inform the parent(s) of the presence of tubes, drains, lines, and equipment before visiting. The intensive care unit environment is frightening, and explanation of sights, sounds, and scenarios is imperative and indicated for managing parental anxiety and fear. Edema and bleeding are usually responsible for airway complications and require careful assessment and attention for the first 48 hours after surgery. The facial and hypoglossal cranial nerves (VII and XII, respectively) should be assessed for motor and sensory function (see Table 11–2). Pain control is initially achieved with narcotic agents that require monitoring oxygen saturation levels and cardiac and respiratory rates. Drains are removed when output is minimal. Wound closure is done in layers with subcutaneous skin closure. Activity is permitted as tolerated with attention to avoid trauma to the operative site. Shock, anger, guilt, fear, depression, rejection, and a sense of loss of a healthy infant are the most common emotions expressed by parents when the infant has a birth defect or requires major

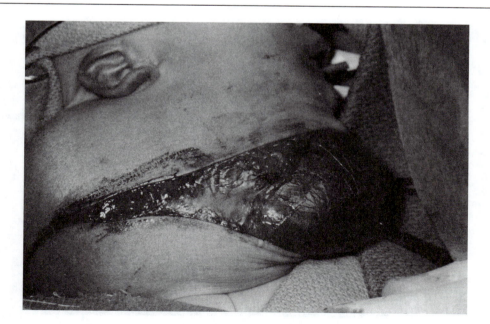

Figure 11–8 Large Cystic Hygroma of Posterior and Anterior Neck Delivered through a Large Transverse Incision

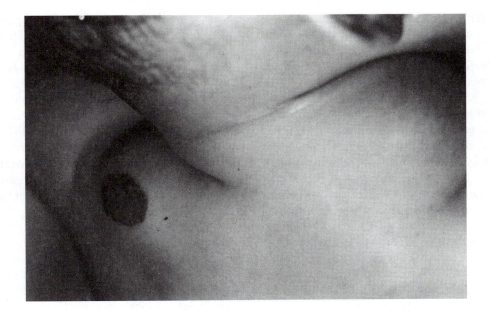

Figure 11–9 Hemangioma on the Shoulder of an Infant

surgery (Mercer, 1990). Nurses are in a position to support and validate the family's emotions while encouraging bonding and adaptation.

HEMANGIOMAS AND VASCULAR MALFORMATIONS

Hemangiomas and arteriovenous malformations (AVMs) are the most common head and neck masses in children. They are the result of faulty embryologic development of peripheral blood vessels. The process is described as unopposed angiogenesis. Hemangiomas appear in the first few weeks of life; are more common in females; and are seen as soft, compressible masses (see Figure 11–9). A bluish hue to the skin over the lesion is common. Hemangiomas progress through two phases: proliferation and involution. Proliferation is characterized by enlargement of the lesion during the first 6 to 8 months of life, followed by growth of the lesion commensurate with the child until the end of the first year. Involution takes place over several years and is characterized by shrinking and color changes from red to bluish purple. Most hemangiomas spontaneously and completely regress by 5 to 10 years of age without intervention. Lesions that threaten facial features or vital structures, or are extremely large, may be treated with steroids to hasten regression. Failure to respond to steroids is the rare indication to excise the lesion (Filston, 1994; Mulliken & Fishman, 1998). Aggressive reassurance and tincture of time are the primary modes of therapy for hemangiomas. The nurse's role is to support

and validate the parents' feelings and promote bonding and attachment to an infant with a disfiguring lesion.

AVMs are less common than hemangiomas and may be evident shortly after birth. These lesions are characterized by a patch of warm, purple skin, a palpable mass, and a bruit or thrill when superficial. Trauma and puberty contribute to enlargement of the malformation. Long term, these lesions produce ischemic skin changes, pain, and intermittent bleeding within the lesion. The most severe effects of AVM are congestive heart failure because of shunting of blood through the AVM and limb hypertrophy when they occur in an extremity. Excision is usually performed in late childhood or adolescence or if the lesion causes life-threatening bleeding, but complete surgical excision is seldom possible. Selective embolization is useful as the first line of palliative therapy during bleeding or painful episodes. Embolization to occlude the nidus is not recommended mainstay therapy because collateral vessels contribute to the reformation of the lesion; however, partially occluding the nidus before surgical excision minimizes bleeding during the procedure (Mulliken & Fishman, 1998).

Venous malformations usually appear as a blue patch anywhere on the body, superficially or deep. They may be local or extensive, nondescript or disfiguring, and grow with the child. Venous malformations are compressible, expand when dependent, and worsen during puberty. Compression garments are required conservative therapy to minimize dependent edema, venous congestion, sequestration of blood in the lesion, and pain. Sclerotherapy with 1% sodium tetradecyl sulfate (small lesions) or absolute ethanol (large lesions) is helpful before surgical resection, which is indicated to reduce the bulk of the lesion or for cosmetic reasons. Sclerotherapy is performed by an interventional radiologist. Venous malformations tend to recur (Mulliken & Fishman, 1998).

Capillary malformation (port wine stain) is a macular, vascular lesion that occurs on the face, trunk, or limbs. During adolescence, it produces skin darkening, soft tissue nodules, and hypertrophy. Capillary malformations in the limbs are associated with Klippel-Trenaunay and Parkes-Weber vascular anomaly syndromes. Klippel-Trenaunay syndrome features a vascular anomaly (usually capillary malformation, varicose veins, or hypoplastic or aplastic deep veins) and pronounced limb hypertrophy. Parkes-Weber syndrome features the same limb hypertrophy, but the vascular anomaly is an arteriovenous fistula. Problems encountered in both syndromes include joint pain, skin ulcerations, and the need for a prosthetic shoe or heel lift for the unaffected leg when the lower extremities are involved. Capillary malformations of the face are sometimes associated with Sturge-Weber sequence, which also features hemangiomata of eye structures and meninges, seizures, paresis, and mental deficiency (Jones, 1988). Flashlamp pulsed-dye laser is the treatment for capillary malformations, and 70% to 80% are significantly lightened with this therapy (Mulliken & Fishman, 1998).

Vascular anomalies are chronic and have an impact on the physical, emotional, and social aspects of the affected child's and family's life. Grotesque and disfiguring lesions affect the child's body image development, self-esteem, and sense of being different. Social isolation, rejection, and feelings of abandonment may dominate the child's behaviors as a result of ridicule and rejection from other children and adults. Limited mobility, pain, and risk for trauma interfere with physical activities for the child with a vascular malformation. The nursing role is largely supportive and should facilitate the child's adaptation to a chronic condition through validation of feelings and reinforcement of positive attributes. Parental bonding and acceptance of the child are crucial to providing a nurturing and supportive environment for the child (Mercer, 1990).

LYMPHADENOPATHY

Lymphadenopathy is enlargement of a lymph node(s), and lymphadenitis is a form of lymphadenopathy with additional symptoms of local pain, tenderness, and fever. Enlarged nodes are a common and normal finding during puberty, and cervical nodes up to 1 cm in diameter are normal in children less than 12 years of age. Nonspecific reactive cervical lymphadenopathy is self-limiting and usually the result of an upper respiratory viral infection or other systemic viral illnesses such as Epstein-Barr virus. Bacterial infections may also cause cervical lymphadenitis (see Figure 11–10). These infections typically respond to a course of antibiotics unless the nodes develop an abscess within them. Abscess requires incision and drainage for treatment. Granulomatous diseases

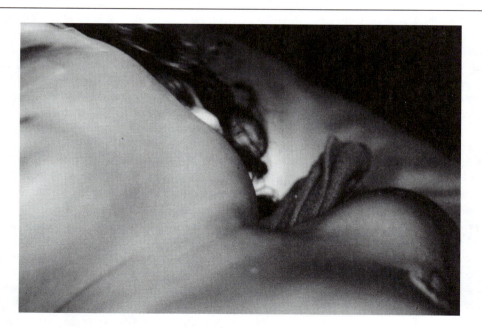

Figure 11–10 Cervical Lymphadenitis Caused by Bacterial Infection of the Node

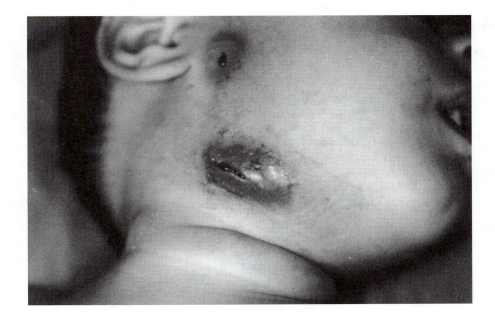

Figure 11–11 Spontaneous Drainage of Lymphadenitis Caused by Atypical Mycobacterium

produce chronic lymphadenopathy and may involve several nodes (see Figure 11–11) (Bodenstein & Altman, 1994; Friedberg, 1989).

Treatment of lymphadenopathy involves several approaches that are based on the history, chronicity, presentation, and differential diagnoses. A summary of common surgical lymphadenopathies is listed in Table 11–3 for brevity and is not intended as an exhaustive list of all lymphadenopathy seen in childhood. Suppurative lymphadenitis is usually benign, self-limiting, and a clinical finding or symptom of a systemic disease rather than a singular disease entity. Suppurative lymphadenopathy may be approached surgically by incision and drainage, whereas nonsuppurative lymphadenopathy requires excision, biopsy, or fine-needle aspiration when indicated. Surgical therapy is intended as diagnostic, curative, palliative, or any combination of these outcomes. The nursing role with surgical treatment of lymphadenitis is educational with regard to hospital-specific ambulatory surgery procedures and process. Instructions for wound care, bathing, activity, complications, and appropriate medical and surgical follow-up should be given before discharge. After incision and drainage, the wound often requires cleaning and packing the cavity on a daily or twice daily basis. Packing prevents early skin closure as the wound heals by secondary intention. The nurse explains the rationale and demonstrates the wound care regimen to the parent(s) and determines whether the parent(s) can safely perform the procedure. Bathing is permitted if the wound needs to be washed out. Clean excisions are closed primarily with subcutaneous skin closure and topical collodion and/or

wound closure strips. Normal activity is resumed with instruction to avoid strenuous activity for 5 to 7 days and trauma to the operative site. Medical follow-up for lymphadenitis includes compliance with the antibiotic regimen and referral or follow-up with the primary care physician or an infectious disease specialist. Surgical follow-up allows assessment of wound healing and assessment for complications.

DERMOID CYST

Dermoids are a type of sebaceous cyst that contain ectodermal elements such as sebaceous glands, hair follicles, and connective tissue. They are most commonly located along the supraorbital palpebral ridge, attached to the bony fascia, are movable, and nontender (see Figure 11–12). Epidermoid cysts have a similar presentation and differ only by their contents, which is sebaceous without skin appendages. Dermoids and epidermoids in the midline of the skull are studied on plain films for penetration to the epidural space; no other diagnostic studies are indicated for dermoids. If the cyst penetrates to the epidural space, a computed tomographic scan and neurosurgery consult are appropriate management. Differential diagnoses include lipoma, lymphangioma, thyroglossal duct cyst, and pilomatrixoma. Calcified epithelioma of Malherbe (pilomatrixoma) is a hamartoma of hair follicle origin and a common type of sebaceous cyst. Pilomatrixoma may occur anywhere except the palms and soles (no hair follicles). Indications for surgical excision are

Table 11–3 Summary of Surgical Indications and Approaches to Lymphadenitis

Classification of Node Inflammation	Most Common Causative Agent[a]	Medical Management[a]	Indications for Surgery[b]	Surgical Approach[b]	Surgical Outcomes[b]
Reactive lymphadenopathy	Upper respiratory viral infection Epstein-Barr virus Kawasaki disease	Observation	None	None	None
Bacterial lymphadenitis	Staphylococcus Streptococcus Hemophilus influenza	Penicillin Cephalosporin	Fluctuance Induration	Incision and drainage	Diagnostic and curative
Fungal lymphadenitis (usually in immuno-compromised patient)	Candida albicans	Amphotericin B	Fluctuance Induration Surgery may be deferred until medical therapy terminated	Incision and drainage	Diagnostic and palliative
Granulomatous infection: Tuberculous lymphadenitis	Mycobacterium tuberculosis	Isoniazid Rifampin Pyrazinamide	Chronicity Diagnosis	Fine-needle aspirate Excisional biopsy	Diagnostic and palliative
Granulomatous infection: Atypical mycobacterium	Mycobacterium scrofulaceum Mycobacterium avium Mycobacterium kansasii	Rifampin Clarithromycin Antituberculosis drugs	Draining tracts with skin involvement	Excision	Diagnostic and curative
Granulomatous infection: Cat scratch disease	Bartonella henselae	Observation	Discomfort because of size	Aspiration	Palliative
Toxoplasmosis	Toxoplasma gondii	Pyrimethamine Sulfadiazine	Diagnosis	Excisional biopsy	Diagnostic

[a] American Academy of Pediatrics, 1997. [b] Bodenstein & Altman, 1994.

cosmetic and risk for infection. Dermoids and other sebaceous cysts are benign and cured with surgical excision (Guarisco, 1991; Knight & Reiner, 1983).

The nursing role is educational with regard to hospital-specific ambulatory surgery procedures and process. Instructions about incision care, bathing, activity, complications, and follow-up are given. Excision of a sebaceous cyst is often perceived by surgical nurses as trivial; however, it is important to approach the family with sincerity and allay their anxiety about the surgical procedure. The incision is closed subcutaneously and covered topically with collodion and/or wound closure strips. Bathing is permitted on POD 1 but soaking the incision should be avoided. Normal activity is resumed with instruction to avoid trauma to the operative site. Regular diet is resumed when the child is fully alert and able to tolerate liquids without aspiration. Pain control is achieved with nonnarcotic agents.

GANGLION CYST

Ganglion cysts originate from the capsule of a joint or from a tendon sheath. They most commonly are seen on the dorsal surface of the wrist, occasionally on the palmar surface of the wrist, and rarely on the foot. Most ganglions are 1 to 2 cm in diameter, round, slightly tender, and may interfere

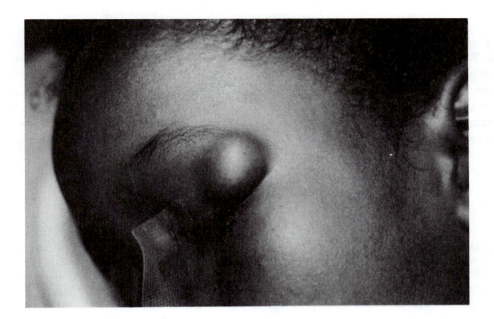

Figure 11–12 Dermoid Cyst on the Palpebral Ridge of the Eye

with function of the wrist or foot (see Figure 11–13). They contain a thick, clear fluid that may be aspirated or injected with steroids as means of treatment. Surgical excision is the best method of treatment and one that offers the lowest rate of recurrence (Smith & Yandow, 1996). The oldest method for treating a ganglion cyst is to hit it with the family Bible; this bursts the cyst, permitting the capsule to scar. Aspiration, injection, and traumatic methods of treatment have a significant recurrence rate.

The nursing role is educational with regard to hospital-specific ambulatory surgery procedures and process. Instructions about incision care, bathing, activity, complications, and follow-up are given. The affected wrist is immobilized in a soft splint for 7 to 10 days postoperatively. The family is

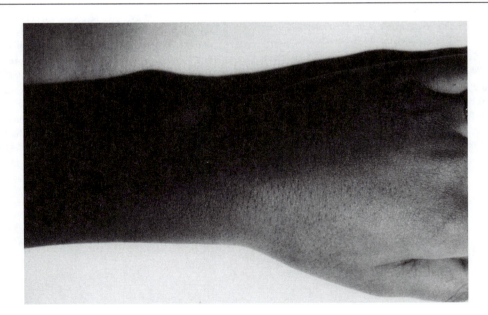

Figure 11–13 Ganglion Cyst on the Dorsal Surface of the Wrist

instructed on removal and replacement of the splint for bathing. Bathing is permitted on POD 2 but soaking the incision should be avoided. The skin is closed with subcutaneous sutures. Normal activity is resumed with instruction to avoid trauma to the operative site. Regular diet is resumed when the child is fully alert and able to tolerate liquids without aspiration. Pain control is achieved with narcotic agents on POD 1 and 2 and nonnarcotic agents thereafter as needed.

CONCLUSION

A simple and straightforward surgical approach is curative for most of the common cysts of childhood. These cases are often clean, straightforward, and carry a low risk and incidence of complications and problems. The safety and efficacy of pediatric anesthesia has also contributed to minimal hospital stays and low complication rates after cyst removal.

REFERENCES

American Academy of Pediatrics. (1997). *1997 Red Book: Report of the Committee on Infectious Diseases* (24th ed.). Elk Grove Village, IL: American Academy of Pediatrics.

Bates, B.M. (1983). *A guide to physical examination* (3rd ed., pp. 370–427). Philadelphia: Lippincott.

Bill, A.H., & Vadheim, J.L. (1955). Cysts, sinuses and fistulas of the neck arising from the first and second branchial clefts. *Annals of Surgery, 142*, 904–908.

Bodenstein, L., & Altman, R.P. (1994). Cervical lymphadenitis in infants and children. *Journal of Pediatric Surgery, 3* (3), 134–141.

Chervenak, F.A., Isaacson, G., Blakemore, K.J., Breg, W.R., Hobbins, J.C., Berkowitz, R.L., Tortura, M., Mayden, K., & Mahoney, M.J. (1983). Fetal cystic hygroma: Cause and natural history. *The New England Journal of Medicine, 309*(14), 822–825.

Filston, H.C. (1994). Hemangiomas, cystic hygromas, and teratomas of the head and neck. *Journal of Pediatric Surgery, 3*(3), 147–159.

Friedberg, J. (1989). Pharyngeal cleft sinuses and cysts, and other benign neck lesions. *Pediatric Clinics of North America, 36*(6), 1451–1469.

Guarisco, J.L. (1991). Congenital head and neck masses in infants and children. *Ear, Nose, and Throat Journal, 70*(2), 75–82.

Jones, K.L. (Ed.). (1988). *Smith's recognizable patterns of human malformations* (4th ed., pp. 456–457). Philadelphia: W.B. Saunders Company.

Knight, P.J., & Reiner, C.B. (1983). Superficial lumps in children: What, when, and why? *Pediatrics, 72*(2), 147–153.

Langer, J.C., Fitzgerald, P.G., Desa, D., Filly, R.A., Golbus, M.S., Adzick, N.S., & Harrison, M.R. (1990). Cervical cystic hygroma in the fetus: Clinical spectrum and outcome. *Journal of Pediatric Surgery, 25*(1), 58–62.

Mercer, R.T. (1990). *Parents at risk* (pp. 169–195). New York: Springer Publishing Co.

Mulliken, J.B., & Fishman, S.J. (1998). Vascular anomalies: Hemangiomas and malformations. In J.A. O'Neill, M.I. Rowe, J.L. Grosfeld, E.W. Folkalsrud, & A.G. Coran (Eds.), *Pediatric surgery* (5th ed., Vol. 2, pp. 1939–1952). St. Louis, MO: Mosby.

Ninh, T.N., & Ninh, T.X. (1974). Cystic hygroma in children: A report of 126 cases. *Journal of Pediatric Surgery, 9*(2), 191–195.

Ravitch, M.M., & Rush, B.F. (1986). Cystic hygroma. In K.J. Welch, J.G. Randolph, M.M. Ravitch, J.A. O'Neill, & M.I. Rowe (Eds.), *Pediatric surgery* (4th ed., Vol. 1, pp. 533–539). Chicago: Year Book Medical Publishers.

Roback, S.A., & Telander, R.L. (1994). Thyroglossal duct cysts and branchial cleft anomalies. *Journal of Pediatric Surgery, 3*(3), 142–146.

Sade, J., & Rosen, G. (1968). Thyroglossal cysts and tracts: A histological and histochemical study. *Annals of Otology, Rhinology, and Laryngology, 77*, 139–145.

Sistrunk, W.E. (1928). Technique of removal of cysts and sinuses of the thyroglossal duct. *Surgery, Gynecology and Obstetrics, 46*, 109–112.

Skandalakis, J.E., Gray, S.W., & Ricketts, R.R. (1994a). The lymphatic system. In J.E. Skandalakis & S.W. Gray (Eds.), *Embryology for surgeons*, (2nd ed., pp. 877–897). Baltimore: Williams and Wilkins.

Skandalakis, J.E., Gray, S.W., & Todd, N.W. (1994b). The pharynx and its derivatives. In J.E. Skandalakis & S.W. Gray (Eds.), *Embryology for surgeons* (2nd ed., pp. 17–64). Baltimore: Williams and Wilkins.

Smith, J.T., & Yandow, S.M. (1996). Benign soft-tissue lesions in children. *Orthopedics Clinics of North America, 27*(3), 645–654.

Solomon, J.R., & Rangecroft, L. (1984). Thyroglossal-duct lesions in childhood. *Journal of Pediatric Surgery, 19*(5), 555–561.

Soper, R.T., & Pringle, K.C. (1986). Cysts and sinuses of the neck. In K.J. Welch, J.G. Randolph, M.M. Ravitch, J.A. O'Neill, & M.I. Rowe (Eds.), *Pediatric surgery* (4th ed., Vol. 1, pp. 539–552). Chicago: Year Book Medical Publishers.

Appendix 11–A

Critical Pathway for Removal of Common Cysts

	Preoperative	Operative	Initial Postoperative (<8 hr)	Late Postoperative (>8 hr)
Nursing intervention	Vital signs Last oral intake History and physical History of recent illness Allergies Laboratory tests Child understands procedure and fears addressed	Appropriate site prepped Venous access obtained OR documentation	Vital signs per PARU routine Observe airway, breathing, circulation, temperature Wound assessment Pain assessment Patient safety Prepare for discharge	Discharge Make follow-up appointment Follow-up phone call Admit if necessary School and P.E. notes
Physician intervention	Surgical consent History and physical Anesthesia consult	Operative procedure performed Anesthesia maintained	Findings reported to parent Notes dictated Postoperative orders and prescriptions written and signed Recovery from anesthesia	Check pathologic findings
Medication	Topical anesthetic to potential IV site(s) Preoperative sedation	Antibiotics if indicated Incisional anesthesia	Narcotic pain management Miscellaneous IV medications	Oral pain medication Oral antibiotics if indicated
Nutrition	NPO 8 hr for solids NPO 6 hr for milk and formula NPO 4 hr for clear liquids	NPO IV fluids	NPO IV fluids Initiate clear liquids when fully alert and able to swallow D/C IV when tolerating oral fluids Advance diet when liquids tolerated	Diet as tolerated
Activity	Ad lib	Anesthetized	As tolerated	As tolerated Avoid trauma to operative area Activity restrictions
Wound care	N/A	Wound closure methods	Observation for bleeding and/or drainage Secure dressing and/or drains	Dressing changes Wound protection

continues

Appendix 11–A continued

	Preoperative	Operative	Initial Postoperative (<8 hr)	Late Postoperative (>8 hr)
Family education	Hospital routine (policy, procedure) Hospital environment (parking, restrooms, food service) Location of waiting room When/where to see child after procedure Importance of NPO orders Indication(s) for operation	Expected length of procedure	Wound care Drain care Activity Bathing Pain management Complications Who and when to call for problems or questions Admit if necessary for observation	Prevention of complications Drug indications, dosing, and side effects Child and family understand restrictions
Expected outcomes	Family present and supportive Family understands need for procedure Child is comfortable, secure, and safe Timely and effective premedication Preoperative health acceptable Child ready for OR on time	Procedure completed Minimal blood loss Proceed to PARU	Parent resumes caregiving Child awake and able to breathe on own Safe and comfortable recovery from anesthesia	Parent able to care for child No complications Tolerating diet Child is comfortable

CHAPTER 12

Tracheostomy

Beverly B. Kelleher

A tracheostomy is a surgical procedure that places a direct opening into the airway below the vocal cords between the second and the fourth tracheal rings (Figure 12–1). A transverse incision is made into the skin, and tissue is dissected downward to the strap muscle. The strap muscle and anterior jugular veins are retracted laterally. A vertical incision is made into the trachea without removing cartilage. Two nonabsorbable stay sutures are placed lateral to the incision to prevent potential loss of the airway should the new tracheostomy tube fall out before a tract has formed (Myers, Stool, & Johnson, 1985).

This surgical procedure was first reported in the second century BC as a method of dealing with acute airway obstruction often caused by infection (Wetmore, 1996). Today, the indications for tracheostomy have been expanded to include a need for improved pulmonary toilet and for prolonged assisted mechanical ventilation (Exhibit 12–1). Improvement in airway management has occurred because of more frequent use of orotracheal or nasotracheal tubes. Fewer tracheostomies are performed today for airway obstruction resulting from acute infection such as epiglottitis or laryngotracheobronchitis. However, for the child with a tracheostomy today, it is more likely that the tracheostomy is placed for airway pathology or prolonged ventilatory support, and the tracheostomy remains in place for a longer period (Arcand & Granger, 1988). This chapter reviews the pre- and postsurgical course for a child undergoing a tracheostomy. Information about suctioning, maintenance, emergency care, and decannulation is included, and a critical pathway is provided in Appendix 12–A.

The child's upper respiratory tract is unique (Figure 12–2). Although it is like the adult airway in that inspired air is warmed, filtered, and humidified as it passes through the nasopharynx, the pediatric airway is smaller and lymphoid tissue in the nasopharynx (adenoids) and oropharynx (tonsils) is often enlarged. The larynx is funnel shaped, positioned higher and more anterior in the pharynx, and the cartilaginous structures are soft and compressible during the first

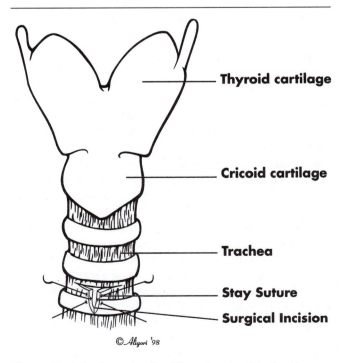

© Aligori '98

Figure 12–1 Tracheostomy Is a Direct Opening into the Airway

Acknowledgments: I thank Thomas R. Weber, MD, Professor and Director, Department of Surgery, Division of Pediatric Surgery, St. Louis University School of Medicine; Gary M. Albers, MD, Assistant Professor, Department of Pediatrics, St. Louis University School of Medicine; and Mary K. Braskin, MSW, and Debbie Kienstra, RN, Cardinal Glennon Children's Hospital, St. Louis, Missouri.

Exhibit 12–1 Indications for Tracheostomy

Airway Obstruction	*Pulmonary Toilet*	*Prolonged Mechanical Ventilation*
Congenital/acquired stenosis	Coma	Spinal cord injury
Vocal cord paralysis	Aspiration	Neuromuscular disease
Trauma	Neuromuscular disease	Bronchopulmonary dysplasia
Airway lesion		
Toxic ingestion		
Laryngomalacia		
Tracheomalacia		
Craniofacial conditions		
Infection		
Obstructive sleep apnea		
Foreign body		
Neoplastic lesions		

year of life. For the child less than 10 years of age, the narrowest part of the airway is at the cricoid cartilage (Chameides & Hazinski, 1997). These differences in the pediatric airway have significant consequences. The smaller airway diameter results in an increased resistance to flow and increased work of breathing. The soft, floppy nature of the larynx results in airway obstruction in some children manifested as laryngomalacia with noisy inspiratory sounds. For the infant requiring intubation, there is an increased risk for placing an endotracheal tube that is too large into the compressible airway. Tight-fitting endotracheal tubes cause damage to surrounding tissues, particularly at the level of the cricoid cartilage, which can lead to stenosis (Jursich & Kennelly, 1987). This results in airway compromise and in some cases requires surgical correction. As the child grows, airway size and support structures change. Lymphoid tissue shrinks, laryngeal position lowers, cartilaginous structures are strengthened, and airway caliber increases.

PREOPERATIVE PREPARATION

The child's age and level of development determine the approach to preoperative preparation. At each stage in development, certain tasks must be accomplished physically, cognitively, and emotionally to move on to the next phase. The child's reaction to the stress of illness and hospitalization is determined by the child's past experiences (Gohsman, 1981). Collaboration with a child life specialist is helpful in developing and implementing a plan for preparing a child for a tracheostomy.

Parent or primary caregivers should be involved at teaching sessions. Caregivers should be provided with written materials to review at their own pace and to serve as a useful resource. A tracheostomy tube like the one the child will receive should be shown to the child and primary caregiver and kept at the bedside for future reference. A teaching checklist should be initiated preoperatively and maintained until the day of discharge (Exhibit 12–2).

Parents should be told to anticipate a stay in the pediatric intensive care unit or a transitional care unit during the im-

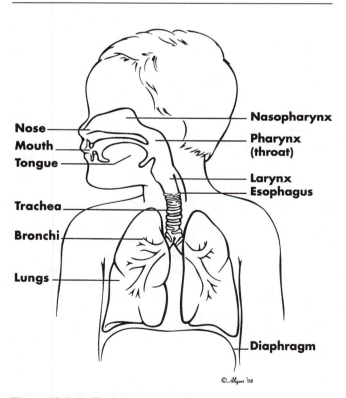

Figure 12–2 Pediatric Respiratory Tract

mediate postoperative period. Many patients with airway management issues may already be in this setting. If this is not the case, arrange a tour of the unit before surgery to familiarize the child/family with a critical care setting, review visiting regulations, and become acquainted with the staff.

OPERATIVE CONSIDERATIONS AND POSTOPERATIVE CARE

Although placement of a tracheostomy is beneficial and sometimes a lifesaving measure, it has a significant associ-

---

Exhibit 12–2 Tracheostomy Discharge Checklist

1. Patient Name _____
2. Tentative discharge date _____   3. Home health agency referral _____
   Name of agency _____
   Phone number of agency _____
4. Caregivers at home _____
5. Trach booklet given to _____
6. Skills to be taught:

Skill	Observed	Performed	Approved
Trach care	Nurse _____ Learner _____ Date	Nurse _____ Learner _____ Date	Nurse _____ Learner _____ Date
Suctioning	Nurse _____ Learner _____ Date	Nurse _____ Learner _____ Date	Nurse _____ Learner _____ Date
Change ties	Nurse _____ Learner _____ Date	Nurse _____ Learner _____ Date	Nurse _____ Learner _____ Date
Change tube	Nurse _____ Learner _____ Date	Nurse _____ Learner _____ Date	Nurse _____ Learner _____ Date
CPR	Nurse _____ Learner _____ Date	Nurse _____ Learner _____ Date	Nurse _____ Learner _____ Date
Other skills	Nurse _____ Learner _____ Date	Nurse _____ Learner _____ Date	Nurse _____ Learner _____ Date

7. Emergency kit
   a. Duplicate trach tube____   e. 250 ml bottle saline ____
   b. Suction catheters (2) ____   f. 2 oz. bulb suction with catheter taped in ____
   c. Box of kleenex ____   g. disposable suture removal set ____
   d. 3cc syringes (no needle) ____
8. Equipment ordered:
   suction machine ____   suction catheters ____
   oxygen (if needed) ____   humidity set-up with trach collar ____
   ambu bag ____   other _____
9. Local M.D. notified of discharge ____   Home health agency notified of discharge ____

ated risk of morbidity in children, particularly in the very young (Arcand & Granger, 1988; Donnelly, Lacey, & Maguire, 1996). Other options for airway management are considered before proceeding with a tracheostomy. Intraoperative complications associated with tracheostomy include cardiac arrhythmias or arrest, hemorrhage, pneumothorax, pneumomediastinum, subcutaneous emphysema, injury to adjacent structures, pulmonary edema, respiratory arrest, mechanical problems with the tracheostomy tube, and death (Wetmore, 1996). Possible postoperative complications include hemorrhage, pneumothorax, pneumopericardium, mediastinal emphysema, subcutaneous emphysema, tracheal lesions, tracheostomy tube problems including obstruction or accidental decannulation, infection, deglutition difficulty, stomal problems, aphonia, delay in decannulation, and death (Wetmore, 1996).

The immediate postoperative period is spent in a pediatric intensive care or transitional care unit to facilitate monitoring. Vital signs and a head-to-toe systems assessment are obtained every 1 to 2 hours for the first 24 to 48 hours. The respiratory effort, specifically, respiratory rate, the presence or absence of retractions, nasal flaring, the quality and intensity of breath sounds, and the patient's ability to cough and clear the airway are carefully evaluated (Lothschuetz Montgomery, 1996). Frequent suctioning is necessary initially because of increased secretions. The increased secretions found in the immediate postoperative period are due to the foreign body (tracheostomy tube) in the airway. Cardiac and respiratory monitors and continuous pulse oximetry to assess oxygen saturation should be used during the immediate postoperative period and thereafter whenever the patient sleeps or is not in direct view of caregivers. A constant source of warm, humidified air must be applied with oxygen supplementation as needed.

The stomal area should be inspected frequently for signs of bleeding, drainage, or crepitus. Crepitus is the coarse, crackling sensation that can be felt near the stomal opening. It results from air that escapes from the lungs into subcutaneous tissue. Tracheostomy tube ties must be secured. Stay sutures should be taped to the chest. After 24 to 48 hours, the child can usually be transferred to a less acute inpatient unit, and while close monitoring continues, a greater effort is made to prepare the child and family for discharge.

CARE OF THE CHILD WITH A TRACHEOSTOMY

Maintenance of the new artificial airway involves interventions related to the following areas: humidity, suctioning, stoma care, tracheostomy tube care, and emergency care (Storgion, 1996). In addition, special attention is given to speech and to other activities of daily living such as playing, feeding, and bathing.

Humidity

The normal functions of the airway to heat, humidify, and filter inspired air are bypassed by a tracheostomy. Because mucociliary clearance of the airway declines without adequate humidification (Davis, 1998; Motoyama, 1985), heat and humidity must be provided either directly through a ventilator circuit, a tracheostomy collar, or in some other effective fashion. A heat and moisture exchanger (HME) is a device that directly attaches to the 15-mm tracheostomy adapter (Burstein, 1995) (Figure 12–3). It serves to a limited degree to trap heat and moisture and to filter inspired air. Using the HME increases patient mobility because for short periods of time the child is not connected to a stationary humidity source such as a high-humidity tracheostomy collar. However, over a prolonged period it will not maintain enough humidity to promote adequate airway clearance and should not be substituted on a permanent basis for a direct humidity source. The HME is removed from the tracheostomy before the application of direct humidity. At a minimum, a direct humidity source should be used during naps and at night while the child is sleeping.

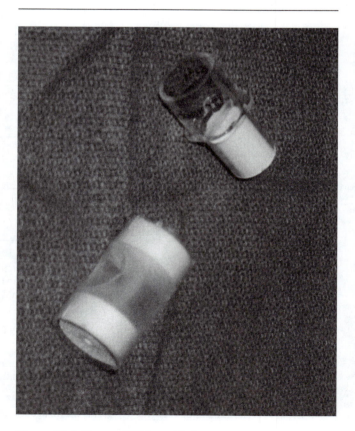

Figure 12–3 Heat and Moisture Exchanger

Suctioning

Normal mucociliary clearance moves secretions to the tracheostomy tube. The purpose of routine suctioning is to remove accumulated secretions from within the tracheostomy tube or at the distal opening, not from deep within the lungs. Shallow suctioning should be performed with a bulb syringe or some other similar device to remove secretions that have been brought up to the top of the tracheostomy tube by coughing. If suctioning is required to remove secretions from the tube, a depth-limited or premeasured technique must be used to avoid trauma to the delicate tracheal mucosa (Hodge, 1991; Kleiber, Krutzfield, & Rose, 1988; Warnock & Porpora, 1994).

With a depth-limited suctioning technique, the depth that the suction catheter is inserted is equal to the length of the tracheostomy tube (as published by the manufacturer) plus 1.5 cm to account for the tracheostomy tube adapter and 0.5 cm for clearance of the artificial airway (Figure 12–4). On determining the depth limit, a sign or card is posted at the patient's bedside indicating the length to be used as a guide by all caregivers for suctioning (Figure 12–5). If calibrated suction catheters are not available, the catheter is measured against the predetermined length indicated on the ruler using the thumb and forefinger as the marker while maintaining cleanliness (Warnock & Porpora, 1994).

Only under unusual circumstances is suctioning beyond the distal end of the tracheostomy tube required. For instance, the child with a weak cough related to an underlying neuromuscular disease might require a deep suctioning technique to clear airway secretions. In this situation, the catheter

DO NOT INSERT SUCTION CATHETER PAST _____ cm

Figure 12–5 Guide for Suction Catheter Measurement

is gently inserted until resistance is met and then is withdrawn 0.5 cm. Suction is applied until the catheter is fully removed from the tracheostomy tube. The decision to use deep suctioning on a routine basis is made after discussion with the managing physician because of the risk of tracheal mucosa trauma, which could result in decreased mucociliary function and the development of tracheal granulomas.

In general, the largest catheter that fits easily should be used for suctioning. The catheter is gently rolled between the thumb and finger. Suctioning is rapid, not exceeding 4 to 5 seconds. Suction vacuum pressures vary from 60 to 80 mm Hg for the neonate to 80 to 100 mm Hg for the older pediatric patient (Pettignano & Pettignano, 1995). Higher suction pressures may lead to excessive trauma. While the child is hospitalized, sterile suctioning is usually used to decrease the incidence of nosocomial infection. However, at home the risk of exposure to pathogens is less than that in the hospital setting and the technique is usually clean. Parents or caregivers need to be aware of this practice variation, particularly as the patient is prepared for discharge. No research exists describing the best solution for cleaning reusable supplies and equipment. In many situations, cleaning a suction catheter for reuse at home involves rinsing through with water or normal saline and reusing if it appears clear. Further research is needed in this area. Good hand washing is emphasized as the best defense against the spread of infection.

Frequency of suctioning depends on many factors, such as effectiveness of patient cough, thickness and volume of secretions, old versus new tracheostomy, presence of a respiratory tract infection, age, level of humidity, level of activity, and underlying diagnosis. Most children require routine suctioning on awakening in the morning and after a nap, after a nebulizer treatment, before a meal, when not feeling well, with increased activity, and after a mucus plug is removed. Parents and caregivers should be taught to assess the need for suctioning on the basis of physical findings. Excessive suctioning can cause unnecessary trauma to the airway, result-

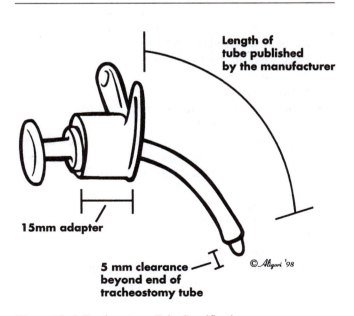

Figure 12–4 Tracheostomy Tube Specifications

ing in an increase in mucus production and a vicious cycle of suctioning (Kleiber et al., 1988; Warnock & Porpora, 1994).

Other aspects of suctioning technique that must be addressed on an individual basis include the need for increased respiratory support before and after suctioning. The mechanically ventilated or severely debilitated child may not be able to tolerate suctioning as well as others. Therefore, hyperoxygenation, hyperventilation, or hyperinflation before and after suctioning is indicated to make the procedure as safe and benign as possible (Hodge, 1991).

Controversy exists around routine use of isotonic saline lavage before suctioning because of the potential harmful effects of saline lavage, such as oxygen desaturation, poor mixing with mucus, and contamination (Davis, 1998). Saline lavage should be used judiciously (Fitton, 1994). Saline lavage is indicated for the evacuation of thick, tenacious secretions.

Stoma Care

The skin surface surrounding the stoma should be inspected and cleaned at least twice a day.

- Cleanse the skin surface with cotton-tipped applicators and an appropriate solution. Initially a normal saline solution is recommended. When the wound is healed, a mild soap and water cleansing is adequate. If crusted secretions accumulate around the site, diluted hydrogen peroxide solution is helpful in their removal. When cleaning, start close to the stoma and work outward until all surfaces are thoroughly clean.
- Pat dry or allow to air dry.
- Inspect the skin surfaces for any sign of irritation from moisture or pressure from the tube flange.
- A dressing is not always required. Dressings may hide trapped secretions, which lead to irritation or maceration of surrounding tissue. However, if desired, an absorbent presplit gauze dressing may be used to provide patient comfort.
- Occasionally, a hydrocolloid dressing such as Duoderm may be helpful in relieving flange pressure, allowing skin surfaces to heal (Bressler, Coladipietro, & Holinger, 1997).

Antibacterial ointments are not routinely applied at the site but are used as indicated for evidence of local skin infection.

Tracheostomy Tube Care: Selecting the Proper Tube, Changing the Tube and Ties

There are many types of tracheostomy tubes. The tracheostomy tube selected for each patient is chosen to best meet that individual child's airway needs and neck anatomy. Three different materials are used for tracheostomy tubes: polyvinyl chloride (PVC), silicone, and metal. Metal tubes do not conform to the shape of the child's airway and are rarely used in the pediatric setting. PVC and silicone tubes are more desirable because they cause minimal tissue reaction, are more flexible, conform to the child's airway without causing pressure, and are more comfortable (Davis, 1998; Wetmore, 1996).

To provide the best fit within the airway without causing pressure to delicate tracheal mucosa, a variety of standard tube sizes are available in different lengths and diameters. Proper tube length positions the distal portion of the tube at 1 to 2 cm above the carina. Customized tubes are also available to meet a child's unique needs. Customized tubes may be ordered from the Shiley or Bivona companies.

Tubes are cuffed or uncuffed. Cuffed tubes are usually not required for the pediatric patient unless the child is being mechanically ventilated or is at risk for aspiration. In most cases, uncuffed tubes provide an adequate airway while allowing phonation. Tubes with removable inner cannulas are infrequently used with pediatric patients.

The first tube change is generally performed by the surgeon on the fifth to seventh postoperative day. This time period may vary, but the purpose for this delay in changing the tube is to allow a tract to form and avoid the creation of a false passage. At the time of the first tube change, the stay sutures are removed. The nursing staff or capable primary caregivers perform subsequent changes on a 1-week to 2-week basis. Although tube changes at a 1-week to 2-week interval seem to be common practice no evidence in the literature supports a standard interval for routine tube change. Routine tracheostomy tube change should be performed in a controlled, calm environment and always with an assistant.

- Assemble all supplies: new tracheostomy tube (and available at the bedside a tracheostomy tube one size smaller), ties, lubricant (a water-soluble gel lubricant or sterile isotonic saline), and scissors.
- Place the child in a supine position with a small roll beneath the shoulders.
- Suction if needed.
- Maintaining sterility, remove new tube from packaging.
- Insert the obturator.
- Thread the ties through one side of the tracheostomy tube wing (cutting the edge of the tie at an angle will ease insertion through the flange opening).
- Apply lubricant and hold the tube with the curve pointing downward.
- Assistant cuts/removes old ties and withdraws the old tube.
- While applying gentle traction to the skin below or on either side of the opening, insert the tube (if child is coughing, wait until cough subsides).
- If some resistance is met, withdraw the tube 3 inches and try to ease the tube in, turning it slightly from side to side.

- When the tube is in place, remove the obturator immediately (keep the obturator at the bedside in a clean container for future use if needed).
- Hold the new tube in place while the assistant secures the ties.
- To secure the ties thread the tie through the other side of the tube wing (use a forceps to grasp the tie if necessary), pull strings to the back, and tie securely so that only one small finger will fit underneath the ties.
- Continue to monitor the child closely immediately after the change to ensure that the procedure was well tolerated.
- Suctioning may be required immediately after the change.
- Auscultate lung sounds ("Home care: Child with a tracheostomy," 1995).

Tracheostomy tube ties are changed on a daily basis or more frequently if they become soiled. A variety of tracheostomy tie materials are available. Twill tape works well and is inexpensive. Each tie is used once and discarded. From time to time the skin surface at the back or side of the neck may become irritated under the twill tape ties. Keeping the skin clean and dry is the best defense against potential breakdown. Moleskin applied to the portion of the twill tape that encircles the neck provides comfort and protection (Figure 12–6).

Velcro ties may also be used and reused as long as they remain clean and functional. They must be used with caution with the younger child who might unfasten the ties and cause accidental decannulation. The most important aspects in terms of selecting tracheostomy ties are that they are secure and comfortable for the child.

Emergency Care: Tube Obstruction, Accidental Decannulation, and Cardiopulmonary Resuscitation

Even with the most meticulous care unexpected situations may arise. Should the tube become obstructed or accidentally fall out, quick deliberate action must be taken to reestablish the child's airway. In the event that a child with a tracheostomy has a cardiopulmonary arrest, the principles that guide cardiopulmonary resuscitation (CPR) are nearly the same, with some adjustments.

A   B

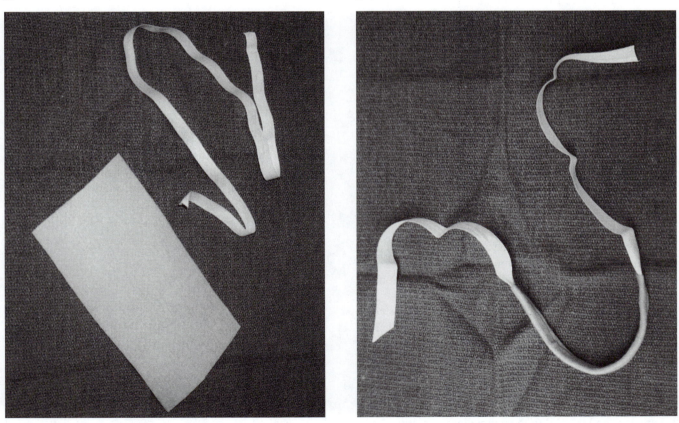

Figure 12–6 Moleskin Applied to Twill Tape Provides Comfort and Protection

Maintain tube patency by using adequate humidity, suctioning, and routine tube changes. Should the child's condition deteriorate suddenly, evaluate tube patency for obstruction caused by secretions, a mucus plug, or a kink in the tube. Children who are active, restless sleepers can kink the tracheostomy tube while sleeping. Keep in mind a well-known motto, "if in doubt, change the trach" (Buzz-Kelly & Gordin, 1993, p. 159).

Accidental decannulation may occur if the tracheostomy ties are too loose or if the tube length is too short. When decannulation occurs, insert a new tube as soon as possible to reestablish the child's airway. Keep an extra tube of the same size and one size smaller at the bedside at all times. If decannulation occurs in the early postoperative period, stay sutures are used to spread the opening to appropriately replace the tube and avoid creating a false passage. If the new lubricated tube does not fit, the next smaller size should be placed. If this is unsuccessful, a smaller endotracheal tube should be attempted. If attempts to place the smaller-sized tube fail, a suction catheter should be used as an obturator in the following manner:

- Pass the suction catheter through the tracheostomy tube.
- Apply lubricant to the catheter tip and the tracheostomy tube.
- Insert the catheter into the stoma approximately 2 cm.
- Gently ease the tube over the catheter, using it as a guide, until the tube is in the proper position.
- Remove the suction catheter.
- Hold the new tube in place while ties are securely fastened.
- Observe the child closely to ensure that procedure was well tolerated.
- Suction if needed.
- Apply additional oxygen as needed.

The CPR process is essentially the same for a child with a tracheostomy except for a few mechanical alterations. Rescue breathing is provided by use of an Ambu bag or by mouth to tracheostomy tube method. Placing a hand over the mouth and nose prevents an upward air leak (Figure 12–7). If for any reason the tube is removed and attempts to replace it are unsuccessful, rescue breathing by means of mouth to nose/mouth should be performed. An air leak at the stoma is controlled by placing a finger over the stoma.

An emergency kit should be assembled and should accompany the child throughout the hospital (Exhibit 12–3). This kit or one similar should be used after discharge when away from home.

Speech

Language and the ability to communicate are critical elements for normal child development. A tracheostomy tube

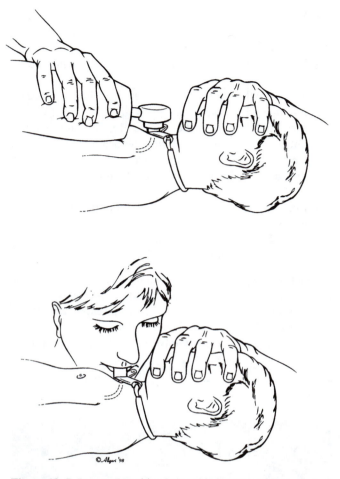

Figure 12–7 Rescue Breathing Is Provided by Use of an Ambubag or by Mouth to Tracheostomy Tube

interferes with normal speech development (Jackson & Albamonte, 1994). The ability to speak is a concern for the parent of a child with a tracheostomy and for the child. Often, the toddler or older child is able to move air around the

Exhibit 12–3 Emergency Kit

- Ambu bag/mask
- Tracheostomy tubes (same size and one size smaller)
- Suction catheter
- Bulb suction
- Suction source
- Water-soluble lubricant
- Preslit dressing
- Scissors
- Emergency phone numbers
- Saline

tube to some degree to vocalize. Or, in some instances the older child places a finger over the tracheostomy tube to redirect the air to speak. A commonly used device is the Passy-Muir speaking valve (Passy-Muir Inc., Irvine, CA) (Figure 12–8). This one-way valve opens during inhalation but closes during exhalation, redirecting air up around the tube through the larynx past the vocal cords allowing speech to occur. Redirecting the flow of air in this manner increases the work of breathing for the infant or small child. Therefore, initial trials must be conducted in a controlled monitored setting.

Some children are not able to redirect air around the tube and past the vocal cords. For these children an alternative form of communication such as sign language is recommended. Every child with a tracheostomy tube must receive an early speech therapy evaluation to assess language capabilities and to develop a plan of treatment.

Playing, Bathing, and Feeding

A child with a tracheostomy is encouraged to participate in all developmentally appropriate activities with some precautions in mind (Figure 12–9). The tracheostomy must be protected from foreign body aspiration by covering with a scarf or the HME, particularly when playing outdoors. Contact sports or activities should be avoided. Water play is possible if careful attention is given to avoid getting water in the tracheostomy. If the child is using the HME and it gets wet

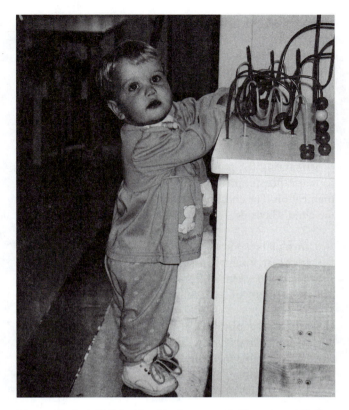

Figure 12–9 A Child with a Tracheostomy Is Encouraged To Participate in all Developmentally Appropriate Activities

during water play, the saturated device will not allow air to pass easily. This results in increased work of breathing. The same water precautions apply for bathing. As long as the tracheostomy is protected, showering or bathing is possible.

On the return of gastrointestinal function postoperatively, the child with a tracheostomy resumes the preoperative diet or an appropriate diet for age. Some children may experience disturbances with feeding. Children at risk for "oral defensive" behavior have a history of multiple endotracheal intubations followed by a surgically created tracheostomy. An evaluation by an occupational therapist is necessary for determining the scope of the problem and for developing a plan of treatment.

DISCHARGE PREPARATION

An interdisciplinary approach by an experienced health care team ensures that the transition from hospital to home is a seamless process. Members of this team should include, but are not limited to, at least two family members, the physician, nurse case manager, clinical nurse specialist, primary staff nurse, social worker, respiratory care practitioner, pastoral counselor, dietitian, speech therapist, physical/occupational therapist, child life specialist, and representatives from

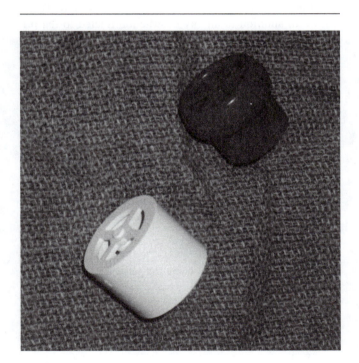

Figure 12–8 Passy-Muir Valve

home care agencies (both nursing and durable medical equipment).

The process begins early. In an ideal situation, no limits are placed on discharge preparations. However, given the financial limitations of the health care industry today, discharge is imminent as soon as the patient is stable. This means that shortly after the first tracheostomy tube change, the child is discharged if no other medical problems require hospitalization.

Monitoring the progress toward discharge in a checklist format is helpful in keeping on target and maintaining communication. The checklist should be kept in a visible place at the child's bedside. It should address the following issues:

- financial resources
- home environment assessment
- competency/skills of primary caregivers
- assessment of additional family and community resources
- school (if applicable)
- home nursing agency
- home durable medical equipment/supply company
- transportation
- telephone communication

Financial resources should be assessed preoperatively. A social worker can help identify potential sources of funding through private insurance, state or federal programs, or services for disabled children. Evaluate the home for electrical and structural safety to accommodate medical equipment. Letters to local power and phone companies are written to ensure that power and phone communication is a priority for the child's home in case of power failure.

The family's readiness to independently manage the tracheostomy at home should be carefully assessed. Providing repeated hands-on care for the child under the direct supervision of the bedside nurse is a necessary approach to ensure mastery of essential skills (Kennelly, 1987). Primary caregivers must be able to provide all routine care and articulate and demonstrate emergency care measures before discharge. Role-playing allows family members the opportunity to rehearse responses to a variety of situations that could occur. Additional family support or community resources should be explored to offer relief to primary caregivers as needed (Kenney, 1987). If the child attends school, notify the school nurse to prepare for the child's return to the classroom. The school nurse should be familiar with the child and family, competent in routine tracheostomy care, and able to establish an emergency action plan in the school setting.

Health care team members must determine how much nursing support is needed. Most financial resources require a tentative plan for decreasing hours of service required over time. A nursing agency experienced in providing care to the child with a tracheostomy should be selected. Home care nurses visit the child early to become familiar with the child's unique needs and demonstrate competency with the care (Kenney, 1987). An experienced durable medical equipment company provides equipment and supplies to the child with a tracheostomy. Any special equipment that is to be used at home is brought to the hospital before discharge so that the primary caregivers can use and become familiar with its proper use (Exhibit 12–4).

Transportation home is arranged for the day of discharge, as well as transport for future follow-up visits. The local emergency medical system or fire department is notified of the presence of a child with a tracheostomy in the community.

Before the day of discharge, a care conference is planned to review the overall plan of care, document progress toward the goal of discharge, and provide a forum for questions or concerns.

DECANNULATION

Ultimately, for most children with tracheostomies, decannulation is the final goal. The timing and method of decannulation depend on the original reason for the tracheostomy, the condition of the airway, and the child's current health status (Runton & Zazal, 1989).

The primary underlying pathologic condition should be addressed before decannulation. Conditions such as acquired or congenital laryngotracheal stenosis require repair or reconstruction (Ochi et al., 1992; Weber, Connors, & Tracy, 1991). In addition to airway obstruction related to the primary pathologic condition, granulation tissue may form within the lumen of the airway over time. This tissue reduces airway diameter and must be removed by the surgeon before decannulation. Laryngotracheoplasty or laryngotracheal reconstruction relieves subglottic stenosis by surgically expanding the airway lumen (Ochi et al., 1992). Tracheal carti-

Exhibit 12–4 Durable Medical Equipment and Other Supplies

- Apnea monitor
- Pulse oximeter
- Humidity source (for in-home and portable use)
- Portable suction
- Suction catheters
- Tracheostomy tubes
- Tracheostomy ties
- Heat and moisture exchange (HME) device
- Bulb syringe

lage may also become soft and collapsible as a result of the incision during the initial procedure or pressure on the cartilage from the tracheostomy tube. This may need to be surgically corrected before attempts to decannulate (Ochi, Bailey, & Evans, 1992; Runton & Zazal, 1989). The suprastomal collapsed tracheal area is hitched forward. This is accomplished by suturing it to the strap muscles on either side (Ochi et al., 1992).

The child must be growing appropriately and be in a good state of health. A history of recent illness, particularly a respiratory tract infection, delays decannulation. To enhance the rate of success, avoiding decannulation attempts just before or during the onset of the cold and flu season is a common practice.

Many children require downsizing of the tracheostomy tube in preparation for decannulation. A child becomes accustomed to the ease of breathing through the tracheostomy tube. As the tube is downsized the child begins to move more air around the tracheostomy and through the nasopharynx. The dead space between the nasopharynx and the tracheal stoma increases the airway resistance and therefore the work of breathing (Runton & Zazal, 1989). This requires a period of adjustment but can be performed on an outpatient basis. When the smallest tube size has been placed, the child is admitted to the hospital. The tube may be capped for a 24-hour period. If tolerated, the tube is then removed, the site covered with a sterile gauze dressing, and the child observed overnight for another 24 hours before discharge. Alternatively, the tracheostomy tube can be removed without first capping and the child observed in the hospital setting for 24 to 48 hours. Primary skin closure is usually not required after removal of the tracheostomy tube. If a laryngotracheoplasty or laryngotracheal reconstruction is performed, a primary skin closure is part of the procedure (Ochi et al., 1992). During hospitalization, instruments for endotracheal intubation should be kept at the bedside in case of recurrent airway obstruction.

CONCLUSION

Tracheostomies in children are usually performed to provide a temporary stable airway. After the initial postoperative period, the focus of care is on educating the primary caregivers in independent management of the tracheostomy tube. The goal is to normalize the child's life by encouraging attendance at school, eating an oral diet, and communicating with family and peers. Support from the multidisciplinary team ensures the family's success in achieving this outcome.

REFERENCES

Arcand, P., & Granger, J. (1988). Pediatric tracheostomies: Changing trends. *Journal of Otolaryngology, 17,* 121–124.

Bressler, K., Coladipietro, L., & Holinger, L. (1997). Protection of the cervical skin in the pediatric patient with a recent tracheostomy. *Otolaryngology–Head and Neck Surgery, 116,* 414–415.

Burstein, L. (1995). Home care. In S.L. Barnhart & M.P. Czervinske (Eds.), *Perinatal and pediatric respiratory care* (pp. 658–679). Philadelphia: W.B. Saunders Company.

Buzz-Kelly, L., & Gordin, P. (1993). Teaching CPR to parents of children with tracheostomies. *Maternal Child Nursing Journal, 18,* 158–163.

Chameides, L., & Hazinski, M.F. (Eds.). (1997). *Pediatric advanced life support.* Dallas: American Heart Association.

Davis, S. (1998). Guidelines for care of the child with a chronic tracheostomy. In *Advances in pediatric pulmonary care: Interdisciplinary approaches to asthma and home care of technology dependent children.* Conference presentation, Memphis, Tennessee.

Donnelly, M.J., Lacey, P.D., & Maguire, A.J. (1996). A twenty year (1971–1990) review of tracheostomies in a major pediatric hospital. *International Journal of Pediatric Otorhinolaryngology, 35,* 1–9.

Fitton, C.M. (1994). Nursing management of the child with a tracheostomy. *Pediatric Clinics of North America, 41,* 513–523.

Gohsman, B. (1981). The hospitalized child and the need for mastery. *Issues in Comprehensive Pediatric Nursing, 5,* 67–76.

Hodge, D. (1991). Endotracheal suctioning and the infant: A nursing care protocol to decrease complications. *Neonatal Network, 9,* 7–15.

"Home care: Child with a tracheostomy." (1995). (Available from Cardinal Glennon Children's Hospital, 1465 S. Grand Blvd., St. Louis, MO 63104).

Jackson, D., & Albamonte, S. (1994). Enhancing communication with the Passey-Muir valve. *Pediatric Nursing, 20,* 149–153.

Jursich, C.E., & Kennelly, C. (1987). Anterior cricoid split: An alternative to tracheostomies in infants with subglottic stenosis. *Neonatal Network, 5,* 7–12.

Kennelly, C. (1987). Tracheostomy care: Parents as learners. *Maternal Child Nursing Journal, 12,* 264–267.

Kenney, M.M. (1987). Hospital to home: Care of the child with a tracheostomy. *Neonatal Network, 5,* 21–24.

Kleiber, C., Krutzfield, N., & Rose, E.F. (1988). Acute histologic changes in the tracheobronchial tree associated with different suction catheter insertion techniques. *Heart and Lung, 17,* 10–14.

Lothschuetz Montgomery, K. (1996). SOP: Care of the patient with a tracheostomy. *NIH Clinical Center Nursing Department* [On-line]. Available: http://www.cc.nih.gov/nursing/trach.html.

Motoyama, E.K. (1985). Physiologic alterations in tracheostomy. In E.N. Myers, S.E. Stool, & J.T. Johnson (Eds.), *Tracheotomy* (pp. 177–200). New York: Churchill Livingstone.

Myers, E.N., Stool, S.E., & Johnson, J.T. (1985). Technique in tracheotomy. In E.N. Myers, S.E. Stool, & J.T. Johnson (Eds.), *Tracheotomy* (pp. 113–124). New York: Churchill Livingstone.

Ochi, J.W., Bailey, C.M., & Evans, J.N. (1992). Pediatric airway reconstruction at Great Ormond Street: A ten-year review. III. Decannulation and suprastomal collapse. *Annals of Otology, Rhinology, Laryngology, 101,* 656–658.

Ochi, J.W., Evans, J.N.G., & Bailey, C.M. (1992). Pediatric airway reconstruction at Great Ormond Street: A ten-year review. I. Laryngotracheal reconstruction. *Annals of Otology, Rhinology, Laryngology, 101,* 465–468.

Pettignano, M.M., & Pettignano, R. (1995). Airway management. In S.L. Barnhart & M.P. Czervinske (Eds.), *Perinatal and pediatric respiratory care* (pp. 239–252). Philadelphia: W.B. Saunders Company.

Runton, N., & Zazal, G.H. (1989). The decannulation process in children. *Journal of Pediatric Nursing, 4,* 370–373.

Storgion, S.A. (1996). Care of the technology-dependent child. *Pediatric Annals, 25,* 677–684.

Warnock, C., & Porpora, K. (1994). A pediatric trach card: Transforming research into practice. *Pediatric Nursing, 20,* 186–188.

Weber, T.R., Connors, R.H., & Tracy, T.F. (1991). Acquired tracheal stenosis in infants and children. *Journal of Thoracic and Cardiovascular Surgery, 102,* 29–35.

Wetmore, R.F. (1996). Tracheotomy. In C.D. Blustone & S.E. Stool (Eds.), *Pediatric otolaryngology* (pp. 425–440). New York: Churchill Livingstone.

Appendix 12–A

Critical Pathway for Tracheostomy

CARDINAL GLENNON CHILDREN'S HOSPITAL
1465 S. Grand Blvd., St. Louis, MO 63104

PATIENT IDENTIFICATION

Pt. Hgt. (cm): _____   Pt. Wgt. (Kg): _____
Primary Tracheostomy Caregiver (MD): _____
Key: N/A = Cross Through and Initial   Completed = Initial   To Be Completed = Circle and Initial
Care Pathway Trach for Patients. Patient's care to follow pathway. Patient-specific modifications noted.

(Physician Signature)

CARE ITEM	Pre-Op	OR	Post-Op Day 1	Post-Op Day 2	Post-Op Day 3
Assessments/ Monitoring	▸ Assessment-Every 4 Hours ∘ Heart Rate (HR), respiratory rate (RR), auscultation, use of accessory muscles, dyspnea, alertness, color, SpO_2, medication side effects. ▸ I&O each shift. ▸ Social Service consult. ▸ Child Life Assessment.	▸ Assessment-Every 2 Hours ▸ Trach ties and stay sutures secure.	▸ Assessment-Every 2–4 Hours	▸ Assessment-Every 2–4 Hours	
Treatment	▸ Peripheral IV (When NPO)	▸ Humidified tracheostomy collar; oxygen to maintain saturation. ▸ Suction PRN	▸ Tracheostomy care BID and PRN		
Medications		▸ Narcotic or non-narcotic analgesia PRN			
Activity	▸ Up ad lib. ▸ Comfort measures.	▸ Bedrest: Supine with head of bed elevated or side lying position. ▸ Change position at least every 2–4 hours.		▸ Up ad lib.	
Diet	▸ NPO 6 hours before procedure		▸ Clear liquids	▸ Advance diet.	▸ Decrease IV rate when tolerating diet.

Each column contains sub-headings: Date / Planned Unit and Time / Actual Unit.

Courtesy of Cardinal Glennon Children's Hospital, St. Louis, Missouri.

CARE ITEM	Pre-Op (Planned Unit / Date / Time / Actual Unit)	OR (Planned Unit / Date / Time / Actual Unit)	Post-Op Day 1 (Planned Unit / Date / Time / Actual Unit)	Post-Op Day 2 (Planned Unit / Date / Time / Actual Unit)	Post-Op Day 3 (Planned Unit / Date / Time / Actual Unit)
Tests	► Chest x-ray →	→	→	→	→
Consults				► Occupational Therapy ► Speech Therapy →	→
Education	► Orient to unit. ► Discuss pre-op preparation and post-op course. ► Provide written teaching materials. ► Show sample tracheostomy tube. →	→	► Demonstrate supplies and routine care. →	→	→
Discharge Planning	► Initiate teaching checklist. ► Identify home nursing agency and equipment company. →	→	→	→	► Plan interdisciplinary care conference prior to discharge.
Evaluation		► VS within normal limits: Yes/No ► Oxygen saturation level acceptable: Yes/No ► Tracheostomy ties and stay sutures secure: Yes/No ► Patent airway: Yes/No		► Tolerating feedings: Yes/No	► Discharge teaching completed: Yes/No ► Home care equipment and home nursing arranged: Yes/No ► Follow-up scheduled: Yes/No
Signature	Signature	Signature	Signature	Signature	Signature

CHAPTER 13

Esophageal Defects

Danuta E. Nowicki

Defects of the esophagus, whether congenital, acquired, or functional, are among the most common anomalies in children. Congenital defects include esophageal atresia (EA), tracheoesophageal fistula (TEF), laryngotracheoesophageal clefts, congenital esophageal stenosis, and esophageal duplication, among others. Corrosive injuries to the esophagus, esophageal strictures, and foreign bodies in the esophagus are among the acquired esophageal defects. Achalasia and gastroesophageal reflux (GER) are examples of functional disorders of the esophagus. Prompt identification of the disorder is necessary for appropriate management. This chapter focuses on EA, TEF, corrosive injuries to the esophagus, esophageal stricture, and esophageal replacement.

CONGENITAL DEFECTS

Esophageal Atresia and Tracheoesophageal Fistula

Of all the potential anomalies involving the esophagus and trachea, EA and the associated TEF are the most common and the most fatal if not promptly diagnosed and treated surgically (Holder, 1993). Before 1939, there was 100% mortality in infants born with EA/TEF (Raffensperger, 1990). Advances in medical and surgical care in the past 40 years have led to a survival rate of near 100% in otherwise healthy infants born with the disorder (Holder, 1993; Randolph, Newman, & Anderson, 1989). The cause of death in the ill infants is attributed to extreme prematurity and associated anomalies. Limited data are available regarding long-term status of children with EA or TEF. The available data have primarily focused on complications such as esophageal motility and pulmonary function (Spitz, 1996).

Often referred to as one condition, EA/TEF is in reality two entities, which may present separately or, more commonly, occur together. EA refers to the condition wherein there has been a disruption in the development of the esophagus, preventing it from becoming a continuous tube. This results in the formation of a proximal and distal pouch. TEF is an abnormal connection, by way of the fistula, between the esophagus and trachea. Most common is a combination between the two in which the esophagus has failed to fuse as a continuous tube, and a fistula connects the proximal, distal, or both pouches to the trachea.

Incidence and Etiology

EA/TEF occurs in approximately 1 in 3,000 births, with a slight male predominance (Bankier, Brady, & Myers, 1991; Holder, 1993; Raffensperger, 1990). Prematurity is common with EA or EA with an associated TEF; 34% of these infants weigh less than 2,500 gm (Holder, 1993). In general, infants with pure TEF are not born prematurely; their average gestational age is 37 weeks.

The origin of these anomalies is not known. They usually occur sporadically, although there are reports of several family members having EA/TEF. The anomaly is found in twins, siblings, and offspring of adults who themselves had the disorder (Bankier et al., 1991; Harmon & Coran, 1998; Holder, 1993; Raffensperger, 1990).

Embryology

The foregut of the embryo is seen as a single cell-layer tube at 19 to 23 days of gestation. This tube gives rise to the esophagus and pharynx. The dorsal foregut, or primitive esophagus, begins to divide from the ventral trachea at the level of the carina by a union between two proliferating ridges of cells composing the epithelial lining. This division

Acknowledgments: I thank Dr. Kathryn D. Anderson for her advice and for proofreading the text and Dr. Nilda Garcia for photographic and technical assistance.

progresses in a cephalad direction and is completed to the level of the larynx by approximately the 26th day. A disruption in this process is thought to result in a TEF (Beasley, 1991a; Holder, 1993; Raffensperger, 1990).

EA is thought to occur as a result of the unavailability of tissue caused by the rapid growth and elongation of the primitive esophagus. An interruption of the vascular supply to the area during development may also play a role in the cause (Beasley, 1991a; Harmon & Coran, 1998; Holder, 1993; Raffensperger, 1990).

Classification

Although EA and TEF occur as isolated entities, a combination is more common. The classification of these defects has marked clinical significance in the treatment, management, and eventual outcome of these children. Following are the most commonly recorded classifications based on the pathologic condition they represent and rate of occurrence. Their alphabetical ranking is based on Gross' (1953) method of classification (Figure 13–1).

Associated Anomalies

Approximately 50% of infants born with EA/TEF have other anomalies that vary in severity and associated mortality (Exhibit 13–1). In addition to surgical correction for EA/TEF, the infant may require corrective repairs of the associated anomalies. Associated cardiac anomalies are the most common and the most lethal. The incidence of cardiovascular anomalies ranges from 14.7% to 28% (David &

O'Callaghan, 1974; Greenwood & Rosenthal, 1976; Mee, 1991). EA/TEF is also a component of the VATER or VACTERL association (Quan & Smith, 1973). This association of anomalies includes defects of the vertebrae, anorectal malformations, cardiac defects, renal defects, and defects of the radius and/or limbs. Although most patients do not exhibit all the associated defects, if one defect is present, others should be suspected. The most common associated gastrointestinal defect found in this grouping is imperforate anus.

Pathophysiology

Swallowing by the fetus begins at about 14 weeks' gestation. By the end of the pregnancy, the fetus swallows several hundred milliliters or half the amniotic fluid volume daily (Stokes, 1991). It is estimated that the fetus may get as much as 10% to 14% of its nutrition from the amniotic fluid (Mulvihill, Stone, Debas, & Fonkalsrud, 1985). Infants with EA have a small stomach because it has not been dilated through swallowing. The size of the stomach may be problematic in the creation of a gastrostomy, gastric fundoplication, and may limit the ability to advance feedings. EA prevents saliva and oral intake from reaching the stomach. Strenuous attempts at swallowing by the fetus cause hypertrophy and distention of the upper pouch. The pooling of liquid or food in the blind upper pouch compresses the trachea, interfering with the development of the tracheal cartilage. This may lead to tracheomalacia, a condition in which the tracheal wall is especially soft and pliable (Filler & Forte,

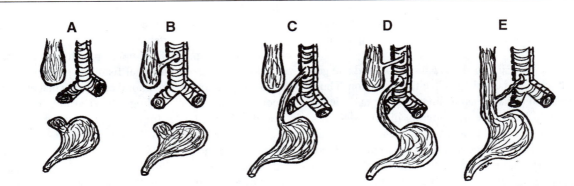

Type A, Isolated EA (3.7%–7%). Almost always found with a long gap between the proximal and distal pouches. Type B, EA with proximal TEF (0.8%). The proximal esophageal pouch is usually short because of tethering by the fistula to the trachea. This results in a long esophageal gap. Type C, EA with distal TEF (86%). This combination is the most common presentation of the anomaly. The upper esophagus usually ends blindly between the seventh cervical and fifth thoracic vertebra. There is usually a short esophageal gap. The upper pouch is larger then the distal esophageal segment because of dilation and hypertrophy, which occur by efforts of the fetus to swallow amniotic fluid. There may be muscular continuity between the esophageal pouches. The distal esophagus, which has its origins from trachea, connects by way of the fistula to a membranous portion of the lower trachea. Type D, EA with proximal and distal TEF (0.7%–6%). Type E, Isolated TEF (4.4%–7%). Not an esophageal atresia but included in the grouping. The continuity of the esophagus is intact. One or multiple fistulas may occur between the esophagus and trachea at any level from the carina to the cricoid but usually occur around the lower cervical to upper thoracic area. The fistula inserts higher on the trachea than on the esophagus. The defect is often referred to as an H-type fistula.

Figure 13–1 Classification of EA/TEF

Exhibit 13–1 Common Associated Anomalies

Cardiac[a]
  ASD
  VSD
  Tetralogy of Fallot
  Truncas Arteriosis
  PDA
  Coarctation of the aorta
  Arch anomalies
  Vascular ring
  Others
Gastrointestinal[b]
  Anorectal (imperforate anus/cloaca)
  Duodenal (atresia/stenosis)
  Pyloric (atresia/stenosis)
  Esophagus (congenital stenosis)
  Hirschsprung's disease
  Others
Urinary Tract[b]
  Renal defects
  Hypospadias
  Others
Orthopaedic[b]
  Vertebral
  Limb
Chromosomal[b]
  Trisomy 21
  Trisomy 18
  Others

[a] Mee, 1991. [b] Myers, Beasley, & Auldist, 1991a.

1998). If there is an associated proximal TEF, the pooled liquid in the upper pouch will cross the fistula, causing respiratory distress.

The presence of a TEF allows the passage of food and gas between the trachea and esophagus in either direction. Thus, air forced across the fistula as an infant cries may elicit a belch. If the child has the more common distal fistula between the lower esophageal pouch and trachea, the stomach may become massively dilated and the diaphragm elevated, causing respiratory compromise. A distal fistula also allows gastric contents to pass along the fistula to the trachea, causing respiratory complications such as tracheobronchitis, pneumonia, and atelectasis.

Clinical Presentation

Often the first sign of EA is polyhydramnios on the prenatal maternal ultrasonographic scan (Harmon & Coran, 1998; Holder, 1993; Stringer et al., 1995). The failure to identify the fetal stomach and/or the presence of a dilated proximal pouch is strongly suggestive of EA. If this anomaly is sus-

pected, the presence of associated anomalies should be investigated. After birth, the pooling of secretions in the upper pouch or the inability to tolerate oral feeding with coughing and choking are suspicious. After effective oral/pharyngeal suctioning, the infant appears normal until fed again. If an associated distal TEF is present, the infant may have a distended abdomen from air being forced through the fistula into the stomach.

TEF without the presence of EA may not be recognized for several months (Andrassy et al., 1980; Crabbe, Kiely, Drake, & Spitz, 1996). The severity of respiratory symptoms depends on the size and number of fistulas present. Abdominal distention, especially after feedings, is common. Often these infants are discharged home. Only after multiple visits to the primary health provider's office for choking episodes is aspiration resulting from a TEF suspected.

Diagnosis

A quick diagnostic test to evaluate for EA/TEF is to attempt to pass a No. 10 to 12 F feeding/Replogle tube down the esophagus. A smaller tube is too flexible and folds on itself. If resistance is met when advancing the tube, usually at about 10 to 12 cm, a radiographic film should be obtained with the tube in position. The presence of EA/TEF can be confirmed with a simple chest/abdominal radiographic film (Holder, 1993; Myers & Beasley, 1991; Raffensperger, 1990). The tip of the feeding tube indicates the length of the proximal pouch. Presence of air in the stomach indicates a distal TEF. Air in the stomach but not in the small intestine is suggestive of associated duodenal atresia. A gasless stomach is diagnostic of pure EA (Figure 13–2), although a distal fistula so small as to not allow the passage of air may rarely be present. This initial radiographic film also reveals information about the child's pulmonary status, cardiac size and contour, and possibly vertebral anomalies.

A contrast study of the upper pouch may be obtained to evaluate whether a proximal fistula is present. With care to avoid aspiration, 0.5 ml of oral contrast is placed in the upper pouch with a small feeding tube (Harmon & Coran, 1998; Holder, 1993). Under fluoroscopic guidance, this may accurately locate the level of the pouch and presence of a fistula. Contrast in the trachea suggests a proximal TEF, although this may also be spillover from the pouch. Because of the risk of aspiration during this test, bronchoscopy can be performed at the time of esophageal repair and replaces the need for these upper pouch studies (Harmon & Coran, 1998).

The isolated TEF may be diagnosed with a limited upper gastrointestinal study or esophagram. A small nasogastric tube is passed into the distal esophagus and contrast media is slowly injected while the tube is gradually withdrawn. The esophagram may show abnormal peristalsis. Failure to identify a fistula radiologically indicates the need for bronchoscopy/esophagoscopy for diagnosis (Andrassy et al., 1980).

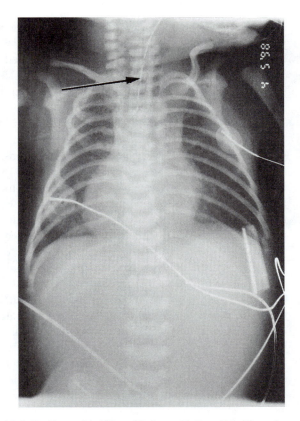

Figure 13–2 Radiographic Film of Infant with Pure EA. Note absence of gas in abdomen. Arrow points to feeding tube in upper esophageal pouch.

Associated anomalies can be excluded with echocardiogram, renal ultrasonography, and radiographic films/ultrasonography of the spine. Because repair of the esophagus is usually performed through a right thoracotomy, the side of the aortic arch must be identified. Approximately 5% of children have an aberrant right aortic arch, which may require the surgeon to approach the esophagus from a left thoracotomy to facilitate exposure during the repair (Harrison, Hanson, Mahour, Takahashi, & Weitzman, 1977).

Preoperative Management

If the diagnosis of EA/TEF is suspected, the infant is transferred to a tertiary care center where pediatric surgeons are available. Once EA/TEF is diagnosed, the goals of preoperative care include the prevention of aspiration pneumonia, provision of respiratory support, and evaluation of associated anomalies. Broad-spectrum antibiotics covering respiratory flora should be started as soon as possible. If respiratory support is needed, the team member with the most experience should intubate the infant. Bag/mask ventilation should be avoided because it may cause massive abdominal distention if a TEF is large.

Management of these often challenging infants can be facilitated through use of a critical pathway (Appendix 13–A).

Infants with EA awaiting primary repair must have their proximal esophageal pouch drained with a small single/double lumen tube on continuous/intermittent low suction (Figure 13–3). The patency of the suction catheter should be

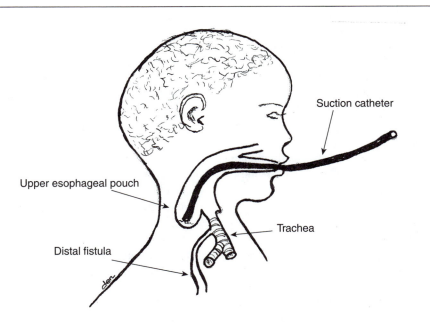

Figure 13–3 Infant with EA and Distal TEF. Suction catheter is draining upper esophageal pouch.

frequently assessed. These infants do better when placed prone or on their sides with the head of the bed slightly elevated. The esophageal pouch has a 1 to 2 ml capacity, and malfunction of the drainage tube can lead to aspiration, desaturation, and bradycardia. Some surgeons advocate irrigating these tubes with 0.5 ml sterile normal saline every 2 hours, although this may increase the risk of aspiration (Roy, 1991).

A decision must be made whether any surgery is indicated for associated anomalies before the repair of the esophagus. The severity of a cardiac anomaly may supersede the need to repair the esophagus (Holder, 1993). A definitive repair of the esophagus may be deferred in the severely ill infant who requires ventilatory support (Raffensperger, 1990). Since 1982, physiologic status has been used as the sole basis for repair without regard to weight, gestation, or pulmonary condition (Randolph et al., 1989).

A gastrostomy tube may be placed at the time of cardiac repair to decompress the stomach (Holder, 1993). The infant with an associated imperforate anus or intestinal atresia will need to have a repair or stoma within the first day of life. If clinically stable, this surgery can be paired with the esophageal repair (Raffensperger, 1990).

Operative Repair

Repair of EA or EA/TEF can fall into three scenarios: primary repair, delayed repair, and staged repair (Exhibits 13–2 and 13–3). Primary repair includes the ability to get the two ends of the esophagus together and ligate and divide any fistula in one surgical procedure. Preservation of native esophageal tissue is superior to anything used to replace it. If a long gap exists between the two segments of the esophagus, primary repair may not be possible. Some surgeons favor frequent stretching of the proximal esophageal pouch at the bedside with a Bougie or similar catheter to gain length for closure (Holder, 1993; Raffensperger, 1990). The distal pouch may also be stretched in a retrograde manner through the gastrostomy, providing a TEF is not present. Elongation of the proximal pouch occurs over 3 to 6 weeks. Others believe that the pouch gains length through growth and does not need stretching (Beasley, 1991b). Infants usually remain in the hospital while awaiting the delayed repair. Depending on clinical condition, the infant may wait several weeks to months before repair is attempted. Improved survival is found in the poor-risk infant if the esophageal repair is delayed, and delaying primary repair has been found to have a better outcome than a staged repair (Raffensperger, 1990). Although now seldom performed, some surgeons create an esophagostomy to drain the proximal pouch while awaiting delayed repair. Indications for cervical esophagostomy include little or no distal esophagus, ultra-long gap between the pouches, life-threatening anastomotic complications,

and long gap without appropriate facility for prolonged upper pouch care (Myers, Beasley, & Auldist, 1991). An esophagostomy allows the infant to be discharged home. However, creation of an esophagostomy may sacrifice much needed esophageal length and commit the surgeon to performing an esophageal substitution (Spitz, 1995).

Primary repair is the preferred operative plan (Figure 13–4). Ideally, the gap between the pouches should be no wider then two to three vertebral bodies to avoid postoperative tension on the anastomosis (Beasley, 1991b; Raffensperger, 1990). This repair is accomplished by means of a posterolateral thoracotomy on the side opposite the aortic arch (Harrison et al., 1977). The tips of the pouches are excised and brought together by end-to-end (Beasley & Auldist, 1991) or end-to-side anastomosis (Poenaru, Laberge, Neilson, Nguyen, & Guttman, 1991; Touloukian, 1992). The anastomosis may be difficult because the proximal pouch may be two to four times larger in diameter than the distal pouch. The esophagus, having no serosal lining, does not hold sutures well. If a considerable gap is present between the two pouches, a circular myotomy may be performed on the proximal pouch to gain esophageal length (Holder, 1993; Raffensperger, 1990). A chest tube or soft drain is usually placed in the retropleural space next to the anastomosis to allow any drainage from the surgical site to be recognized. Some surgeons favor not leaving a drain at the site and identify anastomotic complications by clinical deterioration and radiologic changes. In one review, only 47% of patients with anastomotic complications were noted to have drainage from the surgical drains. Of these, 80% required additional drains placed (McCallion, Hannon, & Boston, 1992). The success of the anastomosis depends on the gentle handling of tissue, the blood supply, and lack of tension on the suture line rather than any particular technique. A gastrostomy tube is placed to assist with feedings and/or decompression, although the trend is to avoid gastrostomies whenever possible (Santos, Thompson, Johnson, & Foker, 1983; Shaul, Schwartz, Marr, & Tyson, 1989). If it is impossible to bring the two ends of the esophagus together, the infant undergoes a staged repair as described in the following.

The infant with isolated EA requires placement of a feeding gastrostomy. Before this procedure the gap length between the pouches can be assessed with contrast media and fluoroscopy. Usually the ends of the pouches are too far apart to be brought together safely. Surgery to anastomose the pouches is delayed, hoping to gain length with time, or planned for eventual esophageal replacement. Staged repair is reserved for those infants with severe respiratory distress, very high proximal pouches, or severe associated anomalies (Raffensperger, 1990; Randolph et al., 1989).

The operative repair of an isolated TEF involves division of the fistula and repair of the esophageal and tracheal de-

Exhibit 13–2 Management of Esophageal Atresia: Gasless Abdomen

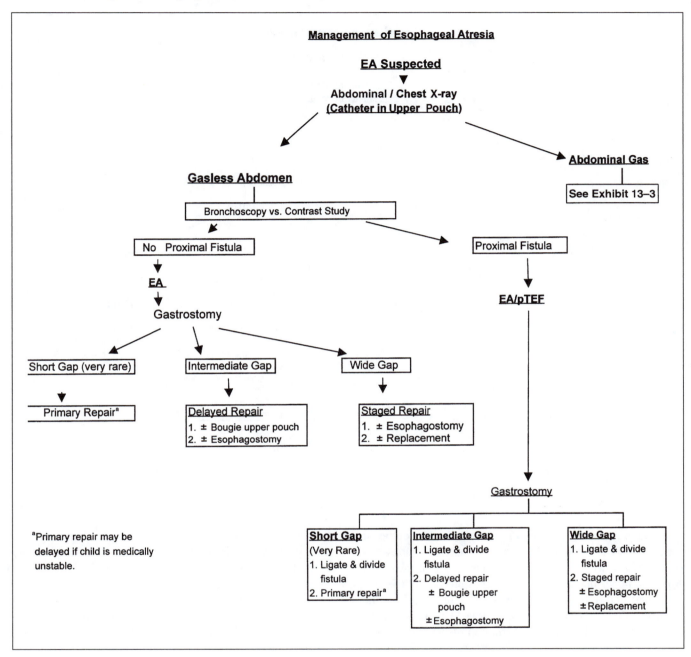

fects. Most of these fistulas are above or at the level of the clavicle and can be reached by a cervical approach (Raffensperger, 1990).

Postoperative Management

Care of the infant after repair of EA/TEF includes effective pain management, evaluation, and support of all organ systems, with focus on the respiratory and gastrointestinal systems and care of surgical wounds and drains.

Pain Management. The level of the infant's pain is assessed by means of physiologic indicators. The infant may be kept on continuous intravenous analgesics or intermittent boluses. Effective pain control is important because the infant risks disruption of the anastomosis as a result of excessive movement and crying from inadequate pain relief.

Respiratory. The healthy infant who has undergone primary repair of an EA/TEF, isolated TEF, or pure EA may be extubated soon after surgery, whereas a smaller, ill infant

Exhibit 13–3 Management of Esophageal Atresia: Abdominal Gas

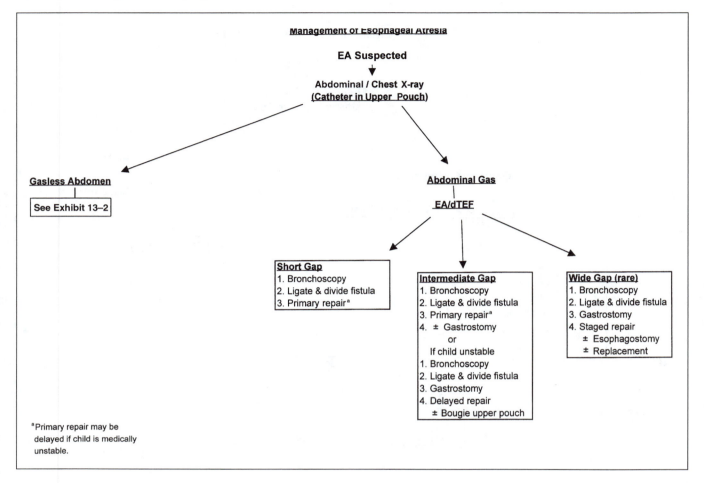

may require prolonged ventilation. Frequent suctioning of the pharynx is needed until the infant is able to swallow his or her own saliva. The suction catheter is often measured from the upper dental ridge to the anastomosis by the surgeon and marked. An approximate measure can be done from the tip of the nose to the earlobe. Deep suctioning should be avoided to prevent disruption of the anastomosis (Beasley & Auldist, 1991; Raffensperger, 1990). The infant should be positioned to reduce strain on the esophageal anastomosis; if placed supine, care must be taken to prevent extension of the neck (Raffensperger, 1990). After 48 hours, gentle chest physiotherapy is provided three to four times daily. Infants with isolated TEF repairs have considerable dissection of the trachea and may be hoarse and stridorous during the postoperative period.

Gastrointestinal.   Traditionally, a contrast esophagram is performed 5 to 10 days after repair to assess for anastomotic leaks (Holder, 1993; Raffensperger, 1990; Santos et al., 1983). If no leak is demonstrated on radiologic examina-

tion, oral feedings are initiated. The chest drains are removed after the infant begins oral feedings without signs of anastomotic leak. Signs indicative of leak include fluid from chest drains resembling saliva or formula/breast milk, respiratory distress, and sepsis. Some surgeons forego the contrast esophagram and feed the infants orally as early as the third day postoperatively (Brown, Eyres, & Myers, 1991). Others do not place drains or chest tubes at the time of repair (McCallion et al., 1992). Those infants are watched for respiratory distress and sepsis before being fed.

If a gastrostomy tube is present, feedings are started as soon as bowel function returns. Because of the possibility of gastric reflux, many elect to delay feeding until the anastomosis is well healed to protect the surgical site (Holder, 1993; Raffensperger, 1990). A jejunal tube may be passed through the gastrostomy for feeding the gut downstream. Patency of enteral tubes should be maintained by irrigating them with 1 to 2 ml sterile normal saline every 3 to 4 hours or per the surgeon's preference. Delay in enteral feedings necessitates the administration of parenteral nutrition. Infants with isolated TEF repair can start oral feeding 4 to 7 days after surgical repair (Holder, 1993; Raffensperger, 1990).

Esophagostomies. Infants that have undergone an esophagostomy need frequent assessment of the patency of the stoma. If the esophagostomy becomes occluded, the infant is at risk for aspiration pneumonia and respiratory compromise. These children may begin gastrostomy feedings as soon as bowel function returns, providing no surgery has been performed on the distal pouch and no fistula ligation has been done. Oral sham feedings (feedings given when there is esophageal discontinuity) should be started as soon as the esophagostomy has healed, usually within a few days. Although messy because the feedings come out the esophagostomy, sham feedings enable the infant to develop and maintain oral skills such as sucking and swallowing. The skills of an enterostomal therapist in fitting a pouch over the stoma are invaluable. The infant who is not sham fed may refuse oral feeding once the esophageal repair is completed.

Dressings/Tube Care. In general, surgical dressings over incisional sites are removed in 24 hours. Wounds are kept clean and dry. Chest tubes should be well secured and dressed. The surgeon should be notified of leakage at the incision or around chest tube insertion sites because this may indicate disruption or leakage at the anastomosis. The patency of the chest tube should be checked and the physician should be informed if blockage is suspected. The gastros-

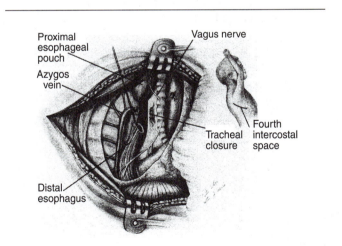

Figure 13–4 Operative Approach for Exposure of Tracheoesophageal Fistula and Repair of Esophageal Atresia. Retropleural approach is made between the fourth and fifth ribs. A rib is not removed. Entry into the mediastinum is gained by division of the azygos vein. The trachea has been closed by interrupted sutures, and the distal esophagus has been prepared by trimming away the fibrotic fistula. The vagus nerve is carefully spared from injury, and the two segments of esophagus are then brought into apposition for reconstruction.

tomy tube should be dressed and secured well. Because these infants may have very small stomachs, the maximum capacity in the reservoir balloon should be clarified with the surgeon if this type of device has been placed. The reservoir balloon should be checked every 4 to 5 days or per institutional protocol.

Complications

The most common and dangerous early postoperative complication after repair of EA/TEF is *anastomotic leak* (Harmon & Coran, 1998; Touloukian, 1992). Small leaks often close spontaneously. Larger leaks, especially those occurring within the first few days after repair, may necessitate reexploration. The area of anastomosis may need to be resutured. However, if complete disruption occurs at the anastomotic site, the proximal esophagus may need to be brought out as an esophagostomy. Some surgeons have reported good results in saving the native esophagus by resuturing the primary repair with or without a pleural patch (Chavin, Field, Chandler, Tagge, & Otherson, 1996). Complications of a leak include sepsis, mediastinitis, and recurrent fistulas.

Recurrent TEFs occur in the early postoperative period but may not be recognized for months or years. Diagnosis is made by contrast esophagram or bronchoscopy. Surgical repair is necessary. There have been reports on the successful use of fibrin glue, a biologic product, injected into the fistula through a bronchoscope as an alternative to tying and dividing the fistula (Gutierrez et al., 1994).

Esophageal *anastomotic strictures* occur frequently. They primarily cause difficulty in swallowing and may lead to choking and respiratory difficulty. Diagnosis is made by barium swallow or esophagoscopy (Raffensperger, 1990). The treatment is esophageal dilation. Opinion varies whether children need routine dilation after repair. Some surgeons elect to dilate infants as early as 2 weeks postoperatively, especially if the anastomosis was done under tension (Raffensperger, 1990; Santos et al., 1983). These dilations may continue monthly for some time. Others may follow the progress of their patients with scheduled esophagrams.

GER is a frequent occurrence in children with EA/TEF repair. It is exacerbated by poor peristaltic clearance of the esophagus caused by intrinsic motor dysfunction (Jolly et al., 1980; Tovar et al., 1995). The incidence of GER is documented in more than 50% of these patients (Holder, 1993; Wheatley, Coran, & Wesley, 1993). Anastomotic tension may cause shortening of the intraabdominal esophagus, deform the gastroesophageal junction, and cause reflux. Treatment, medical or surgical, is generally the same as for GER not associated with EA/TEF. Many surgeons favor not doing a fundoplication because of the poor pumping action of the esophagus (Curci & Dibbins, 1988; Wheatley et al., 1993); however, GER may be severe enough to require fundoplication in 6% to 45% of patients (Snyder et al., 1997). A partial wrap fundoplication (Thal/Toupet) may be performed or the reflux managed through the use of jejunal rather than gastric feedings.

Children with esophagostomies need frequent evaluation for *esophagostomy stenosis* or obstruction of the tract that may lead to respiratory distress. The child may need gentle dilation of the esophagostomy tract on a daily or twice-daily basis by the caregiver. Obstruction of the tract may require removal of a foreign body. Skin around the esophagostomy may become macerated, preventing the fit of an appliance device over the site in infants who sham feed.

Tracheal obstruction caused by *tracheomalacia* and/or pressure of the innominate artery or aorta is not uncommon. Tracheomalacia affects 10% to 20% of children after repair of esophageal atresia (Harmon & Coran, 1998). These infants are predisposed to anterior-posterior collapse of the trachea. The onset occurs at approximately 2 to 3 months of age and resolves in 1 to 2 years as the cartilage becomes more firm. Those with severe obstruction may exhibit "dying" (apneic) spells (Filler & Forte, 1998). These spells are most common during or immediately after eating and are thought to be caused by obstruction of the trachea by the food-filled esophagus. Surgical correction by aortopexy is reserved for children with life-threatening attacks.

At various stages throughout their management, children with EA/TEF may present a nutritional challenge. Severely ill infants require total parenteral nutrition by means of a central venous catheter. Others may be dependent on gastrostomy or jejunostomy feedings. Weight gain should be carefully monitored in all infants. The transition to oral feedings may be slow and difficult for some infants. These infants may expend excessive energy in the effort to feed. Infants with EA/TEF require a higher caloric intake to grow well (Holder, 1993). It is not until they reach early adolescence that they begin to catch up with their peers (Holder, 1993). Once table foods are introduced, children should be encouraged to eat slowly and wash their food down with substantial liquid. Lifelong esophageal dysmotility is present in 95% of these children (Holder, 1993). Parents should be advised to cut table foods into small pieces and to avoid hot dogs, ends of french fries, and other sharp foods. All children should adhere to GER precautions. Many times consultation with a speech or occupational therapist is indicated if the infant shows difficulty in coordinating suck and swallow. Nutritional management should be continued on an outpatient basis, especially with those infants who are waiting for delayed or staged repair.

Discharge Criteria

Discharge planning is initiated at the time of the infant's arrival at the hospital but facilitated when the surgical plan has been established. Discharge criteria include an extensive list of potential needs (Exhibit 13–4). The child's primary caregiver should begin to learn the care of the child as early as possible. The home environment should be assessed to identify specific infant and caregiver needs. Home nursing visits should be arranged after discharge to assess growth and respiratory progress of the infant.

Infants with primary repair may be discharged within 2 weeks of surgery. Infants who require staged repair may be sent home between surgical procedures. Criteria for discharge include tolerating feedings. The plan for discharge includes scheduled appointments, radiologic tests, scheduled dilations, and future surgical procedures. Chronically ill children are at risk for developmental delay, and all attempts should be made to frequently assess skills and milestones.

Laryngotracheoesophageal Cleft

A rare anomaly, laryngotracheoesophageal cleft (LTEC) is related to and may be associated with EA/TEF. With this defect, closure of the tracheoesophageal septum is completely lacking. A cleft exists in the midline, between the posterior aspect of the trachea/larynx and the anterior portion of the esophagus. In its more severe presentations, it is highly lethal (Donahoe & Gee, 1984; Dubois, Pokorney, Harberg, & Smith, 1990; Lipshutz, Albanese, Harrison, & Jennings, 1997; Robie, Pearl, Ronsales, & Hoffman, 1991; Ryan, Muehrcke, Doody, Kim, & Donahoe, 1991). The cause of the disorder remains unclear. Approximately 0.3% of children with congenital anomalies of the larynx have LTEC (Dubois et al., 1990). Treatment of the anomaly is an orchestrated effort between the pediatric surgery and oto-

---

Exhibit 13–4 Discharge Criteria

- CPR training
- Oxygen
- Pulse oximeter
- Cardiac monitor
- Apnea monitor
- Suction machine and accessories
- Enteral pump and accessories
- Intravenous infusion pump and accessories
- Enteral formula
- Total parenteral nutrition
- Medications
- Gastrostomy/jejunostomy supplies
- Home nursing
- Respite care
- Resource phone numbers
- Referral to support groups

laryngology departments. The postoperative goal is to prevent the formation of fistulas and granulation tissue while maintaining a patent airway. The infant is paralyzed, sedated, and ventilated for 1 to 2 weeks to minimize movement and coughing, thus protecting the suture lines. A tracheostomy is left in place for months, sometimes years.

Congenital Esophageal Stenosis

Rossi first described isolated congenital esophageal stenosis (CES) in 1826 (Murphy, Yazbeck & Russo, 1995). In 1987, Nihoul-Fekete et al. defined the entity as "an intrinsic stenosis of the esophagus present although not necessarily symptomatic at birth, which is caused by congenital malformation of the esophageal wall architecture" (Murphy et al., 1995). Although CES may be found anywhere along the length of the esophagus, it is most often found in the distal end.

The incidence of CES is approximately 1 in 25,000 to 50,000 live births (Murphy et al., 1995). Diagnosis includes evaluation with a contrast esophagram and esophagoscopy. The stenotic area is usually short and amenable to repeated dilations. Resection is the best treatment for severe cases where there is circumferential involvement of the esophagus (Murphy et al., 1995; Ohkawa, Takahashi, Hoshino, & Sato, 1975). Complications include esophageal perforation at the time of dilation that may or may not require surgical repair.

ACQUIRED DEFECTS

Corrosive Injury to the Esophagus

Children are by nature curious creatures and do not hesitate to put various substances in their mouths. Parental negligence, ignorance, or child abuse are potential causes for ingestion (Raffensperger, 1990). In the older child, suicidal intent must be considered. A high degree of family stress, such as the loss of a family member, physical illness, or mental illness, is associated with corrosive ingestion (Raffensperger, 1990).

Corrosive substances come in various liquid, gel, and crystal forms. Liquids tend to be gulped rapidly by children and primarily cause injury to the mouth, hypopharynx, esophagus, stomach, and occasionally the small intestine. Little evidence of oral injury may exist because the substance may have been swallowed too rapidly. Solid substances tend to stick to the oral mucosa and are spit out by the child as they begin to cause pain. These agents primarily cause injury to oral structures and surrounding skin. However, they may cause damage to the esophagus as well (Shikowitz, Levy, Villano, Graver, & Pochaczevsky, 1996). Alkaline chemicals are the most damaging. They cause liquefaction necrosis of the esophagus, which can involve the

mucosa, submucosa, and muscular wall (Shikowitz et al., 1996). Liquefaction continues until dilution is sufficient to alter the caustic agent to a near neutral pH. Acid injuries most often involve the antrum of the stomach.

The effect of caustic injury depends on the extent of damage to the wall of the esophagus (Figure 13–5). The depth of injury predicts the amount of stricture formation. Mucosal erythema alone is usually without significant sequelae. Full-thickness injury may lead to perforation of the esophagus, mediastinitis, and injury to mediastinal structures.

Clinical Presentation

Ingestion of a caustic substance should be suspected if the child is found drooling and refusing foods. The child may have a hoarse cry or respiratory distress (Millar & Cywes, 1998; Raffensperger, 1990).

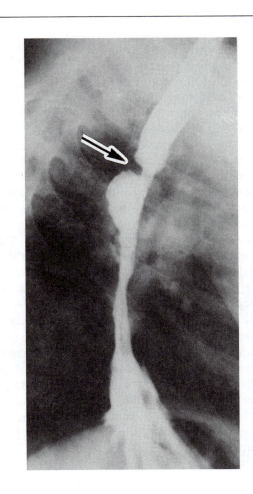

Figure 13–5 Injury to Esophagus after Ingestion of Oven Cleaner. Arrow points to area of stricture. Note ragged appearance of esophageal mucosa distal to stricture.

Diagnosis

Diagnosis and treatment are contingent on identification of the ingested substance. Caregivers are encouraged to bring the container of the suspected substance to the hospital with the child. The child remains NPO during the evaluation phase. The oral cavity should be carefully examined under strong lighting and suction equipment should be kept available. The amount of damage to the oral mucosa does not predict the extent of injury to the esophagus. Injury to the esophagus after ingestion is immediate. What passes into the stomach is most often in such a dose that it is buffered with gastric acid to neutrality, thereby halting further injury.

With the exception of household bleach, a mild irritant that does not require extensive evaluation (Anderson, Rouse, & Randolph, 1990), ingestion of most substances, particularly those that contain either sodium or potassium hydroxide, call for endoscopic evaluation. Esophagoscopy to evaluate the extent of injury should be carried out within 24 hours of ingestion.

Treatment

Initial treatment involves supportive care with intravenous fluids before determination of the extent of injury. Vomiting should not be induced because this returns the substance to the esophagus, where it can do further damage. Ingestion of large amounts of fluid should also be avoided because this may also lead to vomiting.

Admission to the hospital is based on the child's clinical condition. An intensive care unit admission should be arranged for the child who has had a massive ingestion of an alkaline substance. Radiologic studies of the chest and neck help determine the extent of tracheal edema, mediastinal widening, and signs of perforation. Esophagoscopy is usually done with the child under general anesthesia. The rigid esophagoscope is passed up to but not through the most proximal observed injury. Flexible endoscopy has the added advantage of allowing the stomach and duodenum to be evaluated (Anderson et al., 1990b).

Depth of injury is graded as first, second, and third degree as with skin burns. First-degree injury is characterized by superficial mucosal hyperemia, edema, and sloughing. Second degree involves transmucosal injury; the entire wall of the esophagus has exudate and ulceration is present. The injury extends into muscle. Third-degree injury involves erosion through the esophagus into the periesophageal tissues, including the mediastinum, or perforation into the pleural or peritoneal cavities (Raffensperger, 1990).

Linear burns are of less clinical significance than circumferential burns, which cause stricture. Tracheostomy placement is indicated for extensive injuries that cause increasing stridor (Raffensperger, 1990). Shock and signs of peritonitis are indicative of necrosis and possible stomach perforation.

Early esophageal perforation indicates almost total destruction of the esophagus. In this case, an esophagostomy and gastrostomy should be placed. Plans should begin for eventual esophageal substitution. Some surgeons advocate immediate esophagectomy and gastrectomy if massive ingestion has occurred to prevent liquefaction necrosis of the mediastinal structures.

The first 4 days after the ingestion constitute the acute inflammatory phase. Children with first-degree injuries are given fluids and allowed to resume a regular diet in 24 to 48 hours (Anderson et al., 1990b). These children do not stricture. The subacute phase lasts up to 15 days. At the end of this phase, the necrotic tissue sloughs and leaves a denuded ulcerated surface. Swelling decreases and swallowing may return to normal function. The child may be re-endoscoped during the subacute phase to evaluate the extent of injury and healing. The third phase takes place during the third to fourth weeks after ingestion; the inflammatory reaction subsides and tissue contraction begins. Normal tissue is replaced by dense fibrous scar tissue. Reepithelialization is usually complete by the sixth week (Shikowitz et al., 1996).

Steroid therapy to decrease the inflammatory response and thus prevent stricture formation has been in use since the 1950s. Dexamethasone, 0.3 mg/kg/day in four divided doses, is begun within the first 2 days of injury (Raffensperger, 1990). Steroids are continued until there is evidence that the mucosa has healed. More recent information has strongly suggested that the use of steroids in the treatment of esophageal injury is ineffective (Anderson et al., 1990b; Millar & Cywes, 1998; Shikowitz et al., 1996). Antibiotics are usually begun immediately after the injury to prevent infection and are continued while the child is receiving steroids.

Some surgeons advocate early esophageal dilation before strictures develop. Others may use esophageal stents or nasogastric tubes to prevent stricture formation. If evidence of stricture formation is present, a gastrostomy may be placed to assist with feedings, as well as retrograde dilations (Millar & Cywes, 1998).

Complications

Complications can be divided into three phases (Shikowitz et al., 1996). The acute phase occurs during the first 72 hours. This is when there is a high risk of circulatory collapse and pulmonary necrosis resulting from aspiration. The latent phase occurs during the first and second week, when infection, perforation, and abscess can occur. The third phase, or delayed complications, result in esophageal stricture. Strictures are the most common sequelae of corrosive injury to the esophagus. These are treated with scheduled dilations and in severe cases may require resection. In severe cases of esophageal stricture, esophageal replacement may be indicated. Severe damage to the hypopharynx, larynx, and cervical esophagus make eventual esophageal substitution challenging (Raffensperger, 1990; Shikowitz et al., 1996).

Other more serious complications include TEF and aorto-esophageal fistula resulting from erosion and damage to the mediastinal structures (Millar & Cywes, 1998).

Follow-up Care

In the event of mild damage to the esophagus, the child may be discharged from the hospital if he or she is asymptomatic and has a normal esophagram. The child should be closely followed clinically and reevaluated with an esophagram as needed.

Suicide attempt should be included in the differential diagnosis in the older child who has ingested a large quantity of a caustic substance. After stabilization of the child's condition, psychiatric evaluation and intervention share an equal role in the ongoing medical management. Even those who have not made a suicide attempt may need such intervention because injuries caused by ingestion may adversely affect the emotional outcome and physical well-being of the child.

Esophageal Stricture

Acquired esophageal strictures in childhood are most likely a result of reflux esophagitis, corrosive injury, or anastomotic scarring (Allmendinger et al., 1996). The scarring across an anastomosis is made worse by the presence of GER. The management of this situation includes treatment of the stricture and the identification, correction, and prevention of reflux.

Clinical Presentation

Presenting signs and symptoms of stricture include drooling, inability to swallow saliva or fluids, ability to take liquids but not solids, and regurgitation of undigested food. Stricture should be suspected if the preceding signs are accompanied by a history of esophageal surgery, injury, or reflux disease (Holder, 1993).

Diagnosis

The diagnosis is established with an esophagram (Holder, 1993). Esophagoscopy is used to evaluate the character and length of stricture, the ability to dilate the defect, and the condition of the mucosa (Millar & Cywes, 1998). Passing a barium-filled Penrose tube down the esophagus at the time of esophagoscopy yields an accurate fluoroscopic view of the length and character of the stricture (K.D. Anderson, personal communication, June 1998).

Treatment

Universal treatment of esophageal strictures involves dilation with various types of dilators. Sedation for dilation varies but may include oral and intravenous sedation or general anesthesia. Methods of dilation vary among surgeons. Ante-grade methods of dilation include the passing of rubber/silicone or balloon dilators through the mouth. Proponents of balloon dilation report that it produces a uniform radial force causing less trauma on the esophagus than Bougie dilators, which exert a shearing axial force (Allmendinger et al., 1996; Ashcraft, 1993). Retrograde dilation with Tucker dilators through an existing gastrostomy is considered one of the safest methods of dilating. The disadvantage of retrograde dilation is that a guide string may be left in the esophagus between dilations. This string, which exits the mouth or nostril, often causes much distress to the older child. Potential complications of dilation include perforation and septicemia. After routine dilation, the child is awakened, allowed to drink, and discharged home.

The number of dilations needed before abandoning the esophagus and committing to the replacement of the organ varies among surgeons. The child's quality of life should be considered when evaluating the response to dilations. Frequency of dilations depends on the child's clinical condition. The child who is able to take modified oral feedings and goes months between dilations may not need to have the esophagus replaced. In contrast, the child who is fed by gastrostomy and needs to be dilated every few weeks because of the inability to swallow oral secretions should have the esophagus replaced in an effort to normalize life as much as possible. The timing of substitution depends on failure of dilation as a primary method of treatment (Pederson, Klein, & Andrews, 1996).

Follow-up

Subsequent dilations are performed at scheduled intervals as required by the patient's symptoms. Esophagrams may not be indicated if the esophagus is routinely visualized during dilation. Occasionally the stricture persists radiographically, but the child compensates by more forceful swallowing and thorough mastication of food.

Foreign Body in the Esophagus

Congenital or acquired esophageal strictures halt the passage of an object that may have otherwise been swallowed without difficulty. Common culprits are fibrous foods, such as meats and stringy vegetables; foods with sharp edges, such as french fries and corn chips; and bulky foods, such as breads and tortillas. In children with normal esophageal anatomy, the areas of physiologic narrowing such as the cricopharyngeus, aortic arch, and cardioesophageal sphincter are often the sites where objects lodge. In this case, the foreign body is usually something in the child's immediate environment such as a small toy, coin, safety pin, or other sharp item (Gans & Austin, 1993). Swallowed batteries from toys or calculators are problematic because they may cause corrosive injury as well.

Clinical Presentation

The child may be initially seen with dysphagia, drooling, choking, or pain. If the swallowed object is large, coughing and respiratory distress may be present as the object distends the esophagus and compresses the trachea. Oftentimes, the caregiver has witnessed the ingestion or has evidence of the ingestion from other items found in the environment. Aspiration pneumonia, fever, cough, signs of perforation, or TEF may develop if the presence of a foreign body has been missed or neglected (Gans & Austin, 1993).

Diagnosis

Diagnostic tests include plain films of the chest and neck. If the item is radio-opaque, the size and location of the object will be evident. If the object is difficult to visualize, a barium swallow may be needed (Raffensperger, 1990).

Treatment

Removal of foreign bodies is best accomplished with the child under general anesthesia. Endotracheal intubation is used to prevent respiratory obstruction by pressure of the foreign body or endoscope. Retrieval of the foreign body is usually successful with the endoscope and forceps (Gans & Austin, 1993; Raffensperger, 1990).

Follow-up

Although difficult to remove all potential objects for aspiration from the environment, parents should be counseled or given written information on how to childproof their environment. Particular emphasis should be placed on the provision of age-appropriate toys for their children.

FUNCTIONAL DEFECTS OF THE ESOPHAGUS

Functional disorders of the esophagus are few but severely limit the ability to eat and thrive when present. They may affect the capacity to attain normal developmental milestones. The most common functional disorder is GER. Chapter 16 is devoted to the management of this condition. Other functional disorders include diffuse esophageal spasm as seen in achalasia, lack of normal peristalsis as evidenced in scleroderma, and impaired function as seen when esophageal diverticula are present. The latter are so rare that they are rarely seen in clinical practice in children.

ESOPHAGEAL REPLACEMENT

Although pediatric surgeons generally agree that the native esophagus is superior to anything used to replace it, there may be a time when substitution is necessary (Stone, Fonkalsrud, Mahour, Weitzman, & Takiff, 1985). Age of replacement varies with condition but it can be performed in early infancy if the child is clinically stable (Vargas-Gomez, 1994). Pederson and associates (1996) reported replacement as early as 36 days after birth in premature infants.

Indications for Replacement

The most common reason for substitution is long-gap esophageal atresia followed by severe caustic injury and benign strictures that are too long for resection and primary anastomosis (Campbell, Webber, Harrison, & Campbell, 1982; Stone et al., 1985). These strictures are caused by reflux esophagitis, corrosive injury, or anastomotic scarring. Barrett's epithelium in the distal esophagus may warrant full replacement. Major disruption of an anastomosis may also lead to esophageal replacement.

Preoperative Care

Children with esophageal disease are a nutritional challenge. Many children with an esophageal defect have a gastrostomy tube in place to provide adequate calories. The child's pulmonary status should be assessed, particularly if aspiration has been a part of the clinical picture. Although these children require aggressive pulmonary care, usually they do not improve until the esophageal defect is repaired.

Options for Substitution

Properties of the ideal esophageal substitute are that it should closely mimic in size and function the native esophagus, particularly in reference to peristaltic activity; it should not occupy a large space in the thorax; and it should have a good blood supply (Table 13–1). In addition, the operative procedure should be relatively straightforward with a low complication rate (Spitz, 1992).

Regardless of technique, the intestinal tract must be thoroughly cleansed before surgery. Various methods of cleansing include elemental diet, laxatives, and rectal irrigations. This preparation may begin several days before surgery, and much of it can be done at home. Older children may begin a liquid diet as early as 3 days before surgery, switching to clear liquids the day before. Most will be admitted to the hospital the day before to ensure that the bowel is adequately cleansed before surgery. Intravenous antibiotics are given on call to the operating room to prevent postoperative infection. Many surgeons advocate the use of oral antibiotics preoperatively to decrease the bacterial flora in the intestine.

Operative Repair

Colon Interposition

The colon remains the most frequently used organ for replacing the esophagus (Campbell et al., 1982; Lindahl,

Table 13–1 Types of Esophageal Replacement—Advantages and Disadvantages

Procedure	Advantages	Disadvantages
Colon interposition	Readily available Good blood supply[a] Easy to mobilize[a] Adequate length usually attained[a,c]	Leaks/strictures at anastomotic sites[a] Redundancy of graft over time[a] Slow transit time/stasis of food[b] GER[d] May have difficulty swallowing[d] May have cervical bulge on swallowing[d] Transient diarrhea[d]
Reversed gastric tube	Ease of procedure[a] Good blood supply[c] Adequate length usually attained[c] Rapid transit of food[c] Readily available	Leaks/strictures at cervical anastomosis[c] May not be long enough to reach proximal esophagus high in neck[a] GER[b,d]
Gastric transposition ("pull-up")	Ease of procedure[a,c] Adequate length usually attained[c] Good blood supply[c] Readily available	Bulk in chest may cause respiratory problems[c] GER[c] May have delayed gastric emptying[c] Poor blood supply if needed high in neck[a] Transient dysphagia[b] May have transient dumping syndrome[b]
Jejunal interposition	Adequate length readily available[a] Caliber of substitution similar to esophagus[c] Peristaltic activity[c]	Precarious blood supply making needed length difficult to attain[a,c]

[a] Otherson, Smith, & Tagge, 1995. [b] Myers, Beasley, & Auldist, 1991b. [c] Spitz, 1991. [d] Anderson, Noblett, Belsey, & Randolph, 1990.

Louhimo, & Virkola, 1983; Spitz, 1992) (Figure 13–6). Right, left, or transverse colon is used per surgeon preference (Figure 13–7). The colon may be placed in the retrosternal position posterior to the left lung by means of a left thoracotomy or by way of the transhiatal route eliminating the need for thoracotomy. The arguments against retrosternal replacement include increased incidence of leakage at anastomosis, higher rate of cervical stricture, dysphagia, and cervical bulge on swallowing (Ahmad et al., 1995). Those who favor this method claim better function with fewer complications (Stone et al., 1985). It is imperative to identify that no cardiac anomaly is present that would require correction by means of a median sternotomy because this approach would be difficult with a retrosternal colon in place. The colon is anastomosed to the cervical esophagus through a separate neck incision. The transposed colon may be placed in an isoperistaltic or antiperistaltic manner. In early studies the colon was described as merely a conduit dependent on gravity to propel food; later research claims that sequential propulsive waves might be present with isoperistaltic placement (Kelly, Shackelford, & Roper, 1983). Additional procedures may include appendectomy, gastrostomy, gastric fundoplication, and pyloroplasty or pyloromyotomy.

Reversed Gastric Tube

A relatively straightforward procedure, the reversed gastric tube has become the favored method of replacement in several major pediatric centers around the world (Anderson et al., 1990a; Lindahl et al., 1983). After determining that the stomach is large enough with a preoperative contrast study, the abdominal cavity is entered by means of a midline or left subcostal incision. A tube is fashioned from the greater curvature of the stomach based on a pedicle of the left gastroepiploic artery. This tube is then tunneled through the native esophageal bed, retrosternally or transthoracically (Figure 13–8). The child should be prepared for a colon interposition if the stomach is found to be unsuitable during surgery. Pyloroplasty is not usually necessary. A small intussuscepted portion of the distal gastric tube at its junction with the stomach can be sutured to prevent reflux (Buras, Jacir, & Anderson, 1986).

Gastric Transposition

A gastric pull-up is technically the simplest replacement procedure. Anatomic variants such as a small stomach, unsuitable colon, or previous failed interpositions may make

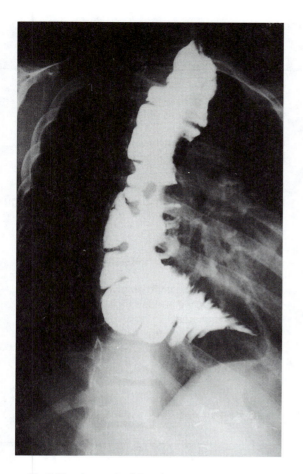

Figure 13–6 Esophagram of Esophageal Replacement with Colonic Interposition

presence of a single surgical anastomosis, an excellent blood supply to the transposed organ, and the fact that adequate length is almost always obtained ensures good results with this procedure (Spitz, 1992). Extended long-term follow-up is not yet available.

Jejunal Transposition

Theoretically, the use of the jejunum as a substitute is ideal because it has the appropriate diameter and peristaltic action (Figure 13–10). There is technical difficulty in attaining length without sacrificing adequate vascularity (Cusick, Batchelor, & Spicer, 1993). Despite extensive reports of Russian experience with the procedure, there is no detailed information on the ages of the children, complications, or long-term functional results (Ring, Varco, L'Heureux, & Foker, 1982). Ring et al. (1982) reported minimal complications in the early and late postoperative periods in 16 children who underwent jejunal replacement surgery. Free jejunal

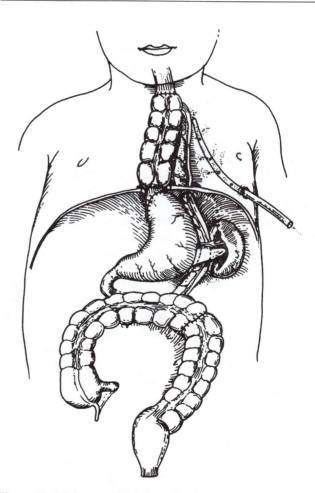

Figure 13–7 Diagram of Esophageal Substitution with Transverse Colonic Segment

this the only available option. In this procedure, the stomach is exposed by means of a midline abdominal incision and the previous gastrostomy site is closed. The stomach is then brought up into the chest through the hiatus and anastomosed to the proximal stump of the healthy esophagus (Figure 13–9). A pyloroplasty usually accompanies the procedure (Spitz, 1992). Early problems reported include gastric reflux, dumping syndrome, and dysphagia. These usually resolve in time. Because many of these children are born with a tenuous respiratory system, there is concern of having a potentially distensible organ in the chest. However, it appears that the stomach tubularizes with time and functions more like a conduit than a reservoir in this position (Davenport et al., 1996). Recently, it has been reported that the denervated stomach as an esophageal substitute is not merely a conduit but a contractile organ that demonstrates increasing motor activity with time (Collard, Romangnoli, Otte, & Kestens, 1998). This activity may aid in the propulsion of food. The

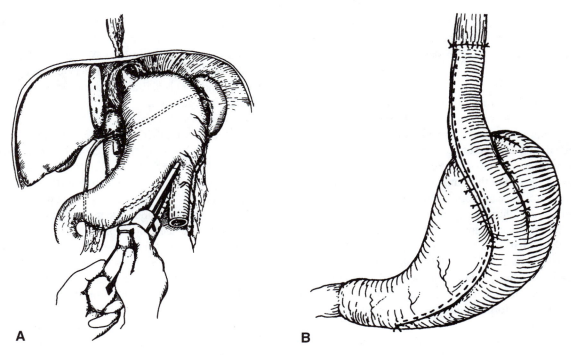

A   **B**

Figure 13–8 Creation of Reversed Gastric Tube. A, Using a stapler, the tube is fashioned from the greater curvature of the stomach. B, It is then tunneled through the native esophageal bed and anastomosed to the upper esophagus.

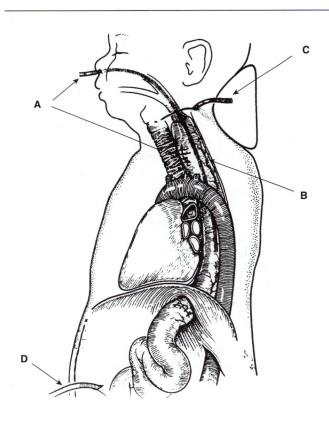

Figure 13–9 Lateral Diagram of Child with Gastric Transposition. A, nasogastric decompression tube; B, pulled-up gastric segment; C, drain at cervical anastomosis; and D, jejunal feeding tube.

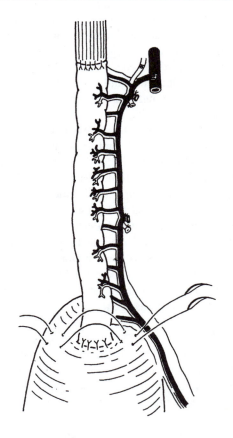

Figure 13–10 Esophageal Substitution Using Piece of Jejunum

grafts with microvascular surgery are routinely done to augment and attain length in colonic and gastric tube interpositions that do not reach a short proximal esophageal pouch.

Postoperative Care

Close monitoring is required in the early postoperative period. The child may remain intubated for several days, depending on the postoperative respiratory status. The head should be slightly elevated to decrease the amount of stress on the cervical anastomosis. A Penrose drain is usually left in the neck at the site of the cervical anastomosis to drain any fluid collection. A gastrostomy tube is present in those children who have undergone a colon interposition, reversed gastric tube, or jejunal transposition. A jejunal tube will be placed in those that have had a gastric pull-up. It is imperative that these enteral tubes are left to gravity drainage until peristalsis commences. Clamping these tubes prematurely may cause reflux into the transposed segment and lead to disruption or stricture formation at the anastomotic sites (Raffensperger, 1990).

If there is no drainage from the neck wound, a contrast study is obtained in approximately 1 week. The cervical drain is removed if there are no radiologically demonstrated leaks at the time of the study. The child is then allowed to eat orally (Ahmad et al., 1995). Commencement of an oral diet as early as 4 days after surgery has been reported, providing there is no leakage from the cervical drain and no indication of disruption of the anastomosis (Marujo, Tannuri, & Maksoud, 1991). The diet is advanced slowly. Soft food cut into small pieces is offered until the child is old enough to understand the principle of thorough mastication. The child should eat upright and remain in this position for at least 1 hour after eating. If there is a demonstrated leak at the cervical anastomosis, the child is kept NPO until resolution of this leak.

Enteral feedings are resumed after intestinal function returns. The feeding tubes are not removed until it is proven that there are no delayed surgical complications and the child is able to eat orally and sustain weight.

Parenteral antibiotics are administered for approximately 7 days to avoid postoperative infections at the anastomotic and incisional sites. As with any major abdominal and thoracic surgery, pain is to be expected. Children should be kept pain free by the use of epidural catheters to deliver analgesia in addition to intravenous agents.

Complications

Low complication rates and good functional results depend on experience with the operative technique rather than on which substitute is used (Campbell et al., 1982). Complications can be grouped as immediate, intermediate, and long term.

Necrosis of the transposed segment is most often seen with colon interpositions and is considered an immediate complication because it is seen mostly in the early postoperative period (Stone et al., 1985). The occurrence is reported to be as high as 18%. When this occurs, the transposed segment is removed, a cervical esophagostomy is placed, and the child is allowed to recover before attempting another interposition.

Anastomotic leak at the cervical esophagocolic/gastric anastomosis is another immediate complication and has been described in 2.8% to 70% of cases (Campbell et al., 1982; Ring et al., 1982; Stone et al., 1985). Most of these leaks close spontaneously. A rare and unfortunate complication is perforation through the cervical anastomosis by a suction catheter. Catheters should be measured from the upper dental ridge before each intervention.

Other early and less common complications include *wound infections, pneumonia, pneumothorax, pericarditis*, and *Horner's syndrome* (Stone et al., 1985).

The list of long-term complications is extensive. *Strictures* may develop at the anastomotic areas and are the most common. Anastomosis to a scarred proximal esophagus, as in corrosive injury, predisposes to stricture formation (Bassiouny & Bahnassy, 1992). Persistent strictures may need to be surgically revised.

Food obstruction in the neoesophagus can be a result of narrowing at the site of stricture and/or ingestion of large amounts or pieces of food without adequate fluid intake (Lindahl et al., 1983). Fibrous foods, such as meats and certain vegetables, can be particularly troublesome and may need to be removed endoscopically.

Over time, these colons may become very boggy and redundant (Lindahl et al., 1983). Food can sit for long periods of time in a patulous colon interposition. Fetid breath can be a social problem. Substantial ingestion of liquid aids in the propulsion of food. *Graft redundancy* may need revision or replacement if causing severe dysphagia (Bassiouny & Bahnassy, 1992).

Dumping syndrome is due to rapid gastric emptying and is usually seen in children who eat a hypertonic meal. It is more common in children who have had a gastric pull-up. This is usually a transient problem. It does not appear to be associated with the presence or absence of pyloroplasty (Ravelli, Spitz, & Milla, 1994).

Transient *diarrhea* may be observed after colon transposition. On average, two to three loose stools daily are reported but with only occasional social inconvenience. Stool incontinence is common in children who have also had repair of high imperforate anus. It is possible that resecting the colon for replacement causes decreased water absorption in the shortened colon, thus aggravating the condition in these children (Anderson et al., 1990a).

Children with a gastric pull-up have been identified as having problems with *anemia* as documented by low serum ferritin levels. Iron absorption is facilitated by presence of acid in the stomach. It is thought that poor absorption is caused by atrophic gastritis and hypochlorhydria (Davenport et al., 1996). It is suggested that these children receive iron supplementation (Davenport et al., 1996).

GER is present in 60% of children who have had colonic interposition. Antireflux procedures can be performed at the time of surgery; however, this may cause problems in a colon that depends mostly on gravity to empty. Some surgeons believe that GER is better controlled when the replacement surgery is delayed until the infant is able to sit up for feedings. The colon is thought to be resistant to peptic ulceration because of its mucus production. Alkaline secretions of the colon neutralize the refluxed gastric acid. However, ulceration with bleeding may occur in the interposed segment and is more common in colon substitution. Food stasis within the colon segment causing ulceration has been reported. These children should be followed for possible dysplastic changes, which may lead to cancer. Reflux is present in children who have had a gastric pull-up or reversed gastric tube procedure. These children should also adhere to reflux precautions. A modified plication at the lower end of the gastric tube is often successful in minimizing reflux (Buras et al., 1986). A comparative study between children who underwent a colon interposition in the United Kingdom and those who had a reversed gastric tube in the United States did not identify GER as a major problem in either population (Anderson et al., 1990). Feeding through an enteral tube in the early postoperative period and continuous or small frequent feedings instead of feeding large boluses minimizes the risk of reflux into the replaced segment.

Postoperative *pneumonia* is almost always caused by aspiration. A transient early *growth delay* is present in those who have had esophageal atresia. This appears to resolve in the early adolescent period. No evidence of growth delay exists in children who have had esophageal replacement for other conditions (Campbell et al., 1982; Stone et al., 1985). Other long-term complications include *small bowel obstruction* from adhesions and *dysphagia*. Death is rare with this surgery and is usually attributable to pulmonary complications (Ahmad et al., 1995).

Discharge Planning

As with any medically fragile child, considerable effort should be devoted to planning for discharge from the hospital. Patients with complications usually have an extensive list of needs. Most of these children do well. Follow-up care should focus on nutritional status. Consult a dietitian to assist the family and medical team in choosing appropriate foods and recommending supplementation by means of an enteral tube when indicated.

These children should be observed for any signs of anastomotic stricture, especially if there was an anastomotic leak in the postoperative period. The surgeon may elect to place the child on a schedule for dilation or decide to follow the child with dilation on an as-needed basis. The family is instructed to call the office if the child is experiencing increased difficulty swallowing or regurgitating food.

If these children are school age, they may find themselves behind in their studies because of missed school days. Efforts should be made to commence studies as soon as possible during hospitalization and convalescence at home. Involving the school nurse is beneficial because he or she can function as the child's advocate once the child returns to school. Copies of discharge instructions and phone numbers of the primary health team should accompany the child back to school.

REFERENCES

Ahmad, S.A., Sylvester, K.G., Hebra, A., Davidoff, A.M., McClane, S., Stafford, P.W., Schnaufer, L., & O'Neill, J. (1995). Esophageal replacement using the colon: Is it a good choice? *Journal of Pediatric Surgery, 31*(8), 1026–1031.

Allmendinger, N., Hallisey, M.J., Markowitz, S.K., Hight, D., Weiss, R., & McGowan, G. (1996). Balloon dilatation of esophageal strictures in children. *Journal of Pediatric Surgery, 31*(3), 334–336.

Anderson, K.D., Noblett, H., Belsey, R., & Randolph, J.G. (1990). Long-term follow-up of children with colon and gastric tube interposition for esophageal atresia. *Surgery, 111*(2), 131–136.

Anderson, K.D., Rouse, T.M., & Randolph, J.G. (1990). A controlled trial of corticosteroids in children with corrosive injury of the esophagus. *New England Journal of Medicine, 323,* 637–640.

Andrassy, R.J., Ko, P., Hanson, B.A., Kubota, E., Hays, D.M., & Mahour, G.H. (1980). Congenital esophageal fistula without esophageal atresia. *American Journal of Surgery, 140,* 731–733.

Ashcraft, K.W. (1993). The esophagus. In K.W. Ashcraft & T.M. Holder (Eds.), *Pediatric surgery* (2nd ed., pp. 228–248). Philadelphia: W.B. Saunders Company.

Bankier, A., Brady, J., & Myers, N.A. (1991). Epidemiology and genetics. In S.W. Beasley, N.A. Myers, & A.W. Auldist (Eds.), *Oesophageal atresia* (pp. 19–27). New York: Chapman & Hall.

Bassiouny, I.E., & Bahnassy, A.F. (1992). Transhiatal esophagectomy and colonic interposition for caustic esophageal stricture. *Journal of Pediatric Surgery, 27*(8), 1091–1096.

Beasley, S.W. (1991a). Embryology. In S.W. Beasley, N.A. Myers, & A.W. Auldist (Eds.), *Oesophageal atresia* (pp. 31–42). New York: Chapman & Hall.

Beasley, S.W. (1991b). Oesophageal atresia without fistula. In S.W. Beasley, N.A. Myers, & A.W. Auldist (Eds.), *Oesophageal atresia* (pp. 137–158). New York: Chapman & Hall.

Beasley, S.W., & Auldist, A.W. (1991). Oesophageal atresia with distal tracheo-esophageal fistula. In S.W. Beasley, N.A. Myers, & A.W. Auldist (Eds.), *Oesophageal atresia* (pp. 119–134). New York: Chapman & Hall.

Brown, T.C.K., Eyres, R., & Myers, N.A. (1991). Anaesthesia and perioperative care. In S.W. Beasley, N.A. Myers, & A.W. Auldist (Eds.), *Oesophageal atresia* (pp. 103–115). New York: Chapman & Hall.

Buras, R.R., Jacir, N.N., & Anderson, K.D. (1986). An antireflux procedure for use with the reversed gastric tube. *Journal of Pediatric Surgery, 21*(6), 545–547.

Campbell, J.R., Webber, B.R., Harrison, M.W., & Campbell, T.J. (1982). Esophageal replacement in infants and children by colon interposition. *The American Journal of Surgery, 144,* 29–34.

Chavin, K., Field, G., Chandler, J., Tagge, E., & Otherson, H.B. (1996). Save the child's esophagus: Management of major disruption after repair of esophageal atresia. *Journal of Pediatric Surgery, 131*(1), 48–52.

Collard, J.M., Romangnoli, R., Otte, J.B., & Kestens, P.J. (1998). The denervated stomach as an esophageal substitute is a contractile organ. *Annals of Surgery, 227*(1), 33–39.

Crabbe, D.C.G., Kiely, E.M., Drake, D.P., & Spitz, L. (1996). Management of the isolated tracheoesophageal fistula. *European Journal of Pediatric Surgery, 6,* 67–69.

Curci, M.R., & Dibbins, A.W. (1988). Problems associated with a Nissen fundoplication following tracheoesophageal fistula and esophageal atresia repair. *Archives of Surgery, 123,* 618–620.

Cusick, E.L., Batchelor, A.A.G., & Spicer, R.D. (1993). Development of a technique for jejunal interposition in long-gap esophageal atresia. *Journal of Pediatric Surgery, 28*(8), 990–994.

Davenport, M., Hosie, G.P., Tasker, R.C., Gordon, I., Kiely, E.M., & Spitz, L. (1996). Long-term effects of gastric transposition in children: A physiological study. *Journal of Pediatric Surgery, 31*(4), 588–593.

David, T.J., & O'Callaghan, S.E. (1974). Cardiovascular malformation and oesophageal atresia. *British Heart Journal, 36,* 559.

Donahoe, P.K., & Gee, P.E. (1984). Complete laryngotracheoesophageal cleft: Management and repair. *Journal of Pediatric Surgery, 19*(2), 143–148.

Dubois, J.J., Pokorney, W.J., Harberg, F.J., & Smith, R.J.H. (1990). Current management of laryngeal and laryngotracheoesophageal clefts. *Journal of Pediatric Surgery, 25*(8), 855–860.

Filler, R.M., & Forte, V. (1998). Lesions of the larynx and trachea. In J.A. O'Neill, Jr., M.I. Rowe, J.L. Grosfeld, E.W. Fonkalsrud, & A.G. Coran (Eds.), *Pediatric surgery* (5th ed., pp. 863–872). St. Louis, MO: Mosby.

Gans, S.L., & Austin, E. (1993). Foreign bodies. In K.W. Ashcraft & T.M. Holder (Eds.), *Pediatric surgery* (2nd ed., pp. 82–88). Philadelphia: W.B. Saunders Company.

Greenwood, R.D., & Rosenthal, A. (1976). Cardiovascular malformations with tracheoesophageal fistula and esophageal atresia. *Pediatrics, 57,* 87.

Gross, R.E. (1953). *The surgery of infancy and childhood.* Philadelphia: W.B. Saunders Company.

Gutierrez, C., Barrios, J.E., Lluna, J., Vila, J.J., Garcia-Sala, C., Roca, A., & Ruiz Company, S. (1994). Recurrent tracheoesophageal fistula treated with fibrin glue. *Journal of Pediatric Surgery, 29*(12), 1567–1569.

Harmon, C.M., & Coran, A.G. (1998). Congenital anomalies of the esophagus. In J.A. O'Neill, Jr., M.I. Rowe, J.L. Grosfeld, E.W. Fonkalsrud, & A.G. Coran (Eds.), *Pediatric surgery* (5th ed., pp. 941–967). St. Louis, MO: Mosby.

Harrison, M.R., Hanson, B.A., Mahour, G.H., Takahashi, M., & Weitzman, J.J. (1977). The significance of right aortic arch in repair of esophageal atresia and tracheoesophageal fistula. *Journal of Pediatric Surgery, 12,* 861–869.

Holder, T.M. (1993). Esophageal atresia and tracheoesophageal malformations. In K.W. Ashcraft & T.M. Holder (Eds.), *Pediatric surgery* (2nd ed., pp. 249–269). Philadelphia: W.B. Saunders Company.

Jolly, S.G., Johnson, D.G., Roberts, C.C., Herbst, J.J., Matlak, M.E., McCombs, A., & Christian, P. (1980). Patterns of gastroesophageal reflux in children following repair of esophageal atresia and distal tracheoesophageal fistula. *Journal of Pediatric Surgery, 15,* 857–867.

Kelly, J.P., Shackelford, M.D., & Roper, C.L. (1983). Esophageal replacement with colon in children: Functional results and long-term growth. *The Annals of Thoracic Surgery, 36*(6), 634–640.

Lindahl, H., Louhimo, I., & Virkola, K. (1983). Colon interposition or gastric tube? Follow-up study of colon-esophagus and gastric tube-esophagus patients. *Journal of Pediatric Surgery, 18*(1), 58–63.

Lipshutz, G.S., Albanese, C.T., Harrison, M.R., & Jennings, R.W. (1997). Anterior cervical approach for repair of laryngotracheoesophageal cleft. *Journal of Pediatric Surgery, 33*(2), 400–402.

Marujo, W.C., Tannuri, U., & Maksoud, J.G. (1991). Total gastric transposition: An alternative to esophageal replacement in children. *Journal of Pediatric Surgery, 26*(6), 676–681.

McCallion, W.A., Hannon, R.J., & Boston, V.E. (1992). Prophylactic extrapleural chest drainage following repair of esophageal atresia: Is it necessary? *Journal of Pediatric Surgery, 27*(5), 561.

Mee, R.B.B. (1991). Congenital heart disease. In S.W. Beasley, N.A. Myers, & A.W. Auldist (Eds.), *Oesophageal atresia* (pp. 229–239). New York: Chapman & Hall.

Millar, J.W., & Cywes, S. (1998). Caustic strictures of the esophagus. In J.A. O'Neill, Jr., M.I. Rowe, J.L. Grosfeld, E.W. Fonkalsrud, & A.G. Coran (Eds.), *Pediatric surgery* (5th ed., pp. 969–979). St. Louis, MO: Mosby.

Mulvihill, S.J., Stone, M.M., Debas, H.T., & Fonkalsrud, E. (1985). The role of amniotic fluid in fetal nutrition. *Journal of Pediatric Surgery, 20* (6), 668–672.

Murphy, S.G., Yazbeck, S., & Russo, P. (1995). Isolated congenital esophageal stenosis. *Journal of Pediatric Surgery, 30*(8), 1238–1241.

Myers, N.A., Beasley, S.W., & Auldist, A.W. (1991a). Associated anomalies. In S.W. Beasley, N.A. Myers, & A.W. Auldist (Eds.), *Oesophageal atresia* (pp. 211–226). New York: Chapman & Hall.

Myers, N.A., & Beasley, S.W. (1991b). Diagnosis. In S.W. Beasley, N.A. Myers, & A.W. Auldist (Eds.), *Oesophageal atresia* (pp. 77–91). New York: Chapman & Hall.

Myers, N.A., Beasley, S.W., & Auldist, A.W. (1991b). Oesophageal replacement. In S.W. Beasley, N.A. Myers, & A.W. Auldist (Eds.), *Oesophageal atresia* (pp. 171–190). New York: Chapman & Hall.

Ohkawa, T., Takahashi, H., Hoshino, Y., & Sato, H. (1975). Lower esophageal stenosis in association with tracheobronchial remnants. *Journal of Pediatric Surgery, 10*(4), 453–457.

Otherson, H.B., Smith, C.D., & Tagge, C.P. (1995). In L. Spitz & A.G. Coran (Eds.), *Rob & Smith's operative surgery: Pediatric Surgery* (5th ed.) (pp. 136–142). New York: Chapman & Hall.

Pederson, J.C., Klein, R.L., & Andrews, D.A. (1996). Gastric tube as the primary procedure for pure esophageal atresia. *Journal of Pediatric Surgery, 31*(9), 1233–1235.

Poenaru, D., Laberge, J.M., Neilson, I.R., Nguyen, L.T., & Guttman, F.M. (1991). A more than 25-year experience with end-to-end versus end-to-side repair for esophageal atresia. *Journal of Pediatric Surgery, 26*(4), 472–477.

Quan, L., & Smith, D.W. (1973). The VATER association: Vertebral defects, anal atresia, T-E fistula with esophageal atresia, radial and renal dysplasia: A spectrum of associated defects. *Journal of Pediatrics, 82,* 104.

Raffensperger, J.D. (Ed.). (1990). *Swenson's pediatric surgery* (5th ed.). Norwalk, CT: Appleton & Lange.

Randolph, J.G., Newman, K.D., & Anderson, K.D. (1989). Current results in repair of esophageal atresia with tracheoesophageal fistula using physiologic status as a guide to therapy. *Annals of Surgery, 209*(5), 526–531.

Ravelli, A.M., Spitz, L., & Milla, P.J. (1994). Gastric emptying in children with gastric transposition. *Journal of Pediatric Gastroenterology and Nutrition, 19*(4), 403–409.

Ring, W.S., Varco, R.L., L'Heureux, P.R., & Foker, J.E. (1982). Esophageal replacement with jejunum in children. *Journal of Thoracic Cardiovascular Surgery, 83*, 918–927.

Robie, D.K., Pearl, R.H., Ronsales, R.D., & Hoffman, M.A. (1991). Operative strategy for recurrent laryngotracheoesophageal cleft: A case report and review of the literature. *Journal of Pediatric Surgery, 26*(8), 971–974.

Roy, R.N.D. (1991). Transport of the neonate with oesophageal atresia. In S.W. Beasley, N.A. Myers, & A.W. Auldist (Eds.), *Oesophageal atresia* (pp. 93–102). New York: Chapman & Hall.

Ryan, D.P., Muehrcke, D.D., Doody D.P., Kim, S.H., & Donahoe, P.K. (1991). Laryngotracheoesophageal cleft (type IV): Management and repair of lesions beyond the carina. *Journal of Pediatric Surgery, 26*(8), 962–970.

Santos, A.D., Thompson, T.R., Johnson, D.E., & Foker, J.E. (1983). Correction of esophageal atresia with distal tracheoesophageal fistula. *Journal of Thoracic Cardiovascular Surgery, 85*, 229–236.

Shaul, D.B., Schwartz, M.Z., Marr, C.C., & Tyson, K.R.T. (1989). Primary repair without routine gastrostomy is the treatment of choice for neonates with esophageal atresia and tracheoesophageal fistula. *Archives of Surgery, 124*, 1188–1191.

Shikowitz, M.J., Levy, J., Villano, D., Graver, L.M., & Pochaczevsky, R. (1996). Speech and swallowing rehabilitation following devastating caustic ingestion: Techniques and indicators for success. *Laryngoscope, 106*, 1–12.

Snyder, C.L., Ramachandran, V., Kennedy, A.P., Gittes, G.K., Ashcraft, K.W., & Holder, T.M. (1997). Efficacy of partial wrap fundoplication for gastroesophageal reflux after repair of esophageal atresia. *Journal of Pediatric Surgery, 32*(7), 1089–1092.

Spitz, L. (1992). Gastric transposition for esophageal substitution in children. *Journal of Pediatric Surgery, 27*(2), 252–259.

Spitz, L. (1995). Cervical esophagostomy. In L. Spitz & A.G. Coran (Eds.), *Rob & Smith's operative surgery: Pediatric surgery* (5th ed., pp. 121–123). New York: Chapman & Hall.

Spitz, L. (1996). Esophageal atresia: Past, present, and future. *Journal of Pediatric Surgery, 31*(1), 19–25.

Stokes, K.B. (1991). Pathophysiology. In S.W. Beasley, N.A. Myers, & A.W. Auldist (Eds.), *Oesophageal atresia* (pp. 59–71). New York: Chapman & Hall.

Stone, M.M., Fonkalsrud, E.W., Mahour, G.H., Weitzman, J.J., & Takiff, H. (1985). Esophageal replacement with colon interposition in children. *Annals of Surgery, 203*(4), 346–351.

Stringer, M.D., McKenna, K.M., Goldstein, R.B., Filly, R.A., Adzick, N.S., & Harrison, M.R. (1995).Prenatal diagnosis of esophageal atresia. *Journal of Pediatric Surgery, 30*(9), 1258–1263.

Touloukian, R.J. (1992). Reassessment of the end-to-side operation for esophageal atresia with distal tracheoesophageal fistula: 22-year experience with 68 cases. *Journal of Pediatric Surgery, 27*(5), 562–567.

Tovar, J.A., Diez-Pardo, J.A., Murcia, J., Prieto, G., Molina, M., & Polanco, I. (1995) Ambulatory 24-hour manometric and pH metric evidence of clearance capacity in patients with esophageal atresia. *Journal of Pediatric Surgery, 30*(8), 1224–1231.

Vargas-Gomez, M. (1994). Esophageal replacement in patients under 3 months of age. *Journal of Pediatric Surgery, 29*(4), 487–491.

Wheatley, M.J., Coran, A.G., & Wesley, J.R. (1993). Efficacy of the Nissen fundoplication in the management of gastroesophageal reflux following esophageal atresia repair. *Journal of Pediatric Surgery, 28*(1), 53–55.

Appendix 13–A

Critical Pathway for Esophageal Atresia with Distal Tracheoesophageal Fistula

	PRE-OP	O.R.	POD #1	POD #2–6	POD #7–10
Monitoring	1. VS q 1 hr 2. Strict I & O 3. Cardiac monitor 4. Pulse oximeter 5. Isolette/radiant warmer	6. Chest dressing dry & intact	1. VS q 2 hr 6. dc chest dressing; Steri-strips dry & intact	1. VS q 4 hr if stable 5. dc isolette/radiant warmer when infant able to maintain stable temp	
Treatments	1. ± ET intubation	2. Suctioning "depth marker at bedside" 3. Suction pharynx gently PRN	1. Extubate if infant stable		
Lines & Drains	1. Peripheral IV 2. Oroesophageal tube to lo-cont. suction	2. dc oroesophageal tube 3. Chest drain to low suction 4. ± Gastrostomy	1. Start TPN	3. POD #5–7 dc chest drain if no clinical/radiographic evidence of anastomotic leak	1. Decrease TPN as oral feedings increase; dc IV before discharge
Medication	1. Vitamin K 2. Antibiotic prophylaxis	2. Antibiotics 3. Analgesics 4. Sedation		2. dc antibiotics at 48 hr postop; per surgeon preference, may continue until chest drain removed	
Activity	1. Position supine/side-to-side 2. Elevate HOB	3. Do not hyperextend neck			

Tests	1. Labwork: CBC, Chem panel, T&C, ABG 2. Radiologic studies: chest, abdomen, spine 3. Ultrasonography: cardiac, renal, spinal ------	1. CBC, PRN blood gas 2. CXR postop	1. CBC, Chem panel, PRN blood gas 2. CXR ------ 3. Complete all ultrasonography	1. Cont. CBC, Chem panel 2x wkly. Cont. PRN blood gases --- 2. CXR after chest tube removal and before discharge 4. POD #5–7 contrast esophagram
Diet	1. NPO ------			1. May start oral feedings if no evidence of anastomotic leak after esophagram. Start with pedialyte, advance to breast milk/formula as tolerated.
Consults	1. Social work 2. As needed: cardiology, urology, orthopaedics, neurosurgery ------		2. Complete medical/surgical consults	1. Complete social services consult and eval of home environment
Teaching	1. Unit orientation 2. Outline pre- and postoperative plan of care 3. Obtain informed surgery consent 4. EA/TEF handout 5. Encourage mother to pump breasts		2. Continue to outline plan of care	6. Begin discharge teaching: ------ ❑ Gastrostomy care ❑ Wound care ❑ S & S infection ❑ Diet ❑ Activity ❑ CPR ❑ Monitors & pumps ❑ Respiratory care
Discharge Planning	1. Begin eval of home environment (see social services consult) 2. Encourage caregivers to visit and stay with infant as much as possible to learn specialized care		3. Provide support group info: ❑ EA/TEF ❑ VATERS NETWORK ❑ PULL-THROUGH NETWORK	4. Arrange F/U appts: ❑ Surgeon/APN ❑ Pediatrician ❑ ± Cardiologist, urologist, neurosurgery, orthopaedics, pulmonary, dietary, social services. 5. Provide resource phone numbers. 6. Arrange for delivery of discharge supplies. 7. Arrange for home nursing visit.

CHAPTER 14

Congenital Lung Malformations

Teri Crawley-Coha

INTRODUCTION

Congenital malformations of the lung are uncommon and make up a small percentage of the pediatric surgical population. The most common anomalies, and the ones that are discussed in this chapter, are congenital cystic adenomatoid malformation, pulmonary sequestration, bronchogenic cyst, and congenital lobar emphysema. These lesions are pathologically distinct but share similar clinical and embryologic characteristics (dell'Agnola, Tadini, Mosca, Colnaghi, & Wesley, 1996). They may become apparent at any age but are typically recognized prenatally, at birth, or during the first 6 months of life.

Because the most significant problem for infants with congenital diaphragmatic hernia (CDH) is development of the lung, CDH is also included in this chapter. However, CDH is a more complex lesion with many possible treatments and therefore is discussed separately.

CONGENITAL CYSTIC ADENOMATOID MALFORMATION, PULMONARY SEQUESTRATION, BRONCHOGENIC CYST, AND CONGENITAL LOBAR EMPHYSEMA

Overall, congenital lung malformations occur at a 1.3 to 1 ratio of males to females. No ethnic or racial predominance has been found. They are rarely familial. Both the right and left lung are equally affected, bilateral involvement is rare, and usually only one lobe on the affected side is diseased. Associated defects occur in approximately one third of these children (Buntain, Isaacs, Payne, Lindesmith, & Rosenkrantz, 1974).

Most of these lesions are recognized in the first 6 months of life. Neonates have symptoms of a space-occupying lesion, tachypnea, cyanosis, and dyspnea. Diagnosis after the neonatal period occurs when the lesion is found on chest radiography obtained for other reasons or when the patient is seen with a fever, cough, or purulent sputum or symptoms of infection or abscess (Buntain et al., 1974). Bronchogenic cysts and intralobar pulmonary sequestrations are more common diagnoses of late presentation. The identification of the exact type of lesion before excision is sometimes difficult, and a definitive diagnoses is determined after excision.

Advances in and increased use of obstetric ultrasonography and prenatal diagnosis have led to an increase in the diagnosis of congenital lung lesions during the antenatal period. The lesions diagnosed before birth are usually congenital cystic adenomatoid malformation and pulmonary sequestration (Carrol, Campbell, Shaw, & Pilling, 1996; Hernanz-Schulman, 1993).

Serial ultrasonography is recommended to monitor the fetus when a lung abnormality is diagnosed in utero. In the absence of fetal hydrops, many of these infants can easily be carried to term and ultimately do well. However, because the fetus may experience respiratory distress at birth requiring admission to a neonatal intensive care unit for ventilatory support, arrangements should be made for delivery at a tertiary care center (Miller, Corteville, & Langer, 1996). When hydrops is present in conjunction with one of these lung abnormalities, the probability of in utero or neonatal death is great and fetal intervention may be indicated (Adzick et al., 1993; Brown, Lewis, Brouillette, Hilman, & Brown, 1995; Bullard & Harrison, 1995).

The prevailing recommendation for treatment, even in the absence of symptoms, is complete surgical excision at or near the time of diagnosis. This practice is based on the belief that a percentage of the lesions will eventually become symptomatic, increasing surgical morbidity.

An understanding of the spectrum of congenital lung malformations is helpful for nurses who may be involved with the care of these families in a variety of settings: during fetal ultrasonography, prenatal counseling, and labor and delivery or in the neonatal intensive care unit, pediatrician's office, or emergency room.

Four congenital lung lesions are discussed in this chapter. For clarity and ease of reading, they are defined first followed by a brief review of lung development.

Congenital Cystic Adenomatoid Malformation (CCAM): a multi-cystic mass of pulmonary tissue in which there is proliferation of bronchial structures at the expense of alveoli. The cysts are lined by cuboidal or columnar epithelium. This disease is considered a focal pulmonary dysplasia, rather than a hamartoma,* since in many cases there is skeletal muscle in the cyst walls.

Pulmonary Sequestration (PS): a mass, usually cystic, of non-functioning pulmonary tissue that lacks normal communication with the tracheobronchial tree and which receives most or all of its arterial blood from anomalous systemic vessels. In extralobar sequestration, the abnormal tissue is separate from the normal pulmonary lobes; intralobar sequestrations are contained within the affected lobe.

Bronchogenic Cyst (BC): a discrete mass of non-functioning pulmonary tissue, the cysts are lined by ciliated columnar epithelium and the tissue often includes smooth muscle, glands, and cartilage. There is usually no communication with the tracheobronchial tree.

Congenital Lobar Emphysema (CLE): a postnatal overdistention of one or more lobes of a histologically normal lung, thought to result from cartilaginous deficiency in the tracheobronchial tree. (Buntain et al., 1974)

Lung Development

The development of the trachea, bronchi, bronchioles, and lungs begins as a laryngotracheal groove in the floor of the foregut at about 26 days (Figure 14–1). The grooves deepen, creating walls that separate the tubes of the trachea and esophagus (Crouch & McClintic, 1976). The bulb-shaped lung bud then quickly divides into two knoblike bronchial buds. During the fifth week, each bronchial bud enlarges to form the primordium of a main bronchus. The main or pri-

*A hamartoma is defined as "a tumor resulting from new growth of normal tissues. The cells grow spontaneously, reach maturity, and then do not reproduce" (Thomas, 1989, p. 777).

mary bronchi subdivide into secondary bronchi. Each secondary bronchus continues to undergo progressive branching. The muscular, cartilaginous, and connective tissue coats begin to form at about 10 weeks (Crouch & McClintic, 1976). By the 24th week, approximately 17 orders of branches have formed, and the bronchioles have developed (Moore & Persaud, 1993).

Diagnosis

Diagnosis of congenital lung disease by serial prenatal ultrasonography is reliable and allows the practitioner to develop management plans based on prognosis (dell'Agnola et al., 1996). Some lesions, both large and small, will shrink, whereas other lesions persist with fetal development of nonimmune hydrops (MacGillivray, Harrison, Goldstein, & Adzick, 1993).

Diagnosis in infants and children can generally be made on the basis of symptoms and chest radiography. Computed tomography, magnetic resonance imaging, or Doppler ultrasonography may also be used to evaluate the lesion (Aktogu, Yunca, Halilcolar, Ermete, & Buduneli, 1996; Hernanz-Schulman, 1993; Schwartz & Ramachandran, 1997). An accurate diagnosis may be of lesser importance for surgical treatment than anatomic definition (dell'Agnola et al., 1996).

Hydrops Fetalis

The incidence of nonimmune hydrops is approximately 1 in 2,500 to 3,500 neonates. Diagnosis of nonimmune hydrops is an indicator of poor fetal and neonatal prognosis, with prenatal mortality rates ranging from 50% to 98%. Hydrops is often associated with fetomaternal hemolytic disease. Nonimmune hydrops fetalis refers to the occurrence of hydrops without hematologic evidence of fetomaternal blood group incompatibility (Seeds & Azizkhan, 1990). A diagnosis of fetal hydrops is made when there is generalized skin thickening and/or two or more of the following: placental thickness enlargement greater that 6 cm, ascites, pleural fluid, and pericardial fluid. Conditions associated with hydrops include infection, cardiac anomalies, renal disease, gastrointestinal disorders, and placental cord and chromosomal anomalies (Seeds & Azizkhan, 1990). The nonimmune type has also been recognized in the presence of congenital pulmonary malformations, most commonly in association with CCAM and pulmonary sequestration (Evans, 1996).

Treatment

In the presence of nonimmune hydrops associated with CCAM and PS, fetal death is almost certain. If the fetus is less than 32 weeks, an intrauterine intervention may be an

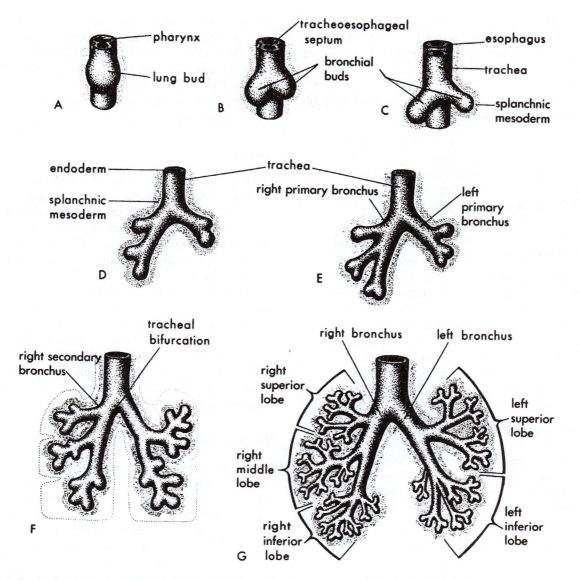

Figure 14–1 Successive Stages in the Development of the Bronchi and Lungs. A to C, Four weeks. D and E, Five weeks. F, Six weeks. G, Eight weeks.

option. Interventions with some reported success include fetal thoracentesis, thoracoamniotic shunting, or surgical resection of the enlarged pulmonary lobe. Thoracentesis has demonstrated some success, but the fluid may reaccumulate (Brown et al., 1995). In centers where thoracoamniotic catheters were used, some were successful whereas others found the catheters difficult to place and reported limited long-term decompression. Resection of the mass in utero is also occasionally successful with resolution of hydrops, return of the mediastinum to the midline, and impressive in utero growth of the lung (Adzick et al., 1993; Bullard & Harrison, 1995).

After confirmation of the diagnosis, additional evaluation includes amniocentesis or percutaneous umbilical blood sampling to exclude chromosomal anomalies and a fetal echocardiogram to assess for fetal heart disease. If the fetus is greater than 32 weeks, early delivery and ex utero resection is advised (Bullard & Harrison, 1995).

In congenital lung malformations diagnosed after the neonatal period, treatment varies. In general, patients who are initially seen with symptoms undergo surgical excision. The treatment for asymptomatic patients, however, is controversial. Many authors express concern over the potential for complications when surgical excision is postponed, including compression of adjacent tissue and organs, infection with risk of rupture and hemorrhage, recurrence in the case of segmental resection, and the development of malignancy (Aktogu et al., 1996; dell'Agnola et al., 1996; Gharagozloo, Dausmann, McReynolds, Sanderson, & Helmers, 1995; Nobuhara, Gorski, LaQuaglia, & Shamberger, 1997; Othersen, 1993; Schwartz & Ramachandran, 1997). However, other authors state that monitoring asymptomatic patients is acceptable, citing cases of infants and children who remain asymptomatic (Bromley, Parad, Estroff, & Benacerraf, 1995).

CYSTIC ADENOMATOID MALFORMATION

Cystic adenomatoid malformation is an abnormal development of pulmonary tissue with failure of the terminal bronchiolus to form channels (Seeds & Azizkhan, 1990). Most (83%) are diagnosed before 6 months of age. Males and females are equally affected. The right and left lung are equally affected, with single lobe disease occurring four times more often than multilobe disease (Cloutier, Schaeffer, & Hight, 1993). Diagnosis of CCAM may be made prenatally on ultrasonography, during the newborn period because of respiratory difficulty, or later in life when the mass becomes infected, presenting as recurrent pneumonia or lung abscess (dell'Agnola, Tadini, Mosca, & Wesley, 1992).

Stocker, Madewell, and Drake (1977) divided CCAM into three distinct pathologic types as follows:

> Type I: Single or multiple cysts (usually numbering between one and four) greater than 2 cm in diameter and lined by ciliated pseudostratified columnar epithelium. The walls of the cysts contain smooth muscle and elastic tissue. Relatively normal alveoli may lie between the cysts. There may be communication between the cyst and the normal bronchial tree.

> Type II: Multiple small cysts, less than 1 cm in diameter lined by ciliated cuboidal or columnar epithelium. Structures similar to respiratory bronchioles and distended alveoli may be present between the cysts. Mucous cells and cartilage are not present. This type is associated with a high incidence of other congenital anomalies.

> Type III: A large bulky, noncystic lesion that often produces a mediastinal shift. Bronchiole-like structures are lined by ciliated cuboidal epithelium and separated by masses of alveolus-size structures lined by nonciliated cuboidal epithelium. The lesion involves the entire lobe or lobes with no normal lung tissue visible (See Figure 14–2).

There are other classifications that separate the lesion into two rather than three anatomic types (Adzick et al., 1985; Seeds & Azizkhan, 1990). Seeds and Azizkhan (1990) define type I as the replacement of normal lung tissue by multiple large cysts in a lobar distribution that varies in size and is anechoic; they define type II as a diffuse lesion that results in replacement of the entire lung with microscopic cysts that enlarge the lung and are echodense. Adzick et al. (1985) proposed two categories on the basis of gross anatomy, ultrasonographic findings, and prognosis. Macrocystic disease consists of single or multiple fluid-filled cystic tumors at least 5 mm in diameter, whereas microcystic lesions are solid and bulky with cysts less than 5 mm in diameter.

Children with CCAM may have minor or severe associated congenital anomalies. Associated anomalies occur in 18% of the patients, with renal agenesis and cardiac anomalies predominating (Cloutier et al., 1993).

Controversy exists over management of children with CCAM. It is unclear whether outcome is determined by ease of resection or absence of fetal hydrops. Seeds and Azizkhan (1990) state that type I carries a good prognosis because it is easily resectable, whereas the diffuse distribution in type II makes resection impossible. Increased mortality is found in infants with concomitant hydrops. Ultrasonography allows serial monitoring. Prenatal counseling, especially related to elective termination of the pregnancy, should acknowledge that these children often have a positive outcome. A discussion of fetal interventions should only occur in the presence of hydrops (Adzick et al., 1985; Brown et al., 1995; Evans, 1996; Miller et al., 1996).

A small percentage of patients with CCAM are not seen until after the newborn period (MacDonald, Forte, Cutz, & Crysdale, 1996). There are also a few reports of CCAM in adults (Lackner, Thompson, Rikkers, & Galbraith, 1996).

PULMONARY SEQUESTRATION

Pulmonary sequestration is an isolated lobe of lung tissue, without parenchymal connection to the bronchial system, supplied by an aberrant artery arising from the aorta or one of its branches and usually drained by the pulmonary veins (Savic, Birtel, Tholen, Funke, & Knoche, 1979; Seeds & Azizkhan, 1990). The isolated area can interfere with the growth and development of adjacent structures (Figure 14–3).

The anomaly originates from the embryonic foregut, making it one of the bronchopulmonary foregut malformations that include enteric cysts, bronchogenic cysts, esophageal duplication, and tracheoesophageal fistulas. It occurs "when there is separation of a segment of the lung or a separate out pouching from the foregut anlage. The timing of the separation is important in that if the sequestered lung tissue arises before pleura formation, the sequestration will be intralobar and surrounded by normal lung tissue. When the sequestra-

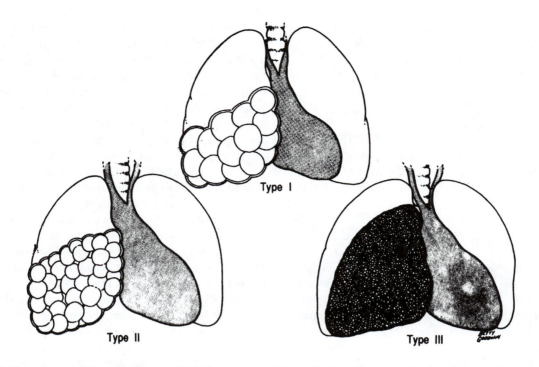

Figure 14–2 Three Types of Cystic Adenomatoid Malformations as Classically Described. Detailed descriptions of the lesion are better than type classifications.

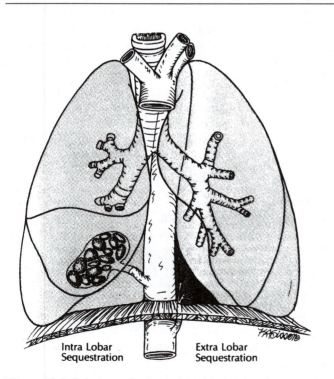

Figure 14–3 Pulmonary Sequestration. A sequestered segment or lobe has no bronchial communication with the trachea or any foregut derivative. Arterial blood supply is from the aorta or other systemic vessel. Venous return is usually through the pulmonary veins. Extralobar sequestrations are isolated and asymptomatic.

tion arises after pleural development, it will be invested by its own pleura and will be extralobar and separate from the remaining pulmonary parenchyma" (Seeds & Azizkhan, 1990, p. 233). Intralobar is more common than extralobar. Although rare, they can present together. They occur most often in the lower lobes and usually only one lobe is involved (Savic et al., 1979).

Pulmonary sequestration is not believed to have a genetic predisposition with only one reported case of two males with PS born to the same parents (Abuhamad, Bass, Katz, & Heyl, 1996). Associated congenital malformations occur approximately 14% of the time (Savic et al., 1979) and increase the mortality rate from 42% to 75% (Chan, Greenough, & Nicolaides, 1996).

The diagnosis of PS is made in the newborn period because of the effect on respiratory function, in older children with chronic respiratory infections, and more commonly today in the antenatal period with ultrasonography (Evans, 1996). Use of prenatal Doppler ultrasonography has helped to identify the anomalous systemic artery indicative of PS (King, Pillling, & Walkinshaw, 1995; MacGillivray et al., 1993). Pulmonary or aortic angiography confirms diagnosis, demonstrates the abnormal vessels, and alerts the surgeon to their location but is only rarely used today (Othersen, 1993).

Intralobar Sequestration

The aberrant artery in 74% of the cases is from the thoracic aorta, and in just less than 15% of cases, more than one anomalous artery is found (Savic et al., 1979). Symptoms generally present in the first decade of life. The most common associated congenital anomalies are esophagobronchial diverticulum, diaphragmatic hernias, skeletal deformities, and heart defects (Savic et al., 1979; Seeds & Azizkhan, 1990).

Children with intralobar sequestrations are predisposed to chronic lung infections, abscess formation, and hemorrhage (Luck, Reynolds, & Rafensberger, 1986). The most common symptoms are cough, expectoration, and recurrent pneumonia. In early series, such as Savic et al. (1979), 15.5% were discovered by chance. They occur slightly more often in the left lung. The lower lobe has a significantly greater occurrence than the upper lobes, specifically the posterior basilar segment (Savic et al., 1979).

Extralobar Sequestration

In 77% of the cases, extralobar sequestrations occur between the diaphragm and the lower lobe. Nearly 80% occur in the left lobe. Arterial supply is provided by a branch of the aorta. Congenital anomalies are more common in intralobar sequestration, occurring 50% to 59% of the time. The most common associated anomaly is diaphragmatic hernia. Less common are congenital heart defects, chest wall abnormalities, and vertebral abnormalities (Savic et al., 1979; Seeds & Azizkhan, 1990).

Treatment is controversial. Seeds and Azizkhan (1990) recommend resection in the neonatal period, projecting a good prognosis for those without severe pulmonary hypoplasia. In a small series, MacGillivray et al. (1993) reported that no resections were performed in infants with PS. Four of five with an antenatal mediastinal shift had no perceptible mass during final prenatal ultrasonographic examination and the fifth was barely perceptible. After delivery, only one had an abnormal chest radiograph examination; four showed lung opacity or sequestration on magnetic resonance imaging or computed tomography scans and were not resected.

BRONCHOGENIC CYST

Abnormal budding from a segment of the tracheobronchial tree is believed to be responsible for the development of bronchogenic cysts (Luck et al., 1986). Small isolated groups of cells form discrete masses of nonfunctioning tissue. They may be centrally located, near the hilum or mediastinum, or located peripherally. Multiple cysts are more likely to occur peripherally, such as in the lung parenchyma, and are also more likely to have bronchial communication.

The occurrence of multiple cysts usually results in respiratory distress at birth. Generally, bronchogenic cysts are spherical and air filled if they communicate with the airway. When no communication exists, they may appear as solid masses (Othersen, 1993). They may have no patent communication with the airway but may be attached to the airway or the esophagus by dense fibrous tissue. Those that occur in the extrathoracic area, such as lower neck or upper chest wall, have no communication or fibrous connection to the airways (Rodgers, Harman, & Johnson, 1986).

The stage of embryonic development determines location of the lesion: the paratracheal or bronchial versus intraparenchymal. Cysts located in the mediastinum near the trachea, esophagus, carina, or main bronchi probably form early during separation of the embryonic foregut. Those that occur later in development, during budding and branching, grow within the lung parenchyma (Nobuhara et al., 1997; St-Georges et al., 1991).

Bronchogenic cysts are generally diagnosed during childhood. No gender predominance and generally no associated malformations exist (Nobuhara et al., 1997; Ribet, Copin, & Gosselin, 1996). Infants and children present with respiratory distress or other symptoms, resulting from compression of the lesion on surrounding structures, or with gastrointestinal complaints of vomiting or poor feeding. Mediastinal bronchogenic cysts produce symptoms by causing airway obstruction, whereas the pulmonary cyst produces symptoms of infection or compression, including cough and hemoptysis (Luck et al., 1986; Nobuhara et al., 1997; Ribet et al., 1996).

Extrathoracic cysts have presented as soft masses over the border of the sternum (Rodgers et al., 1986), over the scapula (Jona, 1995), or as neck masses (Nobuhara et al., 1997). Diagnosis is confirmed with chest radiograph examination, barium esophagram, or chest computed tomography scans (Nobuhara et al., 1997; Rodgers et al., 1986).

The literature supports surgical excision at the time of diagnoses even in asymptomatic patients. Left untreated, prognosis is unpredictable and late complications are frequent, including the threat of bacterial or fungal infection and malignancy (Nobuhara et al., 1997; Ribet et al., 1996; St-Georges et al., 1991). Segmentectomy is an option for small cysts (Ribet et al., 1996).

CONGENITAL LOBAR EMPHYSEMA

CLE is the postnatal overinflation of one or more lobes occurring in a histologically normal lung (Buntain et al., 1974). The etiology of CLE is unclear. One theory is that overinflation occurs when a congenital deficiency of bronchial cartilage is present. Air enters the affected area on inspiration and is trapped when the abnormally flaccid bronchial walls collapse on expiration (Hendren & McKee,

1966). A second theory is that a lesion, such as a redundant bronchial fold or mucus plug, acts as an intraluminal obstruction, again allowing air to enter but not to leave (Kravitz, 1994). In approximately 50% of the cases, the cause is never discovered (Stigers, Woodring, & Kanga, 1992).

Massive air trapping and overdistention leave the lobe physiologically useless and cause compression atelectasis of the ipsilateral lobe or lobes. The overdistended lobe also pushes the mediastinum toward the opposite side, causing compression atelectasis of the other lung, and interferes with venous return to the heart. Profound mediastinal displacement causes almost total collapse of the opposite lung (Hendren & McKee, 1966). Early studies indicated a left upper lobe predominance and single lobe involvement. More recent reports of smaller series describe multilobar and right lung involvement occurring more frequently (Hugosson, Rabeeah, Al-Rawaf, Bakheet, & Banjar, 1995; Stigers et al., 1992).

Congenital lobar emphysema is primarily a condition of early infancy, rarely seen after 6 months of age. Symptoms may be mild to severe, ranging from slight wheezing and increased respiratory rate to respiratory distress (Hendren & McKee, 1966). Cardiac defects are the most common congenital anomaly associated with lobar emphysema (Buntain et al., 1974; Hendren & McKee, 1966). In infants old enough to crawl and put objects in their mouth, aspiration of a foreign body is considered in the differential diagnosis.

A plain chest film demonstrating hyperexpanded and hyperlucent areas in the lung may be all that is needed for diagnosis (Hendren & McKee, 1966). Computed tomography or ventilation/perfusion scans, sometimes technically difficult in a neonate, may help identify additional involved lobes and rule out other conditions such as a vascular ring or thoracic mass as the cause (Markowitz, Mercurio, Vahjen, Gross, & Touloukian, 1989; Stigers et al., 1992).

Controversy exists about the timing and necessity of surgery. Excision of the affected lobes allows normal expansion and ventilation of adjacent lobes previously compressed (Hendren & McKee, 1966; Othersen, 1993). In the absence of persistent or progressive respiratory distress, some patients are managed conservatively and gradually become asymptomatic (Stigers et al., 1992).

NURSING CONSIDERATIONS FOR CHILDREN UNDERGOING THORACIC SURGERY

Correction of congenital lung malformations requires thoracic surgery. When the decision is made for an infant or child to undergo surgery for any congenital lung malformations, the parents and the child, when appropriate, should receive an explanation of what to expect.

The infant has an endotracheal tube placed in the operating room if he or she does not already have one. This allows the lungs to expand and function while subjected to atmospheric pressure. The incision used to gain access to the thoracic cavity may be anterior, lateral, or posterior, depending on the surgeon's preference and the exposure needed to perform the surgery. Entrance below the rib cage is gained by separating the ribs. To close, the ribs are approximated, intercostal muscles are sutured, the pleura is closed, muscles are approximated and sutured, and subcutaneous tissue and skin are closed. During thoracic surgery air enters the pleural space. To restore and maintain negative pressure postoperatively, chest tubes are inserted through a stab wound and secured to the chest wall with suture and tape. When caring for patient's with chest tubes, remember to keep connections tight, maintain the system components below the level of the patient's body to prevent reentry of air or fluid into the pleural cavity, maintain a secure dressing over the insertion site of the tube into the chest, and keep a clamp taped to the child's bed.

If stable, the infant is extubated in the operating room. If extubated, the nasogastric tube is also usually removed. The infant has intravenous lines to administer analgesia during the postoperative period and maintain fluids and electrolytes until able to consume a diet. Unrelieved pain prevents adequate rest and may interfere with ventilation. Discharge instructions include care of the incision and follow-up visits with the surgeon and pediatrician. The caremap reflects the needs of the infant and the family (Appendix 14–A).

CONGENITAL DIAPHRAGMATIC HERNIA

Historical Overview

The first case of CDH was recorded in the English literature in 1701 by Sir Charles Holt. He wrote of attending the postmortem examination of a 2-month-old infant. The mother reported that the child had been restless with labored breathing since his birth. She had observed an odd sort of working in his breast and "could perceive a crawling around the ribs and breast, on both sides, as if a knot of small eels or large earthworms had been penned up within the cavity" (Irish, Holm, & Glick, 1996, p. 628). Only the liver, kidney, and bladder were found in the abdomen. The mesentery was located in the cavity of the thorax lying on the heart and the lungs, and no omentum was found (Irish et al., 1996).

In 1761, Giovanni Battista Morgagni published descriptions of various types of diaphragmatic hernias, including the anterior diaphragmatic hernia, which bears his name. Victor Alexander Bochdalek, professor of anatomy at Prague in 1848, described CDH occurring through both right and left posterolateral diaphragmatic defects. Bettman and Hess performed the first successful repair in a child in 1929 (Irish et al., 1996).

Anatomy and Physiology

The diaphragm is a dome-shaped fibromuscular sheet that separates the thoracic and abdominal cavities. Normally, there are three openings in the diaphragm: the vena cava, the esophagus, and the aorta.

Congenital diaphragmatic hernias occur when the diaphragm does not form completely, leaving an opening between the thorax and the abdomen and allowing stomach, liver, and/or intestines to enter the thoracic cavity. The defect may be a small slit or a total absence of the diaphragm and may occur in several areas of the diaphragm. Eighty percent occur on the left side (de Lorimier, 1993). The most common congenital diaphragmatic hernia is the left posterolateral hernia or Bochdalek hernia. When the defect is located on the left, the small and large bowel, stomach, spleen, and left lateral segment of the liver may migrate into the thoracic cavity.

A small gap, called the foramina of Morgagni, forms in the musculature of the diaphragm on both sides of the xiphoid process between the attachments of the diaphragm to the xiphoid process and the seventh costal cartilage. Hernias, known as Morgagni hernias, may occur through this foramina but are extremely rare (Skandalakis, Colborn, & Skandalakis, 1997). When the defect is on the right, the small and large bowel may be in the chest, but more often it is the liver that enters the thoracic cavity (Bohn, Pearl, Irish, & Glick, 1996).

The pathogenesis of CDH remains unclear. After the description of diaphragmatic development by Broman in 1902, the occurrence of CDH was generally believed to result from failure of the pleuroperitoneal canals to close at the end of the embryonic period at 8 to 10 weeks. It was thought that this allowed bowel loops to herniate through the defect, resulting in pressure on the developing lung bud and lung hypoplasia (Kluth, Losty, Schnitzer, Lambrecht, & Donahoe, 1996). However, it later became clear that both lungs may have fewer bronchial divisions than normal. Also there is a deficiency in the alveolar number with an accompanying decrease in pulmonary vessels. The pulmonary arteries have an abnormally thick muscularis (de Lorimier, 1993). The lungs are also biochemically immature and deficient in surfactant (Breaux, Simmons, & Georgeson, 1995). From this knowledge, a second theory developed, suggesting that lung hypoplasia is the primary pathologic condition and that herniation of the intestine results in additional hypoplasia (Wilcox, Irish, Holm, & Glick, 1996). Research to study the development of the diaphragm and diaphragmatic hernias by creating the hernia with a herbicide in rats is ongoing (Kluth et al., 1996).

Incidence and Diagnosis

CDH occurs in 1 in 3,300 live births (Katz, Wiswell, & Baumgart, 1998) and 1 in 2,200 births when stillbirths are included (de Lorimier, 1993). CDH may be diagnosed during prenatal ultrasonography, which alerts the clinician to look for associated malformations and chromosomal abnormalities. Prenatal diagnosis allows for early consultation with the family regarding therapeutic options and expectations and planning for delivery at a tertiary care center.

Presentation

Infants with CDH generally have symptoms of respiratory distress develop in the first 24 hours of life. Infants with symptoms in the first 6 hours are considered high risk. Inspiration is difficult because the diaphragm is critical to the process. The negative pressure generated during inspiration produces additional herniation of the bowel into the thorax. Also, infants in respiratory distress swallow air, which further distends the bowel and compresses more of the lung (de Lorimier, 1993). Those with extreme pulmonary hypoplasia and atelectasis from surfactant deficiency develop hypoxemia, hypercarbia, and acidosis leading to a cycle of pulmonary vasospasm, pulmonary hypertension, right-to-left shunting of blood and worsening hypoxemia, hypercarbia, and acidosis. This cycle results in pulmonary hypertension of the newborn and death if it is not quickly interrupted (Breaux et al., 1995).

As the gastrointestinal tract fills with air, a mediastinal shift with pressure on the contralateral lung may occur, resulting in increased respiratory distress. The abdomen, void of abdominal viscera, is often scaphoid, and bowel sounds may be heard in the chest.

Late diagnosis, occurring after the newborn period, has been reported and usually is seen before 3½ years of age. These children exhibit symptoms of respiratory infection, fever, and cough or shortness of breath. They may also have gastrointestinal symptoms such as abdominal pain, nausea, and vomiting from obstruction caused by herniation of the bowel through the defect (de Lorimier, 1993).

Outcome

Reported survival averages 60%. Generally, the survival rate is highest for those infants born with an isolated diaphragmatic lesion, lower for those with CDH associated with other nonchromosomal anomalies, and approaching zero in infants with chromosomal defects (Langham et al., 1996). No relationship appears to exist between early diagnosis and survival. Wilson, Fauza, Lund, Benacerraf, and Hendren (1994) reviewed 183 cases of CDH and found no correlation between prenatal diagnoses of *isolated* CDH and outcome, even when the diagnosis occurred before 25 weeks' gestation. Infants with CDH and an associated congenital anomaly, especially a cardiac anomaly, fared poorly. The authors believe that infants with an associated anomaly are more likely to be diagnosed early because of the accompanying congenital malformation and that these additional risk factors lead to a poor outcome.

Treatment

Repair of the defect immediately after birth was one of the first approaches used for the treatment of CDH. The assumption was that the presence of abdominal viscera in the thorax caused compression of the lung bud, resulting in poor development of the ipsilateral lung. In addition, it was believed that compression of the contralateral lung occurred from pressure on the mediastinum from the abdominal organs (Bohn et al., 1996). Therefore, it seemed logical that adequate ventilation required removal of the abdominal viscera from the thoracic cavity. However, although infants often improved immediately after surgery, demonstrating normal blood gases on low ventilator settings, within a period of hours to days they progressively deteriorated. This deterioration probably results from numerous factors, including increased abdominal pressure with impaired visceral and peripheral perfusion, limited diaphragmatic excursion, overdistention of the alveoli and diminished alveolar-capillary blood flow in the hypoplastic lungs, release of vasoactive cytokines, and decrease in pulmonary compliance (de Lorimier, 1993). Various methods of ventilation can provide adequate oxygenation in a paralyzed infant without reducing the hernia. Postponing repair until the infant is physiologically stable is a common approach for CDH today. There may be no significant difference in survival between infants who undergo immediate repair and those who have delayed surgery (Nio, Haase, Kennaugh, Bui, & Atkinson, 1994).

For operative repair, a subcostal, oblique incision is made and the abdominal organs are gently removed from the chest. A primary repair is performed when possible, and a muscle flap or synthetic patch is used when the defect is too large for primary repair. The repair is influenced by the size of the infant, the size of the defect, and the size of the abdominal cavity (Bohn et al., 1996).

CDH is a complex problem of pulmonary hypoplasia and pulmonary hypertension. Infants with CDH often have persistent pulmonary hypertension of the newborn (PPHN). A variety of respiratory therapies are used to manage PPHN and pulmonary hypoplasia associated with CDH, including conventional ventilation, ECMO, oscillation, and nitric oxide. The traditional treatment for PPHN in all infants, including those with CDH, was hyperventilation. This treatment often resulted in significant pulmonary barotrauma (Bohn et al., 1996). In 1985, Wung, James, Kilchevsky, and James published a study that demonstrated successful treatment of persistent pulmonary hypertension of the newborn with pressure-limited ventilation, more commonly known as permissive hypercapnia. The goal is to maintain preductal oxygen

saturation at greater than 90%, ignoring postductal saturations and hypercarbia (Katz et al., 1998). Wung et al. (1985) used this approach successfully, demonstrating a decrease in pulmonary barotrauma.

Extracorporeal life support is a treatment that allows rest for the heart and lungs by allowing oxygen and CO_2 exchange to occur mechanically outside the body. It is indicated for "acute severe reversible cardiac and respiratory failure when the risk of dying from the primary disease despite optimal conventional treatment is high (50 to 100%)" (Zwischenberger & Bartlett, 1995, p. 13). Its use in the treatment of CDH was based on the assumption that the primary cause of deterioration is due to a reactive pulmonary vascular bed with abnormally muscularized vessels and right-to-left shunting across the ductus arteriosus and that these changes could reverse if the infant was supported on extracorporeal membrane oxygenation (ECMO) (Bohn et al., 1996). The Extracorporeal Life Support Organization reports a 58% survival rate in infants with CDH treated with ECMO. Infants with CDH are on ECMO longer and have a greater risk of complications than infants with other respiratory illnesses placed on ECMO (Breaux et al., 1995).

Nitric oxide has also been used in the treatment of CDH. Nitric oxide is a vasodilator that is highly selective to the pulmonary vasculature. It has not been very effective on infants before ECMO but has been used to speed the weaning process from ECMO. It also results in a significant improvement in some infants who continue to experience oxygenation difficulties after ECMO (Bohn et al., 1996; Katz et al., 1998).

High-frequency oscillation ventilation is another mode of treatment for infants with respiratory distress. Although infants with respiratory distress syndrome or pneumonia respond favorably, the benefit of high-frequency oscillation ventilation in the treatment of infants with CDH is unclear (Bohn et al., 1996).

In some situations, CDH is amenable to fetal surgery. Refer to Chapter 9 for more information.

Long-Term Problems

The follow-up studies on infants with CDH reveal a multitude of problems that vary in severity and frequency. It is often difficult to evaluate whether these problems occurred as the result of the disease or the result of the treatment. The most common problems associated with CDH are gastroesophageal reflux, chronic lung disease, and failure to thrive. Other complications include adhesive bowel obstruction, recurrence of the hernia particularly in patients with patch repairs, and neurodevelopmental delays (Katz et al., 1998).

Gastroesophageal reflux is evident in 62% to 80% of infants at the time of discharge (D'Agostino et al., 1995; Kieffer et al., 1995). The etiology of GER in children with CDH is multifactoral, including esophageal dilation, malposition of the stomach with a widened angle of His, a shorter intraabdominal portion of the esophagus, and an increased intraabdominal pressure resulting from reintroduction of the herniated viscera into the infant's abdominal cavity (Kieffer et al., 1995). Prolonged artificial ventilation and residual lung hypoplasia are the cause of persistent lung problems (D'Agostino, 1997; Ijsselstijn, Tibboel, Hop, Molenaar, & de Jongste, 1997).

Persistent feeding problems are also common. These infants tire easily, have inefficient suck, and may completely refuse oral feedings. Chronic lung disease, chest deformity, GER, esophagitis, and hypotonia all play a role in prolonged feeding difficulties (D'Agostino, 1997).

Chronic lung disease has been described in approximately one third of children with CDH. Artificial ventilation and residual lung hypoplasia seem to be the cause of persistent lung problems (D'Agostino, 1997; Ijsselstijn et al., 1997).

Routine developmental assessments are necessary to identify developmental delays early, and primary care physicians should refer these children for treatment. Delays in gross motor skills are more common than problems with cognitive skills (D'Agostino, 1997).

CONCLUSION

Congenital lung malformations are an uncommon finding in the pediatric population but a very interesting one for the surgeon and the nursing staff. The outcome for the family is based on the surgical care and the treatment, teaching, and support the family receives from the nursing staff.

REFERENCES

Abuhamad, A., Bass, T., Katz, M., & Heyl, P. (1996). Familial recurrence of pulmonary sequestration. *Obstetrics and Gynecology, 87*(5), 843–845.

Adzick, S., Harrison, M., Flake, A., Howell, L., Golbus, M., Filly, R., & The UCSF Fetal Treatment Center. (1993). Fetal surgery for cystic adenomatoid malformation of the lung. *Journal of Pediatric Surgery, 28*(6), 806–812.

Adzick, S., Harrison, M., Glick, P., Golbus, M., Anderson, R., Mahony, B., Callen, P., Hirsch, J., Luthy, D., Filly, R., & deLorimier, A. (1985). Fetal cystic adenomatoid malformation: Prenatal diagnosis and natural history. *Journal of Pediatric Surgery, 20*(5), 483–488.

Aktogu, S., Yunca, G., Halilcolar, H., Ermete, S., & Buduneli, T. (1996). Bronchogenic cysts: Clinicopathological presentation and treatment. *European Respiratory Journal, 9,* 2017–2021.

Bohn, D., Pearl, R., Irish, M., & Glick, P. (1996). Postnatal management of congenital diaphragmatic hernia. *Clinics in Perinatology, 23*(4), 843–872.

Breaux, C., Simmons, M., & Georgeson, K. (1995). Management of infants with congenital diaphragmatic hernia with ECMO. In J. Zwischenberger & R. Bartlett (Eds.), *Extracorporeal cardiopulmonary support in critical care.* Ann Arbor, MI: Extracorporeal Life Support Organization.

Bromley, B., Parad, R., Estroff, J., & Benacerraf, B. (1995). Fetal lung masses: Prenatal course and outcome. *Journal of Ultrasound in Medicine, 14,* 927–936.

Brown, M., Lewis, D., Brouillette, R., Hilman, B., & Brown, E. (1995). Successful prenatal management of hydrops, caused by congenital cystic adenomatoid malformation, using serial aspirations. *Journal of Pediatric Surgery, 30*(7), 1098–1099.

Bullard, K., & Harrison, M. (1995). Before the horse is out of the barn: Fetal surgery for hydrops. *Seminars in Perinatology, 19*(6), 462–473.

Buntain, W.L., Isaacs, H., Payne, V.C., Lindesmith, G.G., & Rosenkrantz, J.G. (1974). Lobar emphysema, cystic adenomatoid malformation, pulmonary sequestration, and bronchogenic cyst in infancy and childhood: A clinical group. *Journal of Pediatric Surgery, 9*(1), 85–93.

Carrol, E., Campbell, M., Shaw, B., & Pilling, D. (1996). Congenital lobar emphysema in congenital cytomegalovirus. *Pediatric Radiology, 26,* 900–902.

Chan, V., Greenough, A., & Nicolaides, K. (1996). Antenatal and postnatal treatment of pleural effusion and extra-lobar pulmonary sequestration. *Journal of Perinatal Medicine, 24,* 335–338.

Cloutier, M., Schaeffer, D., & Hight, D. (1993). Congenital cystic adenomatoid malformation. *Chest, 103*(3), 761–764.

Crouch, J., & McClintic, J.R. (1976). *Human anatomy and physiology* (2nd ed.). New York: John Wiley & Sons.

D'Agostino, J. (1997). Congenital diaphragmatic hernia: What happens after discharge? *Maternal Child Nursing, 22*(5), 263–266.

D'Agostino, J., Bernbaum, J., Gerdes, M., Schwartz, I., Coburn, C., Hirschl, R., Baumgart, S., & Polin, R. (1995). Outcome for infants with congenital diaphragmatic hernia requiring extracorporeal membrane oxygenation: The first year. *Journal of Pediatric Surgery, 30*(1), 10–15.

dell'Agnola, C., Tadini, B., Mosca, F., Colnaghi, M., & Wesley, J. (1996). Advantages of prenatal diagnosis and early surgery for congenital cystic disease of the lung. *Journal of Perinatal Medicine, 24*(6), 621–631.

dell'Agnola, C., Tadini, B., Mosca, F., & Wesley, J. (1992). Prenatal ultrasonography and early surgery for congenital cystic disease of the lung. *Journal of Pediatric Surgery, 27*(11), 1414–1417.

de Lorimier, A. (1993). Diaphragmatic hernia. In K. Ashcraft & T. Holder (Eds.), *Pediatric surgery* (2nd ed.). Philadelphia: W.B. Saunders Company.

Evans, M. (1996). Hydrops fetalis and pulmonary sequestration. *Journal of Pediatric Surgery, 31*(6), 761–764.

Gharagozloo, F., Dausmann, M., McReynolds, S., Sanderson, D., & Helmers, R. (1995). Recurrent bronchogenic pseudocyst 24 years after incomplete excision. *Chest, 108*(3), 880–883.

Hendren, H., & McKee, D. (1966). Lobar emphysema of infancy. *Journal of Pediatric Surgery, 1*(1), 24–39.

Hernanz-Schulman, M. (1993). Cysts and cystlike lesions of the lung. *Radiologic Clinics of North America, 31*(3), 631–649.

Hugosson, C., Rabeeah, A., Al-Rawaf, A., Bakheet, S., & Banjar, H. (1995). Congenital bilobar emphysema. *Pediatric Radiology, 25,* 649–651.

Ijsselstijn, H., Tibboels, D., Hop, W., Molenaar, J., & de Jongste, J. (1997). Long-term pulmonary sequelae in children with congenital diaphragmatic hernia. *American Journal of Respiratory Critical Care Medicine, 155,* 174–180.

Irish, M., Holm, B., & Glick, P. (1996). Congenital diaphragmatic hernia. *Clinics in Perinatology, 23*(4), 624–653.

Jona, J. (1995). Extramediastinal bronchogenic cysts in children. *Pediatric Dermatology, 12*(4), 304–306.

Katz, A., Wiswell, T., & Baumgart, S. (1998). Contemporary controversies in the management of congenital diaphragmatic hernia. *Clinics in Perinatology, 25*(1), 219–248.

Kieffer, J., Sapin, E., Berg, A., Beaudoin, S., Bargy, F., & Helardot, P. (1995). Gastroesophageal reflux after repair of congenital diaphragmatic hernia. *Journal of Pediatric Surgery, 30*(9), 1330–1333.

King, S.J., Pilling, D.W., & Walkinshaw, S. (1995). Fetal echogenic lung lesions: Prenatal ultrasound diagnosis and outcome. *Pediatric Radiology, 25,* 208–210.

Kluth, D., Losty, P., Schnitzer, J., Lambrecht, W., & Donahoe, P. (1996). Toward understanding the developmental anatomy of congenital diaphragmatic hernia. *Clinics in Perinatology, 23*(4), 655–669.

Kravitz, R. (1994). Congenital malformations of the lung. *Pediatric Clinics of North America, 41*(3), 453–472.

Lackner, R., Thompson, A., Rikkers, L., & Galbraith, A. (1996). Cystic adenomatoid malformation involving an entire lung in a 22-year-old woman. *Annals of Thoracic Surgery, 61,* 1827–1829.

Langham, M., Kays, D., Ledbetter, D., Frentzen, B., Sanford, L., & Richards, D. (1996). Congenital diaphragmatic hernia: Epidemiology and outcome. *Clinics in Perinatology, 23*(4), 671–688.

Luck, S., Reynolds, M., & Rafensberger, J. (1986). Congenital bronchopulmonary malformations. *Current Problems in Surgery, 23*(4), 245–314.

MacDonald, M., Forte, V., Cutz, E., & Crysdale, W. (1996). Congenital cystic adenomatoid malformation of the lung referred as "airway foreign body." *Archives of Otolaryngology and Head and Neck Surgery, 122*(3), 333–336.

MacGillivray, R., Harrison, M., Goldstein, R., & Adzick, S. (1993). Disappearing fetal lung lesions. *Journal of Pediatric Surgery, 28*(10), 1321–1325.

Markowitz, R., Mercurio, M., Vahjen, G., Gross, I., & Touloukian, R., (1989). Congenital lobar emphysema: The roles of CT and V/Q scan. *Clinical Pediatrics, 28*(1), 19–23.

Miller, J., Corteville, J., & Langer, J. (1996). Congenital cystic adenomatoid malformation in the fetus: Natural history and predictors of outcome. *Journal of Pediatric Surgery, 31*(6), 805–808.

Moore, K., & Persaud, T.V.N. (1993). *The developing human.* Philadelphia: W.B. Saunders Company.

Nio, M., Haase, G., Kennaugh, J., Bui, K., & Atkinson, J. (1994). A prospective randomized trial of delayed versus immediate repair of congenital diaphragmatic hernia. *Journal of Pediatric Surgery, 29*(5), 618–621.

Nobuhara, K., Gorski, Y., LaQuaglia, M., & Shamberger, R. (1997). Bronchogenic cysts and esophageal duplications: Common origins and treatment. *Journal of Pediatric Surgery, 32*(10), 1408–1413.

Othersen, B. (1993). Pulmonary and bronchial malformations. In K. Ashcraft & T. Holder (Eds.). *Pediatric surgery* (2nd ed., pp.176–187). Philadelphia: W.B. Saunders Company.

Ribet, M., Copin, M., & Gossselin, B. (1996). Bronchogenic cysts of the lung. *Annals of Thoracic Surgery, 61,* 1636–1640.

Rodgers, B., Harman, K., & Johnson, A. (1986). Bronchopulmonary foregut malformations: The spectrum of anomalies. *Annals of Surgery, 5,* 517–524.

Savic, B., Birtel, F., Tholen, W., Funke, H., & Knoche, R. (1979). Lung sequestration: Report of seven cases and review of 540 published cases. *Thorax, 34,* 96–101.

Schwartz, M., & Ramachandran, R. (1997). Congenital malformations of the lung and mediastinum: A quarter century of experience from a single institution. *Journal of Pediatric Surgery, 32*(1), 44–47.

Seeds, J., & Azizkhan, R. (1990). *Congenital malformations: Antenatal diagnosis, perinatal management, and counseling.* Rockville, MD: Aspen Publishers.

Skandalakis, L., Colborn, G., & Skandalakis, J. (1997). Surgical anatomy of the diaphragm. In L. Nyhus, R. Baker, & J. Fischer (Eds.), *Mastery of surgery* (Vol. I., pp. 649–670). Boston: Little, Brown and Company.

St-Georges, R., Deslauriers, J., Duranceau, A., Vaillancourt, R., Deschamps, C., Beauchamp, G., Page, A., & Brisson, J. (1991). Clinical spectrum of bronchogenic cysts of the mediastinum and lung in the adult. *Annals of Thoracic Surgery, 52,* 6–13.

Stigers, K., Woodring, J., & Kanga, J. (1992). The clinical and imaging spectrum of findings in patients with congenital lobar emphysema. *Pediatric Pulmonology, 14,* 160–170.

Stocker, J.T., Madewell J.E., & Drake, R.M. (1977). Congenital cystic adenomatoid malformation of the lung. *Human Pathology, 8,* 155–171.

Thomas, C. (Ed.). (1989). *Tabors cyclopedic medical dictionary.* Philadelphia: F.A. Davis.

Wilcox, D., Irish, M., Holm, B., & Glick, P. (1996). Pulmonary parenchymal abnormalities in congenital diaphragmatic hernia. *Clinics in Perinatology, 23*(4), 771–779.

Wilson, J., Fauza, D., Lund, D., Benacerraf, B., & Hendren, H. (1994). Antenatal diagnosis of isolated congenital diaphragmatic hernia is not an indicator of outcome. *Journal of Pediatric Surgery, 29*(6), 815–819.

Wung, J., James, S., Kilchevsky, E., & James, E. (1985). Management of infants with severe respiratory failure and persistence of the fetal circulation, without hyperventilation. *Pediatrics, 76*(4), 488–493.

Zwischenberger, J., & Bartlett, R. (1995). An introduction to extracorporeal life support. In J. Zwischenberger & R. Bartlett (Eds.), *Extracorporeal cardiopulmonary support in critical care.* Ann Arbor, MI: Extracorporeal Life Support.

Appendix 14–A

Critical Pathway for Thoracic Surgery

	Preoperative	Postoperative Day 1	Postoperative Day 2	Postoperative Day 3	Postoperative Day 4
Assessment/monitoring Monitor per NICU protocol Assess per NICU protocol	Instruct parents on operative procedure	Lung sounds Chest tube dressing intact All chest tube connections secure Chest tube drainage system below chest Clamp at bedside	Lung sounds Chest tube dressing intact All chest tube connections secure Chest tube drainage system below chest Clamp at bedside	Lung sounds	Lung sounds
Activity		Up in parents' arms			May have bath
Tests	CBC, T&C, CT, or ultrasonography	ABGs, CXR, CBC	CXR	Chest tube removal CXR 4–6 hr after removal	
Medications		Antibiotics—d/c after 3rd dose Narcotics q2–4h Tylenol for fever	Narcotics q2–4h Tylenol for fever	Narcotics—Tylenol	Tylenol q4h
Lines/drains		Check IV q1h Chest tube to suction	Check IV q1h Chest tube to seal	Remove IV if tolerating fluids and PO pain meds Remove chest tube	
Dressings		Chest tube dressing intact Monitor chest incision dressing for bleeding	Chest tube dressing intact Monitor chest incision dressing for bleeding	Monitor chest incision dressing	Change dressing over incision
Treatments		Respiratory care and suction Maintain sats >92%	Respiratory care and suction Maintain sats >92%	Respiratory care and suction Maintain sats >92%	
Diet	Solids until __ AM Liquids until __ AM Encourage/facilitate pumping of breast milk	NPO—Clears	Formula/breast milk	Formula/breast milk	Formula/breast milk
Teaching	Orientation to NICU	Chest tube Feeding			Instruct on dressing changes, leaving Steri-strips intact until they fall off or 10 days
Consult	Social work Anesthesia	Nutrition Pain service			

CHAPTER 15

Chest Wall Defects: Surgical Interventions and Nursing Issues

Louise Flynn

Chest wall defect refers to a variety of structural malformations of the chest wall. This chapter discusses some of the more common chest wall deformities and the care of the patient postoperatively. It also reviews some of the less commonly occurring anomalies. Most of the chest wall deformities are structural problems with little if any impact on function. Although some suggestion of mild restrictive lung disease exists with these defects, only extreme cases may result in pulmonary or cardiac compromise. The impact of a deformity is often more psychological, affecting the child's perception of self and body image. A visible defect such as a chest wall deformity can be difficult for many children. Surgical correction, when warranted, can help these children greatly.

PECTUS EXCAVATUM

Pectus excavatum is a chest deformity that presents with a sunken appearance of the chest wall, leading people to refer to it as a "funnel chest." The exact etiology of pectus excavatum is unknown. This sunken chest is the result of overgrowth of the anterior costal cartilages. The defect is often present at birth, indicating that the overgrowth of the cartilages begins in utero, late in fetal life (Skandalakis, Gray, Ricketts, & Skandalakis, 1994). It usually is a symmetric defect, affecting the lower half of the sternum and involving ribs 4 through 7 bilaterally. No genetic or chromosomal link is associated with pectus excavatum. It is the diagnosis in 90% of all chest wall deformities, making it the most common chest wall deformity seen. It occurs more often in males than in females with a ratio of 3:1 (Haller, 1988; Haller, Scherer, Turner, & Colombani, 1989; Haller & Turner, 1981; Kandel & Haller, 1997). Pectus excavatum occurs in approximately 1 of 125 children (Lane-Smith, Gillis, & Roy, 1994). A high incidence of pectus excavatum is seen in chil-

dren with Marfan syndrome, occurring in approximately two thirds of these children (Pyeritz & McKusick, 1979).

The primary care provider usually evaluates children who have pectus excavatum initially before referring them to a pediatric surgeon. The primary care provider generally finds these children to be normal, healthy, active children who have a visible, structural deformity of the chest. Occasionally, a child with pectus excavatum complains of a vague, nonspecific discomfort, not necessarily associated with any specific activity. The older child and adolescent may report having shortness of breath with exertion. They will state that they are able to participate in all types of physical activity but tend to become winded before most of their friends and teammates. Adolescents and older children also may express a desire to have the defect repaired because of concerns of body image and physical appearance. The chest deformity makes the posture of children with pectus excavatum distinctive. They all have a stoop shoulder/slouch to their stance and a protuberant or "pot belly" abdomen. A significant decrease in the size of the chest cavity is the result of the sternum being restricted, resulting in the heart being shifted to the left hemithorax. On examination, the pulse of maximal impact is lateral to the areola (Kandel & Haller, 1997). Occasionally, an audible murmur results from compression of the heart.

The breathing pattern for children with pectus excavatum is abnormal. Normal inhalation results in the expansion of the chest cavity, allowing the lungs to fill with air. Inhalation for a child with pectus excavatum consists of paradoxical movement of the sternum. This results in lateral expansion of the rib cage as a means of chest cavity expansion. The sternum retracts deeper during inhalation, making the defect appear worse. These physiological abnormalities are reversible with surgery. No documented evidence of long-term damage to the heart or lungs exists as a result of having a pectus excavatum (Kandel & Haller, 1997).

The actual deformity itself falls within a spectrum of severity that ranges from mild to severe. This rating is mostly subjective in nature. Surgery is an option, depending on the severity of the child's defect. Children with a moderate to severe defect often have complaints of shortness of breath with exertion. This defect also has psychological impact. These children have a poor body image because their chests appear to be so drastically different from their peers. Children with pectus excavatum defects in the mild to moderate severity category only require yearly follow-up examinations to reassess the defect. This is necessary to ensure that a mild defect does not develop into a severe defect during a growth spurt. Often, school-age children will have no change in the measurements until they reach the adolescent growth period.

Various measurements help to determine the severity of the pectus excavatum defect in a more objective way. In addition to the general appearance of the chest, caliper measurements of the depth of the defect (measuring from the deepest point of the defect to the spinal column) and the width of the chest are made. The use of an equation that divides the transverse diameter (width) by the anteroposterior diameter (depth) results in a number that is the pectus index. The ratio between these two distances gives the provider an index of severity. In children without this defect, the index of severity is never greater than 2.5 (Kandel & Haller, 1997).

Haller, Kramer, and Lietman (1987) proposed the use of a single computed tomography (CT) scan image through the deepest part of the defect as an additional way of measuring the chest wall deformity. The CT image accurately measures the transverse diameter and the anteroposterior diameter. In their study a CT scan was performed on patients in whom the decision to proceed with surgery was made. The findings indicated that all the patients had a pectus index of greater than 3.25. Children who had normal chests or mild pectus excavatum had an index less than 3.25. Their conclusion was that any child who has an index greater than 3.25 should have the deformity repaired. The CT scan, in addition to defining the severity of the defect, can also document more accurately the degree of cardiac compression and displacement and lung compression (Nuss, Kelly, Croitoru, & Katz, 1998). If a cardiac murmur is present, a cardiac evaluation with an echocardiogram is necessary to identify any undiagnosed significant cardiac lesion (Shamberger et al., 1988).

The most widely used surgical approaches for correction of pectus excavatum are modifications on the procedure initially performed by Dr. Ravitch in 1949. The procedure has undergone modifications over the past several decades but remains the standard in the United States. Surgical repair is performed through a transverse incision below the nipple line and centered through the deepest part of the defect when possible. The sternum and involved ribs are exposed and all of the abnormal costal cartilages are removed, leaving the perichondrium intact. The sternum is mobilized and an anterior transverse cuneiform osteotomy (removal of wedge piece of bone) is performed on the sternum above the highest abnormal rib. This allows elevation of the sternum to a neutral position. The sternum is supported in this new position by dividing the lowest intact costal cartilages obliquely, which displaces the medial portion anteriorly. This creates an internal tripod suspension that eliminates the use of additional traction (Figure 15–1). In older children and adolescents, additional support is provided by placing a steel strut (Adkins bar) under the sternum. The weight of the pectoral muscle mass in this population is too much for the sternum alone to support during the healing process. The strut prevents recurrence while the cartilages regenerate. Substernal and subcutaneous drains are placed to eliminate fluid collection at the surgical site. The incision is closed with subcuticular sutures below the skin level and sterile adhesive strips. Blood loss is minimal and it is rare that a child requires a blood transfusion for this procedure (Haller et al., 1989; Kandel & Haller, 1997).

Complications of the procedure include pneumothorax, serosanguinous fluid collection either substernally or subcutaneously, and wound infection. Later occurring complications include shifting of the substernal bar and recurrence. The incidence of recurrence is less than 5% (Haller et al., 1989; Kandel & Haller, 1997). In children with Marfan syndrome, the incidence of recurrence is as high as 40%. This is attributed to the fact that the initial surgical correction was performed at a younger age and without the additional support of a substernal strut (Arn, Scherer, Haller, & Pyeritz, 1989). Golladay, Char, and Mollitt (1985) reported a higher frequency of wound separation and a delay in wound healing in children with Marfan syndrome than in children with isolated pectus excavatum. This is most likely related to the connective tissue defect associated with Marfan syndrome.

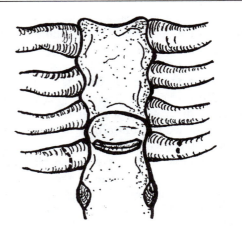

Figure 15–1 Mobilization and Stabilization of the Sternum in the Repair of Pectus Excavatum

This procedure is currently being performed as a same-day admit surgery. The patient arrives the day of surgery and is admitted from the postanesthesia care unit to the general inpatient unit. The average length of stay is 4 to 5 days. Postoperatively, the patient receives intravenous antibiotics for 48 hours. Clear liquids begin when the patient is fully awake after anesthesia, with the advancement to a regular diet as tolerated. Removal of the substernal drain (a chest tube connected to water suction is frequently used) occurs 48 hours postoperatively, provided that the drainage has decreased to <20 ml in an 8-hour period. Removal of the subcutaneous drain occurs 12 to 24 hours after the substernal drain if the quantity of drainage is minimal. The incision is open to air 48 hours postoperatively, and a small bandage or dressing covers the drain site until the wound has formed a scab.

Restriction of the child's activity is for 6 to 8 weeks after discharge from the hospital. During this time, the costal cartilages regenerate and stabilize the sternum in the new position. A protective vest is not required postoperatively, and normal activity resumes once the cartilages have regenerated. For older children and adolescents who received a strut during surgery, removal of the bar is an additional procedure. It occurs 6 to 12 months after the initial surgery as an outpatient procedure with general anesthesia.

Lane-Smith et al. (1994) describe a similar procedure using a modified Ravitch repair. A Dacron vascular graft strut provides the additional support instead of using a steel strut. The use of the Dacron strut eliminates the complications that result from the use of a more rigid strut, and removal of the Dacron strut is unnecessary. This eliminates the need for a second surgery.

A minimally invasive technique is now being performed for repair of pectus excavatum. The Nuss procedure attempts to remodel the chest wall in children by inserting one or two steel pectus bars through transverse lateral thoracic incisions. The surgeon bends the pectus support bar(s) into a convex shape to the configuration of the desired anterior chest wall curvature and places it under the sternum and sutures it into place. A stabilizer bar positioned over the ribs and under the muscle flaps maintains the position of the pectus bar. A 24-hour stay in the intensive care unit is an option for pain management purposes. Patients are discharged from the hospital in 4 to 5 days. Rest and quiet activity are prescribed for the first 2 weeks postoperatively. Gradually mild exercise is resumed and full activity is permitted 4 weeks postoperatively. The bar(s) removal occurs 2½ or more years after the initial surgery. The bars remain in place longer if the child is older than 14 years of age. The removal of the bar(s) is an outpatient surgical procedure, and general anesthesia is used (Nuss et al., 1998). Review the critical pathway (Appendix 15–A) for an overview of the hospital course.

It is important to consider the advantages and disadvantages of the Nuss procedure and the modified Ravitch procedure. The Nuss procedure is less invasive and does not involve opening the chest cavity. Both procedures have a similar length of stay. All patients who have the Nuss procedure require a second surgery for the removal of hardware. Only older children who have the modified Ravitch procedure performed require hardware. The patients who have the Nuss procedure need to have the struts in place for a more extended period of time than the patients having a modified Ravitch procedure. Both indicate equal numbers of recurrence at this time (Kandel & Haller, 1997; Nuss et al., 1998).

The long-term evaluation of outcomes for patients after a repair of a pectus excavatum are similar and are independent of the surgical approach. All series indicate that most patients have excellent results. Retrospective studies using both chart review and patient follow-up demonstrated these results repeatedly (Actis Dato et al., 1995; Haller et al., 1989; Lane-Smith et al., 1994; Nuss et al., 1998).

PECTUS CARINATUM

Pectus carinatum, often called "pigeon breast," refers to deformities of the chest wall that result in the protrusion of the sternum. An overgrowth of the costal cartilages causes the sternum to jut out anteriorly. Children and parents recognize this defect later in childhood because it often becomes more prominent during the adolescent growth period. The defect is usually a symmetric defect but can occur asymmetrically in selected cases (Kandel & Haller, 1997). The cause is unknown and there are no associated anomalies with pectus carinatum. The incidence is higher in males than in females and accounts for less than 10% of all chest wall deformities (Shamberger & Welch, 1987). The defect does not cause any known physiologic damage to the thoracic organs or musculoskeletal system. The impact is more psychological in nature, affecting the child's body image and possibly his or her self-esteem. Thus, the surgical repair to correct pectus carinatum is primarily a cosmetic procedure (Haller & Turner, 1981).

Surgical correction is recommended near the end or after the completion of adolescent growth (late teens to early twenties). There is a higher risk of recurrence for surgical corrections performed before the adolescent growth spurt because of cartilage overgrowth occurring during the adolescent growth spurt (Haller & Turner, 1981; Kandel & Haller, 1997; Pickard, Tepas, Shermeta, & Haller, 1979). However, some surgical practices have found that correction at an earlier age has not led to recurrence in many of their patients. The earlier timing of the surgery allows for quicker recuperation because the procedure is tolerated better at a younger age. Earlier surgery also alleviates the psychological impact of poor body image sooner for these patients (Shamberger & Welch, 1987).

The surgical repair is performed through a transverse incision made just below and between the nipple line (Figure 15–2). The involved overgrown cartilage is resected subperichondrially, and when needed, a transverse wedge osteotomy is performed to allow placement of the sternum in a more neutral position. Suction drains are placed under the skin flaps before wound closure. The risk of bleeding is minimal during the procedure; therefore, it is unnecessary for the patient or family member to donate blood before surgery. The patients receive prophylactic antibiotics for 24 to 48 hours postoperatively. The drains are removed 48 hours postoperatively. Postoperative complications are uncommon but include wound infection, pneumothorax, and subcutaneous fluid collections (Haller & Turner, 1981; Kandel & Haller, 1997; Pickard et al., 1979; Shamberger & Welch, 1987). Restriction of patient activity is mandatory postoperatively. Contact sports and heavy lifting are to be avoided until the cartilage has regenerated and the sternum is once again in a fixed position. It takes 8 to 10 weeks for this to occur (Haller & Turner, 1981).

JEUNE SYNDROME

Jeune syndrome is a congenital anomaly referred to as newborn asphyxiatic thoracic chondrodystrophy. It is a rare autosomal recessive disorder causing disturbance of endochondral bone formation in utero. Clinical presentation at birth consists of a small thoracic cavity and pelvic and phalangeal deformities.

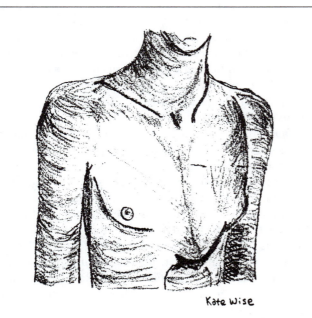

Figure 15–2 Transverse Incision Made during Repair of Pectus Carinatum

The lack of chest wall growth in utero causes secondary pulmonary hypoplasia. Recurrent pneumonia and pulmonary hypertension contribute to a high morbidity and mortality. Consequently, death usually ensues soon after birth. Infants that do survive for a few months have increasing dyspnea and respiratory failure because the chest cavity does not grow. On the basis of pathologic studies, the lung growth potential in these children is normal. Surgical expansion of the chest cavity in these children should allow for the normal growth of the lung tissue. Several techniques are used to achieve thoracic expansion. These procedures involve splitting the sternum, resection of the costochondral cartilages, and lateral rib expansion (Davis, Ruberg, Leppink, McCoy, & Wright, 1995, Kandel & Haller, 1997).

Recently, an acquired form of Jeune syndrome has been described. It occurs in patients who have had a correction of pectus excavatum performed at an early age (less than 4 years of age). The physical findings in this patient population include "a small, immovable anterior chest wall, a very long torso, primary diaphragmatic breathing, and no evidence of recurrence of the excavatum deformity" (Haller, Colombani, Humphries, Azizkhan, & Loughlin, 1996, p. 1618). Surgical correction for these patients provides expansion of the anterior chest wall, resulting in an increased volume of the chest cavity. Modified Rheibein splints act as elevated bridges to hold the sternum in the new position and provide the expansion to the anterior chest wall. The postoperative course is similar to the recuperation period after repair of pectus excavatum. Preliminary results of surgical correction indicate that there is an improvement in pulmonary function in these patients (Haller et al., 1996).

STERNAL CLEFTS

Bifid or sternal cleft is a chest wall deformity that results from the failure of the two sternal halves to fuse in the midline. This normally occurs early in gestation, around the seventh week of fetal development. The cause is unknown and the incidence is extremely rare. This defect is usually apparent in early infancy, with the mediastinal contents protruding through the defective area when the child coughs, cries, or strains. Potential injury to the underlying heart and lungs can occur as a result of their mechanical movement against the two edges of the sternal cleft or from external trauma. The spectrum of the defect ranges from incomplete to complete. If the sternal cleft is small and does not expose any mediastinal contents, surgical correction is not necessary. For the larger partial cleft and the complete cleft, the optimal time for surgery is in the newborn period. The incidence of associated anomalies is extremely low, and these patients tend to do well postoperatively without any complications. A variety of surgical procedures are available to repair a sternal cleft. It is corrected primarily, with the two halves of the sternum being brought together. Secondary bony healing completes the repair (Haller, 1988; Haller & Turner, 1981; Kandel & Haller, 1997; Knox, Tuggle, & Knott-Craig, 1994).

POLAND SYNDROME

Poland syndrome is a congenital chest wall deformity that was first described by Alfred Poland in 1841 during an autopsy (Poland, 1841). It is characterized by hypoplasia or absence of the breast and/or nipple, absence of the costosternal portion of the pectoralis major muscle, absence of the pectoralis minor muscle, absence of the costal cartilages and/or ribs (two through five on the involved side), and a forearm and hand abnormality often consisting of brachysyndactyly (i.e., abnormally shortened, fused fingers) (Clarkson, 1962; Haller, Colombani, Miller, & Manson, 1984; Kandel & Haller, 1997).

The etiology of Poland syndrome is unknown. One theory suggests that a vascular malformation resulting in insufficient blood supply to the limb bud during the critical development of the shoulder girdle and limb causes the syndrome. This occurs at approximately 7 weeks' gestation. Other theories include an abnormal migration of the embryonic tissues forming the pectoral muscles and in utero injuries from attempted abortions (Lord, Laurenzano, & Hartmann, 1990; Shamberger, Welch, & Upton, 1989).

The incidence is between 1 in 30,000 to 1 in 32,000 live births and rarely has familial association (Lord et al., 1990; Urschel, Byrd, Sethi, & Razzuk, 1984). The defect is most often unilateral and occurs on the right side in 75% of the cases (Lord et al., 1990). Associated diagnoses include renal hypoplasia, certain leukemias, thrombocytopenia, spherocytosis, lymphoma, and Möbius syndrome (Lord et al., 1990; Seyfer, Icochea, & Graeber, 1988).

The clinical manifestations of Poland syndrome vary greatly. Children may present in early childhood if the chest wall defects cause lung herniation. This may be evident with crying or coughing. The underlying lung tissue is, in fact, normal tissue. However, if the absence of ribs creates a large enough defect, a functional flail chest may result, causing respiratory compromise. This could require immediate surgical intervention to stabilize the chest wall (Kandel & Haller, 1997). Little disability is associated with Poland syndrome. The involved shoulder function is normal and muscle weakness is rare. Some patients develop scoliosis. In patients who have hand deformities, few report any great degree of disability. Some patients complain of decreased strength of grip (Kandel & Haller, 1997; Seyfer et al., 1988). A child who has syndactyly (fusion of digits) should be referred to a plastic surgeon within the first year of life. Surgical bony separation performed in the first year of life results in a better functional outcome (Lord et al., 1990). The surgical recon-

struction of the chest wall occurs during adolescence as an elective procedure. The surgical methods depend on the extent of chest wall deformity. Autologous rib grafts are used when necessary to replace absent or short ribs. Often, a latissimus muscle flap is performed to provide more adequate chest contour. Adolescent females also have a breast prosthesis placed, either submuscularly or subcutaneously, for symmetry (Haller et al., 1984; Kandel & Haller, 1997; Lord et al., 1990; Seyfer et al., 1988; Urschel et al., 1984).

NURSING CONSIDERATIONS

Chapter 1 of this text discusses the concerns of children and parents preparing for surgery. It is important to take the time to explain the entire process to the family and answer all their questions. The families should be provided with a family version of the critical pathway, if available, and any other written information pertaining to the diagnosis and procedure. When possible, families benefit from verbal communication with children and parents who have already had the procedure performed.

Postoperatively, the challenges of providing care to these children are as variable as the individual patients. Emotional and cognitive developmental levels are important to consider when planning care for the pediatric patient. Table 15–1 outlines the postoperative responsibilities of the nurse.

Respiratory/pulmonary complications are common postoperatively. Symptoms of pulmonary complications include elevation in temperature, dyspnea, tachycardia, altered breath sounds, restlessness, and changes in sputum (Black & Matassarin-Jacobs, 1993). A common postoperative respiratory problem is atelectasis. Atelectasis occurs when the alveoli collapse in sections of the lung. Children who have undergone chest wall surgery are prime candidates for atelectasis. It is difficult for many of them to take the deep breaths required to keep the alveoli open. This is usually a result of discomfort with chest expansion and may also result from sedation. Pulmonary toilet is a key component to the care of these children.

Often children who undergo chest wall reconstruction require a chest tube in the postoperative period. Frequent assessment and proper management of chest tubes are essential to the management of these patients. It is important to know the type of chest tube that is in place, whether it is a mediastinal tube or a pleural tube. A chest tube located in the chest cavity to drain blood and serous fluid is a mediastinal tube. This tube prevents complications of fluid collection and promotes healing (Carroll, 1993). Surgeons use this chest tube placement during the modified Ravitch procedure for repair of pectus excavatum. Chest tubes placed in the pleural space are pleural tubes. This tube allows any fluid or air to escape from the pleural space, which assists in reestablishing negative pressure needed for respiration (Carroll,

Table 15–1 Postoperative Responsibilities in Caring for the Patient after Chest Wall Reconstruction

Preferred Outcomes	Nursing Interventions
1. Adequate airway and respiratory function	a. Monitor temperature. b. Assess breath sounds. c. Encourage coughing and deep breathing (with use of incentive spirometer or blow glove). d. Pulmonary toilet.
2. Adequate cardiac function and tissue perfusion	a. Monitor cardiac rhythm. b. Assess skin color.
3. Adequate fluid and electrolyte balance	a. Monitor intake and output. b. Maintain IV fluids until adequate PO taken.
4. Satisfactory comfort level	a. Assess pain level. b. Provide appropriate pain management.
5. Adequate nutrition and elimination	a. Encourage PO intake when patient able to tolerate diet. b. Provide support if difficulty with voiding (may require catheterization).
6. Infection-free wound	a. Keep chest dressing dry and intact for first 48 hr postoperatively. b. Clean incision and drain sites with normal saline as needed. (Soap and water can be used when child is discharged home.)
7. Appropriate ambulation and mobility	a. Encourage progression of ambulation and mobility.
8. Appropriate coping with hospital experience	a. Support child and family, providing comfort and reassurance. b. Encourage patient and family involvement in decisions and provision of care.
9. Adequate preparation for discharge	a. Review information needed for home care. b. Instruct patient/family in incision care. c. Reinforce activity level allowed.

1993). Management of a pneumothorax, which can occur with any chest wall reconstruction, is an example of use of a pleural chest tube. Pleural chest tubes also manage tension pneumothorax, hemothorax, hemopneumothorax, mediastinal shift, thoracostomy, pleural effusion, empyema, and chylothorax (Smith, Fallentine, & Kessel, 1995).

Chest tubes drain because of the principles of gravity, positive expiratory pressure, and application of suction. A chest tube drainage system is a one-, two-, or three-bottle system. The most commonly used system is the self-contained three-chamber underwater chest drainage system. The first chamber collects fluid or air draining from the patient. The chest tube connects to the tubing that enters this chamber. The purpose of the second chamber is to prevent air from entering the patient. This chamber contains a set amount of water that acts as a water seal or a one-way valve. Air from the system (or the atmosphere) cannot pass through the water into the patient. The third chamber acts as the air vent for the system and provides the control for suction. The level of fluid (usually water) in this chamber determines the amount of suction applied to the system to promote drainage (O'Hanlon-Nichols, 1996; Smith et al., 1995).

Assessment of the chest tube drainage system needs to include the patient, the tubing, and the collection system. Check the tube insertion site: is the dressing clean, dry, and occlusive; is there any bleeding or drainage on the dressing; is subcutaneous emphysema felt around the insertion site? Next, assess the drainage tubing: are the connections securely taped to prevent air leaks; is the tube free of kinks and twists; are there any dependent loops? Gordon, Norton, and Guerra (1997) found that no difference exists in the effect of drainage if the tube is coiled on the patient's bed or is straight. However, they documented that tubing with dependent loops eliminated any drainage from the chest tube. Finally, the collection system should be examined: measure the level of drainage; make sure the water levels in the waterseal chamber and the suction control chamber are appropriate; and assess for any air leak. Some fluctuation occurs with normal inspiration and expiration (Mergaert, 1994).

One of the greatest concerns of both the child and parents when considering a surgical procedure is the amount and severity of pain postoperatively. The source of pain for these patients is more from movement than from incisional pain. Often, it is the chest tube, placed as the substernal drain, that provides the greatest element of discomfort to the child. Most of the children indicate relief of the discomfort once the drain is removed. It is important to stress with the patient and the family that, as with all surgeries, the pain decreases the further out from surgery the patient is. However, it is necessary to administer the appropriate medications to help lessen the intensity of the child's pain.

Pain management has evolved over the years with vast improvements in controlling pain. This has been a wonderful addition to the care of patients who have undergone chest wall reconstruction. Patient-controlled analgesia, offered in many centers, allows the patient to administer his or her own dose of intravenous pain medication with a push of a button. Pain management for these patients might also be through a continuous thoracic epidural catheter. This method of analgesia has proven to be effective and safe while eliminating the potential of sedation and respiratory compromise (McBride, Dicker, Abajian, & Vane, 1996). For more detailed information on current pain management practice, refer to Chapter 6.

CONCLUSION

This chapter has presented an overview of the more common chest wall defects and some of the rarer congenital anomalies, as well as the surgical interventions for these diagnoses. Great advances have been made in the field of pediatric surgery over the years, many of which have made an impact on the surgical approach to chest wall reconstruction. Laparoscopic techniques have made surgeries less invasive. Innovative equipment has decreased blood loss during procedures. Development of new materials provides better supports for reconstructive surgeries with fewer complications for the patient. Better control of pain postoperatively has been a great improvement to the care of the surgical patient.

Most children who undergo a chest wall reconstruction have a successful outcome. It is important as nurses caring for these children to understand the physiology of the defect and the basic principles of the corrective surgical techniques. Changes in surgical technique have an impact on nursing care preoperatively and postoperatively. Nurses have the potential and the responsibility to make the experience a positive one by providing education, reassurance, and nurturing care before, during, and after chest wall reconstruction. Support for the patient and the family at all times, on all levels, throughout the continuum of care is the challenge.

REFERENCES

Actis Dato, G.M., De Paulis, R., Actis Dato, A., Bassano, C., Pepe, N., Borioni, R., & Panero, G.B. (1995). Correction of pectus excavatum with a self-retaining seagull wing prosthesis: Long term follow-up. *Chest, 107*(2), 303–306.

Arn, P.H., Scherer, L.R., Haller, J.A., & Pyeritz, R.E. (1989). Outcome of pectus excavatum in patients with Marfan syndrome and in the general population. *The Journal of Pediatrics, 115*(6), 954–958.

Black, J.M., & Matassarin-Jacobs, E. (Eds.). (1993). *Luckman and Sorenson's medical-surgical nursing: A psychophysiological approach* (4th ed.). Philadelphia: W.B. Saunders Company.

Carroll, P. (1993). Technical update brief: The child with a chest tube. *Pediatric Nursing, 19*(4), 370–371.

Clarkson, P. (1962). Poland's syndactyly. *Guy's Hospital Reports, 111,* 335–346.

Davis, J.T., Ruberg, R.L., Leppink, D.M., McCoy, K.S., & Wright, C.C. (1995). Lateral thoracic expansion for Jeune's asphyxiating dystrophy: A new approach. *Annals of Thoracic Surgery, 60*(3), 694–696.

Golladay, E.S., Char, F., & Mollitt, D.L. (1985). Children with Marfan's syndrome and pectus excavatum. *Southern Medical Journal, 78*(11), 1319–1323.

Gordon, P.A., Norton, J.M., & Guerra, J.M. (1997). Positioning of chest tubes: Effects on pressure and drainage. *American Journal of Critical Care, 6*(1), 33–38.

Haller, J.A. (1988). Operative management of chest wall deformities in children: Unique contributions of southern thoracic surgeons. *Annals of Thoracic Surgery, 46*(1), 4–12.

Haller, J.A., Colombani, P.M., Humphries, C.T., Azizkhan, R.G., & Loughlin, G.M. (1996). Chest wall constriction after too extensive and too early operations for pectus excavatum. *Annals of Thoracic Surgery, 61,* 1618–1625.

Haller, J.A., Colombani, P.M., Miller, D., & Manson, P. (1984). Early reconstruction of Poland's syndrome using autologous rib grafts combined with a latissimus muscle flap. *Journal of Pediatric Surgery, 19*(4), 423–429.

Haller, J.A., Kramer, S.S., & Lietman, S.A. (1987). Use of CT scans in selection of patients for pectus excavatum surgery: A preliminary report. *Journal of Pediatric Surgery, 22*(10), 904–906.

Haller, J.A., Scherer, L.R., Turner, C.S., & Colombani, P.M. (1989) Evolving management of pectus excavatum based on a single institutional experience of 664 patients. *Annals of Surgery, 209*(5), 578–583.

Haller, J.A., & Turner, C.S. (1981). Diagnosis and operative management of chest wall deformities in children. *Surgical Clinics of North America, 61*(5), 1199–1207.

Kandel, J., & Haller, J.A. (1997). Chest wall and breast. In K.T. Oldham, P.M. Colombani, & R.P. Foglia (Eds.), *Surgery of infants and children: Scientific principles and practices* (pp. 871–881). Philadelphia: Lippincott-Raven Publishers.

Knox, L., Tuggle, D., & Knott-Craig, C.J. (1994). Repair of congenital sternal clefts in adolescence and infancy. *Journal of Pediatric Surgery, 29*(12), 1513–1516.

Lane-Smith, D.M., Gillis, D.A., & Roy, P.D. (1994). Repair of the pectus excavatum using Dacron vascular graft strut. *Journal of Pediatric Surgery, 29*(9), 1179–1182.

Lord, M.J., Laurenzano, K.R., & Hartmann, R.W. (1990). Poland's syndrome. *Clinical Pediatrics, 29*(10), 606–609.

McBride, W.J., Dicker, R.J., Abajian, J.C., & Vane, D.W. (1996). Continuous thoracic epidural infusions for postoperative analgesia after pectus deformity repair. *Journal of Pediatric Surgery, 31*(1), 105–108.

Mergaert, S. (1994). S.T.O.P. and assess chest tubes the easy way. *Nursing, (24)*2, 52–53.

Nuss, D., Kelly, R.E., Croitoru, D.P., & Katz, M.E. (1998). A 10 year review of a minimally invasive technique for the correction of pectus excavatum. *Journal of Pediatric Surgery, 33*(4), 546–552.

O'Hanlon-Nichols, T. (1996). Commonly asked questions about chest tubes. *American Journal of Nursing, 96*(5), 60–64.

Pickard, L.R., Tepas, J.J., Shermeta, D.W., & Haller, J.A. (1979). Pectus carinatum: Results of surgical therapy. *Journal of Pediatric Surgery, 14*(3), 228–230.

Poland, A. (1841). Deficiency of the pectoral muscles. *Guy's Hospital Reports, 6,* 191–193.

Pyeritz, R.E., & McKusick, V.A. (1979). The Marfan syndrome. *New England Journal of Medicine, 300,* 772–777.

Seyfer, A.E., Icochea, R., & Graeber, G.M. (1988). Poland's anomaly. Natural history and long-term results of chest wall reconstruction in 33 patients. *Annals of Surgery, 208*(6), 776–782.

Shamberger, R.C., & Welch, K.J. (1987). Surgical correction of pectus carinatum. *Journal of Pediatric Surgery, 22*(1), 48–53.

Shamberger, R.C., Welch, K.J., Castaneda A.R., Keane, J.F., & Fyler, D.C. (1988). Anterior chest wall deformities and congenital heart disease. *Journal of Thoracic and Cardiovascular Surgery, 96*(3), 427–432.

Shamberger, R.C., Welch, K.J., & Upton, J. (1989). Surgical treatment of thoracic deformity in Poland's syndrome. *Journal of Pediatric Surgery, 24*(8), 760–766.

Skandalakis, J.E., Gray, S.W., Ricketts, R., & Skandalakis, L.J. (1994). The anterior body wall. In J.E. Skandalakis & S.W. Gray (Eds.), *Embryology for surgeons: The embryological basis for treatment of congenital defects.* Baltimore: Williams & Wilkins.

Smith, R.N., Fallentine, J., & Kessel, S. (1995). Underwater chest drainage: Bringing the facts to the surface. *Nursing, 25*(2), 60–63.

Urschel, H.C., Byrd, H.S., Sethi, S.M., & Razzuk, M.A. (1984). Poland's syndrome: Improved surgical management. *The Annals of Thoracic Surgery, 37*(3), 204–211.

Appendix 15–A

Critical Pathway for Nuss Procedure

	O.R.	Postoperative Day 1	Postoperative Day 2	Postoperative Day 3	Postoperative Day 4
Monitoring/assessment	Vital signs per unit routine with pain assessment	-------------------------	-------------------------	-------------------------	-------------------------
	Strict I + O	-------------------------	-------------------------	I + O	-------------------------
	Assess surgical site	-------------------------	-------------------------	-------------------------	-------------------------
Treatments	C & DB	-------------------------	-------------------------	-------------------------	-------------------------
	Pulmonary toilet per routine	-------------------------	-------------------------	-------------------------	-------------------------
	O$_2$ as needed to maintain sats >93%	-------------------------	-------------------------	D/C O$_2$	
Lines/drains	IV	-------------------------	-------------------------	Hep lock IV with adequate PO intake	D/C Hep lock
	Epidural catheter	-------------------------	D/C		
	Foley catheter	-------------------------	D/C		
Medications	Prophylactic antibiotic x 3 doses	D/C after 3 doses			
	Epidural/PCA pain medication	-------------------------	D/C epidural	D/C PCA Convert to PO/IV pain medication as needed	PO pain medication as needed
	Docusate sodium when taking PO	-------------------------	-------------------------	-------------------------	-------------------------
Activity	BR	OOB to chair with assistance	-------------------------	OOB to chair bid	
	Elevate HOB 6 hr postoperatively	-------------------------	-------------------------		
		No log rolling	-------------------------	-------------------------	-------------------------
		No bending at waist	-------------------------	-------------------------	-------------------------
			Ambulate with assistance as tolerated	-------------------------	-------------------------
Diet	Ice chips advance to clear liquids as tolerated	Clear liquids advance as tolerated to regular	-------------------------	Regular as tolerated	-------------------------
Tests	CXR	CXR	CXR	CXR	
Consults	Pediatric pain service	-------------------------	D/C when epidural/ PCA d/c'd		
	Intensivist	-------------------------	D/C when transferred out of ICU		
Patient teaching	Orientation to unit		Orientation to unit (if patient transferred from PICU)		
	Review family pathway				
	Begin D/C teaching	-------------------------	-------------------------	-------------------------	Assess learning
Discharge planning					Schedule follow-up appointment
Outcomes evaluation	Surgical incision D + I	Surgical incision D + I	Breath sounds clear	Breath sounds clear	Afebrile
	O$_2$ sats >93% on room air	O$_2$ sats >93% on room air	Effective pain management	Afebrile	Incisions clean
	Effective pain management	Effective pain management	Bar(s) in good position	Incisions clean	Bar(s) in good position
	Discharge needs identified	Bar(s) in good position	OOB with assistance	Bar(s) in good position	Discharge teaching completed, with actual learning documented
				Regular diet	
				Ambulating	

CHAPTER 16

Gastroesophageal Reflux Disease: Recognition and Management

Frances N. Price and Maureen Smith

Gastroesophageal reflux (GER) is a physiologic occurrence in all individuals. It is a normal event in which gastric contents regurgitate into the esophagus. It is especially prevalent in infants because of the immaturity of the lower esophageal sphincter (LES). Three categories of GER have been described in the literature. The first of these, physiologic reflux, is often silent; that is, emesis occurs infrequently or not all. The second category of reflux, functional reflux, may be accompanied by emesis that occurs either immediately or after a prolonged period of time. The third type of reflux, pathologic reflux, is characterized by an infant or child who demonstrates detrimental physical problems as a result of the reflux. This type of reflux, called gastroesophageal reflux disease (GERD), is the focus of this chapter. To assess and treat the child with GERD correctly, it is important that the practitioner understand the physiologic basis for the disease and the treatment modalities available. Appendix 16–A summarizes the postoperative care of a child undergoing a Nissen fundoplicationn with gastrostomy tube insertion.

PATHOPHYSIOLOGY

The esophagus resides in the thoracic cavity. The intrathoracic pressure is lower than the pressure within the abdominal cavity, where the stomach is located. Were it not for certain anatomic and physiologic barriers, reflux would occur continuously from contents flowing from an area of higher to lower pressure. These anatomic and physiologic barriers to reflux include the LES, esophageal motility, and gastric emptying (Boix-Ochoa & Rowe, 1998; Hyman, 1994; Orenstein, 1992).

The LES is an anatomic area formed by the confluence of muscle fibers from the esophagus and the stomach (Figure 16–1). Release of acetylcholine from the vagal nerve pro-

vides a normal resting pressure sufficient to act as a sphincter, preventing reflux of stomach contents into the esophagus. Although LES pressure in infants may be low, less than 5 mm Hg, infants usually develop a normal pressure (15 to 20 mm Hg) by age 15 months. Infants with GER typically outgrow the reflux between the ages of 9 and 24 months caused in part by the maturation of the LES (Armentrout, 1995; Hillemeier, 1996). In children with GERD, LES pressure is inadequate, allowing gastric contents to continue to reflux up into the esophagus.

Esophageal motility is another barrier to reflux. The peristaltic action of the esophagus provides timely clearance of

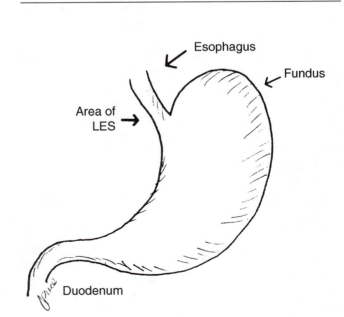

Figure 16–1 Anatomy of Stomach including Area of LES

substances through the esophagus. In the case of GERD esophageal motility is compromised, allowing irritating gastric acids to be in contact with esophageal mucosa for longer periods of time. This leads to inflammation of the mucosa and causes ulceration and scarring leading to potential strictures.

Delayed gastric emptying may also play a role in GERD (Boix-Ochoa & Rowe, 1998; Foglia, 1997; Tunell, 1989). If the stomach empties poorly, feedings accumulate and are not emptied normally. This leads to an increase in stomach volume that places more pressure on an already incompetent LES, resulting in reflux.

Although the specific cause of GERD is unknown, it is theorized that some or all of the barriers to reflux are compromised, resulting in an adverse effect on the patient (Orenstein, 1992; Tunell, 1989). Several groups of children are especially prone to pathologic GER. These include children with neurologic impairment, cystic fibrosis, bronchopulmonary dysplasia, repaired esophageal atresia, and children who require gastrostomy feedings (Hillemeier, 1996; Orenstein, 1992).

CLINICAL PRESENTATION

The clinical presentation of GERD varies according to the severity of the child's disease, and symptoms range from mild to severe. Often, reflux may be "silent" for a time, that is, no obvious symptoms until esophageal inflammation becomes severe enough to cause strictures or dysphagia. Most signs of GERD are caused by excessive or prolonged contact of acid on esophageal mucosa. GERD is a common cause of failure to thrive in infants, with vomiting being the most frequent clinical sign (Armentrout, 1995; Boix-Ochoa & Rowe, 1998). Vomiting can lead to aspiration pneumonia and failure to thrive if the infant cannot retain a sufficient amount of calories for growth. Irritability caused by esophagitis from acid irritation is another common symptom of GERD. GERD can lead to dysphagia and esophageal strictures. Five percent of children with reflux experience esophageal strictures. Severe esophagitis is associated with hematemesis, anemia, and esophageal strictures. Also associated with GERD is Sandifer's syndrome, a rare syndrome of torticollis, an abnormal contracture of the neck muscles, and opisthotonos, a form of spasm in which the head and heels are bent backward and the body is bowed forward (Armentrout, 1995).

Respiratory symptoms associated with GERD may be as mild as coughing or wheezing or as severe as recurrent pneumonia or apnea, which may be associated with sudden infant death syndrome (Foglia, 1997; Jolley, 1992; Jones, 1992; Sterling, Jolley, Besser, & Matteson-Kane, 1991). Aspiration of gastric contents can occur in children with GERD, especially if they are positioned horizontally. Gastric acid in

Exhibit 16–1 Clinical Manifestations of GERD

Constitutional	Failure to thrive[a]
	Weight loss[a]
Gastrointestinal	Irritability associated with feedings[b]
	Vomiting[a]
	Dysphagia[a]
	Esophageal stricture[a]
Respiratory	Recurrent pneumonia[a]
	Apnea spells[a]
	Reactive airway symptoms[a]
Hematologic	Anemia[b]
	Hematemesis[b]

[a] Foglia, 1997. [b] Jolley, 1995.

the tracheobronchial tree can lead to apnea, pneumonia, bronchitis, and reactive airway disease (Foglia, 1997). Exhibit 16–1 summarizes common clinical manifestations of GERD (Armentrout, 1995, Berube, 1997; Sondheimer, 1994).

DIFFERENTIAL DIAGNOSIS

The symptoms associated with GERD can be caused by other processes. Therefore, it is important to eliminate disease processes outside the gastrointestinal tract that might cause the child's complaints. The patient should be evaluated to be certain that no metabolic, infectious, anatomic, or neurologic cause for the vomiting is evident. For instance, bilious vomiting signifies obstruction, whereas projectile nonbilious emesis can indicate pyloric stenosis or a central nervous system cause. Some metabolic disorders can present with vomiting in infancy. The respiratory symptoms associated with GERD may also be caused by asthma, cystic fibrosis, central apnea, seizures, central nervous system trauma or malformations, congenital heart disease, allergies, or primary lung disease. Symptoms of esophagitis may be due to peptic ulcers or nonspecific irritability (Jolley, 1992; Orenstein, 1992). Care must be taken to consider the differential diagnosis of these symptoms before attributing them to GERD.

DIAGNOSTIC STUDIES

Once the need for further evaluation has been established, diagnostic studies are indicated. Diagnostic evaluation for GERD should provide information regarding the presence or absence of reflux, severity of reflux, reflux as the identified cause of symptoms, and evidence of normal gastrointestinal function except for the reflux (Tunell, 1989). Although no single study can consistently identify children with GERD, careful choice of the diagnostic tools available can provide sufficient information to allow the practitioner to determine the appropriate treatment.

The primary diagnostic tools in the workup of GERD in the pediatric population are barium swallow followed by upper gastrointestinal (UGI) series, 12- to 24-hour pH probe monitoring, and radionucleotide gastric emptying study. Other studies such as bronchoscopy and esophageal biopsy can also be obtained. Esophageal manometry is another tool available but not commonly used in pediatric populations (Jolley, 1992; Shannon, 1993).

The "gold standard" for diagnosing GERD is the 12- to 24-hour pH monitor (Armentrout, 1995; Hillemeier, 1996; Shannon, 1993; Sterling et al., 1991). This study involves positioning a thin antimony probe in the child's esophagus and leaving it in place for 12 to 24 hours. During this time, the child is fed normally and feedings are recorded. At the end of the study period, three main parameters are measured: number of reflux episodes per day, number of episodes lasting longer than 5 minutes, and total percent of time that esophageal pH is less than 4. These parameters, along with normal values, are shown in Table 16–1 (Sondheimer, 1994). If the child's pH probe study results exceed the normal values, GERD is confirmed.

The barium swallow with UGI is a radiographic examination that is capable of demonstrating reflux fluoroscopically and showing the presence of a stricture, hiatal hernia, and variations in esophageal motility (Boix-Ochoa & Rowe, 1998). Figure 16–2 depicts an UGI that demonstrates reflux. Note that the barium looks as if it is traveling uphill into the esophagus. Although the barium swallow is helpful and explanatory, it is not the definitive tool for diagnosis of GERD.

Upper gastrointestinal studies should be obtained in all children with a history of recurrent pneumonia because this can be caused by GERD. In addition, it is imperative to determine whether the child with GERD also has a dysfunctional swallow. The treatment for GERD will not rectify a swallowing disorder. It is important that the practitioner and the parents be aware of this fact and use occupational or speech therapy to address problems of swallowing dysfunction.

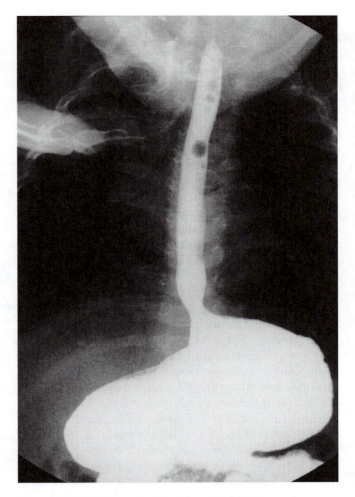

Figure 16–2 UGI Showing Gastroesophageal Reflux

Some centers are now using scintigrams, or radionucleotide gastric emptying studies (GESs), to determine whether the stomach empties at a normal rate. The child either drinks or is gavaged a radiopaque liquid meal, and gastric emptying is monitored. A normal range for gastric emptying is approximately 40 to 60 minutes (Foglia, 1997). Some children with reflux disease, primarily those with neurologic deficits, may have prolonged emptying times that can have deleterious effects on the child if not rectified. These effects include persistent retching despite fundoplication and gas bloat syndrome (Fonkalsrud et al., 1995). Gas bloat syndrome occurs when gas is trapped in the stomach and results in distention and discomfort.

Esophagoscopy can be useful in determining the degree of esophageal irritation and the presence of Barrett's esophagus, a precancerous esophageal dysplasia associated with severe acid reflux. Bronchoscopy is another test sometimes

Table 16–1 Extended pH Study: Normal Values

Parameter	Normal Value (per day)
No. reflux episodes/day	<35
No. reflux episodes >5 minutes	<7
Percent time with esophageal pH <4	<6

used. The presence of lipid-laden macrophages on bronchoscopy is an indication of aspiration of gastric contents.

MEDICAL MANAGEMENT

Once the diagnosis of GERD has been established, treatment can begin. The goal in the treatment of GERD is to control reflux symptoms and prevent sequelae. Medical antireflux therapy is effective in approximately 80% of children with reflux disease (Foglia, 1997). However, it is important to note that medical management is not indicated for those children who have severe symptoms such as esophageal strictures or near-death episodes from aspiration. These children should be referred directly for surgical treatment (Tunell, 1989).

The cornerstones of medical management are upright, prone-elevated positioning, thickening feedings, delivering smaller volumes of feedings at more frequent intervals, and use of pharmacologic agents such as histamine receptor blockers and prokinetic agents (Armentrout, 1995; Jolley, 1992; Shannon, 1993; Tunell, 1989).

Reflux can be exacerbated by supine, seated, or head-down position. For this reason, it is recommended that parents either hold infants upright or place them in a prone position with head elevated at a 30-degree angle for at least 30 minutes to an hour after feeding and while asleep. The head of the infants crib can be elevated to about 30 to 45 degrees. Devices such as sandbags and specially designed harnesses are used to keep the infant from sliding down in the bed when the head of the crib is elevated. The bed elevation, along with gravity, helps decrease the risk of stomach contents refluxing into the lungs (Foglia, 1997; Jolley, 1992). The 1992 American Academy of Pediatric guidelines recommend that infants be laid supine or in a side-lying position to avoid the risk of sudden infant death syndrome; however, for infants with diagnosed GERD, the prone position with head-up 30 degrees is a position accepted by most pediatric gastroenterologists (Armentrout, 1995; Gibson, Cullen, Spinner, Rankin, & Spitzer, 1995).

Thickening the infant's formula can help reduce reflux (Hillemeier, 1996). A common technique for thickening feedings includes adding rice cereal, approximately 1 tablespoon of cereal per 4 to 6 ounces of formula, to the infant's bottle. The nipple of the bottle should be widened so the infant can suck easily, being careful not to make the opening so wide that the child receives too large a bolus. In some cases, jejunal or duodenal feedings may be effective ways to increase nutrient absorption and decrease symptoms while the infant outgrows reflux (Armentrout, 1995; Berube, 1997).

Feeding volumes can be decreased to allow the infant's stomach to empty thoroughly between feedings. If the stomach contains large volumes of formula, the tendency for contents to reflux is greater. Allowing the stomach to empty helps alleviate pressure and decreases the chance of reflux. Parents should be instructed to give smaller, frequent feedings and use proper positioning techniques.

Pharmacologic interventions in the pediatric population include H_2 blockers such as ranitidine, cimetidine, and famotidine and prokinetic agents such as cisapride. Ranitidine and cisapride are frequently used because they have fewer side effects than other drugs in their class. Ranitidine acts to decrease acid production by blocking acid secretion from the parietal cells. Cisapride, a prokinetic agent, stimulates esophageal and gut peristalsis. Cisapride must be used with caution because it does interact adversely with certain antibiotics such as erythromycin. It also interacts with antifungal agents such as fluconazole. As with any drug, it is important to know the actions, effects, and interactions of each medication the child takes (Jolley, 1992; Orenstein, 1992).

Nonoperative treatments are successful in managing reflux in most children. However, some children have disease that is refractory to medical management. Infants and children experiencing complications related to reflux, children with severe neurologic impairment, or children with anatomic abnormalities of the gastrointestinal tract in addition to reflux are more likely to have medical management fail. It is these children who are candidates for surgical intervention.

SURGICAL INTERVENTION

Surgical correction is indicated for those children in whom medical management fails. Indications for operation include unremitting emesis with failure to thrive after 2 to 3 months of intensive medical therapy, recurrent pneumonia, apnea, a near sudden infant death syndrome event, refractory airway disease, severe esophagitis, stricture, or Barrett's metaplasia (Boix-Ochoa & Rowe, 1998; Foglia, 1997; Shannon, 1993).

The most widely used antireflux procedure in pediatric populations is the Nissen fundoplication (Boix-Ochoa & Rowe, 1998). The Nissen fundoplication (Figure 16–3) is a circumferential 360-degree wrap of the greater curvature of the stomach around the intraabdominal esophagus. Other commonly used antireflux procedures are the Thal fundoplication and the Toupet fundoplication. In contrast to the Nissen, the Thal and Toupet procedures entail a partial, 180- to 270-degree wrap of the esophagus. The Thal fundoplication is a partial anterior wrap around the esophagus, and the Toupet is a partial posterior wrap. The goal of fundoplication is to create an area of high pressure at the LES, which acts as a one-way valve when intragastric pressure increases. After antireflux surgery, the portion of the stomach that is wrapped around the esophagus temporarily acts as a one-way valve when gastric pressure increases, thereby preventing reflux into the esophagus. When gastric pressure returns to normal,

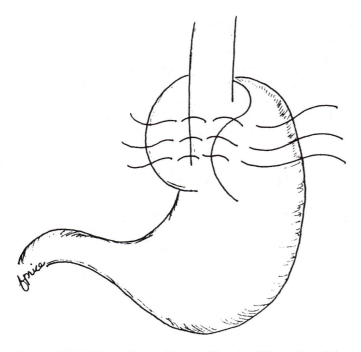

Figure 16–3 Nissen Fundoplication Showing Circumferential Wrap of Lower Esophagus

the wrap relaxes and does not impinge on resting esophageal function (Foglia, 1997; Rowe, O'Neill, Grosfeld, Fonkalsrud, & Coran, 1995).

The surgeon chooses the complete or partial wrap depending on the patient's condition. The Nissen fundoplication is chosen for children with neurologic impairments because these children are less able to protect their airway and need the additional protection that a circumferential wrap offers. The Thal or Toupet may be indicated if the child has respiratory symptoms but does not have any neurologic involvement. Both procedures involve a midline or left subcostal incision. Both the full and partial wrap procedures can be performed open or laparoscopically with satisfactory outcomes (Hunter, Trus, Branum, Waring, & Wood, 1996). Centers report 80% to 90% favorable results with an antireflux procedure for an infant or child in whom medical management has failed. Pulmonary symptoms often improve, the children gain weight, and esophagitis substantially resolves in children who have undergone antireflux procedures (Foglia, 1997).

Some children with delayed gastric emptying may require a pyloroplasty. This is a procedure in which the pylorus muscle is partially divided, thereby enlarging the outlet of the stomach and facilitating gastric emptying. This can be done in conjunction with the antireflux procedure.

Many children who require antireflux procedures also require a gastrostomy for feeding access or for temporary pro-

tection of the wrap. A gastrostomy is a surgically created tract that allows direct access to the stomach for feeding and decompression. A gastrostomy tube or skin level device (SLD) is placed by the surgeon by means of an open or laparoscopic approach. Gastrostomies are discussed in greater detail later in this chapter.

Although antireflux procedures prove beneficial in most children, they are not without complications. Complications of the antireflux procedure include small bowel obstruction, wrap failure, gastric perforation, dumping syndrome, gastric outlet obstruction, damage to the vagus nerve, bloating, diarrhea, dysphagia, choking, or a paraesophageal hernia. The child with developmental delay is particularly at risk for these complications, in part because of the combination of poor esophageal motility and greater propensity for delayed gastric emptying (Armentrout, 1995; Broscious, 1995; Eisenberg, 1994; Raffensperger, 1990; Rowe et al., 1995; Shannon, 1993; Sterling et al., 1991; Tunnell, 1989).

PREOPERATIVE CARE

When the decision is made to intervene surgically, the nurse is vital in helping prepare the child and family for the upcoming surgery. The preparation is twofold: physically preparing the child and mentally preparing the child and family. Much of the physical preparation will be completed throughout the diagnostic evaluation. In the immediate preoperative period laboratory tests may be indicated. Routine preoperative laboratory studies are no longer indicated. However, children with respiratory or other medical conditions may require chest radiograph examination, complete blood count, or electrolytes. Children who have had hematemesis or anemia require additional blood tests (Liebert, 1989).

During the parent and child portion of the preoperative tour, it is ideal to encourage the child to manipulate the nasogastric (NG) tube, gastrostomy devices, masks, or other surgical paraphernalia. If appropriate, it is helpful to allow the older child who is capable of making decisions to participate in the choice of gastrostomy devices if one is indicated. Chapter 1 addresses preoperative preparation in more depth.

POSTOPERATIVE CARE

Routine interventions for a postoperative patient include monitoring for return of gastric function, gastric decompression by means of NG or gastrostomy device, pain management, and care of the incision and tubes (Broscious, 1995). For those children who have an antireflux procedure without gastrostomy, an NG tube is placed in the operating room for gastric decompression until gastric function returns. The patency of the tube is maintained by regulating the suction and irrigation/aspiration of the tube. Manipulation of a surgically placed tube is not recommended. If the NG tube malfunctions, the nurse should notify the surgeon rather than reposition the tube and risk damage to the wrap. If a gastrostomy is performed in conjunction with the antireflux procedure, the gastrostomy device may be used for stomach decompression, obviating the need for a NG tube (Armentrout, 1995; Shannon, 1993).

GASTROSTOMY DEVICES

If a gastrostomy is performed, the surgeon may decide to place a tube or SLD. Before the development of the SLD in 1984 (Steele, 1991), silicone or latex catheters were the only gastrostomy tube options. At present, a variety of SLDs exist. These include the Button and the Genie made by the Bard Corporation and the Mic-Key developed by Kimberly-Clark (formerly Ballard), among others. Figure 16–4 shows these three devices. SLDs have become popular because of their cosmetic appeal, comfort, close proximity to the skin surface, and ease of care. In addition, these devices interfere less with developmental tasks, such as crawling, than do the long gastrostomy tubes. There is also less likelihood of accidental dislodgement of the SLD by the patient or siblings. The choice of device depends on the child's specific circumstance. Figure 16–5 depicts a child with an SLD.

As with any procedure, complications may arise with gastrostomy. Potential problems associated with gastrostomy device placement include dislodgement, stomach perforation, exacerbation of gastroesophageal reflux, skin or stoma infection, granulation tissue, gastric outlet obstruction, and intestinal obstruction (Coldicutt, 1994; Eisenberg, 1994; Tunell, 1989). The general care of the gastrostomy is discussed in greater detail in Chapter 21.

POSTOPERATIVE FEEDING

Whether the child has a gastrostomy as part of the antireflux procedure or not, feeding concerns remain a primary focus in the postoperative period. Feedings are initiated slowly in response to the return of gastric function. It is important to refrain from feeding the child large amounts to regain caloric losses. The child's stomach needs to adjust to the larger, desired volume that initially can be quite uncomfortable. Balancing the volume needs with the discomfort is challenging. Input from the nurse and family is vital in adjusting the feedings. Once the child adjusts to feedings, average-sized meals should be well tolerated.

Some children, such as those with neurologic impairments, are fed exclusively by means of the gastrostomy. For

A   B    C

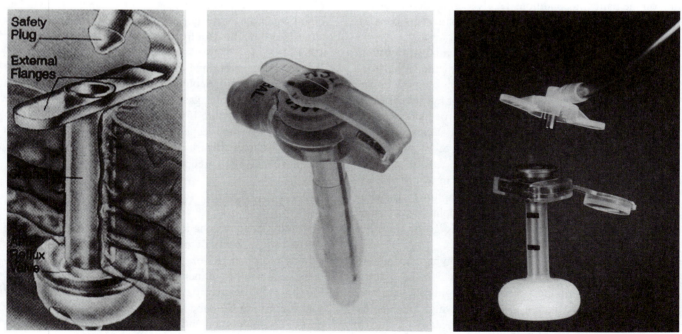

Figure 16–4 Skin Level Devices Currently Available: A, Bard Button; B, Mic-Key; C, Genie

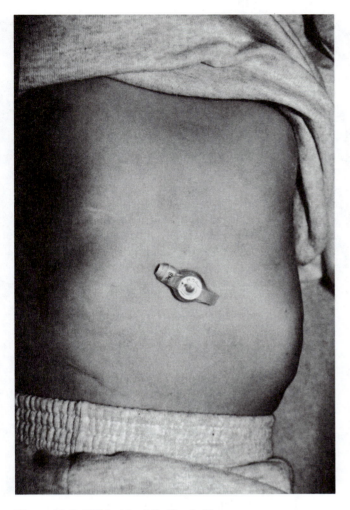

Figure 16–5 Child with a Mic-Key in Place

these children, feeding, developmental, and social considerations must be addressed.

Feeding considerations include warming the formula to a comfortable temperature and simulating normal feeding patterns. Formula that is not at room temperature can cause cramping (Steele, 1991). The presence of a feeding device is not a license to fast feed with little or no time spent nurturing the child. Feed the child over 30 to 45 minutes, just like a child being fed orally (Paarlberg & Balint, 1985). Feeding times should be appropriate to the age of the child. For example, feed a toddler three meals and two snacks (Paarlberg & Balint, 1985). Sometimes the feedings are started as continuous by means of an enteral feeding pump. The child can later transition to larger volume bolus feedings once the stomach becomes acclimated to larger volumes. Bolus feedings are more similar to a normal feeding pattern, but not all children tolerate them. For those children who cannot burp or vomit, it may be necessary to decompress the stomach through the gastrostomy. This can be done with the feeding

tube of the Genie or Mic-Key and with the decompression tube of the Bard SLD. Allowing the stomach to decompress after a few ounces of formula helps maintain the child's comfort during feedings. The gastrostomy device should remain vented for approximately 30 minutes to allow gas to escape from the stomach (Paarlberg & Balint, 1985). An easy way to vent the device is to elevate the feeding/decompression tube. Attach a large syringe in which the plunger has been removed. Tie the syringe to the crib, or, if the child is being held, pin the syringe to the shirt of the caregiver.

Developmental considerations related to gastrostomy feedings are also important. Offering the child a pacifier helps to stimulate sucking and develop oral function skills (Paarlberg & Balint, 1985). When medically safe, allowing the child to eat some food by mouth provides oral stimulation and is important for reinforcing to the child the connection between eating and a full stomach. It is important to verify the ability of the child to swallow with normal function. This can be done by obtaining a modified barium swallow examination before oral feedings are started. Children who aspirate will need further intervention before they begin oral feedings, and in some cases oral feeds will be contraindicated.

Normal interactions between the child and the siblings should be encouraged. Siblings should be included in the care of the child with a gastrostomy to foster sibling bonding. Mealtime provides a rich environment for learning. Having the child receive a tube feeding at the table with the rest of the family enables him or her to learn mealtime rituals and rules (Paarlberg & Balint, 1985; Rubin, 1967; Steele, 1991).

NURSING INTERVENTIONS

The success of the surgical intervention is greatly influenced by the instructions provided to the parents. It is important for staff and families to understand the surgical procedure and the effect it has on the child. After the antireflux procedure, the child and/or parent should be taught not to induce vomiting because initially the child may not be able to vomit and the act of vomiting puts increased pressure on the repair. Use the NG or g-tube for gastric decompression (Paarlberg & Balint, 1985).

If feedings are sluggish, flush the gastrostomy device with water three to four times a day to keep the gastrostomy device patent. In addition, extra water may be necessary to meet the child's fluid requirements.

Accidental dislodgement of the device can result in rapid closure of the tract. Both nursing staff and families should be aware that rapid replacement of the device is imperative to maintain patency of the tract. A Foley catheter can be inserted into a well-established tract in the event of dislodgement. However, in a new gastrostomy, less than 4 to 6 weeks from time of operation, the Foley catheter should be replaced by the surgeon and correct position verified with fluoroscopic examination.

Rapid infusion of formula into the stomach may cause discomfort to the child. Remember if feeding by gravity, the higher the tube, the faster the feeding infuses (Paarlberg & Balint, 1985). Positioning the child right side down helps with emptying of the stomach and can decrease cramping. A bloated or distended abdomen may indicate obstruction or feeding intolerance and should be reported to the physician (Sterling et al., 1991). Monitoring stool patterns in the postoperative period can help identify complications such as dumping syndrome or intestinal obstruction.

Knowing the feeding device is key in minimizing complications and enhancing problem solving (Coldicutt, 1994). Of the SLDs discussed earlier, only the Bard requires a decompression tube to aspirate gastric contents. This is an important distinction. If the feeding tube is used, the nurse cannot aspirate contents. If the decompression tube is used all the time for feedings, the life of the valve within the button is shortened. The other devices use the same tube to feed or decompress the stomach without the risk of harm to the valve. When using the Bard feeding device, the nurse needs to match the feeding tube to the French size of the button. For the other devices, one feeding tube fits all the devices. Additional information regarding the most common causes for gastrostomy devices to malfunction and troubleshooting solutions can be found in Table 16–2 (Coldicutt, 1994; Eisenberg, 1994; Paarlberg & Balint, 1985; Steele, 1991).

TRANSITIONING TO HOME

Despite mastering the tasks of gastrostomy care in the hospital, families become anxious and overwhelmed at the prospect of managing gastrostomy devices at home. The following tips can help to smooth the transition to home. First, a certain area in the house should be designated for storing necessary medical equipment. Supplies should be kept in a clean dry place close to where they will be used and away from other children or pets. A place near the kitchen is best. The family gathers for meals in the kitchen and the sink can be used to clean the feeding tubes. Second, gathering all supplies before a feeding or skin care task decreases the time to do the task. Third, parents should keep emergency phone numbers handy, as well as an emergency travel kit with feeding device replacement supplies and dressings. This kit should be readily available to parents or other caregivers. The parents should instruct babysitters and school personnel, when applicable, on use of the device and how to handle complications such as accidental dislodgement.

In the event the device is inadvertently dislodged within 4 to 6 weeks of the surgery, recommendations are to have the device replaced by medical personnel. Many times the placement is confirmed by a radiologic study because the tract is not well established at this time. Parents can be instructed on device replacement per the institution protocol once the tract is well established. Clothing that does not interfere with the device is recommended. It may be necessary to keep the child in a one-piece outfit to prevent tugging, pulling, or potential dislodgement.

The goal of making the home routine as normal as possible should be reinforced with the parents. Skin care around the feeding device site includes cleaning the site daily with soap and water. Parents can use cotton-tip applicators to get in those hard-to-reach areas under the device. No special cleaning solution is required (Coldicutt, 1994; Paarlberg & Balint, 1985; Steele, 1991). The child can bathe and swim with the device as long as the skin is dried thoroughly afterward to prevent irritation. The cap to the device should be checked routinely to ensure it is secure. The parents should be instructed to rotate the SLD daily to prevent skin ulceration. Turning also allows proper inspection of all the areas of the skin.

Detachable feeding tubes used with SLDs can be cleaned using warm soapy water. For tubes with significant buildup of residue, carbonated water, half-strength vinegar, cranberry juice, or cola can be used to remove debris. The tube is detached from the button and the solution is infused; the tubing is rinsed with water and hung to air dry.

Last, whenever possible, liquid medications are preferred because they are less likely to clog the tube. If the medication is available only in tablet form, the tablet should be crushed and dissolved in water. The gastrostomy should be flushed well to remove particles from the tube. The key to keeping a tube patent is to flush well after medications or feedings. Warm water, cranberry juice, diluted lemon juice, or cola are all used to flush the tube. The appropriate solution should be chosen on the basis of the age and needs of the child. Often a flush of 10 ml is needed (Coldicutt, 1994; Steele, 1991). Smaller amounts are indicated for premature infants and children with fluid restriction. The well-cared-for tube can often last up to a year or more with daily use. In general, the tubes last anywhere from 6 months to a year, depending on use.

RESEARCH

Dealing with a chronic disease such as GERD can be taxing to families and staff. If the child is hospitalized frequently for GERD complications, he or she may fall farther and farther behind in reaching development milestones. Further research needs to be done to assess the effect this disease has on children's development. Identifying which children within this group are most at risk and identifying early intervention strategies that parents can take would be helpful. Early identification of these children may decrease physical and intellectual deficits that result from repeated hospitaliza-

Table 16–2 Troubleshooting Gastrostomy Devices

Presenting Problem	Probable Causes	Solution
Dislodgement	• Tube/button snags on clothing • Child pulls on the device • Poor healing at the exit site	• If the device was placed within 4–6 wk or the dislodgement was traumatic, the tube should be replaced by medical personnel and placement should be confirmed by fluoroscopy. • If the tract is well established, replace the device with the appropriate size Foley or button device. • Wear loose-fitting clothing around abdomen to prevent snagging.
Leaking around the tube onto the skin surface causing skin excoriation	• Improper fit of device • Frequent tugging or pulling of the device causing widening of the tract	• Use gauze or spacer to help get snug fit. • Tape feeding tube securely to the skin surface to prevent rotation in the tract.
Valve incompetence	• Improper feeding attachment placed repeatedly in the button/tube causing stretching of the tube or weakening of the valve (syringes or decompression tubes used for feedings) • Sticky fluids or particles of medicine preventing proper valve closure	• Flush well after medications with 5–10 ml of lukewarm water. (Soda, tonic water, or cranberry juice can be used as a substitute for water, diet permitting.) • Give liquid medications when possible. • Avoid sticky or nonpureed foods.
Bleeding	• During tube change • Rotation of the tube in the tract can irritate the skin surface	• Small amount of bleeding is not uncommon with tube change and it stops quickly with pressure to the site. • Secure the device snugly to the skin surface.
Clogged tube	• Medications or food that is not liquified • Kink in the tube • Inadequate flush after feedings	• Flush well after medications with 5–10 ml of lukewarm water. (Soda, tonic water, or cranberry juice can be used as a substitute for water, diet permitting.) • Give liquid medications when possible. • Avoid sticky or nonpureed foods. • Secure the device adequately.
Vomiting/diarrhea	• Device migration in the tract causing gastric outlet obstruction or dumping syndrome	• Use gauze or spacers to help get a snug fit. • Tape as needed.
Granulation tissue build-up	• Improper fit of device • Tugging or repeated rotation of device	• Use gauze or spacers to help get a snug fit. • Tape as needed. • Apply silver nitrate to granulation tissue qd or qod until resolved—be sure to rinse skin with water after application. • Apply triamcinolone cream 0.5% to granuloma until resolved.
Gastric erosion	• Rapid weight gain leading to inadequate shaft length	• Remeasurement and replacement of device with longer shaft length.
Cellulitis	• Narrow diameter of the shaft of the 18 F mushroom-type SLD allows the mushroom tip to be pulled up into the tract	• Quick recognition of pain with turning of button. • Replacement with appropriate larger-sized tube.

tions and surgeries (Berube, 1997). Quality of life issues related to the morbidity of antireflux procedures warrant further investigation. Finally, continued research into the benefits of positioning in light of the American Academy of Pediatrics recommendations need to be explored for the child with GERD.

In summary, nursing plays an integral role in assisting with the diagnosis and treatment of children with GERD. The families require information and emotional support to follow the medical and/or surgical treatment plan. Both the medical approach and the surgical approach are time intensive for the families. The success of each child's plan is based on parental involvement and commitment to the plan. Consistent, clear instructions given to the parents and reinforced by the staff provide the best method for optimal results. With timely diagnosis and proper intervention, children with GERD can have good outcomes with optimal quality of life.

REFERENCES

Armentrout, D. (1995). Gastroesophageal reflux in infants. *Nurse Practitioner, 20*(5), 54–63.

Berube, M. (1997). Gastroesophageal reflux. *Journal of the Society of Pediatric Nursing, 2*(1), 43–46.

Boix-Ochoa, J., & Rowe, M.I. (1998). Gastroesophageal reflux. In J.A. O'Neill, M.I. Rowe, J.L. Grosfeld, E.W. Fonkalsrud, & A.G. Coran (Eds.), *Pediatric surgery* (5th ed., pp. 1007–1028). St. Louis, MO: Mosby.

Boyle, J.T. (1989). Gastroesophageal reflux in the pediatric patient. *Gastroenterology Clinics of North America, 18*, 315–337.

Broscious, S.K. (1995). Preventing complications of PEG tubes. *Dimensions of Critical Care Nursing, 14*(1), 37–41.

Coldicutt, P. (1994). Children's options. *Nursing Times, 90*(13), 54–56.

Eisenberg, P.G. (1994). Gastrostomy and jejunostomy tubes. *RN, 57*(11), 54–59.

Foglia, R.P. (1997). Gastroesophageal reflux. In K.T. Oldham, P.M. Colombani, & R.P. Foglia (Eds.), *Surgery of infants and children: Scientific principles and practice.* Philadelphia: Lippincott-Raven.

Fonkalsrud, E.W., Ellis, D.G., Shaw, A., Mann, C.M. Jr., Black, T.L., Miller, J.P., & Snyder, C.L. (1995). A combined hospital experience with fundoplication and gastric emptying procedure for gastroesophageal reflux in children. *Journal of the American College of Surgeons, 180*, 449–455.

Gibson, E., Cullen, J.A., Spinner, S., Rankin, K., & Spitzer, A.R. (1995). Infant sleep position following new AAP guidelines. *Pediatrics, 96*(1), 69–72.

Hunter, J.G., Trus, T.L., Branum, G.D., Waring, J.P., & Wood, W.C. (1996). A physiologic approach to laparoscopic fundoplication in gastroesophageal reflux disease. *Annals of Surgery, 223*(6), 673–687.

Hyman, P.E. (1994). Gastroesophageal reflux: One reason why baby won't eat. *The Journal of Pediatrics, 125*(6), S103–S109.

Jolley, S.G. (1992). Current surgical considerations in gastroesophageal reflux disease in infancy and childhood. *Surgical Clinics of North America, 72*(6), 1365–1390.

Jolley, S.G. (1995). Gastroesophageal reflux disease as a cause for emesis infants. *Seminars in Pediatric Surgery, 4*(3), 176–189.

Jones, S. (1992). Relationship between apnea and GER: What nurses need to know. *Pediatric Nursing, 18*(4), 413–418.

Liebert, P.S. (1989). *Color atlas of pediatric surgery.* New York: Elsevier.

Orenstein, S.R. (1992). Gastroesophageal reflux. *Pediatrics in Review, 13*(5), 174–183.

Paarlberg, J., & Balint, J.P. (1985). Gastrostomy tubes: Practical guidelines for home care. *Pediatric Nursing, 11*(2), 99–102.

Raffensperger, J.G. (1990). *Swenson's pediatric surgery* (5th ed. pp. 811–822). Norwalk, CT: Appleton & Lange.

Rowe, M.I., O'Neill, J.A., Grosfeld, J.L., Fonkalsrud, E.W., & Coran, A.G. (1995). *Essentials of pediatric surgery* (pp. 422–427). St. Louis, MO: Mosby.

Rubin, R. (1967). Food and feeding: A matrix of relationships. *Nursing Forum, 6*, 195–205.

Shannon, R. (1993). Gastroesophageal reflux in infancy: Review and update. *Journal of Pediatric Health Care, 7*(2), 71–76.

Sondheimer, J.M. (1994). Gastroesophageal reflux in children: Clinical presentation and diagnostic management. *Gastrointestinal Endoscopy Clinics of North America, 4*(1), 55–74.

Steele, N.F. (1991). The button: Replacement gastrostomy device. *Journal of Pediatric Nursing, 6*(6), 421–424.

Sterling, C.E., Jolley, S.G., Besser, A.S., & Matteson-Kane, M. (1991). Nursing responsibility in the diagnosis, care, and treatment of the child with gastroesophageal reflux. *Journal of Pediatric Nursing 6*(6), 435–441.

Tunell, W.P. (1989). Gastroesophageal reflux in childhood: Implications for surgical treatment. *Pediatric Annals, 18*(3),192–196.

Appendix 16–A

Critical Pathway for Nissen/Gastrostomy

for addressograph plate

	Day 1	Day 2	Day 3	Day 4
Monitoring/assessment	□ Dressing dry and intact □ VS q4° □ Monitor GI output q4° □ Strict I & O □ Weight qd	□ VS per floor routine □ Dressing change PRN if saturated	□ Nursing may remove dressing	
Treatments	□ CR monitor □ Pulse oximetry	□ D/C if patient stable □ D/C if patient stable		
Lines/drains	□ GT to gravity □ PIV—1½ x maintenance	□ Elevate GT □ IV fluid maintenance	□ Begin GT feeds □ PIV—½ maintenance, decrease fluids as GT feedings increase	□ D/C IV if tolerating GT feedings
Medications	□ MSO₄ (.05–.1 mg/kg), q 2–3° PRN □ Tylenol (15 mg/kg), q4° PRN	□ D/C MSO₄ □ Continue Tylenol	□ PO/GT meds if tolerating GT feedings □ Continue Tylenol	
Activity	□ HOB raised 30–40° □ Turn q2° □ Incentive spirometer	□ As tolerated	□ As tolerated	

continues

Appendix 16–A continued

	Day 1	Day 2	Day 3	Day 4
Diet	❑ NPO		❑ Begin GT feedings 1. Pedialyte → ½ strength formula, advance as tolerated 2. Decompress stomach as needed	
Consults/ referral	❑ Home care consult ❑ Nutrition consult initiated ❑ Pain service consult			
Patient teaching	❑ GT video ❑ GT booklet	Postoperative teaching ❑ GT site care ❑ GT feeding protocol ❑ Potential GT problems	Assess D/C needs ❑ Finalize home care needs ❑ Review nutrition goals with parents	❑ Parents demonstrate GT feeding and care of GT
Discharge planning	❑ Home care consult		❑ Obtain supplies for D/C ❑ Schedule follow-up appointment ❑ Provide family with replacement device	❑ Obtain GT supplies, enteral pump ❑ D/C if child tolerating feedings
Evaluation of outcomes	❑ GT teaching started ❑ Wound care ❑ Pain management ❑ Nutrition consult ❑ Home care consult	❑ Teaching continued ❑ CR monitor D/C'd	❑ Family verbalizes understanding of D/C instruction ❑ Home care ❑ Nutrition	❑ Family verbalized readiness for D/C ❑ Tolerating feedings
Signature/ title	Night P Day A Evening	P A	P A	P A

PART IV

Nursing Care of Children with Congenital Abdominal Conditions

CHAPTER 17

Abdominal Wall Defects

Beth Zimmermann

INTRODUCTION

Congenital abdominal wall defects are found in many forms. All the defects are related to the development of the umbilical cord. Abdominal wall defects include gastroschisis, omphalocele, bladder and cloacal exstrophy, prune-belly syndrome, urachal remnants, and omphalomesenteric duct malformations such as patent urachus and Meckel's diverticulum, among others. Congenital malformations are an imbalance between cell proliferation and apoptotic cell death (Keers, Hartwig, &VanDerWerff, 1996). This chapter reviews the operative and nursing care of infants born with omphalocele and gastroschisis, both of which are defects that allow herniation of the intraabdominal contents through the abdominal wall.

Gastroschisis is a Greek word that translates as "belly rent" and is classified as an abdominal wall defect (Moore, 1977). The defect is located lateral to the umbilical cord, commonly to the right. Typically, the defect is small, less than 4 cm. It is seen as a herniation of intestine and other abdominal contents through the rent. The cause of this defect is unknown. Possible theories are ruptured omphalocele in utero, premature obliteration of the umbilical ring, deficiency of embryonic mesenchyme, thrombosis of the omphalomesenteric artery, and accidental tear at the base of the cord from an unknown cause (Tunell, 1993). The uncovered bowel is exposed to amniotic fluid, including urine, leading to thickening and shortening of the bowel and development of a fibrous outer peel, resulting in greater damage to the intestine. This exposure of the bowel is the precursor to prolonged paralytic ileus and hypomotility. Exposure of the bowel affects long-term feeding and prognosis. Constriction of the bowel at the defect can cause twisting or ischemia, leading to stenosis, atresia, or volvulus. See Figure 17–1 for

a photograph of a newborn with gastroschisis. Note the defect to the right of the umbilicus.

Omphalocele results from failure of the intestines to return to the abdomen during the second stage of rotation of the midgut loop occurring during the eighth to tenth week of gestation (Moore, 1977). The covering of the hernia sac is the amnion of the umbilical cord, with the arteries and veins inserted into the defect's apex. Sizes differ; large defects may involve stomach, liver, spleen, and intestines. In con-

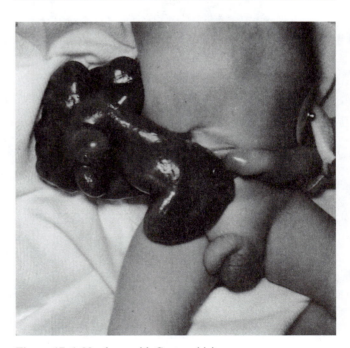

Figure 17–1 Newborn with Gastroschisis

211

trast to gastroschisis the presence of the covering provides protection for the intestine, decreasing the likelihood of long-term feeding problems. Rupture of the omphalocele sac gives an impression of gastroschisis. See Figure 17–2 for a photograph of a newborn with omphalocele prepped for surgery. Note the umbilicus at the apex of the defect.

INCIDENCE

Omphalocele carries an incidence of 1 in 3,200 to 10,000 births (Molenaar & Tibboel, 1993). The cause of omphalocele is unknown. A teratogenic effect has been suggested by some authors based on the association of omphalocele with multiple other related anomalies (Alexander, 1993). Cardiac anomalies occur in 30% to 50% of infants and chromosomal

anomalies in 10% to 40% of infants with omphalocele (Alexander, 1993). Structural, renal, limb, and facial anomalies may be present. Syndromes such as Beckwith-Wiedemann and pentalogy of Cantrell may also be present (Langer, 1996).

Gastroschisis carries an incidence of 1 in 4,000 to 10,000 births, with a low incidence of extraabdominal malformations. However, intestinal atresia is seen in approximately 10% of these infants (Langer, 1996). The low incidence of associated defects suggests a mechanical rather than a teratogenic cause (Alexander, 1993). The recurrence risk of gastroschisis is low in families with this single congenital defect. In families of children with multiple defects, the risk of recurrence increases as a familial cluster effect (Yang et al., 1992). One explanation of the cause of gastroschisis is an early tear of the umbilical cord before complete closure of the umbilical ring, occurring between the fourth to eighth week of gestation. A tear explains the lack of associated defects (Alexander, 1993). The intestinal atresia that occurs with gastroschisis is a result of ischemia secondary to the abdominal wall pinching on the mesentery. Atresias associated with gastroschisis may be singular or multiple involving the large or small intestine (Alexander, 1993).

DIAGNOSIS

Abdominal wall defects are often diagnosed prenatally. Maternal alpha-fetoprotein (AFP) levels are significantly elevated over normal levels in gastroschisis and omphalocele and are a useful diagnostic indicator (Touloukian & Hobbins, 1980). Elevated AFP levels signal the need for thorough ultrasonographic examination of uterine contents. Prenatal diagnosis leads to tertiary center delivery with surgeons and neonatologists in attendance at the birth. The specification of the defect is important because of the increased risk of associated anomalies with omphalocele. Amniocentesis is indicated to identify chromosomal anomalies. The results of chromosomal studies are used for parental counseling, including prognosis for the infant with an isolated anomaly and the possibility of pregnancy termination in the presence of lethal malformations (Dykes, 1996). Highly unusual umbilical cords seen at delivery should be clamped high or remain unclamped until the presence of an abdominal wall defect is ruled out.

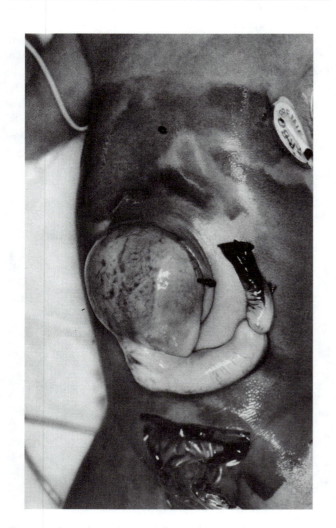

Figure 17–2 Newborn with Omphalocele Prepped for Surgery

PARENTAL COUNSELING

Prenatal diagnosis allows for preparation and care of the family and infant. Continuing controversy exists regarding vaginal versus Caesarean and/or early delivery of these infants. To date, specific benefits of early or Caesarean delivery are unidentified (Dykes, 1996; Howell, 1998). Regardless of the defect, arrangements are made for delivery in a Level III center, facilitating immediate surgical care. Predelivery consultations with the neonatal care team (pediatric surgeon, neonatologist, and advanced practice nurses) are arranged. Tours of the neonatal intensive care unit decrease family stress and begin preparations for the infant's care. The consultation outlines complications of the defect, surgery, and long-term outcomes. Additional discussions regarding hospitalization, breastfeeding, insurance, discharge planning/home care, and general pediatric care are advisable. These infants may spend from 1 week to 3 months in the hospital before discharge. A collaborative relationship among the family, surgeon, advanced practice nurses, and primary pediatrician is important for quality care.

TRANSPORT AND ADMISSION

Infant transport is preferentially in utero. If the child is delivered at an outlying center, the guidelines for transport developed by the American Academy of Pediatrics (1993) and the National Association of Neonatal Nurses should be followed. Interventions for delivery room care of infants with gastroschisis and omphalocele are essentially the same, with the addition of specific care of the exposed bowel of the child with gastroschisis. Nursing care is to maintain the airway, obtain and support vital signs, obtain intravenous access, and prevent hypothermia. Key interventions include placing an orogastric or nasogastric tube for decompression, wrapping the omphalocele in plastic wrap, placing the gastroschisis in a transparent surgical bowel bag to prevent heat loss from the exposed bowel and infection, and positioning the bowel so that it will not kink and compromise the blood supply during transport (Howell, 1998; Strodbeck, 1998).

Admission care includes calling the surgical team for introductions and consent, explanation of the surgery, and orientation of the family to the neonatal intensive care unit. The family is informed of the date, time, and location of surgery. Optimally, the parents have experienced bonding time with the infant before transport, including touching and caressing. Information regarding blood (directed donor), visiting hours, and family amenities is provided. If the mother is at another location, she is contacted and her phone number is documented for future communication.

Nursing care of the surgical neonate requires ongoing assessment and timely interventions (Harjo, 1998). Major considerations include oxygenation, acid-base balance, thermoregulation, fluid and electrolyte balance, and pharmacologic support (Kenner, Amlung, & Flandermeyer, 1998). Refer to Exhibit 17–1 for specific preoperative nursing care of the infant with an abdominal wall defect. For additional information about the management of the surgical neonate, refer to Chapter 33.

Exhibit 17–1 Preoperative Nursing Care

Prevent infection
- Use sterile barriers.
- Use sterile gloves.
- Administer antibiotics as ordered.

Prevent hypothermia
- Cover/protect exposed bowel with bowel bag.[a]
- Warm all solutions.
- Maintain temperature above 36.5°.[a]
- Use warmed humidified O_2.

Protect bowel
- Use bowel bag.[a]
- Prevent kinking of bowel.
- Use large-lumen soft Silastic decompression tube.

Fluid therapy
- Weigh infant.
- Obtain laboratory work (complete blood count, arterial blood gases, electrolytes, glucose, calcium, type and cross-match).
- Maintain patent intravenous access by means of peripheral line (immediately), central access later.
- Provide fluids—maintenance plus 1.5–2X may be required.
- Monitor blood pressure and urine output (fluid loss is common with gastroschisis).
- Measure intake and output and replace as needed.

Respiratory support
- Keep Sao_2 ≥95%.
- Avoid bag and mask because it will distend bowel.[b]
- Auscultate and suction as needed.

[a] Strodtbeck, 1998. [b] Kenner, Amlung, & Flandermeyer, 1998.

OPERATIVE PROCEDURE

In the infant with gastroschisis, the defect is repaired, if possible, within the first 24 hours because of the risk of fluid loss, temperature instability, and infection. The infant with omphalocele is stabilized, and additional tests are completed to rule out cardiac, renal, limb, and chromosomal anomalies as needed (Langer, 1996). In both gastroschisis and omphalocele, a small defect is repaired in one stage; larger defects require two stages of repair. Infants with additional anomalies (more common in omphalocele) require additional tests, consultations, and interventions before surgery occurs. The severity of accompanying anomalies determines the timing and type of surgery. The size of the defect, preoperative respiratory distress, and other coexisting congenital anomalies influence the surgical procedure chosen for the infant.

Primary closure is the preferred treatment of an abdominal wall defect. The bowel is decompressed of meconium from top to bottom to ease closure. Stretching of the abdominal wall and skin flaps to cover the defect without closing the fascia may be necessary (Vegunta, Cooney, & Cooney, 1993). If a ventral hernia is created by the inability to close the fascia, skin flaps are used to cover the area and the hernia is repaired several years later. Skin grafts may be used to cover the defect (Dillon & Cilley, 1993). Abdominal closure accomplished under tension requires close observation for vascular compromise of abdominal contents, decreased renal perfusion, and urine output. Respiratory compromise occurs because of immobilization of the diaphragm and inability to properly ventilate the infant as a result of increased intraabdominal pressure (Howell, 1998).

Intraabdominal pressure is identified as a cause of intestinal and renal ischemia in humans and animals (Lacey, Carris, Beyer, & Azizkhan, 1993). Current technology includes the use of bladder pressure (BdP) monitoring as a means to measure intraabdominal pressure (Tracy, 1997). The surgeon measures the BdP intraoperatively and uses 20 mm Hg as the critical number to decide whether to close the defect primarily or in a staged procedure. In addition, BdP measurements may be used postoperatively to guide the use of analgesics, sedatives, and paralytics depending on the condition of the infant as exhibited by the BdP pressure readings (Lacey et al., 1993).

Nursing care focuses on the set up and use of a Foley catheter connected to a transducer as a BdP device. Connection, calibration, bladder emptying, maintenance, and reporting of the pressures are nursing responsibilities (S.R. Lacey, personal communication, January 19, 1999). Centers that use BdP should establish nursing care policies and procedures.

Staged reduction, the two-staged repair, occurs over a period of days. Definitive closure should take place within 7 to 10 days to decrease the incidence of infection. This time frame allows the exteriorized contents to recede back into the abdomen under the least amount of tension possible. The first stage of repair requires placement of a silicone elastomer (Silastic) pouch around the exposed abdominal contents. Gravity and the mounting pressure from the pouch force the viscera to slowly move back into the expanding abdominal cavity. The pouch is folded/stapled down daily, carefully avoiding pulmonary and bowel compression. When there is room in the abdominal cavity to accommodate the viscera, the infant is returned to surgery and second stage closure is completed (Langer, 1996). See Figure 17–3 for an illustration of the staged silo technique for closing an abdominal wall defect.

Additional surgical procedures may include the placement of a central venous catheter, a gastrostomy tube, and the creation of a diverting stoma in the presence of bowel atresias (Dillon & Cilley, 1993). The need for long-term nutrition

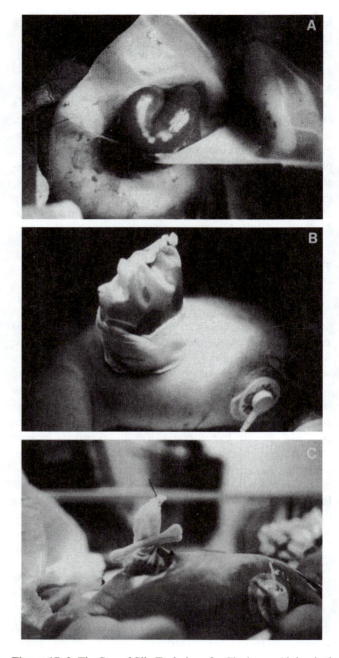

Figure 17–3 The Staged Silo Technique for Closing an Abdominal Wall Defect. A, A sheet of reinforced silicone elastomer (Silastic) is sutured around the fascial defect and over the viscera. B and C, The silo is gradually reduced over 3 to 6 days. The amount reduced each time can be gauged by monitoring intragastric or bladder pressure. Once the viscera are completely reduced, the Silastic is removed, and the fascia are closed in a second operation.

support is a possibility in gastroschisis because of the presence of hypomotility (Dillon & Cilley, 1993; Langer, 1996; Taylor, 1994). Refer to Exhibit 17–2 for nursing responsibilities after surgery.

Exhibit 17–2 Nursing Responsibilities after Surgery (references to silo are first stage only)

Respiratory support (distress may develop at any point, but is likely to worsen as the staged reduction progresses and always occurs after a primary closure)
- Observe pulse oximetry and arterial blood gases closely and frequently
- Increase O_2 as needed to maintain documented parameters
- Give paralytic (intubation required) and sedation agents as needed to maximize relaxation[a]
- Auscultate, suction, and provide chest therapy as needed

Prevent infection (silo integrity and care often require two people to avoid difficulties with tension)
- Administer antibiotics as ordered
- Bathe silo with warmed antibiotic solution/antibiotic ointment at base (surgeon's preference)
- Use strict sterile technique for dressing changes
- Monitor/report base of silo and suture site for separation, redness, or drainage[b]
- Monitor complete blood count/differential daily and report abnormal results
- Provide meticulous central venous access care to prevent infection, clogging, and loss of line

Fluid therapy (large amounts of fluid are lost into the silo from third spacing and pressure on the vena cava or renal artery)[c]
- Replace plasma proteins with Plasmanate/albumin to prevent edema as needed
- Maintain sterile patency of Foley catheter, document hourly urine output (adequate urine output is 1 ml/kg/hr)
- Give renal dose of dopamine as ordered
- Maintain decompression tube patency on low continuous suction, document aspirate and irrigant
- Monitor, record, and replace glucose and electrolytes as needed

Pain management (assessment of signs and symptoms of pain should be completed and documented hourly decreasing in fre-

quency with elapsed time from the procedure)
- Note increasing heart rate, decreasing Sao_2, changes in blood pressure or behavior[d]
- Administer narcotics to effect adequate dose response
- Use behavioral interventions such as pacifier, parent touch, vocalization, and decreased stimulation
- Wean from narcotics when appropriate[e]

Skin care (increased abdominal pressure may impede circulation to the lower extremities)
- Observe pulses, temperature, and color
- Use specialized mattress to decrease pressure
- Keep infant and all linens warm and dry
- Remove povidone-iodine and other solutions from skin with warmed normal saline to avoid chemical burns
- Use pectin-based barriers under all tape to avoid epidermal stripping[f]
- Note the normal reddened appearance of the suture line, report drainage or dehiscence immediately
- Keep sutured area clean with warmed normal saline and thoroughly dried

Gastrointestinal decompression (a nonfunctioning decompression tube fails to decrease pressure, causing pain, aspiration, and possible rupture)
- Irrigate decompression tube with air through the air port and normal saline through the succus port
- Maintain dual-lumen decompression tubes on low constant suction
- Clarify whether nurses or surgeons replace nonfunctioning decompression tubes

Plan of care: anticipate and plan for a daily silo reduction until the final closure
- Document expected time of daily intervention
- Gather requested supplies
- Medicate infant to prevent increased discomfort

[a] Kenner, Amlung, & Flandermeyer, 1998. [b] Howell, 1998. [c] Tunell, 1993. [d] Johnston & Stevens, 1990. [e] Franck & Vilardi, 1995. [f] Lund, Kuller, Tobin, & Lefrak, 1986.

NUTRITION

Hyperalimentation is started early because bowel function returns slowly, particularly in the infant with gastroschisis. Enteral feedings are begun when there is full bowel function including stool passage. Continuous nasogastric, gastrostomy tube, or measured oral feedings begin with clear liquids and advance as tolerated to breast milk or elemental formu-

las in cases of malabsorption. Formulas vary, and additives may be needed depending on the type and brand of formula and the individual infant's nutritional needs. The infant should demonstrate consistent weight gain before discharge. Full enteral feedings are desirable but may not be attainable before discharge. Many children with abdominal wall defects are discharged home on total parenteral nutrition (Taylor, 1994). The importance of breast milk is twofold: (1) the decreased incidence and severity of necrotizing enterocolitis in breastfed infants (Covert, 1995) and (2) the mother's observation that providing breast milk is the mother's unique contribution to her infant's welfare (Zimmermann, 1995). Breastfeeding dyads should be carefully followed and the lactation specialist should be consulted if necessary. Feedings should be advanced slowly; changing either concentration or volume one at a time. Bilious vomiting, residuals greater than 10 ml/kg, guaiac-positive stools, and Clinitest greater than 2% may be signs of necrotizing enterocolitis or obstruction and are reported to the surgery service. Encourage nonnutritive sucking early and often during tube feedings to develop and maintain oral skills. Sucking and swallowing difficulties are managed by the pediatric speech therapist.

DISCHARGE PLANNING AND PARENT CARE

The goal of discharge planning is a well-bonded family with the ability, desire, and knowledge to provide proper care for their infant. Home care needs vary depending on the presence of other anomalies and the condition of the infant. Financial and insurance status should be verified and the possibility of home nursing care should be investigated early. The family should be referred to social services as necessary to obtain needed financial support. The pediatrician should be provided with a discharge summary and phone numbers of specialists involved in the child's care. If the child requires enteral or parenteral feedings at discharge, the family requires extensive education and support at home. Equipment is ordered as early as possible to facilitate delivery and family education. Complex social and educational needs may be minimized if identified and addressed early in the planning process.

COMPLICATIONS AND LONG-TERM OUTCOMES

Families should be educated early as to the signs of complications, such as bilious emesis, abdominal distention, poor appetite, elevated temperature, constipation, diarrhea, and changes in behavior because these may be signs of obstruction or midgut volvulus. Most of these infants lead healthy normal lives with few complications. The most common complications are bowel obstruction and ventral hernias. A ventral hernia is defined as a loop of bowel protruding through the abdominal musculature and may occur in the area of the surgical scar. Surgical repair of ventral hernias or adhesive obstructions are required in approximately one third of cases (Langer, 1996). If complications occur, they are more common in children less than 7 years of age (Tunell, Puffinbarger, Tuggle, Taylor, & Mantor, 1995). It is imperative that parents know their child's "normals" to recognize complications in a timely manner. Parents should be encouraged to visit frequently for long periods of time at various times of the day. "Make parents experts on their baby's wants and needs" (J. Harjo, personal communication, March 1995). Infants without coexisting anomalies, who survive the surgical repairs (approximately 80% to 90%), have a normal quality of life (Vegunta et al., 1993; Tunell et al., 1995).

CONCLUSION

Omphalocele and gastroschisis are abdominal wall defects that require specialized nursing care provided by nurses in the special care nursery at a tertiary center. The infants' long-term survival and quality of life depend on early interventions and care. Nurses have the opportunity to provide surgical patients and their families elegant multidisciplinary care leading to optimal short-term and long-term outcomes.

REFERENCES

Alexander, F. (1993). Anterior abdominal wall defects. In R. Wyllie & J.W. Hyams (Eds.), *Pediatric gastrointestinal disease: Pathophysiology, diagnosis, and management* (pp. 506–514). Philadelphia: W.B. Saunders Company.

American Academy of Pediatrics. (1993). Task force on interhospital transport: Guidelines for air and ground transport of neonatal and pediatric patients. Elk Grove, IL: Author.

Covert, R. (1995). The effects of breastmilk: Incidence of NEC. Paper presented at the society of pediatric research. San Diego, CA.

Dillon, P.W., & Cilley, R.E. (1993). Newborn surgical emergencies: Gastrointestinal anomalies, abdominal wall defects. *Pediatric Clinics of North America 40*(6), 1307–1314.

Dykes, E.G. (1996). Prenatal diagnosis and management of abdominal wall defects. *Seminars in Pediatric Surgery 5*(2), 90–94.

Franck, L.S., & Vilardi, J. (1995). Assessment and management of opioid withdrawal in ill neonates. *Neonatal Network, 14*(2), 39–48.

Harjo, J. (1998). The surgical neonate. In C. Kenner, J.W. Lott, & A.A. Flandermeyer (Eds.), *Comprehensive neonatal nursing* (2nd ed., pp. 781–787). Philadelphia: W.B. Saunders Company.

Howell, K.K. (1998). Understanding gastroschisis: An abdominal wall defect. *Neonatal Network, 17*(8), 17–25.

Johnston, C., & Stevens, B. (1990). Pain assessment in newborns. *Journal of Perinatal and Neonatal Nursing, 4*(1), 41–52.

Keers, N.G., Hartwig, & VanDerWerff, J.F.A. (1996). Embryonic development of the ventral body wall and its congenital malformations. *Seminars in Pediatric Surgery, 5*(2), 82–89.

Kenner, C., Amlung, S.R., & Flandermeyer, A.A. (1998). *Surgical neonate:*

Protocols in Neonatal Nursing (pp. 575–589). Philadelphia: W.B. Saunders.

Lacey, S.R., Carris, L.A., Beyer, J. III, & Azizkhan, R.G. (1993). Bladder pressure monitoring significantly enhances care of infants with abdominal wall defects: A prospective clinical study. *Journal of Pediatric Surgery, 28*(10), 1370–1375.

Langer, J.C. (1996). Gastroschisis and omphalocele. *Journal of Pediatric Surgery, 5*(2), 124–128.

Lund, C., Kuller, J., Tobin, C., & Lefrak, L. (1986). Evaluation of a pectin-based barrier under tape to protect neonatal skin. *Journal of Obstetric, Gynecologic, and Neonatal Nursing, 15*(1), 39–44.

Molenaar, J., & Tibboel, D. (1993). Gastroschisis and omphalocele. *World Journal of Surgery, 17*(3), 337–341.

Moore, K.L. (1977). *The developing human: Clinically oriented embryology* (2nd ed.). Philadelphia: W.B. Saunders Company.

Strodtbeck, F. (1998). Abdominal wall defects. *Neonatal Network, 17*(8), 51–53.

Taylor, D.V. (1994). The infant with gastroschisis. *Suture Line, 2*(3), 1–2.

Touloukian, R.J., & Hobbins, J.S. (1980). Maternal ultrasonography in the antenatal diagnosis of surgically correctable fetal abnormalities. *Journal of Pediatric Surgery, 14*, 373–377.

Tracy, T. (1997). Abdominal wall defects. In K.T. Oldham, P.M. Colombani, & R.P. Foglia (Eds.), *Surgery of infants and children: Scientific principles and practice* (pp. 1083–1093). Philadelphia: Lippincott-Raven.

Tunell, W.P. (1993). Omphalocele and gastroschisis. In K.W. Ashcraft, & T.M. Holder (Eds.), *Pediatric surgery* (2nd ed., pp. 546–556). Philadelphia: W.B. Saunders Company.

Tunell, W.P., Puffinbarger, N.K., Tuggle, D.W., Taylor, D.V., & Mantor, P.C. (1995). Abdominal wall defects in infants: Survival and implications for adult life. *Annals of Surgery, 221*(5), 525–530.

Vegunta, R.K., Cooney, D.E., & Cooney, D.R. (1993). Surgical management of abdominal wall defects in infants. *AORN Journal, 58*(1), 53–63.

Yang, P., Beaty, T., Khoury, M.J., Chee, E., Stewart, W., & Gordis, L. (1992). Genetic-epidemiologic study of omphalocele and gastroschisis: Evidence of heterogeneity. *American Journal of Medical Genetics, 44*, 668–675.

Zimmermann, B.T. (1995). The maternal impact of breastfeeding a preterm infant in the post-discharge period. Paper presented at the National Association of Neonatal Nurses: International Research Conference. Seattle, WA.

CHAPTER 18

Intestinal Atresias, Duplications, and Meconium Ileus

Judith J. Stellar, Kelli M. Burns, and Susan K. Von Nessen

INTRODUCTION

Intestinal obstruction in the neonate is most often due to congenital anomaly rather than to an acquired condition. These patients present a clinical challenge. Symptoms may be acute, as with intestinal atresia, or gradual in anomalies that result in partial obstruction. In addition to the wide scope of clinical presentation, many of these anomalies are associated with other life-threatening and/or genetic conditions that require thorough evaluation and meticulous nursing care. Because intestinal atresias, duplications, and meconium ileus all have the potential for associated anomalies, good understanding of anatomy, physiology, and embryonic development is required. Although most of these conditions unto themselves have a good prognosis overall, the high association with other anomalies and diseases contributes to potentially greater morbidity and mortality. The nurse provides expert clinical care, offers the family support and education, and provides continuous case management through discharge and along the life continuum. (See Appendix 18–A for a caremap for jejunoileal atresia.)

INTESTINAL ATRESIAS

Atresia of the intestinal tract is characterized by total obstruction of the intestinal lumen. A stenosis, on the other hand, is an incomplete obstruction or narrowing of the intestinal lumen. Excluding esophageal atresia and anorectal malformations, small bowel atresias account for 20% of all neonatal obstructions (Skandalakis & Gray, 1994). Overall, the incidence of intestinal atresia (all types) is reported as 1 in 3,000 (Touloukian, 1993). Of all intestinal atresias, duodenal atresia accounts for 40% of the cases, followed by ileal atresia, 35%; jejunal atresia, 20%; and colonic atresia, less than 5% (Skandalakis & Gray, 1994). Sex distribution is equal (Skanadalakis & Gray, 1994; Touloukian, 1993). Duodenal

atresia is far more likely to be associated with other anomalies (Harris, Kallen, & Robert, 1995; Stauffer & Schwoebel, 1998). No true familial tendency has been identified, but there have been reports of intestinal atresias occurring in twins and siblings (Gross, Armon, Abu-Dalu, Gale, & Schiller, 1996; Moore, de Jongh, Bouic, Brown, & Kirsten, 1996; Rothenberg, White, Chilmonczyk, & Chatila, 1995; Yokoyama et al., 1997). Table 18–1 outlines the distinctions between various intestinal atresias.

Embryology

It is theorized that duodenal atresia has a different embryologic mechanism than jejunal-ileal and colonic atresia. Skandalakis and Gray (1994) group the embryogenesis of intestinal atresia as follows.

Primary Atresia

Primary atresias are due to a defect in fetal development. During the second month of gestation there is tremendous growth of epithelial lining cells of the intestine, so much so that the intestinal lumen is obliterated. By the end of the eighth to tenth weeks, the lumen undergoes recanalization. Failure of recanalization is theorized to be the cause of duodenal atresia and esophageal and rectal atresia. Another defect in the developmental process that results in atresias is the resorption of a segment of ileum during the assimilation of the vitelline duct at the fifth week of gestation.

Secondary Atresia

Secondary atresias are thought to be the result of an intrauterine ischemic event. In normal fetal development, bile secretion and swallowing of amniotic fluid begin at the 11th to 12th week of gestation. Autopsies of fetuses with jejunoileal atresia revealed bile and lanugo hairs in the intestinal seg-

Table 18–1 Distinctions between Various Intestinal Atresias

Type of Atresia	Etiology/Embryology	Incidence	Associated Anomalies
Duodenal—40%	Primary atresia Failure of recanalization of lumen during late 8th to 10th wk	1:6,000–1:10,000	High rate of associated anomalies include 1. Trisomy 21 (30% of cases) 2. Malrotation 3. Annular pancreas 4. Congenital heart disease 5. VACTERL association 6. Abdominal wall defects 7. Preduodenal portal vein 8. Biliary tree anomalies 9. Immunodeficiency
Jejunal—20% Ileal—35%	Secondary atresia Result of fetal accident or ischemic event at 10 wk to 4 mo (intra-uterine thrombosis, intussusception, volvulus)	1:750–1:5,000	Low rate of associated anomalies include 1. Cystic fibrosis 2. Meconium ileus 3. Malrotation 4. Renal dysplasia 5. Ocular anomalies 6. Hirschsprung's disease 7. Microcephaly 8. Immunodeficiency
Colonic <5%	Secondary atresia Ischemic event as above	Rare 1:20,000–1:40,000	Moderate rate of associated anomalies include 1. Limb anomalies 2. Hirschsprung's disease 3. Ocular anomalies 4. Cardiac anomalies

ments distal to the atresia, thus indicating that the event causing these atresias occurred later than the recanalization period as described previously. In addition, defects in the arteriomesenteric arcade were also identified, supporting an ischemic event. In experimental models, in utero ligation of a mesenteric vessel leads to an intestinal atresia. Causes of secondary atresias include scar formation after an intrauterine intestinal perforation in meconium ileus, intrauterine intussusception and volvulus, and intestinal snaring through the umbilical ring during bowel reentry into the abdominal cavity. Secondary atresias can also be the result of bowel herniation through various mesenteric defects or localized infarction/thrombosis of the vascular supply to a segment of bowel, resulting in necrosis and subsequent atresia. Jejunal-ileal atresia and colonic atresia are considered the secondary result of an ischemic event, usually occurring much later in fetal development than duodenal atresia.

Classification

Intestinal atresias are classified as follows (Skandalakis & Gray, 1994; Stauffer & Schwoebel, 1998; Touloukian, 1993) (see Figure 18–1).

1. Type I: Intraluminal web, membrane, or diaphragm consisting of mucosa and submucosa, completely obstructing the lumen. Muscularis is intact. This is the most common type of duodenal atresia. The "windsock anomaly" is a type I atresia in which the mucosal membrane has elongated or stretched out into the distal segment because of peristalsis.
2. Type II: Proximal and distal blind ends connected by a fibrous cord with mesentery intact. Type II anomalies occur in both duodenal atresia and jejunal-ileal atresia.
3. Type IIIa: Proximal and distal blind ends separated by a defect, usually V shaped, in the mesentery.
4. Type IIIb: Proximal blind end with distal segment coiling around single ileocolic vessel (apple peel or Christmas tree anomaly).
5. Type IV: Blind proximal end with multiple, isolated, distal segments (string of sausages).

Types III and IV are most often found in jejunal and ileal atresia. Multiple atresias of the duodenum are extremely rare. Type III and IV jejunal anomalies commonly result in short bowel syndrome; types I and II usually result in normal

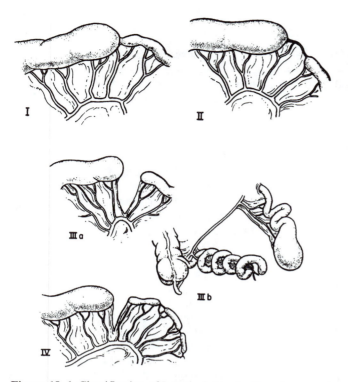

Figure 18–1 Classification of Intestinal Atresia. Type I, mucosal (membranous) atresia with intact bowel wall and mesentery. Type II, blind ends are separated by a fibrous cord. Type IIIa, blind ends are separated by a V-shaped (gap) mesenteric defect. Type IIIb, "apple-peel" atresia. Type IV, multiple atresias (string of sausages).

intestinal length (Skandalakis & Gray, 1994). Type III and IV anomalies of the ileum may not result in short bowel syndrome because of the ileum's ability to adapt to the shortened length.

Specific Types of Atresias

Duodenal Atresia

In a recent review, Stauffer and Schwoebel (1998) reported duodenal atresia occurs in 1 in 6,000 to 1 in 10,000 live births. They reported the first documented case in the literature in the 18th century, but it was not until 1914 that the first successful repair was performed by Danish surgeon Ernst. One third of these cases have associated Down syndrome, and of these, there is a significant incidence of congenital heart disease. There is also an association with Hirschsprung's disease. Because this is a proximal intestinal obstruction, there is usually a history of polyhydramnios. As high as 50% to 65% of cases of duodenal atresia have associated prematurity because of the onset of premature labor as a result of severe polyhydramnios (Nakayama, 1997a; Ross, 1994; Skandalakis & Gray, 1994).

Pathophysiology.   Duodenal obstruction occurs as a result of stenosis, atresia, or extrinsic causes such as annular pancreas, malrotation with volvulus, preduodenal portal vein, or duplications. A preduodenal portal vein is a condition in which the portal vein lies anterior to the duodenum. This anomaly is frequently associated with rotational abnormalities and situs inversus, which are, in turn, associated with duodenal obstruction (Ross, 1994). Annular pancreas is a condition that results from abnormal development of the pancreas during the second month of gestation, resulting in thin, flat segments of the pancreas surrounding the duodenum and causing a partial or complete obstruction. Stenosis and extrinsic causes result in partial obstruction and in some cases symptoms may not appear until later in life. Atresia, on the other hand, results in a complete obstruction and is seen with an acute onset of symptoms within hours after birth. The exception to this is the case of a type I atresia in which an intraluminal membrane or diaphragm perforates, resulting in a partial duodenal obstruction. Approximately 80% of duodenal atresias occur in the first and second portions of the duodenum, below the level of the bile ducts (Skandalakis & Gray, 1994). The proximal duodenum is greatly dilated with thickened, hypertrophied walls. The stomach and pylorus are also dilated. The distal duodenal segment is narrowed (because of disuse) and thin walled. Occasionally, the discrepancy in circumference of proximal and distal segments can be great, with the proximal segment measuring as much as 10 times that of the distal segment. Duodenal atresia rarely occurs above the level of the ampulla of Vater, with the most common site being at the ampulla. Occasionally, anomalies of the ducts and biliary tree are present.

Prenatal Diagnosis.   Duodenal and proximal jejunal obstruction often result in maternal polyhydramnios. This finding, therefore, necessitates fetal ultrasonography. Ultrasonography demonstrates a dilated, fluid-filled stomach and proximal duodenum. Absence of these findings does not necessarily rule out duodenal atresia, but patients with these findings should be closely monitored with subsequent ultrasonography. Amniocentesis is indicated in cases of severe polyhydramnios. An amniotic fluid reduction may be performed for severe polyhydramnios. If this procedure is performed, an aliquot of amniotic fluid is usually sent for karyotyping to rule out trisomy 21. Duodenal stenosis is more difficult to diagnose prenatally because the amniotic fluid passes through the stenotic segment and is absorbed in the distal ileum. In cases in which duodenal atresia is suspected before birth, the family should be prepared for a transfer to a tertiary care center for the genetic workup and postnatal surgical management and intervention (Nakayama, 1997a; Ross, 1994; Stauffer & Schwoebel, 1998).

Clinical Presentation.   Infants with duodenal atresia exhibit signs of an acute, proximal obstruction in the first few hours after birth. This is in contrast to more distal intestinal atresias in which the development of obstructive signs may occur gradually over the first 24 to 48 hours of life. Table 18–2 contrasts the history and presentation of infants with intestinal obstruction. Infants with duodenal stenosis may not have any signs of obstruction develop until months or years later. Occasionally, signs of obstruction develop when there is a change in the consistency in feedings from liquids to pureed, soft, or semisolid foods. In this scenario, the previously liquid feedings were able to pass beyond the stenotic segment, but the newly introduced solid foods cause or reveal a partial obstruction. Infants with complete obstruction caused by duodenal atresia exhibit bilious emesis soon after birth or with the first feeding or have a bile-stained gastric aspirate. Exceptions to this are cases in which a high-level web occurs proximal to the ampulla, where emesis would be nonbilious. Gastric aspirate in excess of 30 ml indicates a high-level obstruction. An abdominal examination may reveal fullness in the area of the epigastrium, and otherwise the belly is flat or scaphoid because of the lack of gas throughout the gastrointestinal (GI) tract. Occasionally, the stomach is so distended that the abdomen appears to have generalized distention. Decompression of the stomach with a vented orogastric/nasogastric (OG/NG) tube, such as a Replogle or Salem sump tube, relieves the distention and leaves the infant with a scaphoid abdomen. Patients with duodenal atresia pass meconium in contrast to those with a more distal obstruction in which meconium is scant. The infant may be jaundiced, with an indirect hyperbilirubinemia. Other abnormal laboratory findings include electrolyte disturbances caused by dehydration and a hypochloremic alkalosis when vomiting occurs.

Diagnostic Workup/Differential Diagnosis. A plain, supine radiograph is indicated as part of the initial diagnostic workup. An abdominal plain film may reveal a dilated, fluid-filled and air-filled stomach and proximal duodenum that appear as the classic "double bubble" sign. The first part of the double bubble is the dilated stomach; the second part is the dilated, atretic duodenum. Beyond the dilated duodenum, the abdomen is gasless. This "double bubble" sign combined with a gasless abdomen are diagnostic for duodenal atresia. Occasionally, a large amount of fluid in the stomach may obscure interpretation of the film. In this situation, an OG/NG tube is placed and gastric fluid is aspirated. Then, 50 to 60 ml of air is instilled into the stomach through the tube. This amount of air usually provides sufficient contrast to demonstrate the double bubble sign more clearly. In cases of complete duodenal obstruction caused by atresia, there is no role for a contrast study. When duodenal stenosis or a partial high-level obstruction is suspected, a double bubble may be seen, but gas is also seen throughout the abdomen. In this case, two views of the abdomen should be obtained: a flat plate and a left lateral decubitus or cross-table lateral. Whenever even a scant amount of gas is seen distal to the obstruction, rotational abnormalities must be ruled out. Malrotation with midgut volvulus can cause compression of the superior mesenteric artery and resultant bowel ischemia within a few hours (see Chapter 24). Because of the possibility of bowel ischemia and necrosis, an upper GI series is performed promptly to rule out rotational abnormalities. Ultrasonography can be helpful in diagnosing an annular pancreas or may reveal a "whirlpool sign," which is characteristic of volvulus (Stauffer & Schwoebel, 1998).

Jejunoileal Atresia

Jejunoileal atresia is a congenital obstruction of either the jejunum or ileum. These small intestinal atresias occur in 1 in 330 (Grosfeld, 1998) to 1 in 5,000 infants (Rowe, O'Neill, & Grosfeld, 1995). The incidence of associated congenial anomalies is lower with jejunoileal atresia, but the associated findings include small for gestational age, meconium peritonitis/ileus, imperforate anus, renal dysplasia, cardiovascular defects, and a 7% association with chromosomal abnormalities (Herman & McAlister, 1995; Kimble, Harding, & Kolbe, 1997; Sanders, Blackmon, Hogge, & Wolfsberg, 1996; Slee & Goldblatt, 1996). Of note, 25% of neonates with jejunal/ileal atresia have cystic fibrosis.

Prenatal Diagnosis. Diagnosis of midgut intestinal atresia may be suspected with maternal polyhydramnios and detected by fetal ultrasonography. Because amniotic fluid is absorbed in the distal ileum, a maternal history of polyhydramnios is less common in jejunoileal atresia than duodenal atresia. Sonography obtained at 24 weeks' gestation demonstrates multiple dilated fluid-filled bowel loops proximal to the stenotic/atretic segment (Sanders et al., 1996) later in gestation than duodenal atresia.

Table 18–2 Gastrointestinal Obstruction in the Neonate

	Proximal	*Distal*
1. Polyhydramnios	Yes	No
2. Prematurity	Frequent	Occasional
3. Onset of symptoms	Early (hours, after first feeding)	Late (24–48 hr)
4. Vomiting		
Character	± Bilious	+ Bilious
Volume	Large	Small
Timing	Early	Late
5. Distention	Mild, localized	Severe, generalized
6. Jaundice	Yes	Yes/No
7. Plain films	Double bubble or few dilated loops	Multiple dilated loops
8. Meconium	Adequate	Scant
9. Microcolon	No	Yes

Clinical Presentation. The classic signs of jejunoileal atresia include bilious vomiting, abdominal distention, and failure to pass normal amounts of meconium. This obstructive picture, associated with jejunoileal atresia, usually does not present until after the first feeding or by 24 hours of life (Ross, 1994). An earlier presentation of obstruction would be suspect for a higher intestinal obstruction. Of note, the presence of bile in gastric aspirates suggests an obstruction distal to the ampulla of Vater, where the bile ducts empty into the duodenum, and is associated to a greater degree with jejunal atresia. The infant exhibits generalized abdominal distention. The greater the abdominal distention, the more distal the intestinal obstruction. In addition, the more distal the obstruction, the passage of meconium becomes more scant. This is due to the lack of succus entericus passing through the distal segment.

Diagnostic Workup/Differential Diagnosis. Abdominal radiographs, flat and erect or lateral decubitus, reveal air-fluid levels and multiple dilated proximal loops of bowel. A contrast enema may be helpful in diagnosing "microcolon." Because the colon never fills with meconium, it remains underexpanded or unused, resulting in a colon smaller in diameter than the normal colon. In addition, a contrast enema helps to differentiate small versus large bowel distention or ileal stenosis, and evaluates intestinal rotation. Hirschsprung's disease should be included in the differential diagnosis of distal ileal atresia and a contrast enema should be obtained to identify a transition zone. Ultrasonography is helpful in distinguishing meconium ileus from ileal atresia. Ileal atresia presents as dilated loops filled with fluid and air (Neal, Seibert, Vanderzalam, & Wagner, 1997). On ultrasonographic examination, meconium ileus is demonstrated by a thick, echogenic fluid in the intestine. This meconium-filled bowel is described as a "soap bubble" or "ground glass" appearance, where air is mixed in with thick, inspissated meconium. These are important radiologic findings because meconium ileus may be treated medically with hyperosmolar enemas, whereas intestinal atresias require surgery.

Colonic Atresia

Colonic atresia is the rarest form of intestinal atresia occurring in about 1 in 20,000 live births and accounting for <5% of all atresias (Oldham,1998; Skandalakis & Gray, 1994). Successful repair with diverting colostomy reportedly was performed in 1922 by Gaub. Dr. Potts was the first to perform successful primary anastomosis in 1947. Colonic atresia is associated with skeletal, ocular and cardiac anomalies, Hirschsprung's disease, and other intestinal atresias (Croaker, Harvey, & Cass, 1997; Oldham, 1998).

Embryology. The embryogenesis of colonic atresia is thought to be the same as jejunoileal atresia: in utero vascular compromise. Possible causes of vascular compromise include incarcerated hernias, colonic volvulus, and intussusception. As described earlier, the classification of small bowel atresia is also applied to colonic atresia (Oldham, 1998; Skandalakis & Gray, 1994).

Clinical Presentation. A prenatal history of polyhydramnios is not usually present in colonic atresia because amniotic fluid is absorbed in the distal ileum. The infant with colonic atresia is seen with signs of a high-grade distal obstruction. These signs include generalized distention, feeding intolerance, and bilious vomiting. Because there is little intestine distal to the atresia, passage of meconium is scant or absent (Oldham, 1998; Ross, 1994; Touloukian, 1993).

Diagnostic Workup. Abdominal plain films reveal multiple, large, dilated loops with a "cut-off sign" and air fluid levels. A cut-off sign is the point at which the intestinal gas pattern abruptly ends. The proximal intestinal loops are distended and no gas is in the rectum or distal colon. Colonic atresia presenting as a perforation is not uncommon. In this case pneumoperitoneum is seen on plain films. A contrast enema, with either barium or a water-soluble agent, demonstrates a microcolon with a cut-off of contrast medium (contrast ends abruptly) at the atretic point and proximal, dilated intraluminal air. The contrast enema establishes a definitive diagnosis of colonic atresia and can help identify an associated distal obstruction, such as short segment Hirschsprung's disease.

Preoperative Management

The infant with a complete proximal intestinal obstruction requires aggressive gastric decompression, fluid resuscitation and replacement, and correction of electrolyte abnormalities. Moderate to severe hypochloremic alkalosis may be present, which, if untreated, can lead to cardiac dysrhythmia. Monitoring of bilirubin levels is indicated because of indirect hyperbilirubinemia. Once stabilized, the infant is a candidate for surgical repair. Associated problems such as congenital heart disease or respiratory distress syndrome should be identified before operative intervention. Malrotation should be ruled out as described earlier. A thorough physical examination is performed before the operation to rule out associated anomalies such as the VACTERL association (V = vertebral, A = anorectal, C = cardiac, T-E = tracheal-esophageal, R = renal, L = limb anomalies) (Skandalakis & Gray, 1994; Touloukian, 1993) and others as listed in Table 18–1. When atresia is associated with an obvious VACTERL anomaly as evidenced on physical examination by findings of radial dysplasia or imperforate anus, further investigation for other associated anomalies within the VACTERL association should be performed.

Preoperative laboratory studies include electrolytes, complete blood count, type and cross-match, and bilirubin levels. Electrolyte imbalances are corrected or communicated to the anesthesia team. Packed red blood cells are available for use during surgery, although the actual need for transfusion is uncommon. Perioperative antibiotics, ampicillin and gentamicin, are given intravenously. Before taking the child to the operating room, a plan for long-term intravenous access should be considered because in some cases progression to full enteral feedings may not occur for some time. The support and education of the family in this preoperative period is crucial. The family is not only adjusting to the arrival of a new infant, but they are also adjusting to the diagnosis, information regarding the upcoming surgery, and perhaps to the concomitant diagnosis of trisomy 21, congenital heart disease, and/or other associated anomalies. Collaboration among surgery, cardiology, genetics, and other subspecialties to provide consistent, timely information to the family at this time is imperative.

Operative Intervention

Once stabilized the infant is a candidate for surgical repair. Options for surgical repair depend on the type of anomaly and the preference of the surgeon. The goal of surgical intervention is to establish intestinal continuity and eliminate or prevent functional obstruction.

Duodenal Atresia Repair

Excision of Duodenal Web (Figure 18–2).   Excision of the duodenal web is performed through a right upper quadrant transverse incision. The dilated proximal duodenum is identified. Because the muscularis is intact, the only finding is that of discrepant size of duodenal segments that are contiguous. A transpyloric tube is passed in the OR in type I anomalies to rule out a windsock anomaly. When gentle pressure is placed on the tube, there is an indentation seen in the outer layer of the bowel at the point of the attachment of the membrane. A longitudinal incision is made at the site of obstruction. The web is identified and the lateral portion is excised. The medial portion of the web is left intact because of the great risk of damaging the ampulla of Vater, which is often located at the site of the web attachment medially. The location of the ampulla can be detected by applying gentle pressure on the gallbladder. After excision of a portion of the web, a catheter is passed distally and saline is instilled until it empties into the colon. This passage of fluid rules out multiple distal webs (Nakayama, 1997a; Ross, 1994; Stauffer & Schwoebel, 1998).

Duodenoduodenostomy (Figure 18–3).   In a duodenoduodenostomy a transverse right upper quadrant incision is made. The hepatic flexure of the colon is mobilized and the proximal, dilated portion of the duodenum identified and freed from its attachments. Careful note is made of the presence of a preduodenal portal vein, abnormal pancreas, or abnormalities in rotation. If malrotation exists, a Ladd's proce-

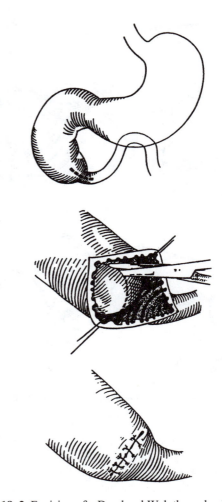

Figure 18–2 Excision of a Duodenal Web through a Longitudinal Incision across the Area of Obstruction. Care must be taken because the opening of the ampulla of Vater is frequently in the medial portion of the web itself. The web is therefore only partially excised along the lateral side, leaving the medial portion intact.

dure is performed (see Chapter 24). The distal duodenal segment is identified and mobilized. A transverse incision is made in the proximal segment carefully placed above the level of the ampulla of Vater. A longitudinal incision is made in the distal duodenal segment. Before closure of the anastomosis, a catheter is passed into the distal segment and saline is instilled until it empties into the colon. This is done to rule out any multiple distal atresias (Cilley & Coran, 1995; Ross, 1994; Stauffer & Schwoebel, 1998). The proximal transverse incision and distal longitudinal incision allow creation of a diamond-shaped anastomosis (Kimura et al., 1990). If an annular pancreas exists, the segment of duodenum and aberrant pancreatic tissue is bypassed with the duodenoduodenostomy. The pancreatic tissue is not divided off the duodenum because of the risk of fistula formation, pancreatitis,

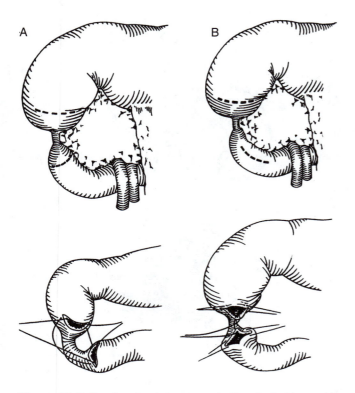

Figure 18–3 Duodenoduodenostomy. A, Standard side to side anastomosis. B, Diamond shaped duodenoduodenostomy.

and possible damage to underlying bile ducts (Cilley & Coran, 1995; Nakayama, 1997a; Stauffer & Schwoebel, 1998).

Duodenojejunostomy (Figure 18–4). Occasionally duodenojejunostomy may be required if the atresia involves the distal portion of the duodenum. A duodenojejunostomy consists of freeing up the proximal dilated duodenal segment and doing a retrocolic end-to-side anastomosis to the jejunum. In performing the duodenojejunostomy, consideration is given to placement of a gastrostomy tube, transanastomotic tube, and central line.

Tapering Duodenoplasty (Figure 18–5). In cases in which the proximal duodenal bulb is extremely dilated and floppy, a tapering procedure is considered to better approximate the proximal and distal portions of the repair. This procedure encourages earlier function of the dilated proximal segment and prevents stasis and dysmotility of the proximal end. This technique consists of autostapling and excising the antimesenteric portion of the dilated proximal segment longitudinally. Plication of the distended segment can also be done over a dilator (Cilley & Coran 1995; Touloukian, 1993). An alternative plication procedure consists of performing an elliptical excision of the seromuscular section of the distended duodenum. The mucosa, which is left intact, is then inverted or imbricated (arranged in a regular pattern

with overlapping edges). This technique avoids a long suture line but still tapers the dilated segment. It has been used to treat both duodenal and jejunal atresia (Kimura, Perdzynski, & Soper, 1996).

Jejunal-Ileal Atresia Repair

Jejuno-jejunostomy. An exploratory laparotomy is accomplished through a right upper quadrant transverse supraumbilical incision. The atresia is identified and the operative choice of procedure depends on the pathologic type of obstruction. In cases of high jejunal atresia, the atonic, atretic segment of proximal jejunum is resected back to the ligament of Treitz, and an end-to-oblique anastomosis performed (Figure 18–6). Leaving an extremely dilated proximal segment of intestine in any type of anastomosis usually results in a functional obstruction (Grosfeld, 1998). This is thought to be due to smooth muscle hyperplasia in the proximal segment, which in turn causes ineffective peristalsis. Inefficient contractions and propulsion lead to a chronic, obstructive state. In extreme cases, this results in decompensation of the segment of intestine and obstruction. Whenever possible, this dilated portion is resected.

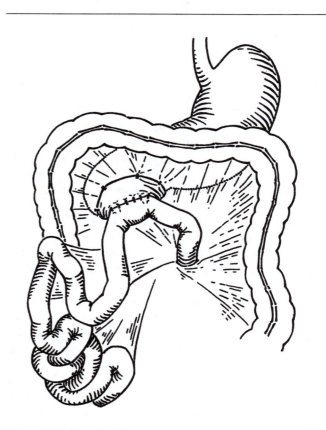

Figure 18–4 Duodenojejunostomy. A loop of proximal jejunum is brought through an opening in the transverse mesocolon and anastomosed to the most dependent portion of the obstructed duodenum.

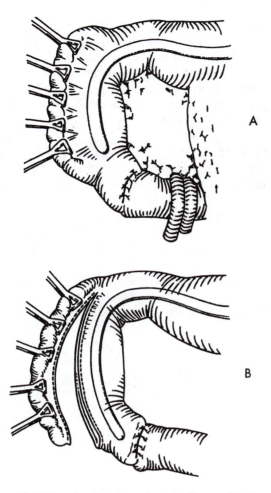

Figure 18–5 Tapering Duodenoplasty in Cases with Excessive Floppy and Distended Proximal Duodenum. A, Plication of the anterior wall with interrupted sutures over a dilator. B, Excision with use of an autostapling device.

remaining bowel is in question, or cases associated with meconium peritonitis, resection of the atretic ileal segment and exteriorization of bowel occurs. Examples of exteriorization procedures are demonstrated in Figure 18–8.

Colonic Atresia Repair. A transverse supraumbilical incision is used to allow the greatest exposure. Resection of the vastly dilated proximal end, with end-to-oblique primary anastomosis, is performed in cases in which no perforation and spillage has occurred and the infant is generally stable. Attention is given to preservation of intestinal length and the ileocecal valve. If the infant is unstable and/or there is significant fecal spillage or peritonitis, a diverting colostomy and a staged repair are performed. If the infant does not have severe cardiac or respiratory disease, prognosis and functional outcome are good. In either approach, the colonic specimen is evaluated for the presence of ganglion cells to rule out coexisting Hirschsprung's disease (Nakayama, 1997a; Oldham, 1998; Ross, 1994).

Nutritional Support

The decision to place a gastrostomy tube is based on the overall condition of the infant and the individual surgeon's preference. Other indications for a gastrostomy tube may include complex congenital heart disease, Down syndrome, and severe prematurity. A transanastomotic nasojejunal or gastrojejunal tube is sometimes placed, with the goal of initiation of earlier enteral feedings. Some surgeons believe that this is not necessary and has not been effective in terms of initiating feedings earlier. For patients who do require a gastrostomy tube and the surgeon prefers a transanastomotic tube, a side-by-side transgastric, transanastomotic tube is placed for early initiation of feedings. Occasionally, a surgical jejunostomy is performed for patients with complex

Tapering Jejunoplasty (Figure 18–7). In cases in which intestinal length is limited, resection may not be possible. Instead, an antimesenteric tapering jejunoplasty may be performed. Alternatively, an imbrication tapering technique can also be done to reduce the caliber of distended intestine and facilitate restoration of function. The advantage of this technique is that mucosa is left intact; the disadvantage is breakdown of the imbrication and recurrent dilation. The goal of either tapering procedure is to decrease the lumen size of dilated segment while preserving intestinal length. Similar to duodenal atresia, some surgeons consider placement of a transanastomotic feeding tube for proximal jejunal atresia to facilitate early enteral feedings.

Ileal Atresia Repair. In cases of ileal atresia, primary anastomosis is preferred. However, in cases of ileal atresia associated with volvulus or where vascular integrity of the

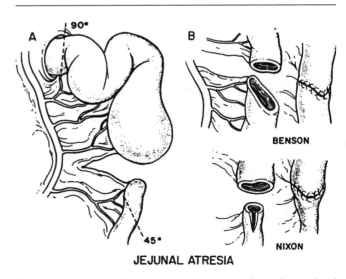

Figure 18–6 Jejuno-jejunostomy. Resection of atretic proximal segment to ligament of Treitz, and end-to-oblique anastomosis.

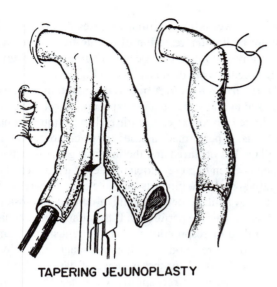

TAPERING JEJUNOPLASTY

Figure 18–7 Tapering Jejunoplasty. The bulbous distal portion of the atresia is resected, and a tube is placed in the antimesenteric side of the lumen; antimesenteric resection with an autostapler device is carried out up to the ligament of Treitz. End-to-end anastomosis completes the procedure. The staple line is also oversewn with interrupted sutures.

anomalies or extreme prematurity. Last, placement of a central line is considered at the time of operation for those patients who may require parenteral nutrition, who have critical associated anomalies, and/or who are small for age (Grosfeld, 1998; Touloukian, 1993).

Postoperative Management

Acute postoperative management includes the following:

1. oronasogastric decompression and drainage
2. intravenous fluid administration, including replacement of gastric output and third space losses
3. administration of intravenous ampicillin and gentamicin for 48 hours postoperatively
4. serial abdominal examinations, including assessment of surgical incision
5. serial laboratory evaluation
6. assessment of return of bowel function as evidenced by
   –presence of bowel sounds, passage of stool (alert surgeon if stool is acholic or if stools are light tan or clay colored because of lack of bile, specifically choleic acid)
   –decreasing NG aspirate
   –"clearing" of NG aspirate color from bilious to "saliva-like" (clear)

7. pain management achieved by judicious administration of intravenous narcotics (morphine) and/or ketorolac, advancing to acetaminophen, as tolerated, or use of an epidural catheter managed in collaboration with the anesthesia pain team (See Chapter 6 for more information about postoperative pain management in the neonate.)

Initiation of enteral feedings occurs when the ileus has resolved, the anastomosis begins to "open up" (GI secretions passing through the anastomosis), and the infant exhibits signs of return of bowel function as described previously. In particular, decreased gastric output that is lightening in color is a sign that the anastomosis has begun to function. Early signs of sepsis, including thrombocytopenia, temperature instability, increased white blood cells, and peritoneal signs herald an anastomotic leak (Nakayama, 1997a). In situations where a transanastomotic feeding tube or surgical jejunostomy are performed, slow continuous feedings can be started on postoperative day 1. Enteral feedings are initiated slowly and with caution, assessing for any signs of obstruction or anastomotic dysfunction. Initial enteral feedings consist of low-volume, clear, oral rehydration solution (Pedialyte) every 2 to 3 hours, with gradual increase in volume. The feeding regimen goal is 150 ml/kg/day of 20 calorie per ounce formula or full-strength breast milk, which translates to 100 kcal/kg/day. Bolus feedings of full-strength 20 calorie per ounce formula or breast milk, given every 2 to 3 hours, are increased by 5 ml each day to goal. Alternatively, continuous feedings of full-strength formula are increased by 1 ml/day to goal. Once goal is reached at 150 ml/kg/day, formula or breast milk can then be concentrated if added calories are

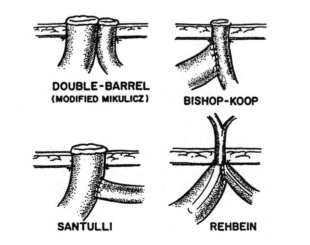

Figure 18–8 Exteriorization Procedures. These are used in instances of severe peritonitis and questionable bowel viability. The double-barrel side-by-side (modified Mikulicz) enterostomy is preferred.

needed. Increased frequency of stools and reducing substances found in stool are signs of intolerance. The most common reason for failure to progress feedings is altered peristalsis through the proximal and distal segments. This results from the size discrepancy in blind ends, especially in cases in which a tapering procedure was not performed. Because of this anatomic problem, some patients may take up to 14 days for anastomotic function and bowel function to return. Another reason for delayed feeding is actual anastomotic dysfunction in which reoperation and anastomotic revision is required. For patients with ileal atresia who have delayed passage of stool, Hirschsprung's disease should be considered if it has not already been ruled out.

Infants with midgut atresias may succumb to associated anomalies or complications of pneumonia, peritonitis, and sepsis. Cases of "apple-peel" deformity (type IIIb) or multiple atresia (type IV) frequently result in short bowel syndrome. This chronic condition is treated with a combination of cycled total parenteral nutrition, continuous elemental enteral feedings, and meticulous monitoring of growth, nutrition, and laboratory values. Unfortunately, the sequelae of short bowel syndrome account for a large percentage of morbidity and mortality in children with severe forms of jejunoileal atresia. Complications of colonic atresia include anastomotic leak, stricture, and dysfunction of the proximal segment. Generally, prognosis is good, with most morbidity and mortality the result of associated cardiac and other disease processes (Grosfeld, 1998; Touloukian, 1993).

GASTROINTESTINAL DUPLICATIONS

The term "duplications" encompasses GI anomalies that are either cystic or tubular in nature and are associated in some way with the GI tract. Three traits are common to duplications: a coating of smooth muscle, an epithelial lining, and an attachment to the GI tract. Cystic duplications are usually closed and do not communicate with the GI tract, whereas tubular duplications usually do communicate with the GI tract, with the communication most often occurring at the caudal end. Duplications may arise anywhere along the GI tract from the base of the tongue to the anus. Seventy-five percent of GI duplications are abdominal, 20% are thoracic, and 5% are thoracoabdominal. Associated anomalies include vertebral anomalies, esophageal atresia, jejunal atresia, anal defects, and genitourinary fistulas. Duplications can occur extensively along a long section of GI tract. Ten percent of GI duplications have more than one duplication.

Embryology

There are varied theories concerning the embryology of GI duplications (Skandalakis & Gray, 1994). One theory is failure of regression of certain embryonic structures. A second theory is failure of recanalization, similar to the duodenal atresia embryogenesis, occurring at about the fifth to eighth week of gestation, where proliferation of epithelial cells obliterate the lumen of the intestine. A third embryologic process theorized to result in duplications occurs during the fourth week of gestation. During this time, the gut endoderm separates from the notochord. This notochord is the precursor of the vertebral column. Abnormal adherence of a cord of gut endoderm to a portion of the notochord results in the formation of GI duplications that are cystic, tubular, or diverticular in nature.

Clinical Presentation

Gastrointestinal duplications typically are seen by 2 years of age. In utero diagnosis of duplication is considered in patients with suspicious fetal ultrasonograms, including signs of proximal bowel obstruction as evidenced by polyhydramnios. Some duplications do not become symptomatic until adulthood, and still others are never symptomatic and are not found until autopsy. Clinical presentation depends on location and size. The symptoms may lead the clinician to suspect the more common diagnoses of intestinal atresia/stenosis, intussusception, volvulus, or Meckel's diverticulum. The typical presentation includes signs of partial intestinal obstruction, abdominal pain, and GI bleeding. Signs of obstruction, including abdominal distention, pain, and vomiting, occur as a result of the duplication compressing the lumen of the adjacent intestine (Ross, 1994; Stauffer & Schwoebel, 1998; Templeton, 1995). Pain is the result of intraluminal distention and bowel necrosis caused by compression of the mesenteric vasculature. GI bleeding is most often caused by ectopic gastric mucosa in the lining of the duplication, which in turn causes peptic ulceration. If ulceration progresses, erosion, perforation, and peritonitis may ensue. Thoracic or thoracoabdominal duplications present with respiratory distress from airway compression, heartburn, and melena. Pyloric or duodenal duplications may mimic hypertrophic pyloric stenosis with emesis and failure to gain weight (Grosfeld, Boles, & Reiner, 1970; Ramsey, 1957). Duodenal duplications, which are rare, present with bleeding, obstruction, and jaundice as a result of obstruction at the ampulla of Vater. Symptoms may range from jaundice to high intestinal obstruction, pancreatitis, and hemorrhage. Colonic duplications may present with signs of constipation, rectal prolapse, and associated perirectal abscess (LaQuaglia et al., 1990).

Diagnostic Workup

Tubular GI duplications are most often identified on contrast studies. Cystic duplications can be identified with ultrasonography. In either situation, further radiographic studies, such as computed tomography (CT) scan with oral and intravenous contrast, may be necessary to rule out multiple duplications. Gastric duplications cause external compression on the greater curvature of the stomach, producing a filling defect on an upper GI examination. The contrast material does not fill that area of the stomach at the point where the duplication impinges on the greater curvature. An intestinal duplication cyst may be distinguished from an abdominal mass/tumor, such as neuroblastoma, because the cyst will only absorb contrast along the wall, whereas a tumor will absorb contrast material throughout the mass. A technetium scan is used to detect ectopic gastric lining (Grosfeld, 1998; Ross, 1994; Stauffer & Schwoebel, 1998; Templeton, 1995).

Operative Management

Treatment depends on symptoms and location. Primary resection and end-to-end anastomosis is attempted whenever possible. Because of the frequent presence of ectopic gastric mucosa in the duplication lining, mucosal stripping is done in all cases to prevent peptic ulceration and carcinogenesis. The goals of surgery are to establish intestinal continuity, relieve obstruction, and preserve intestinal length.

Thoracic and thoracoabdominal duplications require excision. This is accomplished by resection and primary anastomosis or staged repair with communication with the GI tract for drainage. For gastric duplications, complete excision is recommended. If this is not possible, partial excision with stripping of the mucosa or excision of the common wall to facilitate drainage is done. Duodenal duplication is the rarest and most difficult to treat primarily because of the proximity to the biliary and pancreatic ductal systems. The compression of the first or second portions of the duodenum requires complete excision of the duplication or duodenotomy for internal drainage. A duodenotomy creates an opening that allows decompression and drainage from the duplication of the duodenum into the true, patent duodenum. Large cystic duplications that occur on the mesenteric side of the bowel or close to the ampulla of Vater may necessitate a drainage procedure, such as a cystoduodenostomy or cystojejunostomy, in which the cyst is drained into the GI tract. This is because excision is not possible because of the location of the duplication along or adjacent to integral structures (Skandalakis & Gray, 1994).

Small intestine duplication is most common and is usually located in the ileum. There is usually a shared common muscular wall and a common blood supply with the native bowel. Treatment includes primary resection with end-to-end anastomosis, segmental resection (along with the adjacent intestine), or partial resection with internal drainage at the distal end. There are situations in which primary resection and end-to-end anastomosis are not possible. These include lengthy tubular duplications where resection would

sacrifice removal of a large portion of adjacent true GI tract. In these cases in which the communication is often at the caudal end, the proximal end can be opened to create a "double-barreled" segment of intestine.

Finally, colonic or rectal duplication has been classified as type I, those occurring above the peritoneal reflection, and type II, those associated with the urinary and genital tracts (Dodds & Kottra, 1971). Type I requires resection with primary anastomosis, whereas type II may not require surgery if internal communication is adequate. Some rectal duplications may benefit from a transanal exposure of the cyst and stripping of the cyst wall.

Postoperative Management

Postoperative care of an infant after repair of GI duplication is similar to the care after atresia repair as outlined earlier. This includes postoperative antibiotics, gastric decompression until ileus is resolved, pain management, and slow advancement of enteral feedings. For older children, early ambulation is instituted, which helps hasten the return of bowel function. In addition, assessment for signs of infection and skin and ostomy care (if needed) are priorities postoperatively.

MECONIUM ILEUS

History, Incidence, and Associated Anomalies

Andrassy and Nirgiotis (1993) and Rescorla (1998) outline the history of the description and treatment of meconium ileus as follows. Meconium ileus was first described in 1905 by Landsteiner. It was considered a fatal condition until 1948 when Hiatt and Wilson performed the first successful enterotomy. Meconium ileus is the third most common reason for bowel obstruction in the neonate. Nearly all infants with meconium ileus have cystic fibrosis (CF). CF is an autosomal recessive disease affecting approximately 30,000 Americans of every ethnic population. In Caucasians it is considered the most common lethal genetic disorder. About 10% to 15% of patients with CF present with meconium ileus as neonates (Andrassy & Nirgiotis, 1993; Rescorla, 1998). Thus, all patients with meconium ileus should be evaluated for CF. This evaluation should include a sweat test and genetic testing.

Pathophysiology/Diagnosis/Classification

CF is the result of mutations in the gene that codes for the cystic fibrosis transmembranes regulator (CFTR) protein. CFTR protein plays a major role in the transport of chloride, sodium, and water across the apical membrane of the epithelial cells (Andrassy & Nirgiotis, 1993). This aberration results in abnormal airway secretions, causing decreased mucociliary clearance, chronic bronchial infections, and abnormal gastrointestinal secretions causing problems with digestion and absorption of food, and blockage in the bowel.

Prenatal ultrasonography after 20 weeks' gestation that reveals an echogenic bowel may indicate a meconium ileus. This same finding before 20 weeks' gestation is considered normal (Rescorla, 1998). Making the diagnosis of CF includes a comprehensive clinical examination because the sweat test and genetic testing can be inconclusive. Initially, a patient with meconium ileus has abdominal distention, bilious emesis, and no passage of meconium. As part of the differential diagnosis, volvulus, intestinal atresias, Hirschsprung's disease, and perforation should be ruled out. In some cases, volvulus or perforation can occur as a result of meconium ileus. The latter is referred to as complicated meconium ileus. Perforation can occur before birth and results in ascites and peritonitis. Perforations that go undiagnosed and thus untreated can result in calcifications and adhesions. If volvulus is present, ischemia and necrosis may result (Andrassy & Nirgiotis, 1993; Nakayama, 1997b; Rescorla, 1998; Ross, 1994).

Radiographically, meconium ileus is characterized by dilated loops of proximal small bowel and a distal ileum packed with meconium. The distal portion of the ileum and ascending colon may be beaded with meconium. In about one third of the cases, air fluid levels will not be present because the meconium sticks to the lumen of the intestinal wall (Rescorla, 1998). The collection of meconium in the bowel has a granular appearance radiographically and thus is referred to as "ground glass" or "soap bubble" appearance (Rescorla, 1998). Distal to the obstruction, the colon is unused or described as a microcolon when visualized with contrast and radiography.

Preoperative Care/Medical Management

When meconium ileus is suspected, an OG/NG tube should be placed and connected to low continuous suction to decompress the stomach. Adequate hydration of the patient should be maintained and antibiotics should be started prophylactically. In an effort to clean out the thick, inspissated meconium, a hyperosmolar solution known as diomethyl atrozate glucamine (Gastrografin) can be delivered by means of an enema (Rescorla, 1998). This solution is radiopaque and therefore the first dose is delivered during a radiographic study to assist in the diagnostic workup. Gastrografin enemas have been successful in breaking up the meconium and resolving the obstruction. Hyperosmolar solutions cause a shift of fluids from the intravascular space into the bowel lumen, thus facilitating clearing of the thick meconium. Because of the hyperosmolar nature of Gastrografin, electrolytes and the hydration status require close monitoring.

Acetylcysteine (Mucomyst), a mucolytic, has also been used successfully to break up meconium and relieve the meconium ileus (Nakayama, 1997b; Rescorla, 1998; Ross, 1994).

Surgical Interventions

In situations when meconium ileus cannot be relieved by medical management, surgical intervention is necessary. There are four methods of surgical intervention for meconium ileus: enterotomy and irrigation or resection and ileostomy by the Bishop-Koop, Santulli and Blanc, or the Mikulicz method (Figure 18–9) (Rescorla, 1998). Survival of patients with meconium ileus who have had the Bishop-Koop procedure has dramatically increased over the last several decades (Del Pin, Czyrko, Ziegler, Scanlin, & Bishop, 1992). Enterotomy and irrigation (Figure 18–10), which is currently the treatment of choice for uncomplicated meconium ileus, is accomplished by placing a purse-string suture on the antimesenteric wall of the dilated ileum near the transition zone. A small rubber catheter is placed through the enterotomy. The bowel is then irrigated with warm saline, acetylcysteine solution, or Gastrografin solution. Most of the meconium is removed through the enterotomy. The remaining meconium is flushed into the colon and then is excreted (Rescorla, 1998).

In situations of complicated meconium ileus or meconium ileus not resolved by enterotomy and irrigation, an ileal resection is necessary. One of the following procedures is performed: the Bishop-Koop resection of the dilated ileal segment and the proximal end-to-distal ileal anastomosis with distal ostomy or Mikulicz resection with a double-barrel ileostomy. These procedures create temporary ileostomies that can be reversed when the meconium ileus is resolved (Rescorla, 1998). Timing for closure of an ostomy depends on the infant's general health, adequate growth, and assessment for a patent distal limb.

Postoperative Management

Postoperative management consists of GI decompression until the ileus resolves, respiratory support, and administration of antibiotics. Once GI function has resumed as described in earlier sections, enteral feedings are initiated. The diagnosis of CF should be made before the initiation of feedings because pancreatic enzyme supplements may be necessary to help with digestion and absorption of nutrients. From a surgical perspective, these patients do very well. Occasionally, older children with CF have a condition termed "meconium ileus equivalent" develop that mimics meconium ileus of the newborn, in which GI obstruction occurs because of thick, viscous stool. Treatment consists of enemas and washouts of solutions that break up the stool.

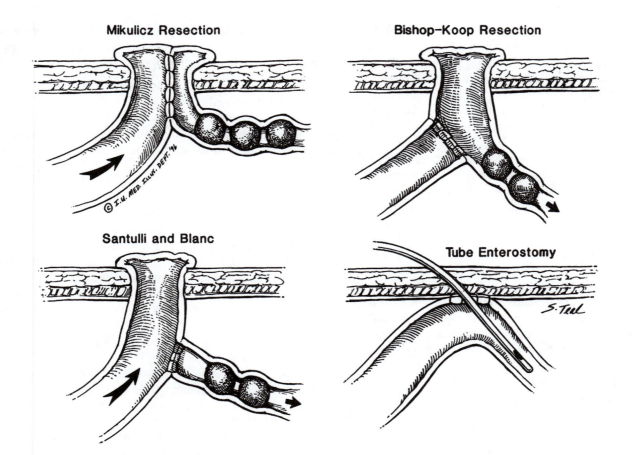

Mikulicz Resection

Bishop-Koop Resection

Santulli and Blanc

Tube Enterostomy

Figure 18–9 Procedures for Treating Meconium Ileus. The Bishop-Koop resection and tube enterostomy are preferred.

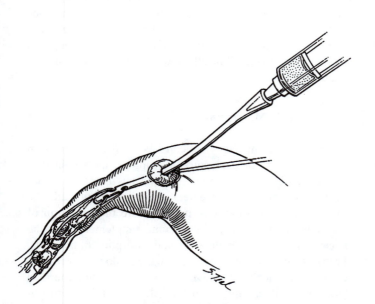

Figure 18–10 Tube Enterostomy and Irrigation. Technique of enterotomy and irrigation that is used preferably in cases of uncomplicated meconium obstruction.

CONCLUSION

Intestinal obstruction in the neonate caused by atresia, stenosis, duplications, or meconium ileus present the nurse with multiple management challenges. Preoperative treatment priorities include establishment and maintenance of respiratory and hemodynamic stability and decompression of a dilated gastrointestinal tract. Because of the high rate of associated anomalies, the nurse must be a strong patient advocate in coordinating care with a variety of subspecialists, including neonatology, genetics, cardiology, and pulmonary medicine. The goals of surgery include relieving the obstruction, establishing intestinal continuity, and maximizing intestinal function. Surgical intervention in a newborn poses a crisis for families. This crisis may be minimized by involving the parents in discussion with the various disciplines, providing prenatal and preoperative teaching and counseling, and referring parents to appropriate support groups. Postoperatively, management strategies include assessment for return of bowel function, slow advancement of feedings, assessment for infection, and assessment and continued education and support of the family. Discharge planning must be comprehensive, especially if coexisting anomalies or disease exists. Most patients with isolated atresias or duplications have a good prognosis. Those with associated anomalies or chronic conditions have a higher morbidity and mortality. These diagnoses may continue to challenge the patient throughout the life span, so early referral to community resources and accessibility to specialized care is imperative.

REFERENCES

Andrassy, R.J., & Nirgiotis, J.G. (1993). Meconium disease of infancy: Meconium ileus, meconium plug syndrome, and meconium peritonitis. In K.W. Ashcraft (Ed.), *Pediatric surgery* (pp. 331–340). Philadelphia: W.B. Saunders Company.

Cilley, R.E., & Coran, A.G. (1995). Duodenoduodenostomy. In L. Spitz & A.G. Coran (Eds.), *Pediatric surgery* (5th ed., pp. 328–332). London: Chapman & Hall.

Croaker, G.D., Harvey, J.G., & Cass, D.T. (1997). Hirschsprung's disease, colonic atresia, and absent hand: A new triad. *Journal of Pediatric Surgery, 32*(9), 1368–1370.

Del Pin, C.A., Czyrko, C., Ziegler, M.M., Scanlin, T.F., & Bishop, H.C. (1992). Management and survival of meconium ileus. *Annals of Surgery 215*, 179–185.

Dodds, W.J., & Kottra, J.J. (1971). Duplication of the large bowel. *American Journal of Roentgenology, 113,* 310.

Grosfeld, J.L. (1998). Jejunoileal atresia and stenosis. In J.A. O'Neill, M.I. Rowe, & J.L. Grosfeld (Eds.), *Pediatric surgery* (pp. 1145–1158). St. Louis, MO: Mosby.

Grosfeld, J.L., Boles, E.T., & Reiner, C. (1970). Duplication of pylorus in the newborn: A rare cause of gastric outlet obstruction. *Journal of Pediatric Surgery, 5,* 365–369.

Gross, E., Armon, Y., Abu-Dalu, K., Gale R., & Schiller, M. (1996). Familial combined duodenal and jejunal atresia. *Journal of Pediatric Surgery, 31*(11), 1573.

Harris, J., Kallen, B., & Robert, E. (1995). Descriptive epidemiology of alimentary tract atresia. *Teratology 52*(1), 15–29.

Herman, T.E., & McAlister, W.H. (1995). Familial type I jejunal atresias and renal dysplasia. *Pediatric Radiology, 25*(4), 272–274.

Kimble, R.M., Harding, J., & Kolbe, A. (1997). Additional congenital anomalies in babies with gut atresia or stenosis: When to investigate, and which investigation. *Pediatric Surgery International, 12*(8), 565–570.

Kimura, K., Mukohara, N., Nishijima, E., Muraji, T., Tsugawa, C., & Matsumoto, Y. (1990). Diamond-shaped anastomosis for duodenal atresia: An experience with 44 patients over 15 years. *Journal of Pediatric Surgery, 25,* 977.

Kimura, K., Perdzynski, W., & Soper, R.T. (1996). Elliptical seromuscular resection for tapering the proximal dilated bowel in duodenal or jejunal atresia. *Journal of Pediatric Surgery, 31*(10), 1405–1406.

LaQuaglia, M.P., Ghavimi, F., Penenberg, D., Mandell, L.R., Healey, J.H., Hadju, S.I., & Exelby, P.R. (1990). Rectal duplications. *Journal of Pediatric Surgery, 25,* 980.

Moore, S.W., de Jongh, G., Bouic, P., Brown, R.A., & Kirsten, G. (1996). Immune deficiency in familial duodenal atresia. *Journal of Pediatric Surgery, 31*(12), 1733–1735.

Nakayama, D.K. (1997a). Duodenal atresia and stenosis. In D.K. Nakayama, C.L. Bose, & N. Chescheir (Eds.), *Critical care of the surgical newborn* (pp. 321–333). Armonk, NY: Futura Publishing.

Nakayama, D.K. (1997b). Meconium ileus, meconium peritonitis, and meconium plug. In D.K. Nakayama, C.L. Bose, & N. Chescheir (Eds.), *Critical care of the surgical newborn* (pp. 347–365). Armonk, NY: Futura Publishing.

Neal, M.R., Seibert, J.J., Vanderzalam, T., & Wagner, C.W. (1997). Neonatal ultrasonography to distinguish between meconium ileus and ileal atresia. *Journal of Ultrasound in Medicine, 16*(4), 263–268.

Oldham, K.T. (1998). Atresia, stenosis, and other obstructions of the colon. In J.A. O'Neill, M.I. Rowe, & J.L. Grosfeld (Eds.), *Pediatric surgery* (pp. 1361–1368). St. Louis, MO: Mosby.

Ramsey, G.S. (1957). Enterogenous cyst of the stomach simulating hypertrophic pyloric stenosis. *British Journal of Surgery, 44,* 643.

Rescorla, F.J. (1998). Meconium ileus. In J.A. O'Neill, M.I. Rowe, & J.L. Grosfeld (Eds.), *Pediatric surgery* (pp. 1159–1171). St. Louis, MO: Mosby.

Ross, A.J. (1994). Intestinal obstruction in the newborn. *Pediatrics in Review, 15*(9), 338–347.

Rothenberg, M.E., White, F.V., Chilmonczyk, B., & Chatila, J.E. (1995). A syndrome involving immunodeficiency and multiple intestinal atresias. *Immunodeficiency, 5*(3), 171–178.

Rowe, M.A., O'Neill, J.S., & Grosfeld, J.L. (1995). *Essentials of pediatric surgery.* St. Louis, MO: Mosby.

Sanders, R.C., Blackmon, L.R., Hogge, W.A., & Wolfsberg, E.A. (1996). *Structural fetal abnormalities: The total picture.* St. Louis, MO: Mosby.

Skandalakis, J.E., & Gray, S.W. (1994). *Embryology for surgeons.* Baltimore: Williams & Wilkins.

Slee, J., & Goldblatt, J. (1996). Further evidence for a syndrome of "apple peel" intestinal atresia, ocular anomalies and microcephaly. *Clinical Genetics, 50*(4), 260–262.

Stauffer, U.G., & Schwoebel, M. (1998). Duodenal atresia and stenosis: Annular pancreas. In J.A. O'Neill, M.I. Rowe, & J.L. Grosfeld (Eds.), *Pediatric surgery* (pp. 1133–1143). St. Louis, MO: Mosby.

Templeton, J.J. (1995). Gastrointestinal obstruction in the neonate. Resident Lecture Series, The Children's Hospital of Philadelphia.

Touloukian, R.J. (1993). Intestinal atresia and stenosis. In K.W. Ashcraft (Ed.), *Pediatric surgery* (pp. 305–319). Philadelphia: W.B. Saunders Company.

Yokoyama, T., Ishizone, S., Momose, Y., Terada, M., Kitahara, S., & Kawasaki, S., (1997). Duodenal atresia in dizygotic twins. *Journal of Pediatric Surgery, 32*(12), 1806–1808.

Appendix 18–A

Caremap for Jejunoileal Atresia

	Preoperative	Operating Room	POD 1	POD 3–20
Treatments	NPO IV fluids D$_{10}$ w/Ca 80 ml/kg (full term) D$_{10}$ w/Ca 100 ml/kg NG/OG decompression	Atresia requires immediate surgery; stenosis can be delayed Exploratory laparotomy: RUQ transverse supraumbilical incision Jejunal —Proximal resection and end-to-oblique anastomosis Antimesenteric reduction —Tapering jejunoplasty —Imbrication technique Resection and exteriorization: rare Ileal End-to-end anastomosis Resection and exteriorization: rare	NPO NG/OG decompression IV fluids: D$_{10}$ .25% NS w/KCl, Ca 100–120 ml/day NG loss replacement D$_5$ .45% NS w/10 mEq KCl/500 ml Rate of: 0.5 cc/cc May require NSS bolus 10 ml/kg for ↓ u/o postoperatively Patients w/transanastomotic tubes Continuous feedings of breast milk or formula, start at 1–2 ml/hr and increase by 1 ml/day to goal	Initiate TPN if return of bowel function delayed beyond POD 3 Initiate enteral feedings w/Pedialyte once NG volume decreases/clears Slow feeding advance Full term: q2–3° bolus—↑ 5ccq feeding to q other feeding to goal: 100 kcal/kg (minimum) Some infants may require slow advance of continuous feedings (i.e., 1 ml q8° →q12° →q24°; use Pregestimal with loss of bowel length Premie: Increase formula no more than 20 kcal/kg/day. Goal: 100–120 kcal/kg/day
Medications	Periop ampicillin/gentamycin		Ampicillin/gentamycin until POD 3–5	
Assessment & monitoring	VS q1–2° I & O q1° NG/OG output q4° Laboratory profile[a] ABD examination—distention Temp. stability ± Stool		VS q1° → q4° I & O q1° NG/OG output q4° Laboratory profile → until tolerating enteral feedings ABD examination—note distention, bowel sounds Temp. stability ± Stool Remove abdominal incision dressing POD 2	VS q4° →8° Assess I & O q shift Feeding tolerance: no emesis; no or low residuals Abdominal assessment: note distention Assess quality and frequency of stools Wound assessment

	Column 1	Column 2	Column 3
Consults	Cardiology ± chromosomes sent to genetics ± prior to transfusion Pulmonary ± R/O CF with meconium ileus		
Tests (diagnostics)	Maternal u/s, postnatal u/s abd. Films flat/erect lat. decubitus Barium enema Laboratory profile[a]	Abd flat plate POD 1 → PRN CXR (if ventilated postop) daily Lab panel (until tolerating enteral feedings) daily Bilirubin first 4 days (longer if elevated or on phototherapy) CBC with diff. POD 1 → PRN Blood cultures PRN	Abd flat plate → PRN CXR PRN Lab profile[a] daily until stable: then 2–3 X/wk Bilirubin first 4 days (longer if elevated or on phototherapy) Blood cultures PRN
Education	Preop care Operative repair ± genetic pulmonary counseling Postop course	Long-term F/U	NG/GT feedings (as necessary) Feeding intolerance Well-baby care Signs of intestinal obstruction Signs of wound infection
Evaluation	Abd. examination: distention? NG/OG output: color, volume Perfusion: adequate intravascular volume? VS q1° R/O sepsis: temp. instability, hypo/hyperglycemia, thrombocytopenia Laboratory values: normalizing?	Abd. examination: distention? NG/OG output: color, volume Perfusion: adequate intravascular volume? VS q1° R/O sepsis: temp. instability, hypo/hyperglycemia, thrombocytopenia Laboratory values: ? normalizing	Tolerating feedings Without signs of wound infection Labs normalized Weight gain (25 gm/day or consistent weight gain x5 days) Readiness for discharge Evaluate previous teaching
Discharge planning	Identify pediatrician Referrals: Early Intervention PRN		Contact DME company for feeding supplies (as needed) Initial nursing visits X1 → X2 → as needed Monitor (cardiac/resp.) if continuous NG feedings overnight

[a] Laboratory profile: electrolytes, glucose, BUN, creatinine, Ca, Mg, Phos, bilirubin, CBC, type and cross-match (preoperatively).

CHAPTER 19

Hirschsprung's Disease

Jennifer Chamberlain and Daniel H. Teitelbaum

INTRODUCTION

Hirschsprung's disease is a form of chronic intestinal obstruction caused by the absence of the intramural ganglia in the distal bowl. The intramural ganglia or ganglion cells are located throughout the gastrointestinal tract from the mouth through the esophagus and intestines down to the rectum. These cells cause the peristalsis of the muscles in the intestine to move food and byproducts down to the rectum. Without ganglion cells the intestine cannot push the waste out of the rectum. Harold Hirschsprung presented his classic description of this disease entity in Berlin in 1886 (McCready & Beart, 1981). An understanding of the pathophysiology of Hirschsprung's disease has been the foundation of the current approach of its diagnosis and treatment.

EMBRYOLOGY

An understanding of the normal embryologic development of the enteric nervous system is necessary to understand the development of Hirschsprung's disease. In normal embryologic development, intestinal ganglion cells originate from neuroblasts that are formed during early fetal development. The cells migrate from the neural crest to the upper end of the alimentary tract and then proceed in the caudal direction. The first nerve cells arrive in the esophagus by the fifth week of gestation. By the 7th week, nerve cells are at the midgut, and migration to the distal colon is achieved by the 12th week. Migration occurs first into the intermuscular layer called Auerbach's (myenteric) plexus, and then these cells subsequently move into the submucosal plexus. How the neural crest cells migrate to the appropriate location in the intestine is an area of active investigation. It has been demonstrated that the neural crest cells are guided in their migration by a variety of neural fibers whose development

precedes the migration of the neural crest cells (Fujimoto, Hata, Yokoyama, & Mitomi, 1989). These fibers progress down the gastrointestinal tract and then move through the bowel, ending up in the muscular layer. This creates a pathway for the neural cells to then migrate.

INCIDENCE

The incidence of Hirschsprung's disease ranges from 1 in 4,400 to 1 in 7,000 births (Ryan, 1995). The male/female ratio in patients with classic Hirschsprung's disease is generally reported as 4:1 (Ryan, 1995). In long segment disease, the ratio approaches 1:1 and may actually favor females to have the higher incidence. Racial incidence seems to be equally distributed over the general population.

There is strong evidence of genetic predisposition to Hirschsprung's disease. According to Passarge (1967), siblings of female patients with Hirschsprung's disease have a 7.5% risk for being born with the disease, and siblings of male patients with Hirschsprung's disease have a 2.5% to 6% higher incidence of Hirschsprung's disease. Other studies also indicate that the longer the segment of aganglionosis, the higher the rate of familial incidence (Ikeda, Ogami, Kume, Konishi, & Konishi, 1968). Parents of children with long segment disease incur a 12% risk of having other affected children.

PATHOLOGY

The physical appearance of the intestine in Hirschsprung's disease varies with the duration of the untreated disease. In the neonatal period, the intestine may appear fairly normal. As the child ages, the proximal, ganglionic bowel hypertrophies and becomes thicker and longer than normal. The transition zone, where ganglionic and aganglionic intestine intersect, may be funnellike and vary in length. Although the distal bowel appears grossly normal, the absence of ganglion cells in the distal intestine is the key feature of the disease. The ganglion cells are absent in both the submucosal (Meissner's) plexus and the intermuscular (Auerbach's) plexus. Associated with this finding is a marked increase in nerve fibers, which extend into the submucosa. Classically, the extent of the aganglionosis is the rectosigmoid region in approximately 80% of cases (Polley, Coran, & Wesley, 1985). In 10% of cases the disease involves a greater length of the colon and in 4% it extends throughout the colon and may also involve a significant part of the small intestine (Figure 19–1). The process of aganglionosis is almost always continuous within the affected intestine and without interruption until the proximal ganglionic

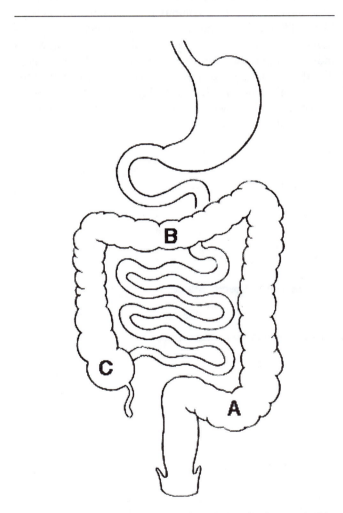

Figure 19–1 The Extent of Aganglionosis in Hirschsprung's Disease. (A) 80% involves rectosigmoid colon; (B) 15% includes colon beyond the sigmoid; (C) 5% involves total colon or more proximal bowel.

segment is reached. A few rare cases have documented ganglion cells to be found intermittently in the colon, but this is extremely unusual.

ASSOCIATED ANOMALIES

Hirschsprung's disease is usually an isolated disorder of full-term, otherwise healthy infants. However, several associated congenital anomalies have been recognized. Down syndrome has been reported to occur in 4.5% to 16% of children with Hirschsprung's disease (Caniano, Teitelbaum, & Qualman, 1990; Goldberg, 1984; Polley & Coran, 1986). Atresias of the large and small intestine have also been noted in Hirschsprung's disease. The cause of this association is unknown, but it may be the result of a vascular accident with a blockage of ganglion cell migration to the distal intestine (Akgur, Tanyel, Buyukpamukcu, & Hicsonmez, 1993). In this instance, the diagnosis of Hirschsprung's disease is often delayed until after intestinal continuity is established and an obstructive pattern develops (Ikeda & Goto, 1984; Moore et al., 1990). Other anomalies associated with Hirschsprung's disease are trisomy 18 and Ondine's curse (Elhalaby & Coran, 1994). A variety of diseases arising from maldevelopment of the neural crest have also been described. These include multiple endocrine neoplasia 2A, congenital deafness, Waardenberg's syndrome, Von Recklinghaussen's disease, and the Smith-Lemli-Opitz syndrome (Clausen, Andersson, & Tommerup, 1989; Kim & Boutwell, 1985; Omenn & McKusick, 1979; Polley et al., 1985).

PATHOPHYSIOLOGY

The intestine contains three neuronal plexi: the submucosal or Meissner's plexus, the intramuscular myenteric or Auerbach's plexus, and a much smaller mucosal plexus (Sharli & Meirer-Ruge, 1981; Yntema & Hammond, 1953). Each contains a finely integrated neuronal network that acts to control many functions of the gut, including absorption, secretion, blood flow, and motility. This occurs with relatively little control from the body's central nervous system. Normal intestinal motility is primarily controlled by these intrinsic neurons in each ganglion. Loss of extrinsic control, as in a spinal cord injury, still allows for adequate function of the intestine (Teitelbaum, Caniano, & Qualman, 1989).

In the normal intestine, a fine balance of contractile and relaxation forces keeps the smooth muscle finely controlled. A normal motility reflex is present in the distal rectum. A mildly distending bolus in the distal rectum initiates a contraction above the bolus and relaxation below the bolus allowing for the passage of the stool. Such a reflex is purely intrinsic to the intestine itself. The absence of this reflex denotes an abnormality, which is seen when there is an absence of intramural ganglion cells.

In Hirschsprung's disease intramural ganglion cells are absent in the distal intestine. The absence of these nerves begins at the anus and continues proximally for a varying extent. The ganglion cells of the intramural plexus in the bowel control the coordination of contraction and relaxation of normal peristalsis. The ganglion cells release nitric oxide, which is critical to the relaxation of the intestinal smooth muscle. If these cells are missing, the bowel appears normal macroscopically, but it is obstructed functionally. Stool is unable to pass through the aganglionic segment and leads to functional obstruction with the secondary result of proximal bowel dilation (Figure 19–2). The dilation occurs in the normally innervated proximal bowel, which leads to the term *congenital megacolon* as a synonym for Hirschsprung's disease.

DIAGNOSIS

Hirschsprung's disease should be considered in any child who has a history of constipation dating back to the newborn period. The differential diagnosis of Hirschsprung's disease should include both mechanical and functional causes for intestinal obstruction (Exhibit 19–1). The age at which children are diagnosed with Hirschsprung's disease has progressively decreased over the past several decades. The usual

presentation of the disease in newborns consists of a history of delayed passage of stool within the first 48 hours of life. Other presenting symptoms include constipation, abdominal distention, poor feeding, and emesis. Older infants may have poor weight gain. Physical examination of a child often demonstrates abdominal distention (Figure 19–3). Assessment for normal anal position on the perineum is important. A low-lying imperforate anus that is displaced in an anterior direction may also be a cause for constipation. Rectal examination of patients with Hirschsprung's disease reveals a tight anus. This may be incorrectly diagnosed as anal stenosis (Swenson, Sherman, Fisher, & Cohen, 1975).

Radiology Studies

Plain Radiographs

Radiologic studies begin with flat and upright or decubitus abdominal films, which commonly show several distended loops of bowel. In the neonate, the initial mode of presentation may be free air on a plain abdominal radiograph, which indicates a perforation of the intestine. It is the periappendiceal area that most commonly perforates proximal to the aganglionic colon (Arliss & Holgersen, 1990; Newman, Nussbaum, Kirkpatrick, & Colodny, 1988). It is important to consider and rule out Hirschsprung's disease with any form

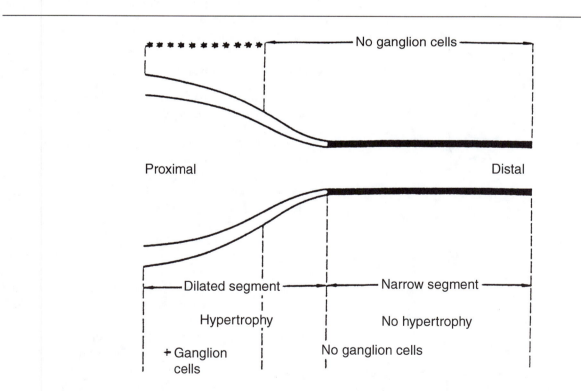

Figure 19–2 The Pathology of Hirschsprung's Disease. The distal, aganglionated segment of intestine transitions through to the dilated, proximal ganglionic intestine. The normal ganglionated bowel is enlarged because of distal obstruction.

Exhibit 19–1 Differential Diagnosis of Hirschsprung's Disease

Mechanical Obstruction	Functional Obstruction
• Meconium ilius	• Prematurity
• Ileal or colonic atresia	• Small left colon syndrome
• Meconium plug syndrome	• Sepsis
• Small intestine stenosis	• Electrolyte imbalance
• Low imperforate anus	• Hypothyroidism
	• Functional constipation

of spontaneous perforation of the small or large intestine in the neonatal period. The morbidity and mortality is high if the diagnosis is delayed or missed (Martin & Perrin, 1967).

Barium Enema

A barium enema may be helpful in making the diagnosis. This study involves the insertion of a small Foley catheter into the rectum. The colon is then filled with barium solution and a series of radiographic films are taken. This allows the radiologist to evaluate the anatomy of the distal bowel and the capacity of the colon. The catheter should be inserted just inside the anus without inflating the balloon because this would also obliterate a low transition zone. In addition, it is important to avoid rectal examinations and enemas before the study, which could also distort a low transition zone (Klein & Philippart, 1993).

A postevacuation film and 24-hour postevacuation film complete the study. This will demonstrate whether the child adequately evacuates the remaining barium or the colon remains dilated. A classic case of Hirschsprung's disease will show a spastic distal intestinal segment with a dilated proximal bowel (Figure 19–4). The barium enema in the first several weeks of life may fail to show a transition zone. A barium enema should not be obtained during a clinical episode of enterocolitis because perforation may result. Parents should be informed that their child might pass chalky white stools for the next 24 to 48 hours. The barium is not absorbed. If the child does not pass any stools in 48 hours, a rectal washout may be necessary because the liquid barium may become firm and difficult to pass if left in the child.

Anorectal Manometry

Anorectal manometry is another method of diagnosing Hirschsprung's disease. A balloon catheter is placed inside the rectum and pressures within the distal colon are measured. The technique relies on the absence of a relaxation

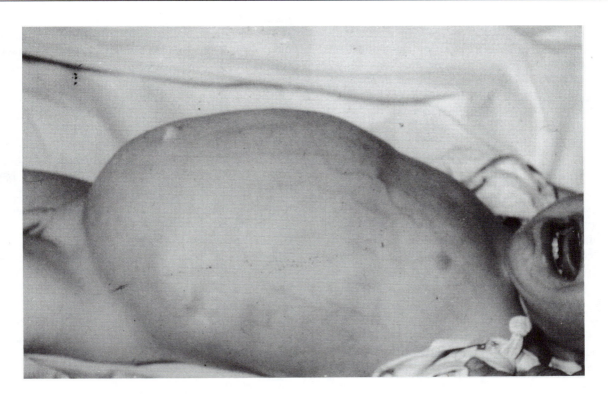

Figure 19–3 Child with Notably Distended Abdomen after Delayed Diagnosis of Hirschsprung's Disease

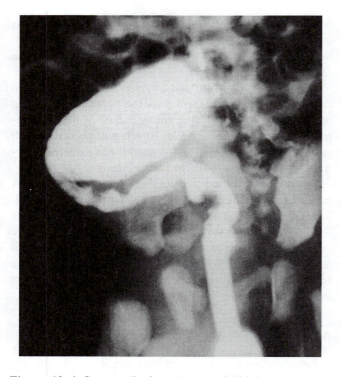

Figure 19–4 Contrast Barium Enema of Child with Hirschsprung's Disease. Note the sigmoid diameter is larger than the distal rectal diameter.

reflex after a distending bolus in the rectal lumen of patients with Hirschsprung's disease. An advantage of this study is that it can be performed at the bedside or as an outpatient procedure and is associated with virtually no complications. Swenson initially advocated the technique as a first approach to children with this disorder (Swenson, 1964; Swenson, Fisher, & Gherardi, 1959; Swenson et al., 1975). Accurate data is obtained from anorectal manometry only when the patient is in a normal physiologic state. Patients examined during an abnormal state such as sepsis or hypothyroidism may yield an inaccurate result (Yunis, Dibbins, & Sherman, 1976). Other limitations include the need for sedation of young children to avoid artifacts that may be created by moving or crying. Reported accuracy rates of anorectal manometry vary widely among reported series (Taxman, Yulish, & Rothstein, 1986; Yunis et al., 1976). The results seem to be most accurate when an experienced operator performs the test. The parent and child should be provided with information about the sensation the child will feel before beginning the test. There will be mild pressure as the balloon is inflated within the rectum, similar to a rectal examination. The test takes approximately 30 minutes. There are few complications or side effects.

Rectal Biopsy

A rectal biopsy is the most definitive method for diagnosing Hirschsprung's disease. Swenson first described the method of a full-thickness rectal biopsy in 1959. The tissue obtained with this technique involves both the submucosal and intermuscular layers. This allowed the pathologist to closely examine the muscle layers of the colon and identify whether ganglion cells are present. In 1960, Gherardi demonstrated that the level of aganglionosis was similar in the submucosa and myenteric plexus. This allowed a submucosal piece of tissue to be used to make the diagnosis. Refinement of the technique led to the development of the suction biopsy by Dobbins and Bill (1965) and Noblett (1969). Use of the suction rectal biopsy has greatly facilitated the diagnosis of Hirschsprung's disease. Biopsies may be performed at the bedside or in a clinic. Although the diagnostic accuracy has been reported to be as high as 99.7%, errors may occur. The most common problem is an inadequate specimen, in which there is an insufficient amount of submucosa, and therefore, an inability to identify if ganglion cells are present. Another problem is performance of the biopsy too close to the sphincter. The normal anus has an absence of ganglion cells at the level of the internal sphincter. The accepted practice is to obtain two or three specimens by suction rectal biopsy at 2 cm above the anal valves. The tissue specimen may be obtained by a rectal forceps, which clips a piece of mucosa from the lining of the colon or a suction biopsy instrument.

The suction biopsy instrument consists of a blunt-ended tube with a 3-mm side hole 1 cm from the tip attached to suction tubing (Figure 19–5). The small capsule with the blade is inserted into the rectum. Suction is then applied by pulling back onto the syringe. A portion of the superficial rectal wall is drawn into the side hole. The circular blade is then triggered, cutting off a biopsy specimen. In Hirschsprung's disease an intense staining of the biopsy specimens reveals hypertrophied nerve fibers throughout the muscle layers and the absence of ganglion cells. When a suction rectal biopsy is inadequate or for an older child, a full-thickness biopsy with the use of biopsy forceps may be performed. A full-thickness biopsy is obtained in the operating room with the child under general anesthesia. This specimen involves all the muscular layers of the colon. It provides a more substantial tissue sample for the pathologist to review. The risks of the procedure include bleeding, scarring, and infection.

Before the test, it is important to discuss with the family the procedure their child will undergo and the sensation that will be experienced. It should be explained that the nerve receptors for pain in the rectum are different than those on the outer surface of the skin. The child will experience pressure, not a painful pinch, when the biopsy specimen is obtained. The family should be instructed to check the child's

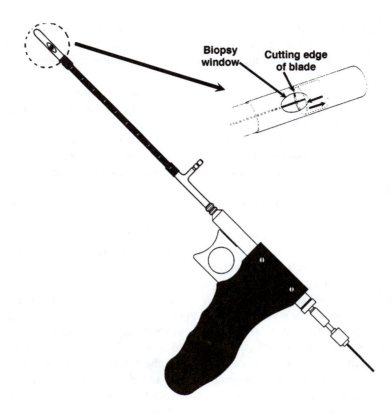

Biopsy window

Cutting edge of blade

Figure 19–5 Suction Rectal Biopsy Instrument

diaper or underpants 30 minutes after the procedure for bleeding. A small amount of blood may be passed with stools, but the staff should be notified if there is persistent bleeding or blood that soaks into the diaper.

DIFFERENTIAL DIAGNOSIS

Total Colonic Aganglionosis

Infants with Hirschsprung's disease that involves the entire length of colon account for approximately 3% to 12% of the patients. These children make a unique subset of patients because of the associated increased morbidity and mortality. Without the colon, the child's ability to reabsorb fluid and store stool is markedly impaired. Many infants with total colonic Hirschsprung's disease require parenteral nutrition for an extended period of time, making catheter sepsis, failure to thrive, stomal dysfunction, electrolyte imbalance, and dehydration commonly encountered complications.

SURGICAL TECHNIQUES

Clinical management of children diagnosed with Hirschsprung's disease is changing as new surgical techniques evolve. The treatment of Hirschsprung's disease involves the surgical resection of the aganglionic bowel, followed by mobilization of the proximal colon and anastomosis of the ganglionic bowel to the distal rectum. Traditionally, the most common approach for correction is a two-staged or three-staged procedure in which a leveling colostomy is first performed for decompression. A staged procedure with a leveling colostomy may need to be used in cases of patients with enterocolitis or those with large dilated loops of bowel at the time of surgery. This occurs more commonly in children who had a delay in diagnosis. The colostomy is left in place for 6 to 12 months before resection of the aganglionic distal bowel and pull-through procedure are performed to allow the dilated bowel to decompress. Recently, many centers have performed the endorectal pull-through without preliminary colostomy in newborns as soon as the diagnosis is made (Teitelbaum & Coran, 1995). The need for a preliminary colostomy is then avoided because the proximal bowel has not become overly dilated. The surgery may take place in the first 24 to 48 hours of life with good results. Three endorectal pull-through procedures with their modifications are being used at present. Each surgeon determines whether a diverting colostomy needs to be performed before the definitive pull-through procedure. At the time of surgery a biopsy specimen is obtained to confirm the presence of ganglion cells at the anastomotic site. Figure 19–6 illustrates the common surgical approaches in the definitive treatment of Hirschsprung's disease.

The three endorectal pull-through procedures follow.

1. Swenson and Bill (1948) first described their curative operation for Hirschsprung's disease in 1948. This is performed through a combined abdominoperineal approach. Essential to this operation is careful dissection immediately adjacent to the rectal wall to avoid injury to the pelvic nerves responsible for rectal and bladder innervation and sexual function. This technique leaves the smallest amount of aganglionic bowel remaining.

2. Duhamel (1960) introduced the retrorectal pull-through technique in 1956. In this procedure the dissection is limited to the retrorectal space, where the dissection avoids potential injury to the pelvic nerves. Normally, the innervated (ganglionic) bowel is brought down posteriorly and anastomosed end-to-end to the aganglionic segment. This creates a neorectum in which the anterior wall is aganglionic and the posterior wall is ganglionic (Duhamel, 1960). An abdominal approach is used for this procedure.

3. Soave (1964) introduced the endorectal pull-through in 1964 in an attempt to avoid injury to the pelvic nerves. The dissection is performed inside the muscular cuff of the aganglionic segment. This preserves the important sensory fibers and the integrity of the internal sphincter. The ganglionic segment is then pulled down through the aganglionic muscular cuff. Although leaving aganglionic muscle to surround nor-

mal intestine would theoretically lead to a high incidence of constipation, this has not been the case (Teitelbaum & Coran, 1995).

A new variation for performing the endorectal pull-through procedure is using a single-stage, primary laparoscopic technique. The actual procedure involves the use of three to four trocars (3.5-mm trocars for infants and 5-mm trocars for older children) for visualization and mobilization of the colon. The transition zone is identified and a liberalized resection is performed to include the entire transition. Georgeson et al. describe a decreased incidence of enterocolitis, a decrease in postoperative pain, a more rapid return of bowel function, and a decrease in hospital stay by the laparoscopic technique (Georgeson, Fuefner, & Hardin, 1995; Wulkan & Georgeson, 1998).

On the basis of the success of the minimally invasive laparoscopic approach, Langer et al. have developed a one-stage pull-through using a completely transanal approach without any intraabdominal dissection (Langer, Minkes, Mazziotti, Skinner, & Winthrop, 1999). Such a procedure has the potential advantages of lower cost, less risk of damage to pelvic structures, and the absence of any abdominal incisions. The long-term outcomes of this procedure have yet to be reported. A critical pathway that describes the pre- and postoperative care of the child with Hirschsprung's disease has been found to facilitate the care of these complex patients (Appendix 19–A).

POSTOPERATIVE MANAGEMENT

The patient is kept from eating or drinking until bowel function returns. Nasogastric suction is used for 24 to 48

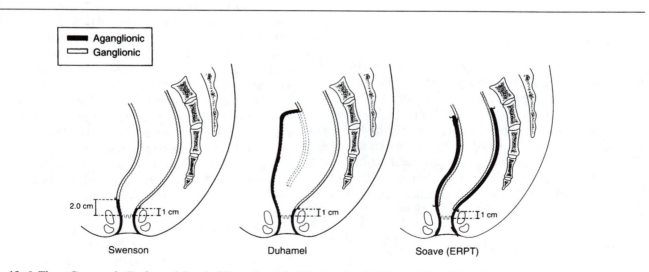

Figure 19–6 Three Commonly Performed Surgical Procedures for Hirschsprung's Disease. Note the variation of remaining aganglionated bowel after each procedure.

hours postoperatively until good bowel sounds are auscultated or the patient passes gas from the rectum. Hydration is maintained with peripheral intravenous therapy.

Clear liquids are started once bowel function has returned. A regular diet is offered in the following 6 to 12 hours once liquids have been tolerated. Pain is managed initially with intravenous narcotics, and acetaminophen (15 mg/kg) is given every 4 hours around the clock for the first 48 hours and then on a PRN basis. Using acetaminophen on a regular basis helps maintain a continuous level of analgesia and reduces the need for narcotic. An oral dose of acetaminophen must be used because suppositories are avoided in the initial postoperative period to prevent disruption of the suture line.

A Foley catheter is left in place for 24 to 48 hours for urinary drainage after extensive pelvic dissection. When a colostomy has been performed, the stoma should be assessed for color, size, and return of function. An enterostomal therapist should be consulted before the procedure to meet with and counsel the family if possible. Stoma teaching should be initiated the first postoperative day because length of hospitalization after the procedures has decreased.

It is important that the patient have nothing placed in the rectum in the initial postoperative period. This includes thermometers, suppositories, or catheters. A sign should be placed to that effect on the patient's bed. In general dilations are withheld for 3 weeks (Marty et al., 1995). Dilations are later performed in the office with each visit. Increasingly, some pediatric surgical practices are performing rectal washouts for the first 3 to 4 months after pull-through (Exhibit 19–2).

Frequent stools that are loose in consistency are expected initially after surgery. Anorectal skin care is important in all patients who have undergone an endorectal pull-through procedure. Initially, after the procedure there can be frequent liquid stools on average of 7 to 12 per day. The most common complication is severe perianal skin breakdown. The loose stool is abrasive, and the skin may become extremely tender despite standard "diaper rash care." The family should be instructed in good perineal care. Frequent tub soaks may be helpful in the weeks after surgery, as well as air drying when possible. It is important that a barrier be placed on the skin to prevent breakdown. Suggested skin barrier products include zinc oxide–based creams such as Desitin (Pfizer, New York) or Critic-aid (Coloplast Corp., Marietta, GA). These should be applied with each diaper change. If the skin is severely broken down and the skin is denuded and moist, Ilex (Medcon, Princeton, NJ), a protective skin barrier, may be applied. When using Ilex, it is necessary to apply the ointment to clean dry skin. After Ilex, a layer of petroleum jelly should be applied so the diaper does not stick to the cream. The cream should not be completely removed with each diaper change because this will cause more irritation to the skin. Instead, wipe away the stool with a soft

Exhibit 19–2 Protocol To Administer Rectal Washouts

The purpose of rectal irrigation is to remove stool and gas from the bowel using small amounts of normal saline every 4 hours until the bowel is clean. Rectal irrigation is different from an enema, where a larger amount of water is given at one time to clear the bowel.

Supplies Needed

1. Red Robinson all-purpose catheter with two additional holes cut in the sides of the catheter.
   Size of catheter used depends on the weight of the child:

Newborn	16 F
5–10 kg	20 F
>10 kg	22 F

2. A 60-ml Toumy syringe for administering the irrigation.
3. Normal saline at room temperature may be used for the irrigation. The volume used is 10 ml/kg. Example, 10 kg child × 10 ml/kg = 100 ml total volume.

Insertion of the Catheter

Position the patient on the left side when possible. An infant may be on his or her back with the legs in a frog position. A water-soluble lubricant may be used to help with the insertion of the catheter. Insert the catheter into the rectum until resistance is met. The normal saline irrigation may need to be instilled into the rectum as the catheter is advanced.

Irrigation

Fill the Toumy syringe with one fourth total volume of normal saline. Push this amount of the saline into the rectum and aspirate back. Disconnect the syringe from the catheter and discard this saline. Repeat three times until the total volume is used. If unable to aspirate, remove the syringe and drain. This procedure may be done every 4 hours.

Example:
10-kg patient, M.D. orders 100 ml NS rectal q4h. Fill Toumy 25-ml normal saline and push into rectum and aspirate back; discard saline and repeat with 25 ml ×3. Then repeat every 4 hours.

moist cloth and use more Ilex to patch the exposed areas. If a yeast-type rash develops, a light dusting of antifungal powder should be applied directly to the skin with a protective ointment on top. If these measures are inadequate to protect the buttocks, consult a wound care specialist for further suggestions.

Continence and the issues regarding toilet training are always the ultimate concern of the child and the family. It is not possible to determine whether the child will have a normal bowel movement pattern or when toilet training should begin. It is recommended that parents try to have a relaxed attitude regarding toilet training. It is unlikely that a child with Hirschsprung's disease will potty train as early as another child or sibling.

Researchers have studied the long-term effects of various procedures for Hirschsprung's disease. Over the past 7 years, 31 primary (one-stage) pull-through procedures were performed at the C.S. Mott Children's Hospital at the University of Michigan Medical Center. Of these, 23 records were available for review. For an accurate history of fecal continence the patients' families of those older than 3 years underwent a detailed interview ($n = 12$). Of these, 10 are completely continent and 2 have occasional soiling. This study concluded that a primary pull-through procedure in the young infant could yield normalization of stooling patterns within 6 months and good levels of continence. It is important to note, however, that after definitive procedures of all types, several children have needed to adopt a bowel training program using enemas to completely evacuate the stool. Families should be aware that surgery is not the end of the disease process. Irregular bowel patterns may persist throughout the child's life. Refer to Chapter 20 for further information on a bowel management program.

COMPLICATIONS

Four major complications associated with Hirschsprung's disease are enterocolitis, anastomic leak, stenosis, and bowel obstruction.

Enterocolitis of Hirschsprung's disease remains the major cause of significant morbidity and mortality. It presents clinically as explosive diarrhea, abdominal distention, and fever (Bill & Chapman, 1962; Elhalaby & Coran, 1994). Pathologically, enterocolitis is defined as an acute inflammatory infiltrate into the crypts and mucosa of the colonic or small intestinal epithelium. As the disease progresses, the mucosal epithelium becomes ulcerated, and the lumen of the intestine becomes filled with fibrinopurulent debris. If this process is left untreated, perforation of the intestine may occur (Teitelbaum, Qualman, & Caniano, 1988). The pathologic process may be seen in ganglionic and aganglionic intestine (Elhalaby, Teitelbaum, Coran, & Heidelberger, 1995; Teitelbaum et al., 1988).

The mortality associated with Hirschsprung's enterocolitis ranges from 6% to 30% (Holschneider, 1982). The diagnosis of enterocolitis is made on the basis of a clinical history of diarrhea (69%), vomiting (51%), fever (34%), and often lethargy (27%) (Elhalaby, Coran, Blane, Hirschl, & Teitelbaum, 1995). On physical examination, the children often have a distended abdomen, hyperactive bowel sounds, and explosive diarrhea after a rectal examination (Bill & Chap-

man, 1962; Caneiro et al., 1992). The odor of the stool may be described as more notably foul smelling than usual. The color of the stool may also change to a darker green or gray. Along with the history and physical examination, the finding of an "intestinal cutoff sign" on abdominal radiographic films has a high degree of sensitivity for enterocolitis. A "cutoff sign" indicates large dilated intestine above or proximal to a markedly narrow, spastic segment of bowel. The incidence of enterocolitis is greater in patients with long segment disease (Teitelbaum et al., 1988; Caneiro et al., 1992). In these patients the enterocolitis is seen after the definitive operative procedure. This form of enterocolitis may be seen with an excessively tight pull-through or may be related to spasm of the internal sphincter. Patients diagnosed with enterocolitis before an operation are more likely to have subsequent episodes (Duhamel, 1964). Patient and family education regarding enterocolitis are extremely important after a definitive operative procedure for Hirschsprung's disease. Often, the family assumes that because the aganglionic portion of intestine has been removed, their child is "cured." By reviewing signs and symptoms of enterocolitis at the time of discharge, parents will seek treatment more quickly. It is important that the family seek medical advice from a physician familiar with Hirschsprung's disease, such as a pediatric surgeon or gastroenterologist.

The treatment of Hirschsprung's disease–associated enterocolitis begins with a series of aggressive washouts using a rectal tube to decompress the colon above the anal sphincter (see Exhibit 19–2). Enemas alone are ineffective because they do not allow for adequate decompression of the colon. Either intravenous antibiotics or oral metronidazole (Flagyl), depending on the clinical presentation, should accompany these serial washouts. A recurrence of enterocolitis may occur and could be due to mucosal changes that occurred early in the life of the child (Fujimoto & Puri, 1988; Lifschitz & Bloss, 1985). Post pull-through enterocolitis can be managed in a similar fashion. The practice of early prophylactic rectal washouts starting 3 weeks after the pull-through appears to decrease the incidence of enterocolitis.

It is imperative that the family is taught to perform rectal washouts by a member of the pediatric surgery service once the rectal anastomosis has healed. Passing dilators, rectal tubes, or thermometers through the rectum in the early postoperative period can damage the rectal anastomosis.

Oral antibiotic therapy may be used in conjunction with rectal washouts to treat mild cases of enterocolitis. Metronidazole has been found effective in the treatment of serious infections caused by susceptible anaerobic bacteria and is effective in the treatment of enterocolitis. It may be dosed at 7.5 mg/kg/dose, given three times daily. The length of therapy is determined by patient symptoms. This drug requires compounding for administration to infants and young children. The addition of a cherry base syrup makes the medication palatable. When prescribing any medication that requires compounding, provide the family with the prescription a few days before it is needed, if possible, and direct the family to a pharmacy that can provide the necessary elixir form. The family should also be educated about the potential side effects of peripheral neuropathy and convulsive seizures when taking metronidazole. Metronidazole should not be taken with acetaminophen (Tylenol) with codeine or cold medicines with an alcohol component.

Another serious complication of Hirschsprung's disease is an anastomotic leak that results from vascular compromise at the pull-through segment of bowel. Presenting symptoms include fever, toxicity, increasing pain, and peritonitis. A water-soluble contrast enema or computed tomography scan can often diagnose this problem. For a mild leak, keeping the child NPO and treating with intravenous antibiotics should suffice. For more severe leaks a diverting colostomy is necessary (Holschneider, 1982).

A third potential complication is stenosis. Mild to moderate stenosis may occur either at the anastomosis or through the length of the cuff. Generally, the anastomotic stenosis is treatable with dilations. To prevent stenosis at the anastomotic site rectal dilations are begun 2 to 3 weeks after the pull-through. In general, these dilations are done without anesthesia. Parents are instructed to perform daily dilations at home. A red rubber catheter or a calibrated dilator may be used to maintain a supple anastomosis and prevent strictures. The dilators are made of stainless steel (Hegar) or a less expensive plastic (Speciality Surgical Products, Hamilton, MT). The dilations are continued until the anastomotic scar is supple, which may take up to 6 months.

Bowel obstruction resulting from adhesions may occur after any abdominal surgery. Obstructive symptoms may occur at any time throughout the child's life. It is important for the patient and family to be instructed to seek medical attention if symptoms of abdominal pain or vomiting persist for longer than 24 hours.

It is important for families, school nurses, and primary care physicians to recognize that although a child has had surgery for Hirschsprung's disease, the disease has not been eliminated. There may continue to be issues regarding stool patterns and constipation. It is common for toilet training to be delayed in children with Hirschsprung's disease compared with siblings or friends. Toilet training is often a trigger for stool retention, which can then lead to constipation, staining of underwear, or gas bloat syndrome. Early symptoms of enterocolitis as previously described should be reported to a specialist immediately; it should not be assumed that they will go away on their own.

A common gastrointestinal virus that may cause mild symptoms of diarrhea or vomiting in a healthy child may have exaggerated effects on a child with Hirschsprung's disease. The symptoms of diarrhea may have increased frequency and persist beyond a few days and should be evaluated if they persist.

CONCLUSION

The increased awareness and improvement of diagnostic techniques has made an important impact on the treatment of Hirschsprung's disease. The average age of diagnosis has shifted from childhood to the infant and newborn age group. This increased awareness has led to a prompt initiation of resuscitation and treatment, resulting in a decrease in mortality. The refinements in surgical treatments and postoperative care have significantly improved the long-term outcome for these patients.

REFERENCES

Akgur, F.M., Tanyel, F.C., Buyukpamukcu, N., & Hicsonmez, A. (1993). Colonic atresia and Hirschsprung's disease association shows further evidence for migration of enteric neurons. *Journal of Pediatric Surgery, 28*(4), 635–636.

Arliss, J., & Holgersen, L.O. (1990). Neonatal appendiceal perforation and Hirschsprung's disease. *Journal of Pediatric Surgery, 25*(6), 694–695.

Bill, J.A.H., & Chapman, N.D. (1962, January). The enterocolitis of Hirschsprung's disease: Its natural history and treatment. *American Journal of Surgery, 103*, 70–74.

Caneiro, P., Brereton, R., Drake, D., Kiely, E., Spitz L., et al. (1992). Enterocolitis in Hirschsprung's disease. *Pediatric Surgery International, 7*, 356–360.

Caniano, D.A., Teitelbaum, D.H., & Qualman, S.J. (1990). Management of Hirschsprung's disease in children with trisomy 21. *American Journal of Surgery, 159*(4), 402–404.

Clausen, N., Andersson, P., & Tommerup, N. (1989). Familial occurrence of neuroblastoma, von Recklinghausen's neurofibromatosis, Hirschsprung's agangliosis and jaw-winking syndrome. *Acta Paediatric Scandinavia, 78*(5), 736–741.

Dobbins, W.O., & Bill, A.H. (1965). Diagnosis of Hirschsprung's disease excluded by rectal suction biopsy. *New England Journal of Medicine, 272*, 990.

Duhamel, B. (1960). A new operation for the treatment of Hirschsprung's disease. *Archives of Diseases of Childhood, 35*, 38–40.

Duhamel, B. (1964). Retrorectal and transanal pull-through procedure for the treatment of Hirschsprung's disease. *Diseases of the Colon and Rectum, 7*, 455.

Elhalaby, E., & Coran, A.G. (1994). Hirschsprung's disease associated with Ondine's curse: Report of three cases and review of the literature. *Journal of Pediatric Surgery, 29*(4), 530–535.

Elhalaby, E.A., Coran, A.G., Blane, C.E., Hirschl, R.B., & Teitelbaum, D.H. (1995). Enterocolitis associated with Hirschsprung's disease: A clinical-radiological characterization based on 168 patients. *Journal of Pediatric Surgery, 30*(1), 76–83.

Elhalaby, E.A., Teitelbaum, D.H., Coran, A.G., & Heidelberger, K.P. (1995). Enterocolitis associated with Hirschsprung's disease: A clinical histopathological correlative study. *Journal of Pediatric Surgery, 30*(7), 1023–1027.

Fujimoto, T., Hata, J., Yokoyama, S., & Mitomi, T. (1989). A study of the extracellular matrix protein as the migration pathway of neural crest cells in the gut: Analysis in human embryos with special reference to the pathogenesis of Hirschsprung's disease. *Journal of Pediatric Surgery, 24*(6), 550–556.

Fujimoto, T., & Puri, P. (1988). Persistence of enterocolitis following diversion of fecal stream in Hirschsprung's disease. A study of mucosal defense mechanisms. *Pediatric Surgery International, 3*, 141–146.

Georgeson, K., Fuefner, M., & Hardin, W. (1995). Primary laparoscopic pull-through for Hirschsprung's disease in infants and children. *Journal of Pediatric Surgery, 30*, 1017–1022.

Gherardi, G.J. (1960). Pathology of the ganglionic-aganglionic junction in congenital megacolon. *Archives of Pathology (Chicago), 69*, 520.

Goldberg, E.L. (1984). An epidemiological study of Hirschsprung's disease. *International Journal of Epidemiology, 13*(4), 479–485.

Holschneider, A.M. (1982). [Complications following surgical therapy of Hirschsprung's disease.] *Chirurgica, 53*(7), 418–423.

Ikeda, K., & Goto, S. (1984). Diagnosis and treatment of Hirschsprung's disease in Japan. An analysis of 1628 patients. *Annals of Surgery, 199*(4), 400–405.

Ikeda, K., Ogami, H., Kume, K., Konishi, Y., & Konishi, T. (1968). [Long segment aganglionosis (Hirschsprung disease) in brothers]. *Shujutsu, 22*(8), 806–813.

Kim, E.H., & Boutwell, W.C. (1985). Smith-Lemli-Opitz syndrome associated with Hirschsprung's disease, 46,XY female karyotype, and total anomalous pulmonary venous drainage [letter]. *Journal of Pediatrics, 106*(5), 861.

Klein, M.D., & Philippart, A.I. (1993). Hirschsprung's disease: Three decades' experience at a single institution. *Journal of Pediatric Surgery, 28*(10), 1291–1293; discussion 1293–1294.

Langer, J.C., Minkes, R.K., Mazziotti, M.V., Skinner, M.A., & Winthrop, A.L. (1999). Transanal one-stage Soave procedure for infants with Hirschsprung's disease. *Journal of Pediatric Surgery, 34*(1), 148–151.

Lifschitz, C.H., & Bloss, R. (1985). Persistence of colitis in Hirschsprung's disease. *Journal of Pediatric Gastroenterology and Nutrition, 4*(2), 291–293.

Martin, L.W., & Perrin, E.V. (1967). Neonatal perforation of the appendix in association with Hirschsprung's disease. *Annals of Surgery, 166*(5), 799–802.

Marty, T.L., Seo, T., Matlak, M.E., Sullivan, J.J., Black, R.E., & Johnson, D.G. (1995, May). Gastrointestinal function after surgical correction of Hirschsprung's disease: Long-term follow-up in 135 patients. *Journal of Pediatric Surgery, 30*(5), 655–658.

McCready, R.A., & Beart, R., Jr. (1981). Classic articles in colonic and rectal surgery. Constipation in the newborn as a result of dilation and hypertrophy of the colon: Harald Hirschsprung, Jahrbuch fur Kinderheilkunde, 1988 Adult Hirschsprung's disease: Results of surgical treatment at Mayo Clinic. *Diseases of the Colon and Rectum, 24*(5), 408–410.

Moore, S.W., Rode, H., Miller, A.J., et al. (1990). Intestinal atresia and Hirschsprung's disease. *Pediatric Surgery International, 5*, 182–184.

Newman, B., Nussbaum, A., Kirkpatrick, J., Jr., & Colodny, S. (1988). Appendiceal perforation, pneumoperitoneum, and Hirschsprung's disease. *Journal of Pediatric Surgery, 23*(9), 854–856.

Noblett, H.R. (1969). A rectal suction biopsy tube for use in the diagnosis of Hirschsprung's disease. *Journal of Pediatric Surgery, 4*(4), 406–410.

Omenn, G.S., & McKusick, V.A. (1979). The association of Waardenburg syndrome and Hirschsprung megacolon. *American Journal of Medical Genetics, 3*(3), 217–223.

Passarge, E. (1967). The genetics of Hirschsprung's disease. Evidence for heterogeneous etiology and a study of sixty-three families. *New England Journal of Medicine, 276*, 138–143.

Polley, T., & Coran, A. (1986). Hirschsprung's disease in the newborn. *Pediatric Surgery International, 1*, 80–83.

Polley, T., Jr., Coran, A.G., & Wesley, J.R. (1985). A ten-year experience with ninety-two cases of Hirschsprung's disease. Including sixty-seven consecutive endorectal pull-through procedures. *Annals of Surgery, 202*(3), 349–355.

Ryan, D. (1995). Neuronal intestinal dysplasia. *Seminars in Pediatric Surgery, 4*(1), 22–25.

Sharli, A.F., & Meirer-Ruge, W. (1981). Localized and disseminated forms of neuronal intestinal dysplasia mimicking Hirschsprung's disease. *Journal of Pediatric Surgery, 16*(2), 164–170.

Soave, F. (1964). Hirschsprung's disease: A new surgical technique. *Archives of Diseases of Childhood, 39*, 116–122.

Swenson, O. (1964). Partial internal sphincterotomy in the treatment of Hirschsprung's disease. *Annals of Surgery, 160*, 540–550.

Swenson, O., & Bill, A.H. (1948). Resection of rectum and rectosigmoid with preservation of the sphincter for benign spastic lesions producing megacolon. *Surgery, 24*, 212–220.

Swenson, O., Fisher, J.H., & Gherardi, G.J. (1959). Rectal biopsy in the diagnosis of Hirschsprung's disease. *Surgery, 45*, 690–695.

Swenson, O., Sherman, J., Fisher, J., & Cohen, E. (1975). The treatment and postoperative complications of congenital megacolon: A 25 year follow-up. *Annals of Surgery, 182*, 266–273.

Taxman, T.L., Yulish, B.S., & Rothstein, F.C. (1986). How useful is the barium enema in the diagnosis of infantile Hirschsprung's disease? *American Journal of Diseases of Children, 140*, 881–884.

Teitelbaum, D.H., Caniano, D.A., & Qualman, S.J. (1989). The pathophysiology of Hirschsprung's-associated enterocolitis: Importance of histologic correlates. *Journal of Pediatric Surgery, 24*(12), 1271–1277.

Teitelbaum, D., & Coran, A. (1995). Hirschsprung's disease. In I. Spitz & A. Coran. (Eds.), *Rob & Smith's operative surgery, pediatric surgery* (pp. 471–494). London: Chapman & Hall.

Teitelbaum, D.H., Qualman, S.J., & Caniano, D.A. (1988). Hirschsprung's disease. Identification of risk factors for enterocolitis. *Annals of Surgery, 207*(3), 240–244.

Wulkan, M., & Georgeson, K. (1998). Primary laparoscopic endorectal pull-through for Hirschsprung's disease in infants and children. *Seminars in Laparoscopic Surgery, 5*, 9–13.

Yntema, C.L., & Hammond, W.S. (1953). Experiments on the sacral parasympathetic nerves and ganglia of the chick embryo. *Anatomy Record, 115*, 382.

Yunis, E.J., Dibbins, A.W., & Sherman, F.E. (1976). Rectal suction biopsy in the diagnosis of Hirschsprung's disease in infants. *Archives of Pathology and Laboratory Medicine, 100*(6), 329–333.

Appendix 19–A

Critical Pathway for Hirschsprung's Disease

Pediatric Surgical Associates, University of Michigan Health Systems, Ann Arbor, Michigan

	Preop Evaluation	*OR*	*POD 1*	*POD 2*
Treatments		1. PIV: D5.045 NS with 20 mEq kcl/L at maintenance 2. NG to LIS if indicated and irrigate with 5 ml normal saline every 6 hours 3. Foley catheter to dependent drain 4. Place sign "NOTHING PER RECTUM" at bedside 5. NPO diet	1. Remove NG 2. Remove Foley 3. Begin clear liquid diet; if vomits, make NPO	1. Advance to regular diet
Medications	1. Bowel prep 2. No bowel prep needed if newborn	1. Cefotetan, 25 mg/kg IV, given in OR then q8h x 3 doses 2. MSO_4 at 0.05–0.10 mg/kg q2–3h PRN 3. Tylenol 10–15 mg/kg q4h A.T.C. PO/NG	1. D/C Cefotetan after third dose 2. MSO_4 PRN 3. Continue Tylenol A.T.C. PO	
Assessment	1. Unprepped barium enema results 2. Suction biopsy results	1. CR monitor if less than 6 months 2. Arm restraints as needed to maintain IV and NG 3. Measure accurate I & O, expect 1 ml/kg/hr urine output		1. D/C monitor
Consults	1. Anesthesia preop evaluation	1. Enterostomal therapist (ET) if indicated 2. Practice management (home care services) 3. Social work as needed	1. Demonstration of stoma teaching by ET or RN	1. Plan for discharge

continues

Appendix 19–A continued

	Preop Evaluation	OR	POD 1	POD 2
Education	1. Provide family with preop bowel prep instructions 2. Provide family with Hirschsprung's education handout	1. Place sign "NOTHING PER RECTUM" above patient bed 2. Keep family updated to patient progress in OR 3. Provide family with rectal skin care sheet if indicated		
Discharge planning		1. Order home discharge supplies 2. Verify if visiting nurse is needed 3. Afebrile 4. Regular bowel movements 5. Perianal skin intact 6. Stoma output less than 20 ml/kg/day		
Evaluation				1. Family demonstrates understanding of patient care and knowledge of symptoms to call MD 2. Arrange follow-up with surgeon and primary care physician

CHAPTER 20

Anorectal Malformations in Children

Kathleen O'Connor Guardino

Expert nursing care of the child born with an anorectal malformation is essential to achieve optimal results in all stages of surgical repair. The natural history of these defects, diagnostic methods, and medical and surgical therapy are reviewed here. The purpose of this chapter is to familiarize the nurse with the assessment and management of children with anorectal malformations. The role of nursing from diagnosis through surgical correction to bowel training and management is emphasized.

Anorectal malformations occur in 1 of every 4,000 newborns (Peña, 1990b). The term "anorectal malformation" encompasses multiple congenital anomalies of the rectum, urinary, and reproductive structures with varying degrees of complexity. Many require different types of treatment with different prognosis for bowel, urinary, and sexual function. Most children with anorectal malformations have an abnormal communication between the rectum, the genitourinary tract, or the perineum. This communication is called a fistula.

Generally, children with complex malformations have poor sphincter tone, a flat perineum, and no clear midline intergluteal groove in addition to an absent anal opening. These children need a three-stage repair: (1) creation of a diverting colostomy, (2) the main repair or pull-through procedure, and (3) colostomy closure. The most frequent surgical repair used is the posterior sagittal anorectoplasty (PSARP). Those children with relatively benign malformations, or "low" defects, simply need an anoplasty, without a colostomy.

Refer to Tables 20–1 and 20–2 for a listing of the different types of defects in both males and females. These defects are described later in this chapter.

PHYSICAL EXAMINATION/WORKUP

The diagnosis of an anorectal malformation is most commonly made in the delivery room on examination of the in-

fant after birth or in the newborn nursery when the nurse attempts to take a rectal temperature and no anus is visible.

Besides the routine nursing examination, the infant with imperforate anus (absent anal opening) should be assessed for the following:

- abdominal distention
- vomiting
- presence of meconium in the perineum of a male infant or in the genitalia of a female infant
- voiding pattern
- presence of meconium in the urine of a male baby as detected by filtering the urine through a gauze pad placed at the tip of the penis or by urinalysis

Once the diagnosis of imperforate anus has been established, the goals of care are as follows:

- provision of general medical support
- evaluation of potential associated defects that require immediate attention
- determination of whether the infant needs a temporary colostomy (high defects) or whether the defect can be treated by a minor operation called anoplasty
- provision of education and emotional support to the parents, including relevant information concerning the diagnosis, tests, treatment, and prognosis

General Support

General support includes administration of antibiotics, keeping the infant NPO (nothing by mouth), insertion of a nasogastric (NG) tube to prevent gastric decompression, administration of vitamin K, administration of intravenous fluids, and strict monitoring of intake and output.

Table 20–1 Types of Male Defects

Diagnosis	Initial Treatment	Final Treatment	Incidence of Associated Defects	Bowel Control (%)	Urinary Control (%)
Perineal fistula	No colostomy	Minimal PSARP	<10%	100	100
Rectobulbar urethral fistula	Colostomy	PSARP	30%	85	100
Rectoprostatic urethral fistula	Colostomy	PSARP	60%	60	100
Rectobladder neck fistula	Colostomy	PSARP with laparotomy	90%	15	100
Imperforate anus without fistula	Colostomy	PSARP	50% Down syndrome	85	100
Rectal atresia and stenosis	Colostomy	PSARP	Undetermined	100	100

Associated Defects

The most frequently associated defects that require immediate attention are those of the urinary tract (Peña, 1997). Therefore, every infant with an anorectal malformation requires an ultrasound examination of the abdomen to detect a urinary obstruction. If the ultrasound examination is abnormal, a more detailed urologic evaluation is indicated. Other associated defects include those of the gastrointestinal tract, including esophageal atresia and tracheoesophageal fistula, and vertebral, cardiac, and skeletal anomalies (Shaul & Harrison, 1997). All infants should have a cardiac evaluation with echocardiogram before surgery (Kiely & Peña, 1998).

The Decision of Colostomy Creation versus Anoplasty

Some minor (low) anorectal malformations can be treated with a one-stage surgical repair called an anoplasty. However, in infants with high defects, the creation of an intestinal diversion called a colostomy is necessary to decompress the bowel. This diversion also helps to prevent infection during the postoperative period after the pull-through procedure. A colostomy is indicated in most malformations as delineated in Tables 20–1 and 20–2. The decision to perform a colostomy is generally made after 24 hours of observation (Wilkins & Peña, 1988).

Traditionally, a study called an "invertogram" or upside-down film (Wangensteen & Rice, 1930) was obtained after 24 hours of life. The radiographic examination was performed at this time so that the infant would have enough intraluminal pressure in the bowel to distend the most distal blind portion of the rectum with gas. Today a cross-table lateral film is obtained with the infant in the prone position with the pelvis elevated (Narasimharao, Prassad, & Katariya, 1983). The gas inside the distended blind rectum gives a radiolucent image. The distance between the radiopaque marker (skin) and the blind rectum is measured to provide objective information concerning the height of the defect and to determine the position of the colon in relationship to the infant's anal sphincter. The infant should be kept wrapped as much as possible to prevent hypothermia during the procedure and should be assessed for vomiting and cyanosis.

Education and Emotional Support

Most parents of a child with an anorectal malformation suffer from emotional stress because of the birth of a child with a congenital defect. The family should be provided with emotional support and information so that they can begin the process of adjustment. Refer to Appendix A at the end of this text for specific resources.

Table 20–2 Types of Female Defects

Diagnosis	Initial Treatment	Final Treatment	Incidence of Associated Defects	Bowel Control (%)	Urinary Control (%)
Perineal fistula	No colostomy	Minimal PSARP	<10%	100	100
Vestibular fistula	Colostomy	PSARP	30%	93	100
Imperforate anus without fistula	Colostomy	PSARP	50% Down syndrome	85	100
Rectal atresia	Colostomy	PSARP	Undetermined	100	100
Persistent cloaca	Colostomy	PSARVUP	90%	70	80

DESCRIPTION OF SPECIFIC DEFECTS

Anorectal Malformations in Male Infants

Perineal Fistula

When the rectum opens into the perineum (Figure 20–1A), it is a low malformation called perineal fistula. This is a benign condition that does not require a protective colostomy and has an excellent prognosis for normal bowel function. Surgical repair involves a limited posterior sagittal anoplasty, which is usually performed during the newborn period. During the first 24 hours of life, these infants usually pass meconium through a small fistula orifice. This orifice is located in the midline, anterior to the anal dimple, in the perineum, at the base of the scrotum or sometimes at the base of the penis. Sometimes the defect is a midline "black ribbon-like" subepithelial meconium fistula. At other times the defect has a prominent midline skin tag located in the anal dimple, below which one can pass an instrument. This last defect is called a "bucket handle" malformation (Figure 20–2; Paidis & Peña, 1997).

Rectourinary Fistulas

About 80% (Rich, Brock, & Peña, 1988) of the male patients with anorectal malformations have an abnormal communication between the rectum and the urinary tract called a rectourinary fistula. The specific location of the fistula has important therapeutic and prognostic implications.

Rectourethral Bulbar Fistula. In a rectourethral bulbar fistula (Figure 20–1B) the rectum communicates with the lower posterior portion of the urethra called bulbar. Usually, meconium can be detected in the urine by filtering it through a gauze pad placed at the tip of the penis. This can be confirmed by urinalysis. The passing of meconium through urine usually occurs after 16 to 24 hours of life, once enough intraluminal bowel pressure has developed to force the meconium through the fistula. A colostomy is indicated followed by a definitive repair. The most common repair performed is the PSARP, which is performed on an elective basis usually within the first year of life (Wangensteen & Rice, 1930).

Rectourethral Prostatic Fistula. In rectourethral prostatic fistula the rectum communicates with the upper part of the posterior portion of the urethra, passing through prostatic tissue (Figure 20–3A). The passage of meconium through the urethra follows the same pattern described for rectourethral bulbar fistula cases. The perineum tends to be flat, with little prominence of the midline groove. Surgical management is the same as described for the bulbar-urethral fistula, but the prognosis for future bowel control is not as good (Wangensteen & Rice, 1930).

Rectobladder Neck Fistula. Rectobladder neck fistula is the highest defect in male patients. The rectum communicates with the bladder neck, and the sacrum is usually abnormal (Figure 20–3B). This indicates the existence of a serious nerve deficiency that translates into a poor prognosis for future bowel control. Children with this defect sometimes experience urinary incontinence. The definitive repair in these cases is generally performed in the first year of life on an

A   B

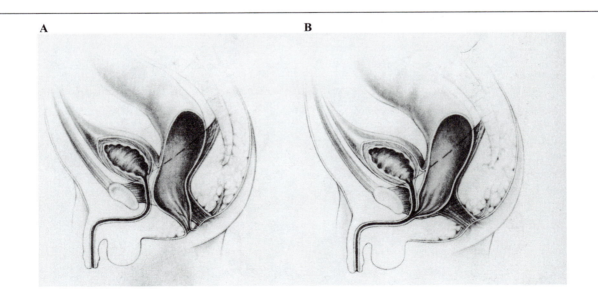

Figure 20–1 Low Malformation in a Male Patient. A, perineal fistula. B, bulbar urethral fistula.

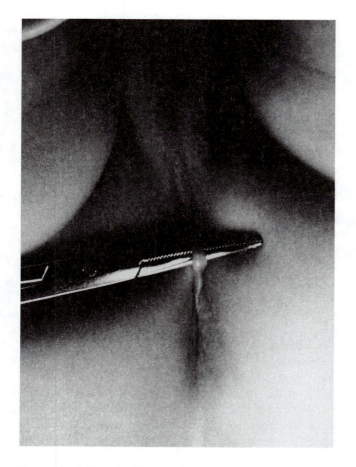

Figure 20–2 Low Malformation in a Male Patient ("Bucket Handle Malformation")

elective basis and includes a PSARP plus a laparotomy to mobilize a rectum that cannot be reached from below. Fortunately, this defect represents only approximately 10% of all the male cases (Peña, 1988).

Imperforate Anus without a Fistula. Imperforate anus without a fistula is an unusual malformation that occurs in less than 10% of all patients (Narasimharao et al., 1983). The rectum is completely blind and ends approximately 2 cm from the perineum. No meconium is present in the urine. Diagnosis is confirmed by a radiologic study to determine the height of the malformation. This defect is frequently associated with Down syndrome (Torres, Levitt, Tovilla, Rodriguez, & Peña, 1998). The treatment, prognosis, perineal appearance, characteristics of the sacrum, and frequency of associated urologic defects are the same as in cases of rectourethral bulbar fistulas.

Rectal Atresia and Stenosis. Rectal atresia and stenosis are unusual defects that occur in approximately 1% of all cases of anorectal malformations. There is no communication with the urinary tract (Peña, 1990b). The perineum looks normal, including a normal-looking anus. Complete obstruction atresia or a decrease in the caliber (stenosis) of the rectum is present approximately 2 cm above the anal opening. These are the cases in which the diagnosis is delayed and established by a nurse while trying to take a rectal temperature. The sacrum and sphincters are normal and therefore the prognosis for bowel function is excellent. A temporary colostomy is indicated followed by a main repair (PSARP) usually performed within the first year of life on an elective basis.

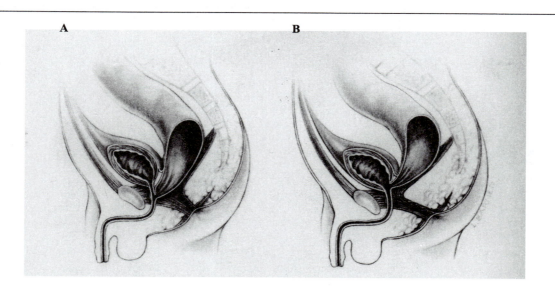

Figure 20–3 A, Prostatic Fistula. B, Bladderneck Fistula.

Anorectal Malformations in Female Infants

Approximately 95% of female infants with imperforate anus have a fistula to the genitalia or to the perineum. Thus, the clinical diagnosis of the specific type of defect and the decision concerning the creation of a colostomy in cases of female patients are usually easier than in male patients (Peña, 1990b).

Perineal Fistula

Perineal fistula is the most benign of all the defects seen in female patients (Figure 20–4A). The rectum opens through an abnormal orifice (fistula) located in the perineum, that is, between the genitalia and the anal dimple (Truffler & Wilkinson, 1962). These patients have an excellent functional prognosis.

Vestibular Fistula

Vestibular fistula is the most frequent defect seen in females (Peña, 1992). The rectum opens through an abnormally narrow orifice located in the vestibule of the genitalia, that is, immediately outside the hymen (Figure 20–4B). Meconium does not pass through the genitalia before 20 hours of life (Peña, 1992). More than 90% of these patients achieve bowel control when adequately managed. Most surgeons believe a colostomy is indicated during the first few days of life.

Vaginal Fistula

Vaginal fistula is an exceptionally rare malformation. Most of the cases reported in the literature as "vaginal fistulas" are cases of vestibular fistulas that have been erroneously diagnosed. To establish this diagnosis, one must see the meconium coming out through the vagina, that is, from inside the hymen orifice. These patients must also receive a colostomy and subsequently a PSARP as in cases of vestibular fistula (Peña, 1992).

Imperforate Anus without Fistula and Rectal Atresia and Stenosis

The characteristics of imperforate anus without fistula and rectal atresia and stenosis, as well as treatment and prognosis, are identical to those previously discussed in male patients.

Persistent Cloaca

Persistent cloaca, a complex malformation, is defined as a defect in which the rectum, vagina, and urinary tract are fused together into a single common channel that communicates exteriorly through a single perineal orifice located at the normal urethral site (Figure 20–5). The diagnosis of persistent cloaca is easily established purely on clinical assessment. The patient's genitalia appears to be smaller than normal (Figure 20–6). Meticulous inspection of the small labia discloses a single perineal orifice, which is the characteristic of this defect. Urologic defects occur at a rate of 90% in children with a cloaca anomaly and may require immediate attention (Rich et al., 1988). These patients represent a potential urologic emergency. An abdominal ultrasound examination must always be performed followed by a urologic workup when necessary before the surgical creation of a colostomy. These infants require a diverting colostomy and

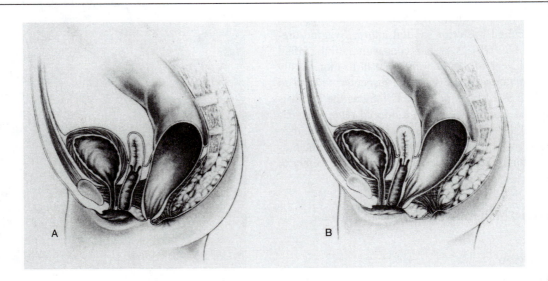

Figure 20–4 A, Low Malformation in a Female Patient (perineal fistula). B, Vestibular Fistula.

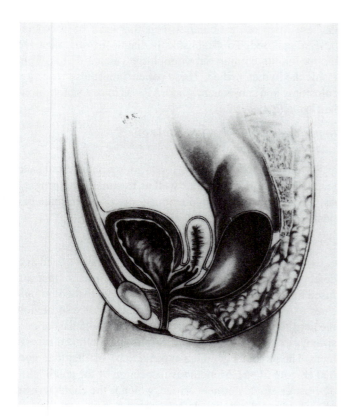

Figure 20–5 Cloaca

anomaly that includes omphalocele, two exstrophied hemi-bladders with cecum between them, imperforate anus, and abnormalities of the sexual structures. Children with this malformation generally undergo multiple surgical procedures throughout their life in an attempt to provide for as normal as possible gastrointestinal, urinary, and sexual functioning (Hendren, 1997).

TREATMENT

Anoplasty

Anoplasty is performed in infants born with low defects or perineal fistulas that do not require a protective colostomy (Peña, 1988). Before the operation, the child remains NPO for 3 to 4 hours. The surgical procedure involves moving the fistula opening into a posterior/anatomically correct position

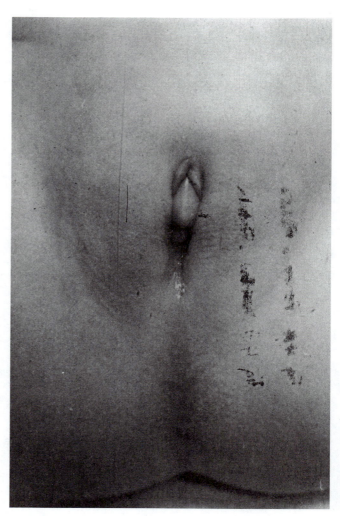

Figure 20–6 Perineum of a Patient with a Persistent Cloaca

concomitant urinary diversion (vesicostomy, ureterostomy) or vaginal diversion (vaginostomy) in cases of obstructed, distended vaginas (Rich et al., 1988). When the infant is older than 3 months, the entire malformation is repaired with an operation called posterior sagittal anorectovagino-ure-throplasty (PSARVUP). Some surgeons wait until the infant is older than 1 year of age or weighs 20 lb to more easily visualize the anatomy. However, some surgeons prefer to do the PSARVUP as early as possible as long as the infant is developing and gaining weight at a normal rate. Approximately 40% of the time, it is necessary to open the abdomen simultaneously with the posterior approach to reach and mobilize a very highly located rectum and/or vagina (Kiely & Peña, 1998).

Rare Anorectal Malformation in Male and Female Infants

Cloacal Exstrophy

Cloacal exstrophy is a rare malformation, occurring about once in every 250,000 births. Cloacal exstrophy is a complex at the center of the sphincter and creating a larger anal opening. The postoperative care consists of application of an antibiotic ointment to the perineum three times per day for 2 weeks. Intravenous antibiotics are administered for 2 to 3 days. Feedings are resumed immediately after surgery. At the 2-week check-up, a program of anal dilations is initiated. The dilation schedule is described in detail later in the text. Breastfeeding is encouraged because it is unlikely to cause constipation. Infants receiving a synthetic formula may require a stool softener and occasionally a laxative.

Colostomy Creation

When a colostomy is needed, usually a descending colostomy is created with a functioning stoma and a mucous fistula (nonfunctioning stoma). It is optimal if there is enough skin between the two stomas to allow an ostomy bag to cover the functional site only (Wilkins & Peña, 1988) (Figure 20–7). This helps to avoid complications from leakage. Creating a colostomy high on the sigmoid loop allows for easy mobilization during the pull-through procedure (Wilkins & Peña, 1988). After the operation, the child has an NG tube for approximately 48 hours and receives intravenous antibiotics to treat enteric pathogens. Colostomy and skin care, as

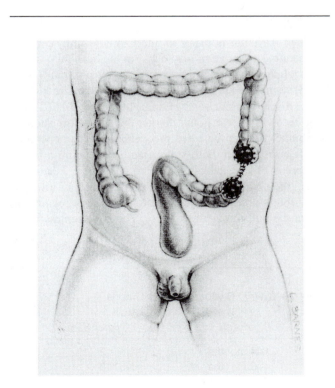

Figure 20–7 Descending Colostomy with Separated Stomas in Left Lower Quadrant of the Abdomen

well as assessment of vital signs, are important during the postoperative care. Postoperative pain is generally managed with intravenous morphine. The expected length of stay is 4 to 5 days.

At this time, the clinical nurse specialist and an enterostomal therapist assess and address the educational and discharge needs of the family. The parents must learn stoma care before the infant's discharge. Some institutions do not use stoma bags in infants with a lower colon colostomy because the stool is more formed and less irritating. Instead, they allow the stool to empty directly into the diaper. Some parents prefer this method. Most parents, however, find that the use of a stoma bag prevents skin breakdown.

The initial reaction from parents who see their infants' colostomy for the first time and are informed that they will be responsible for the care of it is usually one of anxiety. They frequently state that there is no way that they can do this. The nurse plays an important role in reassuring and teaching the parent. With patience, support, understanding, and clinical expertise from the nurse, the parents learn stoma management and become experts in their child's care in a short period of time.

Pre-PSARP Care

Nursing care and assessment are essential during the preoperative stage. A distal colostogram is obtained before the PSARP to determine the location of the most distal part of the bowel and document the presence and location of a fistula between the bowel and the urogenital tract. This test is obtained in an outpatient setting (Gross, Wolfson, & Peña, 1991).

Preoperative preparation may occur in the hospital or home setting. Visiting nurses may assist the family in the home setting. Bowel preparation includes irrigation of the distal stoma (nonfunctional, mucous fistula) with warm normal saline solution with the aid of a Foley catheter. The purpose of this irrigation is to remove all the fecal matter left in the colon distal to the colostomy to avoid contamination at the time of the pull-through. Irrigations are continued until the return is clear.

Posterior Sagittal Anorectoplasty

The posterior sagittal anorectoplasty is more commonly referred to as the PSARP (Peña, 1992), or the "Peña procedure." Generally, this second stage of the surgical repair is performed in patients older than 1 month of age, provided the infant is growing and developing normally. Some surgeons, however, prefer to wait until the baby is 6 to 12 months old. The operation is performed in the prone position (face down) with a Foley catheter inserted in the bladder. It entails a midline posterior sagittal incision running from the middle portion of the sacrum to the anterior edge of the external sphincter. The sphincter mechanism is divided in a midline incision, thereby preserving the nerve fibers and decreasing the amount of postoperative pain. The back of the child's buttocks is opened like a book, and all internal structures are exposed. The rectum is then meticulously separated from the genitourinary tract, dissected, and freed enough to reach its normal site without tension. The fistula site is then closed. With the use of an electrical muscle stimulator, the limits of the sphincter mechanism are determined and the rectum is placed in its optimal location to achieve the best functional results. If the child is known to have a very high defect or the child's rectum is not able to be reached with this approach, the abdomen must also be opened (laparotomy).

The postoperative course for this surgical procedure is relatively benign. If a laparotomy was not needed, the child may drink fluids after the surgery and have a regular diet the next day. The intravenous line must be preserved for the administration of antibiotics (ampicillin, gentamicin, clindamycin) for 2 to 3 days. Some surgeons continue antibiotics for several more days. In males and in females with cloaca, the Foley catheter remains in place 5 to 10 days. This protects the suture line in the urethra, where the communication between the bowel and urethra is located. The surgeon should be notified if the catheter comes out inadvertently. If the infant is unable to void, a suprapubic tube is inserted. The children do not need to be positioned in any particular way; they may simply find the best position for themselves. Instruct the parents to apply antibiotic ointment to the perineum with every diaper change to prevent local infection. Continue the antibiotic ointment for 2 weeks until the child's first postoperative visit. The expected length of stay is 2 to 3 days.

Postoperative Care in Cases of PSARP Plus Laparotomy

Children experience more postoperative pain and a longer hospital stay if a laparotomy is needed with the PSARP (Peña, 1992). A laparotomy is generally performed if the rectum is too high to be visualized and mobilized from a posterior approach. These children return from the operating room with an intravenous line and an NG tube. The NG remains in place for 3 to 4 days or until active bowel sounds are heard. The children are managed with intravenous morphine for their pain. The skin care of the perineum remains the same, with antibiotic ointment as described earlier.

Two-Week Postoperative Visit

Two weeks after surgery the stitches are removed and the antibiotic ointment is discontinued. At this time, the process of anal dilations is initiated (Paidis & Peña, 1997). The dila-

tions prevent anal strictures from forming because of the scar tissue around the anus. It is imperative for the family to adhere to the guidelines given to them. The surgeon generally passes the first dilator and then the surgeon or pediatric surgical nurse teaches the parents the dilation process. Position the child with the knees flexed close to the chest. Lubricate the tip of the anal dilator and insert it 3 to 4 cm into the rectum. Repeat this procedure twice a day for approximately 30 seconds each time. Every week advance to the next size dilator. After 6 to 8 weeks the "desired size" is reached (Table 20–3). Then, colostomy closure is planned.

Dilation Schedule (after the Desired Size Has Been Reached)

Dilations continue, with decreasing frequency, after the PSARP for a total period of approximately 6 months. The parent must continue passing the last desired size dilator twice per day until the dilator passes easily and without pain. Then, the parent can begin decreasing the frequency of dilations as listed below (Peña, 1992):

- one time a day for 1 month
- every other day for 1 month
- two times a week for 1 month
- once a week for 1 month
- once a month for 3 months

Colostomy Closure

When the child is ready to undergo colostomy closure, preoperative preparation may occur in the hospital or home setting. Irrigations are now necessary for the proximal (functional) stoma and are performed in the same manner as those for the distal (nonfunctioning) stoma before the PSARP. The child receives a clear liquid diet on the day before surgery. Antibiotics are administered preoperatively. The operation entails taking down both stomas and performing a bowel anastomosis to reestablish the colon continuity. Postoperatively, the child may experience more pain than after the pull-through procedure if a laparotomy was not required as part of the pull-through procedure. The child returns to the

Table 20–3 Anal Dilator Selection Criteria

Child Age	Hegar Dilator Size
1–4 months	No. 12
4–8 months	No. 13
8–12 months	No. 14
1–4 years	No. 15
>4 years	No. 16

floor with intravenous fluids and an NG tube. Intravenous antibiotics are routinely given for 2 to 3 days followed by oral ampicillin to complete a 1-week course. Pain medication is administered as needed. The child remains NPO and with an NG tube for 1 to 3 days or until bowel sounds are heard. Intravenous fluids are administered during the time that the patient remains NPO. The expected length of stay is 4 to 5 days. Children are not discharged until they pass a stool from the anus at approximately 1 to 3 days postoperatively. A frequent complication is perianal excoriation caused by frequent bowel movements. As the number of bowel movements per day decreases over the next several weeks, the skin begins to heal nicely.

Discuss skin care with the family several weeks before the colostomy closure. One relatively natural preparation to toughen the skin before the colostomy closure is to coat the perineum with a paste and then add a small amount of stool from the colostomy for 15 minutes three times a day for approximately 2 weeks. Because the child is expected to have a rather severe diaper rash after colostomy closure, recommend a variety of "butt pastes" to protect and heal the perineum. For example, one useful paste consists of vitamin A & D ointment, aloe, zinc, and Mylanta (to help the ointment stick to the skin and help form a paste). Add an antifungal cream or powder (only with a prescription) if a yeast infection occurs (Paidis & Peña, 1997). Eventually, the number of bowel movements decreases, and the diaper rash is no longer a concern (Peña, 1992). However, at that point, constipation becomes a concern. Constipation is the most frequent sequela in children born with anorectal malformations (Peña & El Behery, 1993). A laxative-type diet is recommended to prevent constipation and fecal impaction. The family is given a detailed list of fiber-rich foods. If the diet does not result in regular soft stools, a laxative medication such as senna, docusate sodium, or mineral oil is prescribed to ensure that the patient empties his or her rectum every day (Poenaru et al., 1997).

POSTOPERATIVE BOWEL FUNCTION

Children who undergo surgical repair of an anorectal malformation experience variable degrees of bowel control. Children with anorectal malformations generally become toilet trained for stool later than children with normal anatomy, usually after 2½ to 3 years of age or later. There are some signs, however, that the surgeon can use before that age to predict the possibility of the child's success with toilet training.

Patients born with good prognostic types of malformations and showing good prognostic signs as described earlier in this chapter are expected to achieve success with toilet training. Alternatively, patients born with poor prognostic malformations or showing bad prognostic signs are offered a

Bowel Management Program (Peña, 1990, 1992; Peña et al., 1998). The goal of a *Bowel Management Program* is social continence for children who are unlikely to become toilet trained.

Toilet Training

Toilet training for stool is the long-term goal for children with anorectal malformations, although this is not always possible. Parents should be encouraged to use the same strategies for toilet training as in children with normal anatomy. Between 2 and 3 years of age, the parents are instructed to sit the child on the toilet after every meal. The parents are encouraged to do it as a game and not as a punishment. The child should sit in front of a little table and play with favorite toys. The parents should be encouraged to sit with the child and not to argue or force the child to remain seated. However, if the child gets up, the parents should put the toys away. The child should be rewarded for a bowel movement or voiding while on the toilet. If the child is not successfully toilet trained by school age, there are two alternatives: (1) do not send the child to school for one more year and continue attempts at toilet training or (2) try the *Bowel Management Program* (Peña et al., 1998) for 1 year, assuming that it will be implemented on a temporary basis. Then, during the next summer vacation, the parents can again attempt to toilet train the child.

It is unacceptable to send a child with fecal incontinence to school in diapers when his classmates are already toilet trained (Peña, 1997). Children who require diapers or who have accidents while in school because of fecal incontinence are exposed to ridicule from their peers that can lead to adverse psychological sequelae (Poenaru et al., 1997).

Bowel Management Program

To achieve fecal continence, three components are necessary: sensation within the rectum, good motility of the colon, and good voluntary muscle or sphincter control (Peña, 1992). Children with anorectal malformations lack all or some of these essential components.

First, children born with anorectal malformations lack the intrinsic sensation to feel stool or gas passing through their rectum. Therefore, many times the child may unknowingly soil.

Second, the child needs to have good motility of the colon. Normally, the rectosigmoid remains quiet for periods of 24 to 48 hours, then a massive peristaltic wave allows the complete emptying of the colon. Patients with anorectal malformations have abnormal peristaltic waves in the rectosigmoid colon that result in stagnant stool or an overactive colon. The child then develops constipation or encopresis (overflow incontinence). Alternatively, a very active colon may provoke a constant passing of stool, which may significantly interfere with bowel continence.

Third, the child needs good voluntary muscles or sphincteric mechanism. These muscles allow for good control and retention of stool

Children who have fecal incontinence after repair of imperforate anus can be divided into two well-defined groups that require individualized treatment plans: (1) children with constipation are mainly children who underwent operations in which the rectum was preserved (anoplasties, PSARP, and sacroperineal pull-throughs), and (2) children with diarrhea are mainly children who underwent operations in which the rectum and sometimes the sigmoid colon was resected (abdominoperineal procedures, endorectal resections). Sometimes the child lost a portion of the colon for some other reason or suffers from a condition that produces diarrhea.

The basis of the *Bowel Management Program* consists of teaching the parents or patient to clean the colon every day by the use of enemas or colonic irrigations followed by finding a method to keep the colon quiet for the following 24 hours. This prevents soiling episodes and involuntary bowel movements. Success of the *Bowel Management Program* is enhanced with specific diets or medications such as Lomotil or Imodium. Success is usually achieved within a week of a process of trial and error (Peña et al., 1998).

Children with Constipation

This section is a guide to help parents manage children with constipation. Identify a quiet, relaxed time of day for the enema program. After dinner often works well. Administer the enemas 1 hour after eating to take advantage of the gastric-colic reflex. Ask the child to sit on the toilet for 30 to 45 minutes. The use of phosphate enemas (Fleet) is most convenient. However, pure saline enemas are often just as effective. Children older than 8 years of age or heavier than 65 lb may receive one adult phosphate enema daily. Children between 3 and 8 years of age or 35 and 65 lb may receive one pediatric phosphate enema a day. Patients should *never* receive more than one phosphate enema a day because of the risk of phosphate intoxication and hypocalcemia and hyponatremia (Peña et al., 1998). Symptoms of hyperphosphatemia are associated with the symptoms of the related hypocalcemia and include tetany, paresthesias, and Q-T wave prolongation. Treatment of hyperphosphatemia includes elimination of any excess intake, use of aluminum hydroxide antacids, and administration of intravenous saline (Weigle & Tobin, 1992). The phosphate enema administered on a regular basis should result in a bowel movement followed by a period of 24 hours of complete cleanliness. If one enema is not enough to clean the colon, then the patient requires a more aggressive treatment, and a saline (only) enema is administered. If the addition of the saline enema still results in inadequate results, then high colonic washings are

indicated with a Foley catheter attached to the tip of the bottle of the Fleet enema. A No. 20 to 24 F Foley catheter is lubricated and gently introduced through the anus as high as possible (Figure 20–8). The Foley catheter is flexible so parents can maneuver it into the colon of severely impacted children. If the catheter will not pass up into the bowel, insert the tube a few centimeters and inflate the balloon with 20 to 30 ml of water. Pull on the catheter, occluding the colonic lumen with the balloon acting as a plug. This enables the enema solution to go up into the bowel with minimal leakage (Figure 20–9). If the child soils at any point during the following 24 hours, the bowel washout was incomplete and a more aggressive technique is required. Parents can increase the volume of the enema or administer a second saline enema 30 minutes later. The program is individualized and the parents and children learn to look at the consistency and amount of stool obtained after the enema to determine whether it was effective.

Position the child to take advantage of gravity. Washing the colon out as high as possible can increase the efficacy of the enema. Position young children over the parent's lap. In older children, instill the enema with the children on their knees, with the buttocks up and their head close to the floor (Figure 20–10). Encourage the child to sit on the toilet for 30 to 45 minutes after the administration of the enema until he or she feels that the colon is empty. A portable television, books, homework, or games can make this time pass faster. Constipated children have a colon and a rectosigmoid with decreased motility. Frequently, all they may need is a good enema or colonic irrigation to remain clean for 24 hours (Peña et al., 1998).

A second group of children who experience severe constipation are those who undergo a surgical repair for an anorectal malformation with an adequate sacrum and sphincters. The operation was performed successfully without complication and the rectosigmoid was preserved. Yet these children have severe constipation associated with a megasigmoid (Peña & El Behery, 1993). Sometimes the interval between bowel movements is greater than a week and then the child is incontinent of stool. A contrast enema demonstrates the presence of a giant sigmoid colon. These children require an aggressive program of enemas to be clean. Another alternative is surgery that involves resecting the most dilated portion of the megasigmoid. The procedure makes them fecally continent and demonstrates that they had severe constipation with secondary encopresis or overflow pseudo-incontinence (Peña & El Behery, 1993). If the constipation is not extreme, administration of laxatives may have the same effect as the operation.

Children with Diarrhea

This section is a guide to help parents manage children with diarrhea. Children with diarrhea have an overactive co-

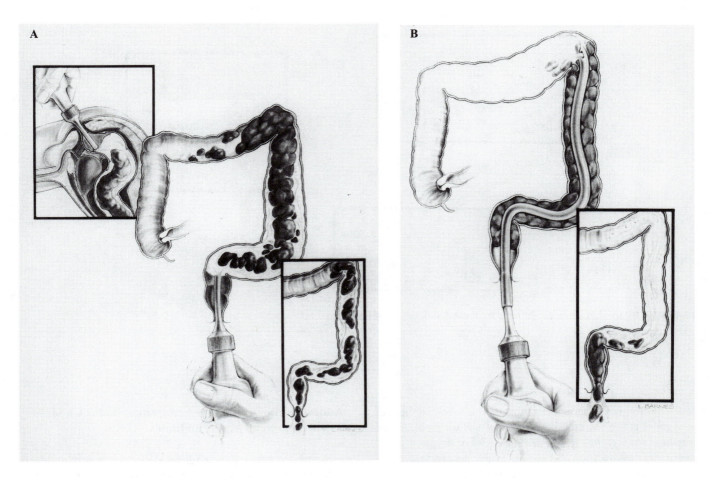

Figure 20–8 Colonic Irrigation Technique. A, without a tube. B, with a tube.

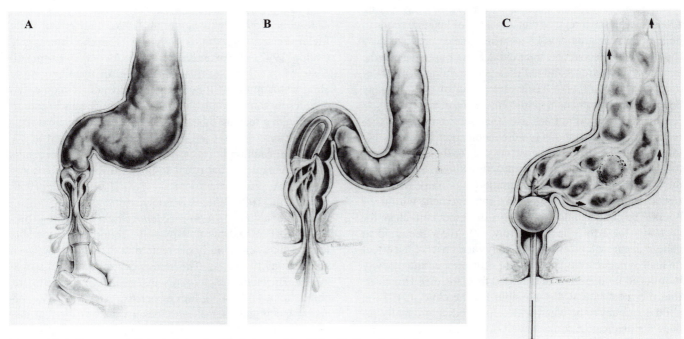

Figure 20–9 Enema and Colonic Irrigation Technique with a Foley Balloon Inflated

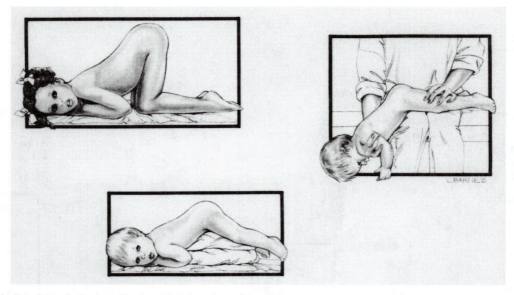

Figure 20–10 Ideal Position for Patients for the Administration of Enemas

lon. Children with anorectal malformations who had the rectosigmoid colon resected have no reservoir for stool. Rapid transit of stool results in frequent episodes of diarrhea. Stool passes so rapidly from the cecum to the descending colon that they are unable to maintain continence even after administration of an enema. A constipating diet and/or medications to slow down the colon, such as loperamide or Lomotil, are recommended. Provide parents with a list of constipating foods to promote a regular diet and a list of laxative foods to be avoided. Most parents know which meals provoke diarrhea and which constipate their child. Sometimes, despite the best efforts of parents and children, some children never develop social continence. This rare group of children may benefit from a permanent colostomy (Peña et al., 1998).

Children who do not achieve successful bowel management with enemas and diet require medication. To determine the combination that will be successful for the child, follow this plan. (1) Start the treatment with enemas, a very strict diet, and a high dose of loperamide (Imodium). Most patients respond to this aggressive management within 24 hours. The child should remain on a strict diet until clean for 24 hours for 2 to 3 days in a row. (2) Allow the child to choose one new food every 2 to 3 days and observe the effect on his colonic activity. If the child soils after eating a newly introduced food, eliminate that food from the diet. However, find the most liberal diet possible for the child. (3) If the child continues to be clean with a liberal diet, gradually reduce the medication to the lowest dose effective to keep the child clean for 24 hours.

Additional Bowel Management Strategies for Children with Anorectal Malformations

Another strategy to manage fecal incontinence in children is the creation of a continent appendicostomy for the administration of an antegrade enema. This procedure is effective in children who experience fecal incontinence despite success with a *Bowel Management Program* (Curry, Osborne, & Malone, 1998; Fukunaga et al., 1996; Graf et al., 1998; Meier, Foster, Guzzetta, & Colin, 1998; Webb, Barraza, & Crump, 1997; Wilcox & Kiely, 1998). A continent appendicostomy involves surgically creating an opening on the child's abdominal wall by using the appendix. Colonic irrigation solution is instilled into the colon by means of cannulation with a feeding tube. This simplifies the cleanout regimen because enemas are needed less frequently, if at all, generally resulting in less trauma to the child. It also results in a predictable period of no soiling, allowing families and children to lead more "normal" lives (Curry et al., 1998; Meier et al., 1998; Wilcox & Kiely, 1998).

Another adjunct to a *Bowel Management Program* is biofeedback. Biofeedback therapy helps children who are able to recognize sensation in the rectum to distinguish between solids, liquids, and gas. The goal is control of bowel movements. Biofeedback involves inserting a probe into the child's anus and asking him or her to perform Kegel exercises. A computer screen provides a visual image that displays periods of contraction and relaxation, the pelvic muscle activity. Continence is improved in children who are able to follow directions, are self-motivated, and are willing to practice the new skills at home in addition to in the training sessions. A carefully planned diet supplements a biofeedback program. Although the use of biofeedback is not widespread in children with anorectal malformations (Paidis & Peña, 1997; Poenaru et al., 1997), it has been shown to be effective in some children (Iwai, Iwata, Kimura, & Janagihara, 1997). It may also be worthwhile to use behavior modification techniques in children who are toilet training, having two to three bowel movements per day, and soiling in between these bowel movements (Paidis & Peña, 1997).

Children with complex or high anorectal malformations require a *Bowel Management Program* (Hendren, 1997; Peña, 1992; Truffler & Wilkinson, 1962) for the remainder of their lives. Children with less severe defects may remain socially continent with a disciplined diet with regular meals to provoke bowel movements at a predictable time. It is never too late to consider a *Bowel Management Program.* Children who initially fail to achieve continence at ages 3 to 5 may successfully achieve continence in the early school-age years. Encourage children with some potential for bowel control to gain control of their bowel movements without enemas over the summer vacation. Parents and children who commit to this process must stay at home, socialize little, and maintain a regular diet and schedule to achieve success. Encourage the child to sit on the toilet after every meal and try to pass stool. In addition, the child must remain alert all day while trying to learn to discriminate the feeling of an imminent bowel movement. Children with constipation may ben-

efit from a daily laxative to provoke a single bowel movement per day. Adjust the dosage of the laxative as needed to avoid uncontrolled diarrhea. Start with a laxative-type diet. Then add a bulk-forming type product such as a stool softener. If these medications do not work, a laxative with an active ingredient is indicated. After a few days or weeks, the family and the child are in a position to decide whether they want to continue with that regimen or whether they would prefer to go back to the *Bowel Management Program.*

The *Bowel Management Program* is an ongoing process that is responsive to individual patient and family needs. The success of the *Bowel Management Program* depends on the dedication, determination, and consistency of everyone involved. Children who have completed the *Bowel Management Program* and remain clean for 24 hours experience a new sense of confidence based on an improved quality of life.

CONCLUSION

A variety of anorectal malformations exist. An understanding of the diagnosis and management of the various types of malformations guides the nurse in caring for these children and their families. Unfortunately, these children may persist with some degree of bowel dysfunction after surgery. A variety of treatment modalities exists to assist the child in achieving continence. The success of any of these strategies (*Bowel Management Program*, biofeedback, or surgical intervention) requires collaboration between the family, the child, and the health care team.

REFERENCES

Curry, J.I., Osborne, A., & Malone, P.S.J. (1998). How to achieve a successful Malone antegrade continence enema. *Journal of Pediatric Surgery, 33*(1), 138–141.

Fukunaga, K., Kimura, K., Lawrence, J., Soper, R.T., & Phearman, L.A. (1996). Button device for antegrade enema in the treatment of incontinence and constipation. *Journal of Pediatric Surgery, 31*(8), 1038–1039.

Graf, J.L., Strear, C., Bratton, B., Housley, H.T., Jennings, R.W., Harrison, M.R., & Albanese, C.T. (1998). The antegrade continence enema procedure: A review of the literature. *Journal of Pediatric Surgery, 33*(8), 1294–1296.

Gross, G.O., Wolfson, P.J., & Peña, A. (1991). Augmented-pressure colostogram in imperforate anus with fistula. *Pediatric Radiology, 21*, 560–562.

Hendren, W.H. (1997). Management of cloaca malformations. *Seminars in Pediatric Surgery, 6*(4), 217–227.

Iwai, N., Iwata, G., Kimura, O., & Janagihara, J. (1997). Is a new biofeedback therapy effective for fecal incontinence in patients who have anorectal malformations? *Journal of Pediatric Surgery, 32*(11), 1626–1629.

Kiely, E.D., & Peña, A. (1998). Anorectal malformations. In J.S. O'Neill, M.I. Rowe, J.L. Grosfeld, E.W. Fonkalsrud, & A.G. Coran (Eds.), *Pediatric surgery* (5th ed., Vol. 2, p. 1425). St. Louis, MO: Mosby.

Meier, D.E., Foster, M.E., Guzzetta, P.C., & Colin, D. (1998). Antegrade continent enema management of chronic fecal incontinence in children. *Journal of Pediatric Surgery, 33*(7), 1149–1152.

Narasimharao, K.A., Prassad, G.R., & Katariya, S. (1983). Prone cross-table lateral view: An alternative to the invertogram in imperforate anus. *American Journal of Roentgenology, 140*, 227–229.

Paidis, C.N., & Peña, A. (1997). Rectum and anus. In K.T. Oldham, P.M. Colombani, & R.P. Foglia (Eds.), *Surgery of infants and children: Scientific principles and practice* (p. 1323). Philadelphia: Lippincott-Raven.

Peña, A. (1988). Posterior sagittal anorectoplasty: Results in the management of 332 cases of anorectal malformations. *Pediatric Surgery International, 3*, 94–104.

Peña, A. (1990a). Advances in the management of fecal incontinence secondary to anorectal malformations. In L.M. Nyhus (Ed.), *Surgery annual* (pp. 143–167). Norwalk, CT: Appleton & Lange.

Peña, A. (1990b). *Atlas of surgical management of anorectal malformations* (p. 1). New York: Springer-Verlag.

Peña, A. (1992). Current management of anorectal anomalies. *Surgical Clinics of North America, 72*(6), 1393–1416.

Peña, A. (1997). Preface: Advances in anorectal malformations. *Seminars in Pediatric Surgery, 6*(4), 165–169.

Peña, A., & El Behery, M. (1993). Megasigmoid: A source of pseudo incontinence in children with repaired anorectal malformations. *Journal of Pediatric Surgery, 28*, 1–5.

Peña, A., Guardino, J.M., Tovilla, M.A., Levitt, G., Rodriguez, G., & Torres, R. (1998). Bowel management for fecal incontinence in patients with anorectal malformations. *Journal of Pediatric Surgery, 33*(1), 133–137.

Poenaru, D., Roblin, N., Bird, M., Duce, S., Groll, A., Pietak, D., Spry, K., & Thompson, J. (1997). The pediatric bowel management clinic: Initial results of a multidisciplinary approach to functional constipation in children. *Journal of Pediatric Surgery, 32*(6), 843–848.

Rich, M.A., Brock, W.A., & Peña, A. (1988). Spectrum of genitourinary malformations in patients with imperforate anus. *Pediatric Surgery International, 3*, 110–113.

Shaul, D.B., & Harrison, A. (1997). Classification of anorectal malformations—Initial approach, diagnostic tests, and colostomy. *Seminars in Pediatric Surgery, 6*(4), 187–195.

Torres, P., Levitt, M.A., Tovilla, J.M., Rodriguez, G., & Peña, A. (1998). Anorectal malformations and Down's syndrome. *Journal of Pediatric Surgery, 22*(2), 1–5.

Truffler, G.A., & Wilkinson, R.H. (1962). Imperforate anus: A review of 147 cases. *Canadian Journal of Surgery, 5*, 169–177.

Wangensteen, O.H., & Rice, C.O. (1930). Imperforate anus: A method of determining the surgical approach. *Annals of Surgery, 92*, 77–81.

Webb, H.W., Barraza, M.A., & Crump, J.M. (1997). Laparoscopic appendicostomy for management of fecal incontinence. *Journal of Pediatric Surgery, 32*(3), 457–458.

Weigle, C.G.M., & Tobin, J.R. (1992). Metabolic and endocrine disease in pediatric intensive care. In M.C. Rogers (Ed.), *Textbook of pediatric intensive care* (2nd ed., Vol. 2, p. 1235). Baltimore: Williams & Wilkins.

Wilcox, D.T., & Kiely, E.M. (1998). The Malone (antegrade colonic enema) procedure: Early experience. *Journal of Pediatric Surgery, 33*(2), 204–206.

Wilkins, S., & Peña, A. (1988). The role of colostomy in the management of anorectal malformations. *Pediatric Surgery International, 3*, 105–109.

CHAPTER 21

Caring for Children with Ostomies and Wounds

Gail Garvin

THE PEDIATRIC OSTOMY PATIENT

The pediatric patient has a gastrointestinal or urinary diversion for one of many reasons. Both congenital and acquired conditions can result in ostomy creation. Some common conditions include Hirschsprung's disease, anorectal malformations such as imperforate anus and cloacal exstrophy, necrotizing enterocolitis, inflammatory bowel diseases, cancer, trauma, bladder exstrophy, spina bifida, midgut volvulus, and malrotation. (Hirschsprung's disease, necrotizing enterocolitis, anorectal malformations, malrotation and volvulus, and trauma are discussed at length in Chapters 19, 23, 20, 24, and 34, respectively). This chapter focuses on the care and management of the infant/child with a traditional ostomy versus a continent diversion. Frequently used terminology to facilitate understanding of the discussion is found in Exhibit 21–1.

The clinical presentation, differential diagnosis, physical examination, diagnostic tests, and operative procedures of a child with an ostomy depend on the individual diagnosis. In general, the infant or child appears with either a visually obvious birth defect or with obstructive symptoms of the affected system, either gastrointestinal or urinary. A series of both laboratory and radiologic tests are performed to determine the exact physical cause of the obstruction, and the appropriate operative procedure is selected. Most commonly, the diseased or problematic portion of the gastrointestinal or urinary tract is either removed or bypassed to create an unobstructed flow of urine, stool, or both if the cause of obstruction requires both.

Most of the time in pediatrics the creation of an ostomy is an emergency event, so rarely is there time before surgery for much preparation of the patient or family. It is also a rare occurrence that preoperative stoma placement can be marked on the patient's abdomen as is frequently done in adults. Many of the ostomies that are created in infants and children are temporary, although some are permanent. Fortunately, most patients requiring an ostomy are infants and no preoperative psychological preparation is required with the infant. For older children play therapy is useful in the preoperative and postoperative periods to help them understand and accept the new ostomy. The parents, however, are usually in a state of shock and disbelief and require considerable postoperative support and nurturing.

POSTOPERATIVE NURSING CONSIDERATIONS

Caremap

A caremap created from a multidisciplinary effort is an efficient way to determine a routine postoperative course for the patient with a newly created ostomy. The length of stay for the patient with a new ostomy varies, depending on the reason for ostomy creation. Some patients are ready for discharge in 3 days; others may take much longer depending on the type and severity of the illness and complications. A generic caremap for the patient with a newly created ostomy is provided here (see Appendix 21–A). Changes can be made to this caremap to adapt it for use at any institution.

Management of the Ostomy

Management of an ostomy depends in part on the type of ostomy created. In infants with very distal colostomies or urinary diversions, the option exists whether to use an appliance or pouch to collect the effluent or to collect the effluent in the diaper. The effluent in either of these situations is generally not caustic to the skin. If the effluent does compromise the skin integrity, pouching may be a better alternative. If the irritation to the skin is mild, the peristomal skin can be satisfactorily protected with topical ointments and creams. Popular topical skin protectants include zinc oxide and petroleum-based ointments.

Exhibit 21–1 Ostomy-Related Terms Related to Intestinal and Urinary Diversions

Cecostomy: Surgical creation of an opening into the cecum to serve as an anus.

Colostomy: Surgical formation of an artificial anus by connecting the colon to an opening in the abdominal wall.

Distal end: The end of the intestine closest to the anus, the nonfunctioning stoma.

Double-barrel ostomy: Two distinct stomas are present, one is the proximal or functional stoma and the other is the distal or nonfunctioning stoma.

Duodenostomy: Surgical formation of an opening through the abdominal wall to the duodenum.

Hartman's pouch: Refers to oversewing of the free end of the distal colon, which is left in the peritoneal cavity when a proximal end stoma is made.

Ileostomy: Surgical formation of an opening into the ileum.

Jejunostomy: Surgical formation of an opening through the abdominal wall to the jejunum.

Loop ostomy: One stoma with two openings; effluent drains from the proximal stoma.

Mucous fistula: The distal nonfunctioning stoma.

Ostomy: An opening into; ostomy is often used interchangeably with stoma, such as colostomy or ileostomy.

Peristomal: The area that surrounds the stoma.

Permanent ostomy: Permanent ostomy implies the stoma will not be closed.

Proximal end: The end of the intestine that is closest to the mouth, functional stoma that produces effluent.

Stoma: Mouth or opening between two cavities.

Temporary ostomy: A temporary ostomy is created with the intention of closing it sometime in the future.

Ureterostomy: Surgical creation of an opening on the surface of the body for the ureters.

Urostomy: An ostomy for elimination of urine from the body.

Appliances for infants and children come in many shapes and sizes. There are one-piece or two-piece configurations, flexible or rigid, and precut or cut-to-fit choices. Ideally, an enterostomal therapy nurse or someone with experience selects an appropriate appliance for the pediatric ostomy patient. In general, if the stoma protrudes nicely away from the abdomen ½ inch or more and the peristomal surface is flat with a nice 1-inch border extending away from the stoma, any type of appliance performs well. If the stoma is flat or recessed below the skin level, an appliance that has a convex surface that adheres to the skin may be necessary to encourage the effluent to flow into the pouch rather than underneath the pouch. If the patient has a peristomal hernia, it may be necessary to experiment with both flexible and rigid types of appliances to see which one performs best for the patient.

Most appliances come with a pectin barrier that adheres to the skin immediately around the stoma. The pectin barrier should extend at least ½ to 1 inch past the stoma opening on all sides to adhere effectively to the skin. This means if the stoma is the size of a pencil eraser (as in the neonate), the pectin portion of the appliance should be about the size of a half-dollar coin. This is not always possible, but it is a nice goal to achieve when possible.

A one-piece pouch has the barrier and the pouch connected as a single unit, whereas a two-piece appliance has a pouch as one piece and a barrier as the second piece. The two pieces are snapped together to form the appliance. The two-piece appliance allows removal of the bag for emptying or replacement without detaching the barrier from the skin. Teenagers in particular find this option appealing when using a closed-end pouch; they can remove the old bag and discard it and then apply the new one. In the hospital, it is strongly recommended to use clear pouches so that the stoma and the effluent are easily visible. Many parents prefer to use clear pouches at home too, so that they can continue to easily visualize the stoma and effluent.

The pectin barrier should be thick enough so that caustic ileostomy or high colostomy effluent does not dissolve the barrier and cause skin breakdown to the immediate peristomal skin. Some of the appliances for infants and neonates come with very thin barriers. The infant with a high ileostomy has effluent that is very caustic and can dissolve the ultrathin barriers in a few hours. This means the pouch must be changed several times a day to prevent peristomal breakdown. A thicker barrier is indicated in this situation. The goal is to get an appliance to stay on for at least 24 hours without peristomal breakdown or leakage. If appliances are changed routinely several times a day, the epidermal skin stripping that occurs with each removal will cause the skin under the appliance to break down. In addition, several reimbursement agencies provide the patient with only one pouch per day at home.

Adhesive enhancers, such as pastes, cements, and spray adhesives, are available to enhance adhesion of the appliance to the skin. The more liquid in the effluent (in a gastrointestinal diversion) the more likely the need for a paste product. One must be cautious, however, when using cements and other adhesive enhancers in the neonate with fragile skin because the bond created between the skin and the ostomy pouch may be greater than the bond between the skin layers (Garvin, 1990a). This combination can result in skin stripping when removing the appliance.

OSTOMY COMPLICATIONS

Many factors are related to ostomy complications. Most patients will have at least one ostomy-related complication during the time that they have an ostomy. It is not uncommon for patients to have more than one complication (Del Pino, Cintron, Osray, Pearl, & Abcarian, 1997). In addition to stomal complications, the patient with an ostomy is also at risk for abdominal adhesions. Adhesions can present with obstructive symptoms such as decreased effluent from the stoma, abdominal distention, pain, and vomiting. The patient with these symptoms needs to be evaluated immediately. The complications discussed here include peristomal denudation caused from effluent, allergy and fungus, stenosis, prolapse, retraction, and peristomal herniation.

Peristomal skin is at risk for impaired integrity or dermatitis because of potential repeated and prolonged contact with a caustic effluent. A common mistake in treating peristomal breakdown that is caused by this prolonged contact with effluent is to cut the hole in the barrier larger so that the barrier is not placed on the irritated skin (Figure 21–1). This is the opposite of what should be done. This irritated skin *must* be covered to heal. If paste is used as an adhesive enhancer, place it on the pectin barrier and let it air dry for a few minutes before applying to the infant. This method allows the alcohol in the paste to dry so it does not sting when placed on the irritated skin.

Contact dermatitis of the peristomal skin is also caused by cleaning products, solvents, cements, and ostomy supplies. All these substances and their components may sensitize the skin and give rise to a form of contact dermatitis that will, at least in the initial stages, reproduce the size and shape of the actual contact. The symptoms are classic: the dermatitis is preceded and accompanied by itching, a bright red erythema appears that may be flat or stand out because of edema, and then vesiculation and serum secretion follow (Franchini, Cola, & d'E Stevens, 1983). The symptoms persist as long as the contact lasts. It is important to take a very thorough history for allergens, and patients should be patch tested with adhesives and cements before use.

Peristomal *Candida albicans* is a commonly occurring dermatitis in the peristomal area. This infection is found around the stoma and sometimes extends into the groin (Figure 21–2). *Candida albicans,* a fungus, establishes itself and multiplies on moist covered skin causing a red shiny macular papular rash that is pruritic (Franchini et al., 1983; Hampton, 1992). An antifungal powder is used to treat this area (Garvin, 1990a). Antifungal medication is most effectively used when applied in powder form (Zuidema, 1991). The powder should be mixed with a small amount of water and the mixture painted on the skin with a cotton swab and allowed to dry before an appliance is applied (Garvin, 1994).

Stomal stenosis, a narrowing and loss of elasticity of the stoma, presents with obstructive symptoms such as increased water content of the effluent, vomiting, cramps, and hypovolemia (Franchini et al., 1983). The stenosis may or may not be visible to the eye. A digital examination of the stoma

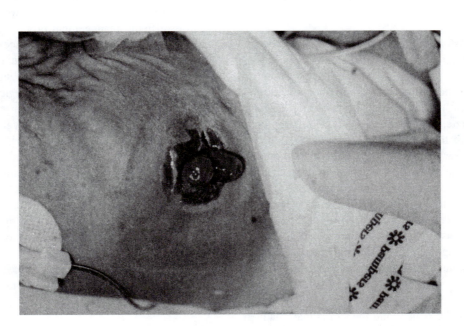

Figure 21–1 Double Barrel Stomas That Are Prolapsed. Note the peristomal denudation from caustic ileostomy output. In this case the hole in the bag was cut larger than the original area of peristomal breakdown, causing the breakdown to increase in size. The correct approach to correction of peristomal breakdown caused by effluent contact with the skin is to cover the area of breakdown with the pectin barrier to protect the skin and allow it to heal.

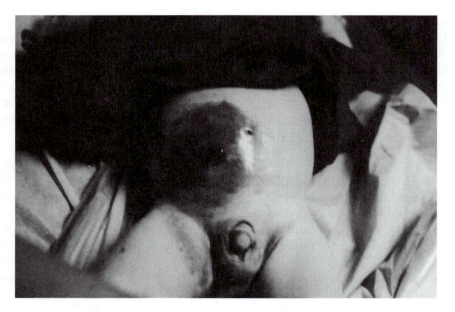

Figure 21–2 Peristomal Denudation Caused by *Candida albicans*. Note the concurrent *Candida* rash in the groin. Examining the pattern of the peristomal skin breakdown helps determine the cause. At first glance this breakdown has many similar characteristics to a contact dermatitis. The rash around the stoma is the same size as the ostomy faceplate. It is possible for a patient to be allergic to the material in the ostomy barrier. Careful examination of this patient's perineum reveals the same type rash in the groin, reducing the suspicion that the rash around the stoma is a contact dermatitis. Note also that the pattern of this rash is different than the skin breakdown in Figure 21–1, which was caused by caustic effluent.

may be diagnostic. In smaller stomas the passage of a catheter or a contrast study may be necessary. Stoma stenosis that significantly obstructs effluent passage requires surgical correction.

A stoma that has prolapsed protrudes away from the skin more than it did when first created. A stoma can prolapse a small amount or several inches. All stomas have the potential to prolapse, but the phenomenon is more frequent in the colostomy, especially those of the double barrel or loop type. Colostomies constructed for obstructive disease of the colon prolapse more easily than others, with a ratio of 5:1 (Franchini et al., 1983). Prolapse alone is not an indication for immediate surgical intervention. From a clinical point of view, the main problems that are associated with stoma prolapse relate to stoma hygiene and containment of the fecal matter (Hampton, 1992). If, however, circulatory compromise of the stoma or obstructive symptoms are present, immediate surgical evaluation is indicated (Figure 21–3). Some patients live with benign prolapsed stomas for years without problems. Caution should be exercised when choosing an appliance for a patient with a prolapsed stoma. It can be difficult getting the entire prolapsed stoma in the pouch, and the stoma may inadvertently be cut (Figure 21–4). A flexible appliance should strongly be considered to avoid trauma to the stoma and to prevent inadvertent strangulation and obstruction of the bowel (Franchini et al., 1983; Hampton, 1992).

Retraction of the stoma occurs when the stoma recedes below the skin level. This is often the result of excessive tension (Franchini et al., 1983; Hampton, 1992). Retraction causes effluent management problems because the effluent leaks under the appliance. One successful pouching technique in this situation is to use a convex rigid faceplate with an adhesive enhancer and a belt to stabilize and secure the pouch to the skin. No immediate surgical intervention is necessary for stoma retraction unless partial or complete detachment of the stoma from the skin layer occurs. If the detachment reaches the fascial layer, the risk of peritonitis is great and immediate surgical intervention is necessary.

Peristomal herniation is the protrusion of colon or ileum into the subcutaneous layers of skin surrounding the stoma. Conditions such as obesity, constipation, and coughing, which tend to produce an increase in intraabdominal pressure, contribute to the formation of a peristomal hernia (Franchini et al., 1983). The presence of a hernia causes problems with pouch adherence but is not considered a surgical emergency unless obstruction or strangulation of the bowel occurs (Franchini et al., 1983; Hampton, 1992).

DIETARY RESTRICTIONS

An infant with an ostomy can be on a regular infant formula unless the infant also has short gut syndrome because

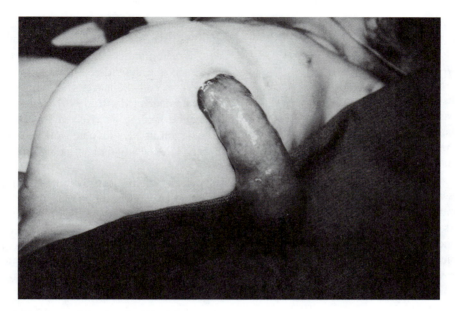

Figure 21–3 Prolapsed Stoma Requiring Surgical Revision

of significant intestinal resection. Dietary restrictions then are reflective of short gut considerations. The parents of infants with short gut syndrome should be taught to measure effluent daily and should be instructed carefully on the signs and symptoms of dehydration. Many clinicians use as a guideline for dehydration effluent that exceeds 20 to 40 ml/ kg/day. Infants, especially those with ileostomies, dehydrate

quickly and intervention must be prompt (Schwarz, Ternberg, Bell, & Keating, 1983). Children with ileostomies are also at risk for dehydration and should be taught to recognize and treat symptoms of dehydration. The child with a urinary diversion to an intestinal segment is at risk for electrolyte imbalance as well (Broadwell & Jackson, 1982). Encourage children with ileostomies who eat table food to

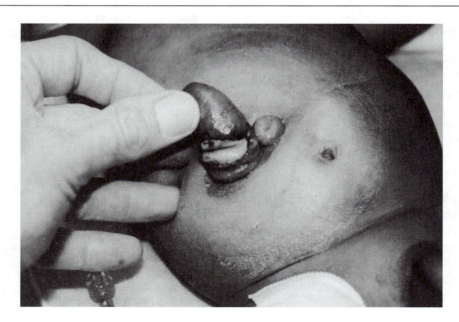

Figure 21–4 Prolapsed Stoma with a Cut in the Mucosa Caused from the Improper Application of the Pouch. The prolapsed stoma is difficult to pouch; care should be taken to include the entire prolapse in the pouch. A flexible rather than a rigid faceplate should be used because the rigid faceplate can cause strangulation of the bowel.

chew their food well to avoid mechanical stomal obstructions.

DISCHARGE TEACHING

A comprehensive discharge teaching plan, a discharge teaching checklist for parents of children with ostomies, and a stoma care plan are helpful when teaching families about ostomy care (see Appendixes 21–B, 21–C, and 21–D). Teaching efforts are directed toward the caregivers for children 6 years and younger. As the child reaches school age, manual dexterity necessary for ostomy care is developing, and the child can be more actively included in the task of changing the pouch. As the child reaches adolescence and the need for independence becomes strong, teaching efforts are focused on the adolescent while also including the parents so that they can provide support to their child.

Nurses involved in teaching pediatric patients ostomy care require a sound working knowledge of normal ostomy care activities and problems that may occur with the ostomy. If well informed, the parent can manage complications successfully as they arise. Most children have at least one complication with their ostomy during the time they have their diversion. Education and support facilitate the best adapting responses for the family.

CARE OF THE PEDIATRIC SURGICAL PATIENT WITH A WOUND

To properly care for the pediatric patient with a surgical wound, it is necessary to have an understanding of the wound-healing process to ensure that the wound care techniques chosen for a specific wound enhance its ability to heal rather than delay healing. It is also important to approach the child in a developmentally appropriate manner to facilitate carrying out wound care procedures. Pain management strategies need to encompass both pharmacologic and nonpharmacologic techniques. Age-appropriate distraction is an important component of nonpharmacologic management.

Closed Surgical Wounds

In a child, the process of wound healing follows the same pathway as it does in adults but at a faster rate (Bale & Jones, 1996). The wound healing process consists of three phases during which the injured tissue is repaired, specialized tissue is regenerated, and new tissue is organized into scar (Martin, 1996). These three major phases are (1) an inflammatory phase (0 to 3 days), (2) a cellular proliferation phase (3 to 12 days), and (3) a remodeling phase (3 days to 6 months) (Jamieson, 1989).

During the beginning of the inflammatory phase, inflammatory cells, predominately neutrophils, enter the wound site followed by lymphocytes, monocytes, and later macrophages (Jamieson, 1989; Jamoff & Carp, 1982). The proliferative phase consists of laying down of new connective tissue, termed granulation tissue, and formation of new blood vessels in the injured area. During the proliferative phase, fibroblasts, endothelial cells, and epithelial cells migrate into the wound area (Martin, 1996). Remodeling, the final phase of wound healing, is affected by both the replacement of granulation tissue with a network of collagen and elastin fibers and the devascularization of granulation tissue (Martin, 1996).

A clean incision heals by primary union after the opposing sides are approximated layer by layer. A sterile dressing is generally applied in the operating room. The epithelial cells migrate from the margins of the incision and regenerate underneath the skin surface to make a continuous layer within 24 to 48 hours (Makelbust, 1996). Frequently the wound is uncovered at this time and left uncovered. By the third postoperative day connective tissue begins to form inside the wound to unite the edges. Granulation tissue develops as macrophages stimulate fibroblasts and vascular endothelial cells to proliferate (Martin, 1996). By the fifth day collagen fibrils are present and capillary channels make this tissue very vascular (Barron, 1983; Norris, Provo, & Stotls, 1990). Fibroblasts continue to grow for 2 to 4 weeks, producing collagen needed to strengthen the wound (Makelbust, 1996).

Open Surgical Wounds

A surgical wound may be open for a variety of reasons. The wound may have been left open to allow visualization. The wound may be contaminated and left open to facilitate cleansing and draining. The wound may have split open or dehisced. Dehiscence can happen at any time but is most common between the 4th and 12th postoperative days (Makelbust, 1996). Often it is preceded by coughing, suctioning, sneezing, or vomiting. Patients who have sutures or staples removed before discharge frequently have adhesive skin tapes placed over the incision line to secure it. Patients should be instructed to leave them in place until they fall off.

Iatrogenic Wounds

Pressure-related wounds require intervention that includes wound care and in some cases surgical intervention. The preferred strategy is identifying the patient at risk and instituting preventive measures. Exhibit 21–2 offers an assessment tool for assessing the pediatric patient at risk and offers suggested interventions for prevention and treatment.

Wound Cleansing

Open surgical wounds need dressing changes and may require cleansing. Refer to Exhibit 21–3 for a dressing change flowchart for surgical wounds. Many practitioners think it is

Exhibit 21–2 Protocol for Assessing Pediatric Patients at Risk for Pressure-Related Breakdown

Day of admission and PRN assess patient for risk of pressure-related breakdown and begin the appropriate level of intervention. For patients receiving Level Two or Level Three interventions, reevaluate Monday, Wednesday, and Friday, or sooner if there is a change in the patient's clinical status.

The following is a scale for predicting pressure sore risk in the pediatric patient. Under each of the four assessment categories choose the number that most closely describes the patient's clinical condition. Add the four numbers together to obtain a total score for the patient. Compare the patient's score to the recommended intervention categories to determine the type of pressure relieving surface the patient should be placed on. (Note: patients who have preexisting pressure-related breakdown should be considered for a Level Three intervention.)

INTERVENTION CATEGORIES

I.   *Level One:* Pressure reduction products, i.e., Spenco Pad, sheepskin pad, etc.
II. *Level Two:* Mattress overlay of 4″ foam, or Hill Rom Critical care bed.
III. *Level Three:* The preferred choice is the RIK fluid mattress (rental fee = $30/day), or a water mattress. A low air-loss mattress (i.e., air beds) are used in some cases; however, some children have developed pressure breakdown *while on* these beds. (Rental fees for air-loss beds are $48–$150/day.) All items MUST BE ORDERED from the Central Processing Department.

Patient risk score/intervention category
4–5   None
6–7   Level I
8–12   Level II   8–14 patients in the Rehab Unit
13–16   Level III

PATIENT ASSESSMENT TOOL FOR ASSESSING PATIENTS AT RISK FOR DEVELOPMENT OF PRESSURE-RELATED BREAKDOWN

A. **Mobility** (ability to control and change position).
1. *No limitations:* Age-appropriate activity: makes major and frequent changes in position without assistance.
2. *Slightly limited:* Makes frequent minor changes in position without assistance, spends majority of day in bed or chair.
3. *Very limited:* Makes occasional slight changes in body or extremity position but unable to make frequent or significant changes independently. Ability to walk severely limited or nonexistent. Cannot bear own weight or must be assisted into chair or wheelchair.
4. *Completely immobile:* Does not make any changes in body position without assistance, confined to bed.

B. **Sensory Perception** (the ability to respond meaningfully to pressure-related discomfort).
1. *No impairment:* Has no sensory deficit which would limit ability to feel or demonstrate pain or discomfort.
2. *Slightly impaired:* Has some sensory impairment which limits the ability to feel pain or discomfort in 1 or 2 extremities.
3. *Very limited:* Has a sensory impairment which limits the ability to feel pain or discomfort over 1/2 the body.
4. *Completely limited:* Unresponsive to painful stimuli due to diminished level of consciousness or sedation, limited ability to feel pain or discomfort over most of the body.

C. **Nutrition** (nutrition to meet growth needs) p.o., tube feeds, or hyperalimentation.
1. *Excellent:* Nutrition intake meets 100% of growth needs.
2. *Adequate:* Nutrition that meets 75% of growth needs.
3. *Probably inadequate:* Receives less than optimum amount of nutrition for an extended period of time, i.e., 3 days in a malnourished patient and possibly up to 7 days for a previously healthy child.
4. *Very poor:* NPO or maintained on clear liquids or IV fluids for more than 5 days.

D. **Moisture** (degree to which skin is exposed to moisture).
1. *Rarely moist:* Skin is usually dry.
2. *Occasionally moist:* Skin occasionally moist, routine diaper changes q 2–4h.
3. *Moist:* Skin is often but not always moist.
4. *Constantly moist:* Skin is kept moist almost constantly by perspiration, urine, medicine, etc. Dampness is detected every time the patient is moved or turned.

Note: IV, intravenous; NPO, nothing by mouth.

Exhibit 21–3 Pediatric Surgical Wound Flowchart

Surgical Wound Assessment

Intact closed incision ⟹ No ⟹	**Open incision**
⇓	⇓
yes	
⇓	Assess and document drainage color, amount, size, and depth of the wound and surrounding skin with each dressing change.
⇓	
⇓	⇓
May uncover after 24–48 hr after surgery and leave open to air.	Obtain order for dressing changes and cleansing. (Preferably with normal saline using a 30-ml syringe and a 19-gauge catheter, the irrigant should be at body temperature or slightly warmer.)
⇓	

Normal cleansing	⇓
⇓	**Deep wound** **Shallow wound**

Observe for signs and symptoms of infection (erythema, pain, swelling, heat) or drainage.

⇓

Yes

⇓

Notify MD of change.

Deep wound	**Shallow wound**
⇓	⇓
Loosely pack with moist saline gauze, protect surrounding skin from maceration, if draining heavily protect with petroleum ointment or a hydrocolloid barrier such as _____.[a] Cover with a moisture-retentive dressing.[b] If frequent dressing changes, consider using Montgomery straps with a hydrocolloid barrier underneath the straps.	Cover with moisture-retentive dressing such as _____.[a] ⇓ Continue dressing changes until the wound closes.

[a] Note blanks may be filled in with dressing choice of a specific institution.
[b] Moisture-retentive dressings allow the wound to remain moist between changes.

---

necessary to use antiseptic solutions in wounds; however, the use of antimicrobials on open wounds is highly controversial, and the results of several studies report adverse effects (Cooper, Layer, & Hansbrough, 1991; Lineweaver et al., 1985; McCauley et al., 1989). The current recommendation is to avoid the use of antiseptics in wounds (Bergstrom et al., 1994; Boynton & Paustian, 1996; Brown & Zitelli, 1995; Doughty, 1994; Garvin, 1997; Makelbust, 1996). The recommendation is that only physiologic agents such as saline be used to cleanse wounds so that tissue defenses are not suppressed by toxic agents (Makelbust, 1996). Normal saline irrigations have been shown to be effective in reducing the bacteria count in wounds (Badia, Torres, Tur, & Sitges-Serra, 1996; Chisholm, Cordell, Rogers, & Woods, 1992; Lawrence, 1997; McDonald & Nichter, 1994; Morse, Babson, Camacco, Bush, & Blythe, 1998). Irrigation pressures of between 4 and 15 psi are considered ideal for cleansing wounds (Bergstrom et al., 1994; Garvin, 1997; Lineweaver et al., 1985; McCauley et al., 1989; Morse et al., 1998). A 35-ml syringe with an 18-gauge blunt needle or Angiocath provides 8.0 psi (Bergstrom et al., 1994). It is further recommended that the temperature of the irrigation fluid be as close to body temperature as possible because it has been noted that it takes 40 minutes for wounds to return to normal temperature after cleansing (Fletcher, 1997). This can be accomplished easily at the bedside in much the same way that one would warm formula. The desired amount of irrigation fluid is placed in a larger cup or bowl and warm water from the sink is run over the fluid until it reaches the proper temperature. Some nurses test a drop or two on the inside of their wrist just as they would formula to make certain the temperature is comfortable to the touch.

The Wound Dressing

For an open wound, a dressing should be chosen that allows the wound bed to remain moist. Studies investigating the mechanisms of reepithelialization have shown that a moist rather than a dry environment provides the optimum condition for healing (Winter & Scales, 1963). Reepithelialization occurs faster in the moist wound bed compared with that of a dry wound bed. The role of humidity has been shown to be of prime importance in affecting both the rate of epithelialization and the amount of scar formation (Field & Kerstein, 1994). Moisture-retentive dressings prevent wound desiccation and promote granulation tissue (Alverez, Mertz, & Eaglstein, 1983). Examples of dressing choices are given in Table 21–1.

Table 21–1 Dressing Options

Dressing Category	Description	Example	Indication	Comments
Gauze dressings	Made of cotton or synthetic fabric that is absorptive and permeable to water, gas, or vapor	Kerlix 2 x 2, 4 x 4, and so forth (Kendall)	As a covering over surgical wounds Nonselective debridement To keep a wound bed that needs frequent inspection moist	Can be used dry Can be used wet-to-dry Can be used moist
Polyurethane film	Transparent adhesive dressing. Allows free flow of oxygen through the pores, impermeable to bacteria	Op-Site (Smith-Nephew) Tegaderm (3M)	To secure and protect intravenous catheter sites On skin that is at risk for abrasion as a prevention dressing Superficial wounds such as blisters	Lacks absorptive capabilities
Hydrocolloids	Water-based nonadherent, polymer-based dressing with some absorptive properties	Duoderm (ConvaTec) Restore (Hollister) Replicare (Smith-Nephew)	Can be used around heavily draining wounds as a skin protector to preserve intact skin Stage I–III pressure sores Some IV infiltrates	Easy to apply Waterproof Dressing must extend 1.5–2 inches past wound to obtain adequate adherence Interacts with wound fluid to form a gel that some misinterpret as infection Do not use around tracheostomy stomas; gel may travel down the tracheostomy tract
Hydrogel	Polyethylene oxide wafers containing 95% water that are sandwiched between two polyethylene films	Vigilon (Bard) Geliperm (Fougera)	Use on dermabrasion-type wounds to enhance reepithelialization	Mild absorption properties Nonadherent so requires a secondary dressing to hold it in place May be used in conjunction with topical antibiotics
Nonadhesive foam	Polyurethane foam	Biopatch (antimicrobial; Johnson & Johnson) Lyofoam (Acme United)	Ideal for use around tracheostomy sites to prevent trauma and absorb moisture	Mild absorption May be used in conjunction with topical antibiotics Needs a secondary dressing to hold it in place
Calcium alginate	Made from a naturally occurring polysaccharide found in brown seaweed; the principal constituent is alginic acid converted to mixed calcium and sodium salts	Kaltostat (Calgon Vestal) Sorbsan (Dow-Hickam)	Heavily exudating wounds	Highly absorptive; will absorb 20 times its weight in exudate Requires a secondary dressing Not appropriate for use in abdominal wounds with large areas of exposed intestinal mucosa because of the potential for systemic absorption of calcium/sodium

Nutrition and Wound Healing

Refer to Chapter 4 for a discussion of nutrition and the surgical patient. Nutritional factors that have been impli-

cated in wound healing include vitamin C, vitamin A, vitamin E, zinc, protein, and individual amino acids (Garvin, 1990b; Mazzotta, 1994; Meyer, Muller, & Herndon, 1994; Thomas, 1997). Some studies have shown positive wound healing effects by supplementation with antioxidants (La-Londe, Nayak, Hennigan, & Demling, 1996; Martin, 1996). In addition, the nutrients arginine, glutamine, and omega-3 fatty acids have been shown to exert a pharmacologic effect that helps to suppress the inflammatory response and enhance the immune response (Bagley, 1996). The effect is positively correlated with reduced incidence of infection and wound complications and subsequent reduction in length of hospital stay (Bagley, 1996).

CURRENT AND POTENTIAL RESEARCH

Wound healing is an area of burgeoning research. Limited studies in burn patients have shown improved wound healing and shortened length of stay with growth hormone therapy (Herndon, Pierre, Stokes, & Barrow, 1996; Martin, 1996; Mayer, Muller, & Herndon, 1996; Ziegler & Leader, 1994). In a study from Spain of 180 patients, improved immune function and resistance to disease were observed with pituitary-derived growth hormone therapy in stable patients after cholecystectomy (Vara-Thorbeck, Guerrero, Rosell, Ruiz-Reguena, & Capitan, 1993). Blinded controlled studies of growth hormone therapy in well-defined patient groups at risk for infection and poor wound healing are indicated to determine whether growth hormone therapy improves immune cell function or reduces the incidence or severity of infection in catabolic patients (Ziegler, 1994; Ziegler & Leader, 1994).

Growth factors have many activities that make them attractive agents for stimulating tissue repair. Growth factors attract cells into the wound, stimulate their proliferation, and have a profound influence on extracellular matrix deposition (Greenhalgh, 1996). Although growth factors have not been the panacea that was originally expected, they have the potential for making significant clinical improvements when targeted for specific problem wounds (Greenhalgh, 1996; Lin & Adzick, 1996; Slavin, 1996).

Cyanoacrylate tissue adhesives such as Histoacryl Blue (Trahacok International, Montreal, Canada) and Dermabond (Ethicon, Somerville, NJ) appear to be an ideal technique for laceration closure in children because they are easy and rapid to apply, are relatively painless, eliminate the need for suture removal, and provide an acceptable cosmetic result (Ameil, Sukhotnik, Kawar, & Siplovich, 1999; King & Kinney, 1999; Liebelt, 1997; Quinn et al., 1997; Saxena & Willital, 1999; Toriumi, O'Grady, Desai, & Bagal, 1998).

Hypothermia can lead to increased risk of infection. Mild hypothermia ($35°$ C or $95°$ F) is common during major surgical procedures because of impairment of thermoregulation by anesthesia (Ovington, 1998). The mechanism for infection involves tissue oxygen levels. Hypothermia causes vasoconstriction and increases hemoglobin's affinity for oxygen, making it less available to tissues and cells. Reduced oxygen availability leads in turn to impaired bactericidal activity by neutrophils (Ovington, 1998). Studies of neutrophils have shown that reduced temperatures decrease both their phagocytic activity and their production of reactive oxygen species (Akriotis & Biggar, 1985; Wenisch et al., 1996). A study of 200 surgery patients demonstrated that 19% of those who experienced hypothermia developed an infection, whereas only 6% of those who received extra warming to maintain normothermia developend an infection (Kurz, Sessler, & Lenhardt, 1996). Future research is necessary to see whether supplying local heat to wounds will optimize wound healing in surgical patients. At present, a wound-warming device is on the market, and studies are being conducted on patients with pressure ulcers (Ovington, 1998).

CONCLUSION

The pediatric patient with wound care benefits from interventions that are developmentally appropriate. Pain management includes both pharmacologic and nonpharmacologic components. Wound care strategies should use moist wound healing techniques. The use of topical antiseptics should be avoided in wounds while the use of physiologic agents such as saline to cleanse wounds is maximized. An optimal nutritional status is positively correlated with reduced incidence of infection and wound complications and subsequent reduction in length of hospital stay.

REFERENCES

Akriotis, V., & Biggar, W.D. (1985). The effects of hypothermia on neutrophil function in vitro. *Journal of Leukocyte Biology, 371,* 51–61.

Alverez, O.M., Mertz, P.M., & Eaglestein, W.H. (1983). The effect of occlusive dressings on collagen synthesis and reepithelialization of superficial wounds. *Journal of Surgical Research, 35,* 142–148.

Ameil, G.E., Sukhotnik, I., Kawar, B., & Siplovich, L. (1999). Use of N-butyl-2-cyanoacrylate in elective surgical incisions: Long-term outcomes. *Journal of the American College of Surgeons, 89*(1), 21–25.

Badia, J.M., Torres, J.M., Tur, C., & Sitges-Serra, A. (1996). Saline wound

irrigation reduces post operative infection rate in guinea pigs. *Journal of Surgical Research, 63*(2), 457–459.

Bagley, S.M. (1996). Nutritional needs of the acutely ill with acute wounds. *Critical Care Nursing Clinics of North America, 8*(2), 159–167.

Bale, S., & Jones, V. (1996). Caring for children with wounds. *Journal of Wound Care, 5*(4), 177–180.

Barron, M.C. (1983, July). The skin and wound healing. *Topics in Clinical Nursing,* 11–21.

Bergstrom, N., Bennett, M.A., Carlson, C.E., et al. (1994). *Pressure ulcer treatment: Clinical practice guidelines. Quick reference for clinicians. No. 15.* (Public Health Service Agency for Health Care Policy and Research [AHCPR] Publication No. 95–0653). Rockville, MD: US Department of Health and Human Services.

Boynton, P.R., & Paustian, C. (1996). Wound assessment and decision options. *Critical Care Nursing Clinics of North America, 8*(2), 125–139.

Broadwell, D.C., & Jackson, B.S. (1982). *Principles of ostomy care.* St. Louis, MO: Mosby.

Brown, C.D., & Zitelli, J.A. (1995). Choice of wound dressings and ointments. *Otolaryngology Clinics of North America 28*(5), 1081–1090.

Chisholm, C.D., Cordell, W.H., Rogers, K., & Woods, J.R. (1992). Comparison of a new pressurized saline canister versus syringe irrigation for laceration cleansing in the emergency department. *Annals of Emergency Medicine, 21,* 1364–1367.

Cooper, M., Layer, J., & Hansbrough, J. (1991). The cytotoxic effects of commonly used topical antimicrobial agents on human fibroblasts and keratinocytes. *Journal of Trauma, 31,* 775–784.

Del Pino, A., Cintron, J.R., Osray, C.P., Pearl, R.K., & Abcarian, H. (1997). Enterostomal complications: Are emergently created enterostomies at greater risk? *American Surgeon, 63*(7), 653–656.

Doughty, D. (1994). A rational approach to the use of topical antiseptics. *Wound Care, 21*(6), 224–231.

Field, C.K., & Kerstein, M.D. (1994). Overview of wound healing in a moist environment. *American Journal of Surgery, 167* (Suppl.), 25–65.

Fletcher, J. (1997). Wound cleansing. *Professional Nurse, 12*(11), 793–796.

Franchini, A., Cola B., & d'E Stevens, P.J. (1983). *Atlas of stomal pathology.* New York: Raven Press.

Garvin, G. (1990a). Skin care considerations in the neonate for the ET nurse. *Journal of Enterostomal Therapy, 17,* 225–230.

Garvin, G. (1990b). Wound healing in pediatrics. *Nursing Clinics of North America, 25*(1), 181–192.

Garvin, G. (1994). Caring for children with ostomies. *Nursing Clinics of North America, 29*(4), 645–654.

Garvin, G. (1997). Wound and skin care for the PICU. *Critical Care Nursing Quarterly, 20*(1), 62–71.

Greenhalgh, D.G. (1996). The role of growth factors in wound healing. *Journal of Trauma, 41*(1), 159–167.

Hampton, B. (1992). Peristomal and stomal complications. In B. Hampton & R. Bryant (Eds.), *Ostomies and continent diversions* (pp. 105–128). St. Louis, MO: Mosby.

Herndon, D.N., Pierre, E.J., Stokes, K.N., & Barrow, R.E. (1996). Growth hormone treatment for burned children. *Hormone Research, 45* (Suppl.) 29–31.

Jamieson, D. (1989). Oxygen toxicity and reactive oxygen metabolites in mammals. *Free Radical Biology and Medicine 7,* 87–108.

Jamoff, A., & Carp, H. (1982). Protease, antiprotease and antioxidants pathways of tissue injury during inflammation. In R.S. Cotvan, N. Kaufman, & G. Majno (Eds.), *Current topics in inflammation and infection.* Baltimore: Williams & Wilkins.

King, M.E., & Kinney, A.Y. (1999). Tissue adhesives: A new method of wound repair. *Nurse Practitioner, 24*(10), 66, 69–70, 73–74.

Kurz, A., Sessler, D.I., & Lenhardt, R. (1996). Perioperative normothermia to reduce the incidence of surgical wound infection and shorten hospitalization. *New England Journal of Medicine, 334,* 1209–1215.

LaLonde, C., Nayak, U., Hennigan, J., & Demling, R. (1996). Antioxidants prevent the cellular deficit produced in response to injury. *Journal of Burn Care and Rehabilitation, 17,* 379–383.

Lawrence, J.C. (1997). Wound irrigation. *Journal of Wound Care, 6*(1), 23–26.

Liebelt, E. (1997). Current concepts in laceration repair. *Current Opinion in Pediatrics, 9,* 459–464.

Lin, R.Y., & Adzick, N.S. (1996). The role of the fetal fibroblast and transforming growth factor: Beta in a model of human fetal wound repair. *Seminars in Pediatric Surgery, 5*(3), 165–74.

Lineweaver, W., MeMorris, S., Saucy, D., et al. (1985). Cellular and bacteriological toxicities of topical antimicrobials. *Plastic and Reconstructive Surgery, 75,* 94–96.

Makelbust, J. (1996). Using wound care products to promote a healing environment. *Critical Care Nursing Clinics of North America, 8*(2), 141–158.

Martin, A. (1996). The use of antioxidants in healing. *Dermatologic Surgery, 22,* 156–160.

Mayer, N.A., Muller, M.J., & Herndon, D.N. (1996, Sept./Oct.). The utilization of nutrient substances during wound healing. *Anestheziologiia I Reanimatologiia, 5,* 29–39.

Mazzotta, M.Y. (1994). Nutrition and wound healing. *Journal of the American Podiatric Medical Association, 84*(9), 456–462.

McCauley, R.L., Linares, H.A., Pelligrini, B.S., Herndon, D.N., Robson, M.C., & Heggers, J.P. (1989). In vitro toxicity of topical antimicrobial agents to human fibroblasts. *Journal of Surgical Research, 46,* 267–274.

McDonald, W.S., & Nichter, L.S. (1994). Debridement of bacterial and particulate-contaminated wounds. *Annals of Plastic Surgery, 33,* 142–147.

Meyer, N.A., Muller, M.J., & Herndon, D.N. (1994). Nutrient support of the healing wound. *New Horizons, 2*(2), 202–214.

Morse, J.W., Babson, T., Camacco, C., Bush, A.C., & Blythe, P.A. (1998). Wound infection rate and irrigation pressure of two potential new wound irrigation devices: The port and the cap. *American Journal of Emergency Medicine, 16*(1), 37–42.

Norris, S.O., Provo, B., & Stotls, N.A. (1990). Physiology of wound healing and risk factors that impede the healing process. *AACN Clinical Issues, 1,* 545–552.

Ovington, L.G. (1998). Warming up the wound can expedite healing. *Wound Care, 3*(4), 41–42.

Quinn, J., Wells, G., Sutcliffe, T., Jarmuske, M., Maw, J., Stiell, I., & Johns, P. (1997). A randomized trial comparing octylcyanoacrylate tissue adhesive and sutures in the management of lacerations. *Journal of the American Medical Association 227,* 1527–1530.

Saxena, A.K., & Willital, C.H. (1999). Octylcyanoacrylate tissue adhesive in the repair of pedatric extremity lacerations. *American Surgeon, 65,* 470–472.

Schwarz, K.B., Ternberg, J.L., Bell, M.J., & Keating, J.P. (1983). Sodium needs of infants and children with ileostomy. *Journal of Pediatrics, 102,* 500–513.

Slavin, J. (1996). The role of cytokines in wound healing. *Journal of Pathology, 178,* 5–10.

Thomas, D.R. (1997). Specific nutritional factors in wound healing. *Advances in Wound Care, 10*(4), 40–43.

Toriumi, D.M., O'Grady, K., Desai, D., & Bagal, A. (1998). Use of octyl-2-cyanoacrylate for skin closure in facial plastic surgery. *Plastic and Reconstructive Surgery, 102,* 2209–2219.

Vara-Thorbeck, R., Guerrero, J.A., Rosell, J., Ruiz-Reguena, E., & Capitan, J.M. (1993). Exogenous growth hormone: Effects on the catabolic response to surgically produced acute stress and on post operative immune function. *World Journal of Surgery, 17,* 530–538.

Wenisch, C., Narzt, E., Seggler, D.I., Parschalk, B., Lenhardt, R., Kurz, A., & Graninger, W. (1996). Mild interoperative hypothermia reduces production of reactive oxygen intermediates by polymorphonuclear leukocytes. *Anesthesia and Analgesia, 82,* 810–816.

Winter, G.D., & Scales, J.T. (1963). Effect of air drying and dressings on the surface of a wound. *Nature, 197*, 91–92.

Ziegler, T.R. (1994). Growth hormone administration during nutritional support: What is to be gained. *New Horizons, 2*(2), 244–256.

Ziegler, T.R., & Leader, I. (1994). Adjunctive human growth hormone therapy in nutrition support: Potential to limit septic complications in intensive care unit patients. *Seminars in Respiratory Infection, 9*(4), 240–247.

Zuidema, G.D. (1991). *Shackelford's surgery of the alimentary tract.* Philadelphia: W.B. Saunders Company.

Appendix 21–A

Caremap for New Ostomy

Expected LOS = _____ days (average LOS is 3–7 days depending on the diagnosis; can be longer if the diagnosis is complicated as in NEC)

	Preop/day of surgery	POD #1	POD #2–discharge
Treatment	• Intravenous fluids @ 1½ mainte-nance • Nasogastric tube to LIWS if indicated • Stoma placement marking by ET if indicated and time allows	• NPO until bowel sounds return • Maintain IV @ maintenance for hydration • Maintain patency of NG tube • Incentive spirometry as appropri-ate • Ambulate as age appropriate	• D/C NG as bowel sounds return • Begin and advance feedings as bowel sounds return • Decrease IV rate as feedings increase • Resume normal nonstrenuous activity
Medications	• Give perioperative antibiotics as indicated, i.e., _____ (drug name) @ ___ mg/kg/day IV q__h • Pain medication per institution protocol, i.e., _____ (drug name) @ ___ mg/kg/day IV q__h PRN	• Postoperative antibiotics as ordered • Pain medication as ordered	• Antibiotics D/C'd • Pain meds reduced then discon-tinued
Assessment and Monitoring	• Weight QD • I & O • Vital signs with BP q4h preop, postop q1h x2 then q4h • Dressing dry and intact or ostomy pouch intact postop	• Vital signs q4h • Assess incision • Assess stoma for viability and character of the mucocutaneous border • Assess for pouch adherence and character of the peristomal skin • Assess for bowel sounds	• Vital signs q4–8h until discharge • I and O until discharge • Assess stoma for function • Assess pouch adherence • Assess and monitor incision
Consults	Anesthesia Enterostomal therapy nurse Social service as necessary Translator as needed Child life Nutrition Pain team		
Tests	• CBC • Other lab tests and x-ray films as indicated for the diagnosis that is requiring the ostomy		
Education	• Preop teaching as appropriate for infant/child development stage if not an emergency surgery	• Begin "Discharge Teaching Plan for Ostomy Care"	• Return demonstration of ostomy care as per the "Discharge Teaching Plan for Ostomy Care"

continues

Appendix 21–A continued

	Preop/day of surgery	*POD #1*	*POD #2–discharge*
Discharge Planning	• Give a copy of the "Discharge Teaching Plan for Ostomy Care" to family (see Appendix 21–B)	• Complete the "Stoma Care Plan" and place at bedside (see Appendix 21–D)	• Procure discharge ostomy supplies • Arrange for home care visits if indicated • Complete "Discharge Teaching Checklist for Ostomy Care" (see Appendix 21–C) • Arrange for follow-up appointments
Evaluation of Outcomes	• Vital signs: Yes ☐ No ☐ • Lab and x-ray tests ordered: Yes ☐ No ☐ • Lab and x-ray results received: Yes ☐ No ☐ • "Discharge Teaching Checklist for Ostomy Care" shared with family: Yes ☐ No ☐ • Pain managed: Yes ☐ No ☐	Verbal understanding of the "Discharge Teaching Checklist for Ostomy Care": Yes ☐ No ☐ • Pain managed: Yes ☐ No ☐ • Incision intact: Yes ☐ No ☐ • Ostomy pouch adhering well: Yes ☐ No ☐	• F/U appointments scheduled: Yes ☐ No ☐ • Antibiotics D/C'd: Yes ☐ No ☐ • Pain managed: Yes ☐ No ☐ • Stoma functioning: Yes ☐ No ☐ • Tolerating feeding: Yes ☐ No ☐ • Discharge supplies ordered: Yes ☐ No ☐ • Return demonstrations of ostomy care: Yes ☐ No ☐ • Home care arranged: Yes ☐ No ☐

Appendix 21–B

Discharge Teaching Plan for Ostomy Care

What is a stoma (ostomy)?

When any part of the intestine is removed because it is not working properly, two open ends remain and can be brought to the surface of the abdomen. Sometimes only one end is brought to the surface. The new opening that brings the end of the intestine to the surface of the abdomen is called a stoma. This opening is created during surgery. Stool will come out of this opening.

If the problem is passing urine through the normal path from the kidneys to the bladder then out of the body through the urethra, surgery may need to be done to direct the urine out of the body through another path. The new opening will be called a stoma.

What does the stoma look like?

The stoma will be round or oval shaped, red, moist, shiny, and will feel soft to the touch. Stomas in children vary in size, the smallest being the size of a pencil eraser and the largest being the size of an orange. The stoma may be raised up from the skin and many times will get smaller during the first 2 months after it is created.

Occasionally, the stoma may bleed a small amount when it is cleaned or when the pouch is being changed. This is normal and will stop. The child cannot feel you touch the stoma. It does not hurt to have urine or stool come out of the stoma.

What is put over the stoma to collect the stool or urine?

In most cases an ostomy bag made for the purpose of collecting a stool or urine will be placed over the stoma to collect the output. This bag is called a pouch or an appliance. Collecting the output in this way helps to protect the skin and allows accurate measuring of what comes out of the stoma each day. If it is important in your child's case to measure the output, you will be taught how to do this. For the specific steps and the supplies needed refer to Appendix 21–D.

When should the pouch be changed?

You will change your child's pouch a few times during the first few days after the operation. This is the time to practice and ask questions. You will become familiar with the normal appearance of the stoma and the skin around it.

For infants and small children expect to change the pouch every 1–4 days. It is important to have the pouch stay on for at least 24 hours to prevent breakdown of the skin that surrounds the stoma. Pouches that are changed several times a day may damage the skin surrounding the stoma. Another consideration for keeping a pouch in place for at least 24 hours without leaking is that many reimbursement sources only pay for one change per day. If the pouch remains in place without leaking for longer than a day (the average is 2–3 days) and the surrounding skin looks good, the changing frequency is good. If the skin surrounding the stoma is irritated from stool or urine leaking on it, you need to change the pouch more frequently. Be sure that you cover all the irritated skin with the barrier to protect it from further damage. The skin breakdown *must* be covered so that it can heal.

Many parents tell us that they like to change the pouch on some sort of a schedule rather than waiting for it to leak and fall off at an inconvenient time.

What other things should you know about the stoma?

- Your infant can bathe with the pouch on or off. Water will not hurt the stoma or be sucked into it.
- To prevent leakage the pouch must be placed on dry skin. The pouch should be emptied when one-third to one-half full.
- Some stomas create gas in the pouch. Opening the pouch and allowing the gas to escape frequently will allow the pouch to stay on longer.
- The infant/child can lie on the stoma; it will not hurt the infant/child or the stoma.
- Carry stoma supplies with you so that you can change the pouch if it should leak.

When should you call for help?

- If you notice an increased amount of output. For your child that is more than _____.
- Your child is unusually sleepy and is not making urine.
- Your child has a fever.

- The stoma changes in size or color.
- Bleeding from the stoma that does not stop.
- No stool comes out of the stoma for 24 hours.
- Crying that will not stop or makes you think that the child is in pain.
- Your child's abdomen becomes firm and bloated.
- Your child vomits green fluid.

Who should you call for help?

_____

_____

_____

_____

_____

Appendix 21–C

Discharge Teaching Checklist for Ostomy Care

Please document who was taught each element of ostomy care. It is preferable to have two return demonstrations for each task for each family.

The person providing instruction should sign at the bottom of the page and initial each instruction that was taught.

Application of pouch	Who was taught	Date	Who was taught	Date
Correctly identifies when to change pouch				
Correctly prepares the pouch for application				
Correctly removes the old pouch				
Correctly applies the new pouch				
Correctly empties the pouch				
Accurately measures and records the amount emptied from the pouch				

Skin care	Who was taught	Date	Who was taught	Date
Correctly cleanses the skin around the stoma				
Correctly verbalizes signs of skin problems around the stoma				
Correctly states how to correct skin problems around the stoma				
Correctly identifies who to contact for skin/stoma problems				

Potential problems	Who was taught	Date	Who was taught	Date
Correctly identifies when to contact M.D.				
Correctly names the M.D. and phone number to contact for problems				
Correctly articulates how to obtain ostomy supplies for use at home				

Signature and date of those providing instruction: _____

_____

Appendix 21–D

Stoma Care Plan

Date _____

Name _____

Reason for stoma _____

Anatomic location of the stoma _____

Drawing of the actual size of the stoma in the box below

Supplies used:

1. (pouch) _____

2. (barrier) _____

3. _____

4. _____

5. _____

Supplies ordered for home:

Date _____

Vendor name _____

Vendor phone number _____

Steps in changing pouch:

_____

_____

_____

_____

_____

_____

_____

_____

PART V

Nursing Care of Children with Acute Abdominal Problems

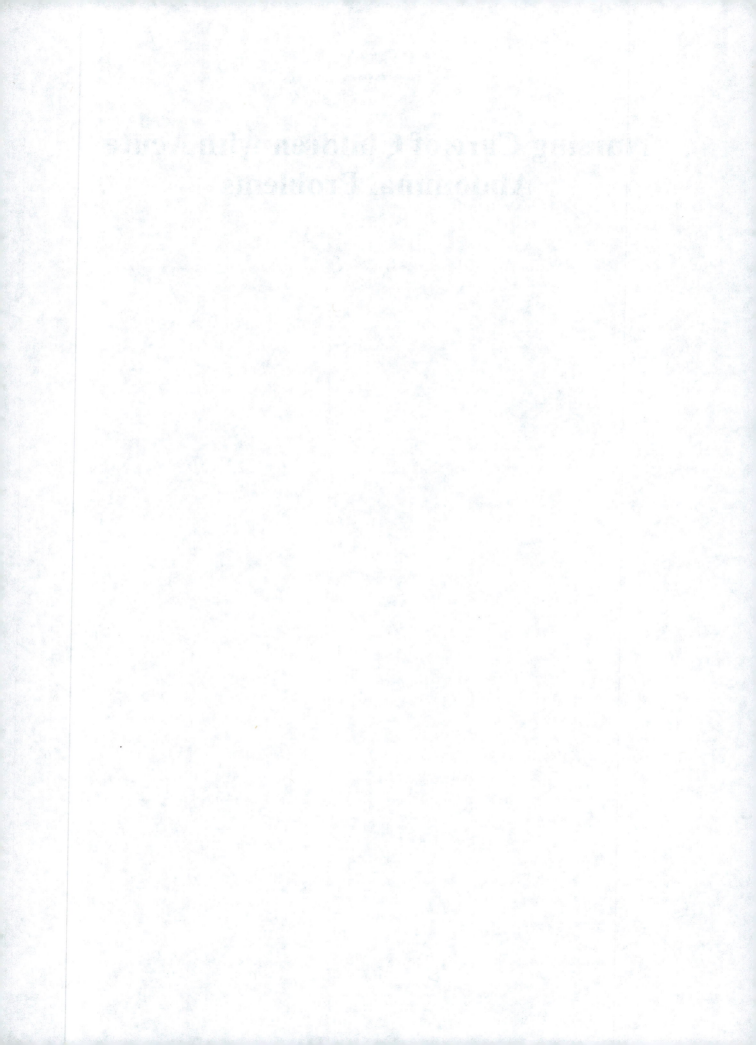

Common Outpatient Pediatric Surgical Procedures: Inguinal and Umbilical Hernias, Hydroceles, Undescended Testes, and Circumcision

Carmel A. McComiskey

INTRODUCTION

Pediatric surgical procedures are performed in a variety of settings: tertiary teaching facilities, children's hospitals, community hospitals, and free-standing surgicenters. Regardless of the site, all children and their families should be offered the same standard of care that is developmentally sensitive and family focused, ensures appropriate pediatric pain management strategies, and causes minimal inconvenience and/or morbidity.

Although most outpatient surgery is considered straightforward and relatively minor by care providers of all levels, parents do not consider any procedure performed on their child minor. For that reason, all children and their families deserve preoperative preparation and education. This results in decreased patient and caregiver anxiety, improved compliance, decreased readmissions, and few postoperative telephone calls. In addition, because the opportunity to provide teaching is limited, it is optimal to provide both perioperative instructions and postoperative educational material at the initial encounter. This chapter reviews the surgical management and nursing care of children undergoing repair of a hernia, hydrocele, undescended testicle, and circumcision.

Preoperative testing is generally not necessary in the pediatric age group, although a recent anesthesia practice survey (Patel, DeWitt, & Hannallah, 1997) reported that hemoglobin testing is still performed by 27% to 48% of the respondents, indicating that policies are slow to change. Many centers do not routinely perform laboratory investigations and have liberalized feeding regimens for both children and adults. Clear liquid diets up to 2 to 4 hours before the induction of anesthesia are usually allowed. Green, Pandit, and Schork (1996) reported that 69% of the anesthesiologists who responded to a preoperative fasting survey allowed a liberal clear liquid pediatric fasting policy without any anesthetic complications.

Minimal physical preparation is necessary beyond these usual anesthetic recommendations. Premedication should be offered to those children older than 6 months of age to decrease separation anxiety. Parent-accompanied anesthetic induction is also offered in some centers where anesthesiologists are comfortable with parental presence and the physical design of the operative area is suited for visitors.

INGUINAL HERNIAS IN CHILDREN

Description/Pathophysiology of the Hernias

A hernia is the protrusion of tissue through an abnormal opening. An indirect inguinal hernia (congenital) exists when the peritoneal contents enter the processus vaginalis through the internal ring and follow the spermatic cord in boys or the round ligament in girls (Figure 22–1). The contents are usually bowel but may include ovary or fallopian tube in girls (Borkowski, 1994; Hutson, Beasley, & Woodward, 1992). The contents emerge at the external ring and extend into the scrotum or the labia. Nearly all inguinal hernias in children are indirect (Hutson et al., 1992). These hernias arise lateral to the inferior epigastric vessels in contrast to a direct hernia, which is medial to these vessels and bulges through a weakened posterior wall of the inguinal canal. Direct inguinal hernias are rarely seen in children. The incidence is 1% of all pediatric hernias. They are seen occasion-

Acknowledgments: I gratefully acknowledge the help of Drs. Roger Voigt and J. Laurance Hill for their advice and review of this chapter.

NORMAL ANATOMY   INGUINAL HERNIA   COMPLETE HERNIA

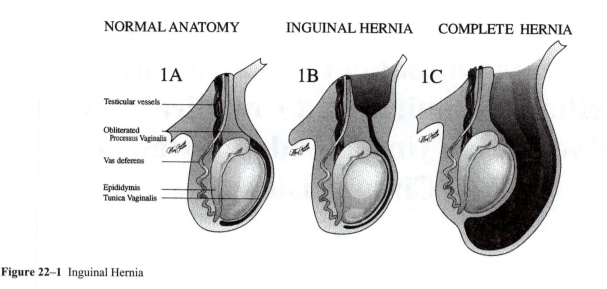

Figure 22–1 Inguinal Hernia

ally in infants with bronchopulmonary dysplasia and in children with cystic fibrosis as a result of prolonged ventilation (Hutson et al., 1992).

Incidence

Although few population-based studies have been done, the incidence of inguinal hernias in children is estimated to be between 10 and 20 per 1,000 live births. The ratio of males to females is 4:1. Approximately 55% to 70% of inguinal hernias are diagnosed on the right side, 30% on the left, and 10% bilaterally (Skinner & Grosfeld, 1993). The higher incidence of right-sided hernias is thought to be related to the later descent of the right testis and delayed closure of the processus vaginalis on the right side. The incidence of inguinal hernia is greater in premature infants. The incidence of hernia in premature infants weighing less than 1,500 g is reported to be as high as 30% (Gill, 1998; Skinner & Grosfeld, 1993). Other conditions that influence the incidence include a positive family history, an undescended testis, hypospadias, ascites, the presence of a ventriculoperitoneal shunt, and ventilatory support increasing intraabdominal pressure. Hernias are also more common in children with connective tissue disorders because of the fragility of the peritoneal tissues (Jones, 1988).

Clinical Presentation of Hernias in Children

Generally, the infant or child has a history of an obvious bulge at the internal or external ring or within the scrotum. The differential diagnosis in males includes hydrocele, retractile testis, undescended testis, varicocele, and testicular tumor. Often the hernia bulge is not present when the child visits the primary care provider and is often difficult to pro-

duce even when the child is crying or straining. Many practitioners attempt to palpate the hernia sac over the cord structures in the inguinal region. The sliding sensation of the sac and cord structures over the pubic bone is known as a positive "silk glove sign." This is a suggestive, but not diagnostic, finding. Occasionally, if the hernia cannot be demonstrated at the surgical office visit, an operation is still planned if the primary care physician has demonstrated the hernia and is a known reliable observer (Rowe, O'Neill, Grosfeld, Funkalsrud, & Coran, 1995).

Surgical Management

Elective surgical repair is recommended for all hernias, with surgery planned as soon as possible (Hutson et al., 1992). Repair of the inguinal hernia is necessary because of the danger of bowel strangulation and ischemic injury to the gonad. Incarceration and potential strangulation can occur when a piece of the bowel extrudes through the ring and cannot be reduced. The term "incarceration" refers to the condition when the bowel is stuck through the ring and cannot be reduced. Strangulation of the bowel occurs when the blood supply is compromised. When the hernia contents are not reducible, surgical intervention is emergent. Strangulation occurs most frequently in the first 6 months of life (Hutson et al., 1992). The incidence of strangulation is reported between 9% and 20%. Children with a strangulated hernia have a firm, hard, and tender mass in the inguinal region. The mass can be erythematous or blue. The children are fussy, often inconsolable, and can have vomiting and abdominal distention.

An incarcerated hernia requires reduction. Parents can be instructed to reduce the hernia at home with gentle pressure on the contents gradually emptying the sac. This procedure is most successful when families administer acetaminophen, elevate the swollen groin, and calm the child. If the hernia sac remains tense, the child should be brought to the emergency room. Often the hernia independently reduces during the ride to the hospital. Sedation can be used to reduce hernias that are still incarcerated on arrival at the hospital. When this is successful, repair is performed in 24 to 48 hours. Emergency surgery is planned once an irreducible hernia is identified because of the risk of strangulation (Hutson et al., 1992; Johnstone, 1998).

Various rationales influence contralateral exploration. To decrease the risks of anesthesia and incarceration, contralateral groin exploration is sometimes recommended. Although age criteria differ slightly, exploration is recommended for all children who have a hernia on either side before the age of 2 years, boys up to 2 years and girls up to 4 years who have left-sided hernias (Hutson et al., 1992; Skinner & Grosfeld, 1993; Wiener et al., 1996).

The procedure to repair a hernia is an inguinal herniorrhaphy. The goal of the operation is a high ligation of the patent processus vaginalis (Borkowski, 1994). Herniorrhaphy performed by open technique is the standard in most pediatric surgery practices. However, laparoscopic repair and laparoscopic exploration of the contralateral side are also performed.

Complications

The hernia repair itself is an uncomplicated operation, with minimal blood loss. Complications include wound infection (1% to 2%), hernia recurrence (less than 1%), and injury to the vas deferens or ilioinguinal nerves (less than 1%) (Skinner & Grosfeld, 1993).

Nursing Interventions and Expected Outcomes

Postoperative Care

Postoperative pain is managed by the use of ilioinguinal nerve blocks or by single-dose caudal or epidural anesthetic, administered during the procedure. Local anesthetic administered as a single dose is reported to manage postoperative pain for at least 6 and as long as 24 hours postoperatively (Fisher et al., 1993). Discomfort at home is managed with the addition of acetaminophen or ibuprofen. Opioids are usually not necessary for postoperative pain control.

Patient education is an important nursing responsibility and has been shown to prevent or at least reduce negative responses to surgery, improve pain management, and achieve an optimum experience for the child and family. Children and parents who are properly educated have decreased anxiety and feel an improved sense of control over the situation (Bar-Mor, 1997; Brewer & Lampert, 1997). Other postoperative concerns are urinary retention and con-

stipation (Linden & Engberg, 1994). Urinary retention is a temporary postoperative concern and does not usually require intervention. It is a side effect of the caudal anesthetic and resolves spontaneously in 6 to 8 hours. Constipation is easily managed with increased clear liquids by mouth and stool softeners or suppository if necessary.

Infants usually return to normal feeding and sleep habits within 24 to 48 hours. Recommendations regarding activity vary by practice. Although school-aged children may return to normal routines after 2 to 3 days, contact sports should be restricted for at least 2 weeks. Yaster, Sola, Pegoli, and Paidas (1994) recommend a full 2-week recovery before toddlers ride tricycles and a full 4- to 6-week recovery period for contact sports.

UMBILICAL HERNIAS IN CHILDREN

Description of the Hernia

Umbilical hernias occur when the fascial ring, which surrounds the umbilical cord and vessels, fails to close after birth. The skin and the peritoneum are intact. A hernia occurs when a loop of bowel protrudes through the ring (Figure 22–2) (Gill, 1998; Rowe et al., 1995).

Umbilical hernias are present in approximately 20% of all newborns. Most umbilical hernias close spontaneously by 3 years of age. In the United States, there is an increased incidence of umbilical hernias found in African-American infants compared with Caucasian infants. The incidence is equal among boys and girls. It is considered an isolated problem in otherwise healthy children, but the incidence is higher in children with Down syndrome, hypothyroidism, and Beckwith-Weidemann syndrome (Gill, 1998; Rowe et al., 1995).

Incarceration occurs when a piece of bowel gets stuck through the opening. This can cause compromise to the

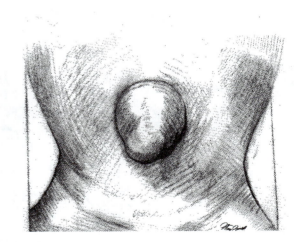

Figure 22–2 Umbilical Hernia

blood supply. Incarceration is rare but is reported (Hutson et al., 1992). Vransky and Bourdelat (1997) reported four cases of incarcerated umbilical hernia over a 5-year period.

Clinical Presentation of Hernias in Children

Umbilical hernias present as a bulging at the umbilicus. The skin becomes stretched. The bulge is more prominent when the infant cries and usually reduces spontaneously when the infant relaxes, leaving the redundant skin.

On physical examination, one can detect the size of the defect by placing a finger into the umbilicus and palpating the fascial ring. The diameter of the hole varies from 1 mm to 3 cm. Because most of these hernias close spontaneously, no treatment is indicated in the first 2 to 3 years of life.

Surgical Management

Surgical repair is performed for the following reasons: incarceration, persistence of a hernia beyond age 3 years, and large defects. The incision is made within an infraumbilical skin crease and is extended down to the rectus fascia and linea alba. The neck of the sac is dissected and then the sac is freed from the overlying skin. The redundant sac is excised, and then the defect in the linea alba is closed transversely, usually in two layers. The umbilical skin is then tacked down to the fascia and the wound is closed. A pressure dressing is placed over the wound (Rowe et al., 1995).

Nursing Interventions and Expected Outcomes

Preoperative Care

Preoperative nursing care emphasizes parental teaching and reassurance that most umbilical hernias spontaneously resolve. Families should be informed that the bulge often becomes larger before the defect closes. In addition, parents may be worried that the skin may rupture. Finally, families should be discouraged from taping coins over the bulge to facilitate early closure because this does not speed closure or prevent incarceration and may cause ulceration and infection to the skin (Rowe et al., 1995).

Postoperative Care

A large sponge dressing is applied with pressure in the operating room to minimize hematoma. The dressing remains intact for at least 48 hours. Children are ready for discharge from the outpatient setting when hemodynamically stable, breathing normally, and tolerating some clear liquids. Pain at home is managed with acetaminophen or ibuprofen. They can resume normal activity and return to day care in 2 to 3 days. Unsupervised play and contact sports should be delayed for 2 weeks.

HYDROCELES

Description of the Hydrocele

A hydrocele (Figure 22–3) is a painless cyst formed by the tunica vaginalis that contains fluid. Hydroceles occur when fluid accumulates in or above the scrotum via a patent processus vaginalis connected to the peritoneal cavity. The hydrocele is usually located in front of the testis. The testis can usually be palpated without difficulty. When the hydrocele is large or tense, the scrotum can be transilluminated (Hutson et al., 1992). Transillumination (shining a small light source through it) differentiates the hydrocele from tumor, varicocele, and blood.

Clinical Presentation of Hydroceles

In male infants, both unilateral and bilateral hydroceles are common in the first few months of life. They are painless,

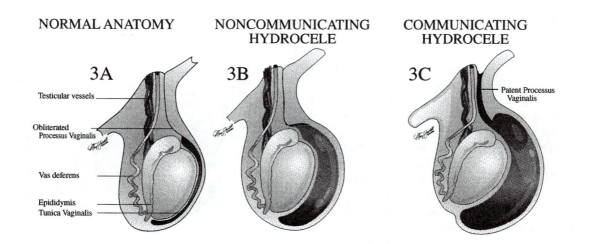

Figure 22–3 Hydrocele

often large, and usually resolve spontaneously by 1 year of age. If the hydrocele persists, there is usually a narrow communication with the peritoneal cavity (communicating hydrocele). The fluid is reabsorbed while the child is lying down and reaccumulates in the scrotum by gravity after ambulation and upright activity during the course of the day. Therefore, caregivers report a change in size, smaller in the morning and after naptime. This type of hydrocele rarely disappears spontaneously and may continue to increase in size. Therefore, surgery is recommended (Hutson et al., 1992). The differential diagnosis includes inguinal hernia, tumor, torsion, and varicocele.

Surgical Management

If the hydrocele is still present at 1 year of age, it is repaired electively. The repair is similar to a hernia repair. In addition to high ligation, a portion of the excess sac down to and around the testis is removed. The fluid may persist for several weeks or months.

Nursing Interventions and Expected Outcomes

Postoperative Care

Postoperative care is the same as discussed previously for an inguinal hernia.

UNDESCENDED TESTIS

Pathophysiology

Cryptorchidism is the failure of the testis to descend into the scrotum during gestation. The mechanism of the descent is not fully understood, although it is generally regarded to be hormonally directed and the level of descent is believed to be related to the long-term quality of the testis (the lower the testis, the more normal the histologic findings) (Hutson, 1998; Kelalis, King, & Belman, 1992). The diagnosis is made on the basis of the physical examination when there is an inability to palpate the testes or to bring them into a normal scrotal position.

Failure of testicular descent by 6 months to 1 year of age requires surgical correction (Hutson, 1998). The testis requires the cooler environment of the scrotum (96° F) to develop and function correctly (produce male hormones and sperm). An increased risk of infertility and cancer is found later in life if the testis is exposed to the warmer environment of the body. It is unclear why males with cryptorchidism are at greater risk for testicular tumors later in life. However, placing the testis in the scrotum and performing regular self-examination in the adolescent years results in early detection of cancer. If the testis is abnormal at the time of surgery, it is removed (Hutson, 1998).

Incidence

Cryptorchidism occurs more commonly in premature males (33%) than in term males (3%). Maternal exposure to estrogens during the first trimester and ordinal rank (first child) are additional risk factors. Descent continues during the first year of life. The postnatal peak in androgen production during the first 6 months of life mediates continued descent of the testis. By age 1, the incidence of cryptorchidism decreases to 0.7% to 0.8% (Kelalis et al., 1992).

Classification

Undescended testes are classified first by whether they are palpable during physical examination. Palpable testes are retractile, ectopic, or truly undescended within the canal. Impalpable testes are either intraabdominal or absent (Figure 22–4). The examination of the testes should take place in a

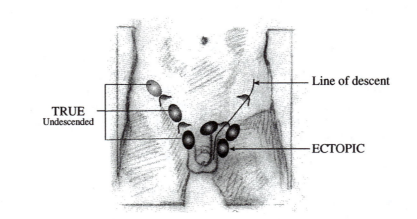

Figure 22–4 Undescended Testes

warm, relaxed examination room. Begin by first placing the thumb and index finger of one hand on the scrotum and palpating gently. Then place the index finger of the opposite hand medial to the iliac spine and move the finger gently over toward the pubis.

Retractile testes are most commonly palpated in the canal or scrotal infundibulum. They are not undescended but rather withdraw secondary to an active cremasteric reflex. Surgical intervention is not indicated unless the testes do not remain in the scrotum (Kelalis et al., 1992). Ectopic testes descend outside the external ring and then are misdirected to the abdominal wall, medial thigh, or perineum. This occurs as a result of a mechanical obstruction of the path of descent (Hutson et al., 1992). Undescended testes may be intra-abdominal, intracanalicular, or emergent (just outside the ring). Both the length and the fixation of the spermatic vessels cause arrest of the descent. The testes may move and intermittently become palpable. The higher the testis, the more severe the degree of maldevelopment (Kelalis et al., 1992). Absent testes are uncommon.

Surgical Management

The treatment of an undescended testis is to surgically fix the testis into the scrotum. This is called an orchidopexy or orchiopexy. Orchiopexy is performed between 6 and 12 months of age. The goal of the procedure is to improve fertility, to reduce the risk of malignancy, to correct associated hernias, to prevent testicular torsion, and for psychological support (Kelalis et al., 1992).

Nursing Interventions and Expected Outcomes

The long-term follow-up of this group of patients is important. Careful testicular examination should be part of the yearly primary care physical. All adolescent males should be taught to perform testicular self-examination.

Postoperative Care

Postoperative care is the same as discussed previously for an inguinal hernia.

CIRCUMCISION

The decision whether to circumcise the newborn boy is greatly debated among family members. It is usually a decision made for either religious or cultural preferences. Many parents make the decision without seeking a medical opinion. When parents' opinions differ, they seek information from other sources. Proper information regarding the foreskin is necessary when advice is given.

In its summary, the American Academy of Pediatrics (1999) offers the following advice: "Existing scientific evidence demonstrates potential medical benefits of newborn circumcision; however, these data are not sufficient to recommend routine neonatal circumcision." All studies that have examined the relationship between urinary tract infection and circumcision have shown an increased incidence in UTI in uncircumcised males. However, the risk is low. In addition, the AAP reviewed the existing literature regarding the incidence of penile cancer and circumcision and found a threefold greater incidence among uncircumcised men related to the development of phimosis in uncircumcised men. However, the studies did not examine whether or not effective hygiene would prevent phimosis. Finally, the relationship between sexually transmitted diseases including HIV and circumcision were reviewed. While there is an increased incidence of STDs in males who are not circumcised, behavioral risk factors were found to be more important.

The AAP recommends providers give unbiased information regarding the risks and benefits of the procedure and suggests that the decision whether to circumcise the normal newborn boy rest with the parents. Ethnic, religious, and cultural traditions are valid factors in the decision making. When circumcision is elected in the newborn period, it should be performed with local analgesia.

The foreskin (prepuce) is the skin that covers the glans. It is lightly adherent to the glans at birth and remains so throughout infancy. Spontaneous separation of the foreskin from the glans occurs with the shedding of normal skin cells (smegma) by the foreskin during infancy. This continues throughout childhood.

The normal foreskin needs no special care other than normal bathing. As the foreskin normally separates from the glans, perform gentle retraction during bathing. This is not recommended before 1 to 2 years of age.

There are three medical indications for circumcision: phimosis, paraphimosis, and balanitis (Hutson et al., 1992). Phimosis is stenosis of the opening of the foreskin. This occurs as a result of forceful attempts at retraction of the foreskin. Paraphimosis occurs in older boys when the foreskin gets pulled behind the glans and cannot be brought back. This causes constriction and swelling of the glans. It is very painful. Local anesthesia and oftentimes general anesthesia are necessary before manual reduction of the foreskin can be performed. A circumcision is then performed to prevent recurrence. Balanitis is an infection of the foreskin. Usually resulting from phimosis, balanitis can also occur when the foreskin is not retracted and contamination occurs. Topical antibiotic ointment or systemic antibiotics are used to reduce inflammation (Hutson et al., 1992). Elective circumcision is planned when the infection and inflammation have resolved.

Surgical Intervention

Circumcision is most commonly performed with local anesthesia in the newborn period. After the dorsal penile nerve block is placed, the circumcision can be performed with the use of a clamp, either a Gomco bell or Plastibell, which is left on for several minutes. The foreskin is then excised and the clamp is removed. When the Plastibell clamp is used, a suture is used to tie off the foreskin and the disposable ring is left on until it falls off. This takes approximately 9 days and occurs when the skin necroses (Cuckow, 1998). The wound is wrapped with petroleum gauze, and antibiotic ointment may be applied for several diaper changes to protect the wound and prevent sticking to the diaper.

Circumcision is considered a more significant surgical procedure in the older boy for a variety of reasons: the need for general anesthesia, increased incidence of postoperative bleeding, and finally, developmental sensitivity to prepare the boy for surgery on his penis. Usually performed in a freehand manner, hemostasis is achieved with cautery and the wound is secured with absorbable sutures.

Complications

Complications are rare. However, the most common is bleeding. Others include meatal ulceration, stenosis, urinary retention, and postcircumcision phimosis.

Postoperative Care

Postoperative care includes the use of petroleum gauze or a transparent dressing to the wound to prevent sticking to the diaper or the underwear. Careful cleansing and antibiotic ointment application to the wound are important for comfort and to prevent infection. Pain control is achieved with oxycodone, ibuprofen, or acetaminophen. Parents are often concerned about the degree of erythema and swelling and should be reassured that this will resolve after 5 to 7 days.

OUTPATIENT SURGERY CAREMAP

Because of the nature of outpatient surgery (short stay, short operating room time, minimal anesthetic risks, and minimal exposure to hospital personnel), many centers have developed practice guidelines or caremaps to standardize the care delivery systems offered to this population. Standardization of care has been shown to minimize laboratory testing, decrease duplication of services, and shorten operating room turnover times (Stewart, Harrill, & Ohlms, 1997).

The caremap described (Appendix 22–A) is a transdisciplinary, transgeographic tool to guide outpatients through all phases of care. In addition, most pediatric surgery sites engage in collecting variance measures to control cost, cancellations, delays in operating start times, discharge delays, and unplanned admissions. Caregivers strive to improve patient satisfaction and improve functional outcome: compliance with instructions and follow-up appointments and loss of time from school, sports, and parents' time from work. This tool collects these data and standardizes the care across each phase of care. Variance information supports modifications of care and practice changes. Every effort should be taken to decrease unnecessary and last-minute cancellations because these have been shown to cause hardship for families. Tait, Voepel-Lewis, Munro, Gutstein, and Reynolds (1997) reported that up to 53% of parents do not get paid for time missed from work and that 25% of children whose surgery was canceled required an additional preoperative appointment or additional testing prior to rescheduling the surgery. Forty-five percent of parents and 16% of the children were disappointed by the last-minute cancellation of the procedure. Cancellation data can be collected directly from the caremap variances and modifications of preoperative preparation, if necessary, can be implemented.

Pediatric outpatient surgery should be both a positive and satisfying life experience for the child and family. Careful attention to preoperative preparation and standardization of the perioperative care achieves cost-effective, efficient, and quality care.

REFERENCES

American Academy of Pediatrics. (1999). Circumcision Policy Statement (RE 9850). Evanston, Illinois. 103, 3, 686–693.

Bar-Mor, G. (1997). Preparation of children for surgery and invasive procedures: Milestones on the way to success. *Journal of Pediatric Nursing, 12*(4), 257–259.

Brewer, S.L. & Lambert, C.S. (1997). Preparing children for same-day surgery: Innovative approaches. *Journal of Pediatric Nursing, 12*(4), 252–255.

Borkowski, S. (1994). Common pediatric surgical problems. *Nursing Clinics of North America, 29*, 551–562.

Cuckow, P.M. (1998). Circumcision. In M.D. Stringer, P.D.E. Mouriquand,

K.T. Oldman, & E.R. Howard (Eds.), *Pediatric surgery and urology: Long term outcomes.* Philadelphia: W.B. Saunders Company.

Fisher, Q.A., McComiskey, C.M., Hill, J.L., Spurrier, E.A., Voigt, R.W., Savarese, A.M., Beaver, B.L., & Boltz, M.G. (1993). Postoperative voiding interval and duration of analgesia following peripheral or caudal nerve blocks in children. *Anesthesia and Analgesia, 76*, 173–177.

Gill, F.T. (1998). Umbilical hernia, inguinal hernias, and hydroceles in children: Diagnostic clues for optimal patient management. *Journal of Pediatric Health Care, 12*(5), 231–235.

Green, C.R., Pandit, S.K., & Schork, M.A. (1996). Preoperative fasting time: Is the traditional policy changing? Results of a national survey. *Anesthesia and Analgesia, 83*(1), 123–128.

Hutson, J.M. (1998). Undescended testes. In M.D. Stringer, P.D.E. Mouriquand, K.T. Oldham, & E.R. Howard (Eds.), *Pediatric surgery and urology: Long term outcomes*. Philadelphia: W.B. Saunders Company.

Hutson, J.M., Beasley, S.W., & Woodward, A.A. (1992). *Jones' clinical paediatric surgery*. Oxford, England: Blackwell Scientific Publications.

Johnstone, M.S. (1998). Inguinal hernia repair. In M.D. Stringer, P.D.E. Mouriquand, K.T. Oldham, & E.R. Howard (Eds.), *Pediatric surgery and urology: Long term outcomes*. Philadelphia: W.B. Saunders Company.

Jones, K.L. (1988). *Smith's recognizable patterns of human malformation*. Philadelphia: W.B. Saunders Company.

Kelalis, P.P., King, L.R., & Belman, A.B. (1992). *Clinical pediatric urology*. Philadelphia: W.B. Saunders Company.

Linden, J., & Engberg, J.B. (1994). Nursing discharge assessment of the patient postinguinal herniorrhaphy in the ambulatory surgery setting. *Journal of Post-Anesthesia Nursing, 9*, 14–19.

Patel, R.I., DeWitt, L., & Hannallah, R.S. (1997). Preoperative laboratory testing in children undergoing elective surgery: Analysis of current practice. *Journal of Clinical Anesthesia, 9*(7), 569–575.

Rowe, M.I., O'Neill, J.A., Grosfeld, J.L., Funkalsrud, E.W., & Coran, A.G. (1995). *Essentials of pediatric surgery*. St. Louis, MO: Mosby.

Skinner, M.A., & Grosfeld, J.L. (1993). Inguinal and umbilical repair in infants and children. *Surgical Clinics of North America, 73*, 439–448.

Stewart, M.G., Harrill, W.C., & Ohlms, L.A. (1997). The effects of an outpatient practice guideline at a teaching hospital: A prospective pilot study. *Otolaryngology Head and Neck Surgery, 10*(4), 388–393.

Tait, A.R., Voepel-Lewis, T., Munro, G.M., Gutstein, H.B., & Reynolds, P.I. (1997). Cancellation of pediatric outpatient surgery: Economic and emotional implications for patients and their families. *Journal of Clinical Anesthesia, 9*(3), 213–219.

Vransky, P., & Bourdelat, D. (1997). Incarcerated umbilical hernia in children. *Pediatric Surgery International, 12*(1), 61–62.

Weiner, E.S., Touloukian, R.J., Rodgers, B.M., Grosfeld, J.L., Smith, E.I., Zeigler, M.M., & Coran, A.G. (1996). Hernia survey of the Section on Surgery of the American Academy of Pediatrics. *Journal of Pediatric Surgery, 31*(8), 1166–1169.

Yaster, M., Sola, J.E., Pegoli, W., & Paidas, C.N. (1994). The night after surgery. Postoperative management of the pediatric outpatient—surgical and anesthetic aspects. *Pediatric Clinics of North America, 41*(1), 199–218.

Appendix 22–A

Critical Pathway for Outpatient Surgery

Date ____/____/____ Page 1 of 2

	Presurgical Evaluation Phase *Date: _____ Time: _____*	*Variance and Actions*
Assessment	◊ Confirmation of diagnosis ◊ Evaluation of concurrent conditions	
Medications and interventions	◊ Operative procedure scheduled	Labs: Add'l Procedure: _____
Documentation	◊ Operative consent signed/pathway faxed ◊ Communication with PCP ◊ Consent faxed to appropriate site	
Patient and family education	◊ Expectations/hospitalization/preop packet ◊ Expectation postop ◊ Anesthesia telephone preop	
Discharge planning	◊ Transportation	
Expected outcomes	◊ Parents to see PCP for H&P ◊ Consent signed ◊ Prep packet given ◊ Diagnosis-specific materials ◊ Consent faxed to appropriate site	

This pathway represents the care for the majority of patients in this case type including resource utilization and outcomes. Variations may occur based upon the clinical progression of individual patients.

_____   _____

Office Staff Signature   Presurgical Phase MD Signature

Courtesy of University of Maryland, Department of Surgery, Baltimore, Maryland.

Date: ___ / ___ / ___   Page 2 of 2   Time in Phase: _____   Time Out: _____   4 Hour/23 Hour

	ASCU Phase — Prep for Surgery	Operative Phase	Recovery Phase I — PACU	Recovery Phase II	Variance and Actions
Nursing assessment	◊ Weight _____ ◊ Last oral intake _____ ◊ Hx of recent URI Yes/No ◊ Vital signs including temperature ◊ T ___ P ___ R ___ ◊ Allergies ◊ Labs reviewed if applicable ◊ Fever history ◊ Premed from anesthesia order		◊ VS q15 min until stable and able to protect airway ◊ Observe respirations ◊ Observe for bleeding	◊ VS on admission then q4° and PRN ◊ Observe hourly comfort, ability to drink and swallow fluid intake, respirations, color, IV site ◊ Observe for bleeding ◊ Pain score assessment	
MS assessment	◊ History and physical ◊ Anesthesia evaluation	◊ Continuous monitoring by anesthesia	◊ Surgeon's assessment as indicated ◊ Anesthesia evaluation prior to close of phase		◊ No H & P
Medications and interventions	◊ EMLA to back of hands ◊ Premedication _____ ◊ Provide safe environment following premedication ◊ Offer age-appropriate diversional activities	◊ Continuous observation ◊ Venous access established ◊ Anesthesia ◊ Surgical procedure ◊ inguinal hernia unilateral side _____ ◊ contralateral exploration ◊ umbilical hernia ◊ hydrocelectomy side _____ ◊ orchiopexy side _____ ◊ circumcision	◊ Continuous observation ◊ Continuous EKG monitoring ◊ Continuous pulse oximetry ◊ Assure minimal stimulation ◊ Bedrest	◊ Tylenol ◊ Ibuprofen ◊ Regular observation ◊ Encourage clear fluids ◊ IV to Hep lock when taking fluids and voiding appropriately for age (Minimal PO requirement _____) ◊ D/C IV prior to discharge	◊ SBE prophylaxis
Nutrition	◊ NPO	◊ NPO ◊ IV hydration per anesthesia	◊ IV fluids	◊ Clear fluids	
Documentation	◊ H & P ◊ Consent signed and verified ◊ Preop orders ◊ Lab results ◊ Anesthesia checklist ◊ OR checklist	◊ Appropriate OR documentation completed	◊ Family present and supporting child by close of phase ◊ Postop consult with surgeon ◊ Operative report on chart ◊ Postop orders on chart	◊ Review what to expect at home ◊ Review education materials ◊ Review pain management strategies ◊ Review signs of complications ◊ Review what to do and phone number to call	
Patient and family education	◊ What to expect today ◊ Where to wait		◊ Interpret child's behavior and experience for family	◊ Parents know when to call ◊ Parents know how to manage pain	
Discharge planning			◊ Parents know criteria for discharge ◊ Prescriptions written ◊ Verify transportation		
Expected outcomes	◊ Family present and supporting child ◊ Family understands what to expect today ◊ Family knows where to wait ◊ Timely, effective medication ◊ Physical condition acceptable for surgery ◊ Ready for OR on time	◊ Procedure complete ◊ Minimal bleeding ◊ Family and child know what to expect ◊ Proceed to PACU	◊ Child awake and able to protect airway ◊ Parents have resumed some caregiving responsibilities ◊ Family and child know what to expect ◊ Admit to ASCU ◊ Admit to Peds/Recovery	◊ Child awake ◊ Child able to protect airway ◊ Child has voided ◊ Parents have resumed caregiving responsibilities	◊ Fever ◊ URI ◊ Child ate ◊ Labs unacceptable ◊ _____

This pathway represents the care for the majority of patients in this case type including resource utilization and outcomes. Variations may occur based upon the clinical progression of individual patients.

CHAPTER 23

Necrotizing Enterocolitis

Betty R. Kasson

Necrotizing enterocolitis (NEC) is a baffling disease that is the source of the most common surgical emergency in the neonate (Kosloske & Musemeche, 1989). It is primarily a disease of prematurity but can affect the term neonate (Andrews, Sawin, Ledbetter, Schaller, & Hatch, 1990). The overall mortality rate for infants with NEC is 25%, with the rate of mortality for more premature infants approaching 66% (Foglia, 1995). NEC has been attributed to perinatal and postnatal factors. The perinatal factors include hypoxia and ischemia (Nowicki, 1990). Postnatal factors involve exchange transfusions through umbilical vein catheters, placement of umbilical arterial catheters, cardiovascular abnormalities, hyperviscosity, ischemia of the intestinal mucosa, feeding of hyperosmolar formulas and medicines, and the cleanliness of the neonatal intensive care unit (Lawrence, Bates, & Gaul, 1982; Rowe, 1986). Infectious agents have also been implicated, including *Clostridia*, *Escherichia coli*, *Klebsiella*, and others (Han, Sayed, Chance, Brabyn, & Shaheed, 1983). After many careful studies over 25 years, no single factor has been demonstrated as the sole cause of NEC. It is now believed that NEC is the common final pathway resulting from a variety of factors (Kleigman & Walsh, 1987).

EPIDEMIOLOGY

NEC is primarily a disease of premature infants who have been fed. NEC occurs in 1% to 2.4% of live births (Rowe, 1986) and accounts for 10% of deaths in very low birth weight infants (Foglia, 1995). In the premature infant, NEC usually occurs within 1 to 4 days of life if feeding starts on day 1 (Andrews et al., 1990). Udall (1990) has described a decrease in the risk of NEC at 34 to 35 weeks' gestational age. He believes this is due to intestinal maturation and the development of an intact intestinal mucosal barrier.

Goldman (1980) reports that NEC is a rare phenomenon in the unfed infant; feeding clearly plays a role in the development of NEC. In one study, NEC was equally distributed between males and females and showed no racial or seasonal distribution (Wilson et al., 1981).

NEC can present as individual or "cluster" cases, and the cause appears to be different for the two types. There are several reports of sudden clusters of cases occurring in neonatal intensive care units (NICUs) in which an infectious viral or bacterial organism was isolated, and appropriate infection control enforcement resolved the epidemic (Han et al., 1983; Moomjian, Peckham, Fox, Pereira, & Schaberg, 1978). Several of the organisms isolated were normal colonic flora, and there was no clear explanation for why they suddenly caused disease.

PATHOGENESIS

General agreement exists that NEC is the result of a cluster of factors. Rowe (1986) classified these factors as indirect (such as perinatal hypoxia or low flow states caused by cardiac disease) and direct (such as bacterial overgrowth in the intestine by a particular organism or feeding). A brief discussion of some factors believed to contribute to NEC follows.

Indirect Factors

Ischemia

Ischemia is the major indirect factor implicated in NEC. Low flow states in the bowel vascular system lead to necrosis of the bowel. Infants at risk for low flow states include children with cardiac defects, umbilical arterial and venous catheters, and hyperviscosity. All these factors cause decreased blood flow in the intestine. Hypoperfusion leads to oxygen deprivation and the buildup of metabolic waste products, resulting in mucosal damage. The evidence for this mechanism is not conclusive. Rowe (1986) matched "at-risk" NEC babies with similar babies without risk factors and found no difference in the incidence of NEC. In this study on ischemia and reperfusion, Rowe noted that it may be the return of blood flow after a period of low flow that results in NEC. During the high-flow (hyperemic) recovery period after an ischemic event, endothelial cells swell and cell membranes are disrupted. Inflammatory cellular mediators such as platelet-activating factor (PAF) and oxygen free radicals are released from the cells. In animal studies, these compounds have caused NEC-like injury (Foglia, 1995; Ford, Watkins, Reblock, & Rowe, 1997; MacKendrick & Caplan, 1993).

Direct Factors

Immature Infant Immunologic Defenses

The neonatal gastrointestinal tract is immunologically immature (Udall, 1990). Premature infants have a limited capacity to defend against bacterial toxins because the intestine in the neonate is actually adapted to absorb whole macromolecules to acquire passive immunity from breast milk. The maternal immune system is part of the neonatal host defense because under normal circumstances, neonates rely on breast milk to provide phagocytes, B cells, T cells, and IgA. The lymphatic tissue in the neonatal intestine is not able to produce B and T lymphocytes at a level that can effectively control bacterial overgrowth without this maternal "boost." Neonatal and premature intestine is also deficient in immunoglobulin A (IgA), which is thought to suppress bacterial growth and keep bacteria from adhering to the intestinal mucosa. The distal ileum and the cecum have increased lymph tissue, decreased secretory function, and immature mucus production in the premature infant. Little mucus is present to protect the bowel mucosa, and the protective lymphoid tissue is not yet functional. This means premature infants have a decreased ability to defend against bacterial toxins that can damage the ileal and cecal mucosa and helps explain why these regions of the bowel are those most commonly affected by NEC.

Neonates may develop abnormal bacterial flora because normal gut colonization is delayed or absent. Most infants establish bacterial colonization from contact with and feeding by their mothers. This mechanism provides a large variety of organisms that colonize the gut in a balanced and competitive fashion. Lawrence et al. (1982) proposed that the physical isolation, the cleanliness of NICU procedures, and the use of antibiotics conspired to produce a situation in which one or two dominant bacterial species might proliferate and produce a large amount of toxin damaging to the neonatal gut. They noted that in germ-free animal models, the

bacteria that proliferated in a similar situation were all toxin producers. It is not yet known whether premature babies undergoing "kangaroo therapy," in which there is skin-to-skin contact between the premature infant and the parent, colonize their intestinal tracts in a balanced way despite not being fed.

Nonimmunologic Defense Mechanisms

Neonates have decreased gastric acid production for the first month of life. Gastric acid is the first line of defense against the introduction of bacteria into the enteric system and is an effective killer of swallowed organisms. Without a high acid environment, large numbers of bacteria travel from the stomach into the bowel (Hyman et al., 1985).

Neonates also produce a lower level of pancreatic enzymes that can attack and break down proteins. Because bacterial toxins are proteins, the secretion of pancreatic enzymes into the duodenum inactivates these toxins. Without an effective pancreatic enzyme system, the neonate is more vulnerable to the effects of these toxins (Lebenthal & Leung, 1988).

Udall (1990) observed that the mucous membrane of the neonate is not "closed." The neonatal gut is able to absorb large macromolecules to achieve passive immunity through breast milk. The premature gut is even more permeable, and the translocation of bacterial and viral particles and toxins across the mucous membrane has been demonstrated histologically (Ballance, Dahms, Shenker, & Kleigman, 1990). The closure of this membrane is thought to be a maturational event, and the decrease in the risk of NEC at 34 to 35 weeks' gestation is consistent with this timing. In one study, it was noted that mothers who had been treated with steroids in the antenatal period had infants with a lower incidence of NEC than a matched control group. The difference was thought to be due to earlier maturation of the bowel because of the steroid treatment (Bauer, Morrison, & Poole, 1984).

Factors characteristic of the premature gastrointestinal tract that have been implicated in NEC include poor motility, a lack of mucus production, and decreased function of lymphoid tissue. MacKendrick and Caplan (1993) describe a condition in which these factors interact. Poor motility for moving bacteria through the bowel, poor mucus production for entrapping bacteria, and a lack of phagocytes and mucosa-protecting IgA combine to make the bowel vulnerable to bacterial toxins and inflammatory compounds.

Feeding

Few unfed infants develop NEC. One theory that connects feeding to mucosal damage involves the overgrowth of intestinal bacteria when provided with a carbohydrate source (Kien, Liechty, & Mullett, 1990). This is supported by the evidence that hydrogen, a product of carbohydrate fermentation, is found in the bowel. Primary digestion of formula in infants takes place in the enzyme-rich environment of the small bowel and is not characterized by hydrogen-producing fermentation. Studies on the digestion of formula by premature infants show that all lactose is not digested by enzymes and that the residual lactose undergoes fermentation in the ileum and colon (Kien et al., 1990). This provides an important second source of nutrition for the infant but also creates a situation that encourages the overgrowth of bowel-damaging bacteria (Cheu, Brown, & Rowe, 1989).

A study of 926 preterm infants by Lucas and Cole (1990) showed that NEC was 6 to 10 times more common in formula-fed than breast-fed babies and that babies fed a combination of breast milk and formula had three times more NEC than those that were breast fed only. They concluded that breast milk significantly decreased the incidence of NEC in preterm infants. However, some infants fed only breast milk have developed NEC. Lucas and Cole's evidence and the presence of phagocytes, B and T cells, and IgA in breast milk support the important role that breast milk plays in the health of the neonatal gastrointestinal system.

Having a premature infant with NEC is a stressful event for parents who frequently feel helpless and exhausted. The nurse plays a vital role in encouraging the mother of an infant with NEC to keep pumping to provide milk. Parents of acutely ill, ventilated infants sometimes feel that there is nothing they can do for their child. The evidence presented by Lucas and Cole shows the importance of producing breast milk for later feedings.

Vasoactive and Inflammatory Cellular Mediators

In animal models, cell mediators such as PAF, inflammatory cytokines, interleukins, and tumor necrosis factor alpha have produced a clinical and histologic picture that looks like NEC. Ischemia-reperfusion injuries and metabolism of carbohydrates by gas-producing organisms also release a burst of these vasoactive compounds. The action of these compounds seems to lead to vasoconstriction and bowel necrosis (Foglia, 1995).

Compounds that block the production of PAF, such as nitric oxide, reduce bowel injury in these animal models (MacKendrick, Caplan, & Hsueh, 1993). Increasing evidence suggests that PAF is a mediator in the final common pathway that creates the clinical picture of NEC, no matter what the causative factors (Caplan & Hsueh, 1990).

THE PRESENTATION OF NEC

Because NEC is the result of many interacting factors, the presentation is also variable. Symptoms of NEC vary from a mild illness that responds to a few days of antibiotics and gastric decompression to a life-threatening condition characterized by thrombocytopenia, respiratory failure, and cardiovascular collapse.

Clinical Signs

Early clinical signs may be nonspecific, including lethargy, poor feeding, bilious emesis, and temperature instability. Abdominal distention, increasing prefeeding gastric residuals, and gross or occult blood in the stools are other frequent findings. This picture has factors in common with the presentation of sepsis, feeding intolerance, and hypomotility of prematurity. Placement of a nasogastric tube can cause gastric bleeding, and stools commonly test positive for occult blood, complicating the picture. Careful observation for abdominal distention and tenderness, increasing gastric residuals, and fecal blood is the key to early diagnosis (Foglia, 1995; Kleigman & Walsh, 1987; Rowe, 1986).

Physical Findings

Physical findings in later NEC include a green or bluish hue to the abdominal wall, labia, or scrotum. The neonatal abdominal wall is thin, and meconium spilled into the peritoneal cavity can sometimes be seen as dark coloration under the skin (see Figure 23–1). Abdominal wall erythema is frequently an indicator of the underlying inflammation of peritonitis. Abdominal wall edema, tenderness, and rigidity usually accompany it. Increasing abdominal girth or a palpable fixed loop of bowel are other physical findings (Rowe, 1986).

Laboratory Findings

Laboratory findings are frequently nonspecific and indicative of generalized sepsis. There may be either an increase or decrease in the white blood cell count. The decrease is more ominous because it indicates that the infant is unable to generate a systemic immune response. A continuing fall in platelets less than 100,000/mm^3 is also ominous and is frequently associated with intestinal perforation and sepsis. Electrolyte abnormalities are indicative of fluid shifts and the capillary leakage associated with infection. An increase in the C-reactive protein is another nonspecific indicator of sepsis (Foglia, 1995).

Radiologic Evaluation

Radiographs are important for noting a change from the normal bowel gas pattern. They can detect free gas in the abdomen, in the venous system of the liver (portal venous gas), and in the wall of the bowel (pneumatosis intestinalis). Radiographs are obtained every 6 hours if NEC is suspected. Plain abdominal films show a change from the normal "honeycomb" gas pattern to distended loops of bowel with thickened, edematous walls. "Fixed" loops, large gas-filled loops that are in the same position from film to film, may indicate

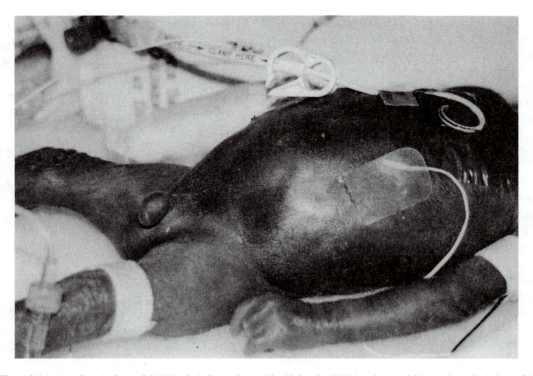

Figure 23–1 The Abdomen of an Infant of 24 Weeks' Gestation with Abdominal Distention and Meconium Staining of the Left Lower Quadrant

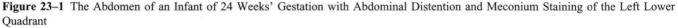

segmental necrosis. Pneumatosis intestinalis is seen early in NEC and can change over a matter of hours as gas pockets in the bowel wall fill and empty (see Figure 23–2). Two forms of pneumatosis occur: a cystic form that appears early and is characterized by pockets of gas in the innermost mucosal layer of the bowel and a linear form indicative of gas in the muscular or outermost (serosal) layer. Cysts and blebs may appear in the serosa as well (Foglia, 1995).

Portal venous gas is seen as a dark, treelike pattern over the light shadow of the liver in the right upper quadrant and indicates that bowel gas is in the capillary system of the mesentery and has traveled into the portal vein. This is an indicator of severe disease, although there is a report of portal venous gas resolving without surgery (O'Neill, Stahlman, & Meng, 1975). Pneumoperitoneum, free gas in the abdomen, is always an indication for surgery because it demonstrates perforation of the bowel wall (Foglia, 1995). Free gas is more difficult to see on a supine film because air rises and the film is taken through the gas with the bowel loops as background. When it is detected on this radiographic view, it forms a round or oval shadow overlying the abdominal contents (football sign) (see Figure 23–3). The free gas can also outline the falciform ligament lying just to the right of the vertebral column. Free gas is best seen on a cross-table lateral or left lateral decubitus film. In a cross-table lateral view, the

film is taken supine from the side so that the free gas that has risen to the anterior abdominal wall appears as a dark shadow above the bowel. The left lateral decubitus film, taken with the infant's left side down and shot from the side allows the free gas to rise to the right side where the air is outlined against the shadow of the liver (Figure 23–4). Small amounts of gas can best be seen on this film because there is no interference from the gas within the bowel. (Foglia, 1995).

Paracentesis is used in some centers when the diagnosis is in question. The baby is placed in a lateral position. This allows the free fluid in the abdomen to sink to a dependent position where a small amount can be aspirated with a fine catheter. The demonstration of stool-stained fluid or bacteria in the peritoneal cavity is diagnostic for perforated NEC (O'Neill et al., 1975).

MANAGEMENT

Appendix 23–A provides a caremap for management of necrotizing enterocolitis.

Medical Management of NEC

More than half of infants with the clinical picture of NEC are managed medically and resolve the NEC without surgi-

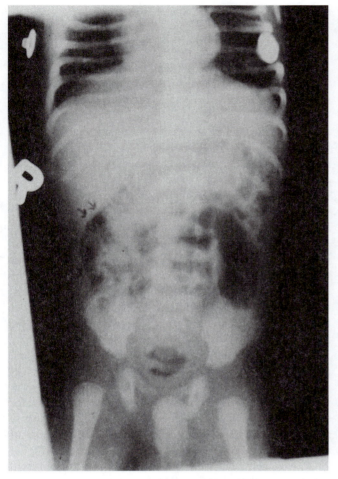

Figure 23–2 A Supine Radiograph of an Infant with a Dilated Loop of Bowel in the Left Lower Quadrant and Bowel Wall Pneumatosis in the Right Upper Quadrant at the Arrows

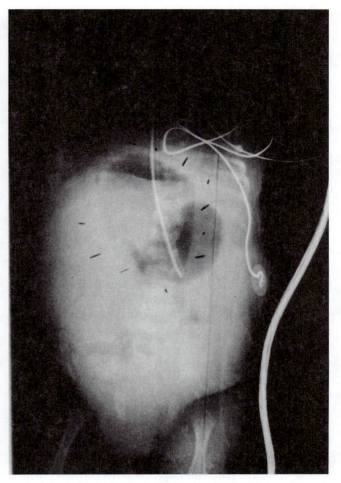

Figure 23–3 A Radiograph Showing Free Gas in the Abdomen Overlying the Stomach Bubble and an Air-fluid Level. The free gas is outlined by hash marks.

cal intervention. Treatment and surveillance consist of the elements listed in Exhibit 23–1. The goals of medical management are to detect and fight infection, to support ventilation and oxygenation, to provide adequate intravascular volume, and to decrease the work of the bowel and its metabolic needs to a minimum. Physiologic management goals support the infant's metabolism and equilibrium. Bowel rest allows the damaged organ to heal.

When the bowel is full of food, its work is increased. It has to meet both its tissue metabolic needs and the needs of digestion and absorption. It requires greater amounts of oxygen and more blood flow to supply nutrients and remove metabolic wastes for these two functions. Feeding also provides fermentable material to fuel the growth of bacteria and the production of bacterial toxins. Bowel rest, decompression, and nasogastric suction remove the substrate for bacte-

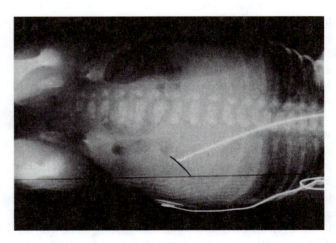

Figure 23–4 Left Lateral Decubitus Radiograph with Free Gas Rising to the Right Side and Outlining the Liver

Exhibit 23–1 Medical Management of NEC

- Aggressive fluid resuscitation
- Gastrointestinal rest with nasogastric drainage to suction
- Peripheral and central blood cultures
- Antibiotic coverage for aerobes and anaerobes
- Close monitoring of abdominal girth
- Correction of volume, and electrolyte abnormalities
- Mechanical ventilation to correct blood gas abnormalities
- Correction of coagulopathies
- Total parenteral nutrition
- Serial physical examinations
- Serial radiographs

rial overgrowth, decrease the work of the bowel, and allow the oxygen and nutrients to be used for metabolism and healing.

Without the enteral route, achieving an adequate level of nutrition is a challenge. Neonates with NEC require 120 to 150 kcal/kg/day, depending on their gestational age and weight. This level of parenteral nutrition requires central venous access or peripherally inserted central catheters (PICCs) that support a major advance in nutrition for these infants (Ryder, 1993).

Infants with NEC can be critically ill, requiring aggressive fluid resuscitation, ventilation, inotropes, diagnostic procedures, and antibiotic coverage. NEC is superimposed on the special needs and problems of prematurity, and this can be a devastating combination, even without a frank bowel perforation.

When feedings are restarted, the initial volumes are very small (1 ml/hr or less) and they are advanced slowly (1 to 2 ml/day). The feedings are given by continuous nasogastric infusion. Breast milk is the preferred formula because of the presence of its immunologically active components. If breast milk is not available, elemental formulas with predigested proteins and fats may be used. The infant must be monitored closely for abdominal girth changes, blood in the stools, increasing gastric residuals, and behavior changes during the feeding advances. Feedings are stopped if there is any sign of recurrence of NEC. Achieving full enteral feedings can be a lengthy process with many interruptions. This is a difficult time for parents. When feedings are begun, they believe that there is real progress. When feedings have to be stopped, parents can become despondent. It is important to let parents know that many increases, decreases, and stops in the feeding regimen are not unusual in an infant who has had NEC and that these changes are not indicative of final outcome. It is not easy for parents to "ride the feeding roller coaster" with NEC. Reminding them that this is an expected part of the disease helps allay anxiety.

Indications for Surgery

Surgery is indicated when medical management fails or when the bowel is perforated. The failure of medical management includes many of the signs listed in Exhibit 23–2. An infant with a clear intestinal perforation or a significant number of other clinical signs requires operation. Bell, Ternberg, and Feigin (1978) developed clinical staging criteria for NEC that define stages of severity and the therapeutic interventions appropriate for each. The Bell criteria are still useful and have been modified by other clinicians (Kleigman & Walsh, 1987).

If the infant is unstable and transport to the operating room would be hazardous, the operation may be performed in the NICU. Anesthesia, scrub and circulating nurses, sterile operating packs, and all necessary equipment are brought to the infant's bedside. Foglia (1995) found that only 50% of infants with intraoperative findings of NEC had radiographs showing free gas that were diagnostic of intestinal perforation before surgery. This leads to the conclusion that in about half of the cases, a multifactorial picture is as diagnostic for NEC as a radiograph showing free gas.

On opening the abdomen, the surgeon may find a swollen, purple bowel with areas of full-thickness or partial-thickness necrosis (white, green, or gray patches) or a skip pattern in which normal bowel is present between areas of pneumatosis, edema, and necrosis. Often visible blisters (pneumatosis) are found on the serosal surface of the bowel. The bowel wall may be thin and friable and is usually hemorrhagic (Figure 23–5). The peritoneal fluid is bloody with necrosis or turbid and brown with perforation. Fibrinous exudate is found over the serosa and areas of mucosal slough (Foglia, 1995; Rowe, 1986; Erik Skarsgard, personal communication, 1998). The most common areas of involvement are the terminal ileum, cecum, and right colon, but any portion of the bowel may be involved. The goal at operation is to remove only the bowel

---

Exhibit 23–2 Signs of the Failure of Medical Management

- Hypothermia
- Apnea
- Hyperbilirubinemia
- Uncorrectable metabolic acidosis*
- Falling platelet counts requiring repeated transfusions*
- Unexplained coagulopathies*
- Increasing rigidity of the abdominal wall*
- Free gas or portal venous gas on radiograph*
- Oliguria
- Bleeding

  * Indications for immediate operation.

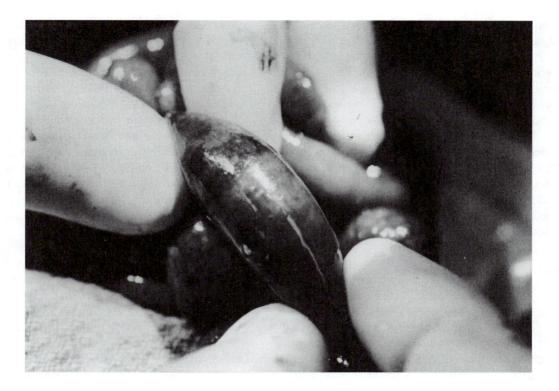

Figure 23–5 Segment of Necrotic Bowel Showing Hemorrhage and Gray Patches

that is fully necrotic and to leave any marginal areas with the hope that they will survive. This can be a difficult decision because studies of the microscopic changes during NEC show that there can be active development of necrosis right next to areas that are healing and building new mucosa (Ballance et al., 1990).

The marginal bowel is brought to the abdominal skin surface (exteriorized) so that leaky internal anastomoses do not contaminate the peritoneal cavity with stool. Fully resected areas may undergo primary anastomosis with good results (Tan, Kiely, Agrawal, Brereton, & Spitz, 1989). Multiple ostomy formation is preferred over the resection of normal bowel that lies between involved areas so as to retain as much bowel as possible. This means that an infant may have several stomas on the abdomen, although stool is only produced by the proximal stoma. The other stomas will be mucous fistulas. These are sections of bowel not connected to the fecal stream. It is also important to save the ileocecal valve. This valve both slows the transit time of nutrients through the small bowel to give time for adequate absorption and prevents the reflux of bacteria-laden colon contents into the small bowel. The remaining bowel adapts by increasing its surface area until maximum enteral absorption is achieved. How much small bowel is necessary to avoid life-

long dependence on total parenteral nutrition is still a matter of opinion and argument. Sondheimer, Cadnapaphornchai, Sontag, and Zerbe (1998) found an inverse relationship between the length of small bowel remaining and the duration of time on parenteral nutrition. There is also current discussion among pediatric specialists as to whether the ileocecal valve is as vital to the outcome of the patient with short-gut syndrome as is currently believed (Kaufman et al., 1997).

At the end of the operation, the viable and marginal bowel is measured, and this information is used to formulate a long-term nutrition plan for the infant. Sometimes the plan includes a repeat operation in 24 to 36 hours to reevaluate marginal bowel (Foglia, 1995).

After the operation, the surgeon describes the findings for the family. Often parents are unable to understand the implications of removing a portion of the bowel. They focus attention on the stoma formation rather than future bowel adaptation and feeding. The full impact of the surgeon's information is processed over the next days and weeks, and the nurse's explanations and interpretations are an important part of this process. Assessing the parents' understanding of the current information and readiness to learn more helps the family adapt to the situation. The use of diagrams, drawings, and articles, as well as providing access to resources on the

Internet and parent support groups, facilitates parental understanding and coping.

In some instances, a peritoneal drain is placed instead of using a more conventional surgical approach. This procedure is performed in very low birth weight (VLBW) and unstable infants who may not tolerate operation. Morgan, Shochat, and Hartman (1994) reported the drainage procedure as definitive in 18 of 29 infants weighing less than 1,500 gm. No further operation was required, and the infants did well. Because VLBW infants have a 66% mortality rate from more conventional management of NEC, this procedure is a reasonable alternative in these infants. If no improvement occurs after 24 hours of drainage, an open procedure is frequently performed.

Long-Term Consequences

The long-term consequences of NEC include short-bowel syndrome, strictures, adhesions, and malabsorption (Foglia, 1995), with short-bowel syndrome being the major complication. Stevenson, Kerner, Malachowski, and Sunshine (1980) studied late morbidity in prematurely born infants and found 81% of children had no problems related to the gastrointestinal tract. They concluded that the long-term prognosis in NEC is encouraging. Rowe (1986) reviewed

several authors who matched VLBW infants with and without NEC and reported no increased problems in developmental, neurologic, growth, nutritional status, or gastrointestinal function 1 to 2 years after NEC. Schwartz, Richardson, Hayden, Swischuk, and Tyson (1980) reviewed 62 patients and found post-NEC strictures in 25% of them. Not all of these strictures were symptomatic, and more recent data would be valuable in evaluating outcomes (see Figure 23–6).

Strictures in the bowel beyond the ostomy are not usually symptomatic because they do not impede stool flow. Before closing the ostomy, a contrast study of this isolated bowel is done to identify strictures that may cause obstruction and bleeding when the continuity of the bowel is restored.

Short-Bowel Syndrome

The most serious consequence of NEC is short-bowel syndrome (SBS). SBS is defined as an inability to meet the nutritional needs of normal growth and development through the enteral route. The definition is functional rather than being either the percentage of bowel resected or the length of the bowel remaining. In North America, more than one third of SBS cases result from NEC (Georgeson, 1998; Georgeson & Brown, 1998). Normal bowel absorbs nutrients, vitamins, and fluids; produces enzymes and hormones; and recirculates bile. The complications of SBS are the result of disrup-

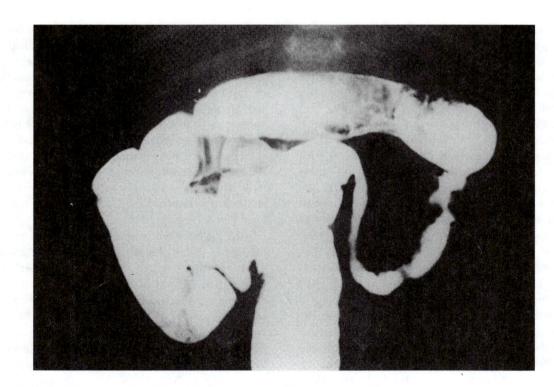

Figure 23–6 Stricture of the Descending Colon at the Splenic Flexure Seen on Barium Enema

tions of these functions. The segment of the bowel resected determines what kind of problems will result because different parts of the bowel have different functions. In NEC, the jejunum, ileum, and cecum are affected most often.

The jejunum has the greatest surface area with long villi, deep crypts between them, and loose junctions between cells. It receives hyperosmotic boluses of food mixed with pancreatic enzymes and bile that cause influxes of fluid into the intestine through the spaces between cells. Most nutrients are also absorbed here. Resection of the jejunum causes malnutrition until the ileum adapts to take over the absorptive function. The ileum reabsorbs fluids secreted into the jejunum; absorbs fat-soluble vitamins, vitamin B_{12}, and bile acids; and secretes the hormones controlling gastric emptying and intestinal transit time. Except for fluid reabsorption, these functions cannot be taken over by other segments of the bowel. If the ileum is resected, fat-soluble and vitamin B_{12} deficiencies result, and gastric emptying and transit time are disordered (Vanderhoof & Langnas, 1997). The ileum also terminates in the ileocecal valve, which controls emptying from the small bowel into the colon and prevents the reflux of bacteria-laden large bowel contents into the ileum. The resection of the ileocecal valve seems to lengthen dependence on parenteral nutrition (Kaufman et al., 1997). Overall, resection of the jejunum is better tolerated than ileal resection. The ileum adapts to increase absorption, while its site-specific functions are not replicable in other bowel segments (Vanderhoof & Langnas, 1997). Resection of the cecum affects water reabsorption and can lead to chronic diarrhea.

Bowel adaptation begins immediately after resection, but it can be months before the enteral route can provide full calories. Survival for infants with SBS increased from 50% to 85% with the advent of total parenteral nutrition (TPN) (Georgeson & Brown, 1998). Prognostic factors for how long a child will remain on TPN and whether he will achieve full enteral feeding are difficult to determine. In a small group of SBS patients, Sondheimer et al. (1998) found that both small bowel length after surgery and the percentage of calories taken enterally at 52 weeks postgestational age were predictive of how long the infants were dependent on TPN. This relationship was essentially linear, with longer small bowel length and a higher percentage of enteral calories varying inversely with length of time on TPN.

In bowel adaptation, villi lengthen and crypts deepen to increase surface area, the bowel dilates and lengthens, and transit time of intestinal contents decreases (Georgeson, 1998). Improvement in nutrient absorption lags behind the increase of surface area (Vanderhoof, 1996). The adaptation process depends on enteral nutrition, and increase of mucosal surface area does not proceed without it. Complex nutrients and long-chain fatty acids appear to be a more powerful stimulant for these adaptive changes than simple sugars and short-chain fats. Formulas high in fats and proteins are preferred because they have a lower osmotic load and cause less diarrhea than those high in carbohydrates. Gastric, pancreatic, and biliary secretions acting directly on the bowel mucosa also stimulate adaptation (Vanderhoof & Langnas, 1997). Therefore, early closure of ostomies and restoration of bowel continuity promote adaptation by providing an uninterrupted route to the bowel mucosa (Georgeson, 1998). Continuous feeding is also beneficial because it keeps the bowel in constant contact with the stimulating nutrients (Vanderhoof & Langnas, 1997). Hormonal secretions such as enteroglucagon, insulin-like growth factor I, and epidermal growth factor are among those being studied to determine their role in adaptation (Georgeson, 1998).

The small intestine is short in the premature infant and nearly doubles its length in the third trimester (Touloukian & Walker-Smith, 1983). Because bowel elongation is also proportional to increase in body length, the capacity for bowel elongation after resection is greatest in the premature infant. As a consequence, premature infants have less time dependent on parenteral nutrition than affected term neonates (Kaufman et al., 1997).

Several surgical interventions may be beneficial in SBS. After resection, the small bowel dilates as its surface area increases during adaptation. This dilation can result in dysmotility, malabsorption, bacterial overgrowth, and sepsis. Children with dilated dysmotile bowel benefit from a tapering enteroplasty in which the bowel is streamlined to increase its functional motility. The intestinal plication achieves the same goal while preserving maximal intestinal surface area. In this procedure a longitudinal fold is made that tapers the bowel by folding the extra tissue inward and stitching the fold along the area where there are no blood vessels (the antimesenteric surface) (Georgeson & Brown, 1998).

Stricture resection for partial small bowel obstruction is important for releasing tight anastomoses, promoting flow of bowel contents, and preventing bacterial overgrowth. Strictures are a common complication of NEC, and the stricturoplasty can improve bowel function substantially (Vanderhoof, 1996).

Bowel dilation also creates extra tissue that can be used in an intestinal doubling (Bianchi) procedure in which the dilated bowel is divided longitudinally into two segments and attached end to end. This improves motility similar to the enteroplasty and increases mucosal surface area over the next 6 to 9 months. Kimura's doubling technique encourages new blood supply for the bowel from the abdominal wall or liver before division of the dilated bowel (Georgeson & Brown, 1998).

Surgical procedures can also decrease intestinal transit time and encourage bowel dilation. In these procedures, intestinal valves are created to slow the progress of enteric contents from one segment to the next. Success requires the right balance of slowing the transit of bowel contents without developing the symptoms of obstruction (Georgeson & Brown, 1998).

Discussion of small intestinal transplantation is beyond the scope of this chapter. See Chapter 31 for a more complete discussion of intestinal transplantation. The outcomes of small bowel transplantation have greatly improved since development of the immunosuppressant drug tacrolimus. Fluid and electrolyte problems and osmotic and secretory diarrhea characterize the postoperative course. Lymphoproliferative disease, sepsis, and cytomegalovirus infections and rejection are also common. Small bowel transplantation is usually performed in conjunction with liver transplantation when TPN-induced cholestatic disease results in liver failure. Success has been limited in small bowel transplant alone (Georgeson, 1998; Vanderhoof, 1996).

There are many complications of SBS beyond malabsorption. Parenteral nutrition–induced liver disease is the most common cause of death from SBS (Vanderhoof, 1996). Liver disease from long-term TPN is frequent, with some degree of cholestasis present in all children on parenteral nutrition. Vanderhoof (1996) reports that an enteral intake of 20% to 30% of calories is effective in preventing liver disease. Gallstones (cholelithiasis) are also common in children on parenteral nutrition. They result from the disordered pathway for bile salt reabsorption and altered bilirubin metabolism. Occasionally, biliary tract disease is silent. A cholecystectomy is recommended when stones are discovered. Renal stone formation from disordered calcium absorption may also occur (Georgeson & Brown, 1998).

Excess secretion of gastric acid caused by overproduction of the hormone gastrin (hypergastrinemia) is the result of a disrupted feedback loop from the small bowel to the stomach. If untreated, gastritis and gastric and duodenal ulcer disease result. Gastric acid production can be managed medically with hydrogen ion and proton pump blocking agents (Vanderhoof, 1996).

Trace mineral and vitamin deficiencies are common once parenteral nutrition is discontinued. Ileal resection predisposes the child to fat-soluble vitamin deficiencies from disordered bile transport and poor fat absorption. Vitamin B_{12} deficiencies also occur because the ileum is the only place where vitamin B_{12} is absorbed. Many trace minerals are poorly absorbed. Routine monitoring of zinc, copper, calcium, magnesium, and iron serum levels is essential in SBS patients. Unexplained skin rashes and hair loss should include trace mineral malabsorption in the differential diagnosis (Vanderhoof, 1996).

Bacterial overgrowth is a major complication in SBS. The motility of the normal small bowel rapidly moves bacteria into the colon. The dilation, dysmotility, and enteral stasis that accompany SBS provide an optimal environment for the growth of bacteria. Feeding regimens that leave undigested nutrients in the bowel provide the nourishment for rapid bacterial growth. Bacterial overgrowth results in enteritis, diarrhea, bacterial translocation with bacteremia, and colonization with unusual organisms such as lactobacilli. Lactobacilli ferment carbohydrate to a product that cannot be metabolized by human cells and causes acidosis and coma (Georgeson, 1998; Georgeson & Brown, 1998). Kaufman et al. (1997) found that bacterial overgrowth and associated inflammation of the enteric tract contribute to prolonged dependence on parenteral nutrition. The treatment of bacterial overgrowth is both medical and surgical. Antibiotics, prokinetic agents that improve bowel motility, adjustment of feeding regimens to decrease nondigested nutrients, and the surgical enteroplasties discussed previously all may play a role (Georgeson & Brown, 1998; Vanderhoof & Langnas, 1997).

Parenteral nutrition requires central venous access, and long-term indwelling catheters have significant management problems. Even with scrupulous care, sepsis and bacteremia are constant threats in children who translocate bacteria across the bowel wall into the bloodstream. Children who are dependent on central catheters for TPN have crises when their catheters occlude, break, become colonized with bacteria, or malfunction. Emboli from clots proximal to the catheter tip may be thrown into the central circulation, and thromboses can occur from partial occlusion of vessels by the catheter itself. Long-term maintenance and care of these catheters is of primary importance to the health of these children (Ryder, 1993).

The nursing care of the SBS child requires expert assessment and intervention. Feeding a baby with diminished absorptive surface requires constant vigilance for evidence of malabsorption as the feedings are advanced. Increasing frequency and volume of stool or a more watery consistency indicate an overload of the bowel's absorptive capacity and potential for dehydration and electrolyte loss. Evaluation of the reducing substances in the stool, a method of monitoring for undigested carbohydrates, is a good objective measure of the degree of carbohydrate malabsorption. If feeding advances are continued in the face of increasing evidence of malabsorption, the intestinal mucosa may be sloughed, resulting in a setback of days or weeks. However, the short bowel increases its surface area substantially over time, and it is important to take advantage of the opportunity to increase enteral feeding. Achieving the balance between malabsorption and adaptation is the art of managing these infants. The nurse's observations and documentation are a vital part of advancing the enteral feedings as safely and rapidly as possible. Helping the parents understand how all these factors interact is an important part of the nursing care of these infants. For further information about the nutritional needs of an infant with NEC refer to Chapter 4.

DEVELOPMENTAL ISSUES

NEC is primarily a disease of the premature infant. An appropriate developmental plan such as the Neonatal Individualized Developmental Care and Assessment Plan (NIDCAP) (Als & Gilkerson, 1995) is important in achieving optimal neurodevelopmental outcomes while enteral problems are being addressed medically and surgically. Appropriate positioning, consistent caregivers, premature skin care, sensitivity to cues for overstimulation, and examination skills using neurodevelopmental guidelines for soothing and calming are important to achieving developmental milestones. Developmental specialists provide the expertise necessary for developing and individualizing plans of care. Neurodevelopmental evaluation should continue at regular intervals through the preschool years to ensure the best outcomes for these children.

Infants who receive nasogastric or gastrostomy feedings and are unable to eat for long periods of time develop an aversion to oral feedings. They lack the practice in coordinating the breathe-suck-swallow sequence that infants need to nipple successfully. The early intervention of a feeding specialist is an important component in the care of these infants.

PLANNING FOR HOME

Many infants with NEC are discharged home with some combination of ostomy care, central venous catheter care, complex feeding regimens, and home parenteral nutrition. While the infant is in the hospital, individualized teaching plans for the parents are crucial. Learning ostomy management, central line care, gavage feeding, or the care of a gastrostomy takes time and commitment on the part of parents and nurses. Other important issues include planning for a backup caregiver, helping siblings respond to a compromised infant, and modifying the home to accommodate equipment and new routines. Intervention by case managers, social workers, primary nurses, and home nurses before discharge is valuable in smoothing the transition from hospital to home.

FUTURE RESEARCH

The cause of NEC is still not known, but the outcome can be a lifetime of chronic bowel, nutrition, and behavior problems. Further research is needed in many areas. The direction of current medical research is to identify the biochemical pathways that lead to NEC in the animal model. In the meantime, many issues of interest to nurses and families remain unstudied. The modification of diet to maximize nutrition, minimize bowel upset, and support normal growth and development in children with NEC has not been fully investigated. Feeding development in NEC children who are not fed orally for long periods of time needs further evaluation. Studies of self-image in children with SBS and ostomies would be a valuable addition to the literature. Studies of the coping behaviors of parents raising a child with a chronic bowel problem would also add information useful in assisting these families. Many opportunities for research exist in physiologic, developmental, and psychosocial areas.

CONCLUSION

Having a child with NEC is a confusing and frightening event for parents. Feeding a child is one of the most basic bonding experiences for a parent. The inability to feed their child may make parents feel inadequate. The multifactorial causes of NEC may engender a parental soul-searching session looking for "what we did wrong." The sense that "you can't do anything but wait and see what happens" once NEC develops also contributes to the feelings of frustration and helplessness. The nurse is a key part of the team providing information and comfort to the parents through this difficult period. A knowledge of what factors are thought to be involved in the development of NEC, an understanding of the diagnostic and therapeutic interventions likely to be used, and a grasp of the actual long-term morbidity from NEC are invaluable in soothing parental fears and helping them understand the realities of their child's situation.

REFERENCES

Als, H., & Gilkerson, L. (1995). Developmentally supportive care in the neonatal intensive care unit. *Zero to Three, 15*(6), 2–10.

Andrews, D.A., Sawin, R.S., Ledbetter, D.J., Schaller, R.T., & Hatch, E.I. (1990). Necrotizing enterocolitis in term neonates. *The American Journal of Surgery, 159*, 507–509.

Ballance, W.A., Dahms, B.B., Shenker, N., & Kleigman, R.M. (1990). Pathology of necrotizing enterocolitis: A ten-year experience. *The Journal of Pediatrics, 117*(1), S6–S13.

Bauer, C.R., Morrison, J.C., & Poole, E.K. (1984). A decreased incidence of necrotizing enterocolitis after prenatal glucocorticoid therapy. *Pediatrics, 73*, 682–688.

Bell, M.J., Ternberg, J.L., & Feigin, R.D. (1978). Neonatal necrotizing enterocolitis: Therapeutic decisions based upon clinical staging. *Annals of Surgery, 187*, 1–7.

Caplan, M.S., & Hsueh, W. (1990). Necrotizing enterocolitis: Role of platelet activating factor endotoxin and tumor necrosis factor. *The Journal of Pediatrics, 117*(1), S47–S51.

Cheu, H.W., Brown, D.R., & Rowe, M.I. (1989). Breath hydrogen excretion as a screening test for the early diagnosis of necrotizing enterocolitis. *American Journal of the Diseases of Childhood, 143*, 156–159.

Foglia, R. (1995). Necrotizing enterocolitis. *Current Problems in Surgery, 32*(9), 759–823.

Ford, H., Watkins, S., Reblock, K., & Rowe, M. (1997). The role of inflammatory cytokines and nitric oxide in the pathogenesis of necrotizing enterocolitis. *Journal of Pediatric Surgery, 32*(2), 275–282.

Georgeson, K. (1998). Short-bowel syndrome. In J.A. O'Neill, M.I. Rowe, J.L. Grosfeld, E.W. Fonkalsrud, & A.G. Coran (Eds), *Pediatric Surgery* (Vol. 2, 5th ed., pp. 1223–1232). St. Louis, MO: Mosby.

Georgeson, K., & Brown, P. (1998). Short bowel syndrome. In M.D. Stringer, K.D. Oldham, P.D. Mouriquand, & E.R. Howard (Eds.), *Pediatric surgery and urology: Long term outcomes* (pp. 237–242). Philadelphia: W.B. Saunders Company.

Goldman, H.I. (1980). Feeding and necrotizing enterocolitis. *American Journal of the Diseases of Childhood, 134*, 553–555.

Han, V.K.M., Sayed, H., Chance, G.W., Brabyn, D.G., & Shaheed, W.A. (1983). An outbreak of *Clostridium difficile* necrotizing enterocolitis: A case for oral vancomycin therapy? *Pediatrics, 71*(6), 935–941.

Hyman, P.E., Clarke, D.D., Everett, S.L., Sonne, B., Stewart, D., Harada, T., Walsh, J.H., & Taylor, I.L. (1985). Gastric acid secretory function in preterm infants. *Journal of Pediatrics, 106*(3), 467–471.

Kaufman, S.S., Loseke, C.A., Lupo, J.V., Young, R.J., Murray, N.D., Pinch, L.W., & Vanderhoof, J.A. (1997). Influence of bacterial overgrowth and intestinal inflammation on duration of parenteral nutrition in children with short bowel syndrome. *The Journal of Pediatrics, 131*, 356–361.

Kien, C.L., Liechty, E.A., & Mullett, M.D. (1990). Effects of lactose intake on nutritional status in premature infants. *The Journal of Pediatrics, 116*, 446–449.

Kleigman, R.M., & Walsh, M.C. (1987). Neonatal necrotizing enterocolitis: Pathogenesis, classification and spectrum of illness. *Current Problems in Pediatrics, 27*, 219–287.

Kosloske, A.M., & Musemeche, C. (1989). Necrotizing enterocolitis of the neonate. *Clinical Perinatology, 16*, 97–111.2.

Lawrence, G., Bates, J., & Gaul, A. (1982, Jan. 16). Pathogenesis of necrotising enterocolitis. *The Lancet*, 137–142.

Lebenthal, E., & Leung, Y.K. (1988). Feeding the premature and compromised infant: Gastrointestinal considerations. *Pediatric Clinics of North America, 35*(2), 215–238.

Lucas, A., & Cole, T.J. (1990). Breast milk and neonatal necrotizing enterocolitis. *Lancet, 336*, 1519–1523.

MacKendrick, W., & Caplan, M. (1993). Necrotizing enterocolitis: New thoughts about pathogenesis and potential treatments. *Pediatric Clinics of North America, 40*(5), 1047–1059.

MacKendrick, W., Caplan, M., & Hsueh, W. (1993). Endogenous nitric oxide protects against platelet-activating factor-induced bowel injury in the rat. *Pediatric Research, 34*(2), 222–228.

Moomjian, A.S., Peckham, G.J., Fox, W.W., Pereira, G.R., & Schaberg, D.A. (1978). Necrotizing enterocolitis: Endemic versus epidemic form [Abstract]. *Pediatric Research, 12*, 530.

Morgan, L.J., Shochat, S.J., & Hartman, G.E. (1994). Peritoneal drainage as primary management of perforated NEC in the very low birthweight infant. *Journal of Pediatric Surgery, 29*, 310–315.

Nowicki, P. (1990). Intestinal ischemia and necrotizing enterocolitis. *The Journal of Pediatrics, 117*(1), S14–S19.

O'Neill, J.A., Stahlman, M.T., & Meng, H.C. (1975). Necrotizing enterocolitis in the newborn: Operative indications. *Annals of Surgery, 182*(3), 274–279.

Rowe, M.E. (1986). Necrotizing enterocolitis. In K.J. Welch, J.G. Randolph, M.M. Ravitch, J.A. O'Neill, & M.I. Rowe (Eds.), *Pediatric surgery* (4th ed., pp. 944–958). Chicago: Year Book Medical Publishers.

Ryder, M.A. (1993). Peripherally inserted central venous catheters. *Nursing Clinics of North America, 28*(4), 937–971.

Schwartz, M.Z., Richardson, J., Hayden, C.K. Swischuk, L.E., & Tyson, K.R.T. (1980). Intestinal stenosis following successful medical management of necrotizing enterocolitis. *Journal of Pediatric Surgery, 15*(6), 890–899.

Sondheimer, J.M., Cadnapaphornchai, M., Sontag, M., & Zerbe, G.O. (1998). Predicting the duration of dependence on parenteral nutrition after neonatal intestinal resection. *The Journal of Pediatrics, 132*(1), 80–84.

Stevenson, D.K., Kerner, J.A., Malachowski, N., & Sunshine, P. (1980). Late morbidity among survivors of necrotizing enterocolitis. *Pediatrics, 66*(6), 925–927.

Tan, C.E.L., Kiely, E.M., Agrawal, M., Brereton, R.J., & Spitz, L. (1989). Neonatal gastrointestinal perforation. *Journal of Pediatric Surgery, 24*(9), 888–892.

Touloukian, R.J., & Walker-Smith, G.J. (1983). Normal intestinal length in preterm infants. *Journal of Pediatric Surgery, 18*, 720–722.

Udall, J.N. (1990). Gastrointestinal host defense and necrotizing enterocolitis. *The Journal of Pediatrics, 117*(1), S33–S43.

Vanderhoof, J.A. (1996). Short bowel syndrome in children and small intestinal transplantation. *Pediatric Clinics of North America, 43*(2), 533–550.

Vanderhoof, J.A., & Langnas, A.N. (1997). Short bowel syndrome in children and adults. *Gastroenterology, 113*, 1767–1778.

Wilson, R., Kanto, W.P., McCarthy, B.J., Burton, T., Lewin, P., Terry, J., & Feldman, R.A. (1981). Epidemiologic characteristics of necrotizing enterocolitis: A population-based study. *American Journal of Epidemiology, 114*(6), 880–887.

Appendix 23–A

Critical Pathway for Necrotizing Enterocolitis

Medical Management	Day of Surgery	Postoperative Day 1–5	Postoperative Day 7	Postoperative Day 8–14	Postoperative Day 15–21
Treatments					
NPO	──				Decrease as feedings increase
NG/OG to suction	────────────────		Remove NG		
Reliable central venous access					
Ventilate to normal arterial blood gases					
Tracheal suction prn		Wean ventilator settings			
Fluid/colloid resuscitation prn		As tolerated			
Correct electrolyte abnormalities					
Replace NG/OG output ml for ml					
Hotbed for temperature instability				Discontinue hotbed if temperature stable	
Total parenteral nutrition 120–150 kcal/kg/day					
GT to gravity if present	────────────────			Use for feedings or clamp	
Replace high ostomy outputs ml for ml		────────────────			
Medications					
Triple intravenous antibiotics with anaerobic and aerobic coverage			Discontinue antibiotics if blood cultures negative		
Diuretics prn transfusions, pulmonary edema					
Mineral supplementation prn prematurity					
Assessment & Monitoring					
Physical examination BID/TID and prn			Physical exams BID		
Constant monitoring of cardiorespiratory O2 saturation, arterial blood pressure, mean arterial pressure, temperature				Discontinue arterial line if off ventilator	
NG/OG output, volume, color					
Stool volume, color, consistency					
Abdominal girth and color					
Ostomy output if present	────────────────				
GT output if present	────────────────				
Consults					
Development specialists					
Occupational therapists for prolonged NPO status					
Social services for family support					
Chaplain if appropriate					
Pediatric surgeons					
			Nutrition		Home Care RN

continues

Appendix 23–A continued

Medical Management	Day of Surgery	Postoperative Day 1–5	Postoperative Day 7	Postoperative Day 8–14	Postoperative Day 15–21
Diagnostics					
Complete blood count with differential		Complete blood count prn instability			
C reactive protein		C reactive protein prn signs/symptoms infection			
Platelet count		Platelet count prn instability			
Serum chemistries		Serum chemistries prn		TPN labs	TPN labs
Hepatic panel per TPN protocol					
Stool Guaiac for occult blood					
Arterial blood gases prn		Arterial blood gases prn ventilator changes			
Peripheral and central blood cultures		Peripheral and central blood cultures if positive	Blood cultures if positive		
Lumbar puncture as indicated		Radiographs prn abdominal change			
Serial abdominal radiographs every 6–24 hours					
Education					
Clinical course of NEC		Begin ostomy teaching			Central line drsg
Developmental guidance for gestational age					
Medical versus surgical management					
Encourage breast pumping	Possible ostomy				
	Prolonged NPO course				
	Possible GT				
Discharge Planning					
Identify primary MD	Ostomy RN if applicable				Formula preparation
Social services for family evaluation					Enteral pumps
Insurance evaluation					Infant care
Referral to supplementary services prn					
Evaluation					
Signs/symptoms of sepsis	Successful resection	Metabolic stability	Stools present	Tolerates ½–1 ml/hr feedings of breast milk or elemental formula	Tolerates feeding advance 1–2 ml per day
Free air in abdomen	Metabolic stability	Soft abdomen	Gains weight		
Portal venous air		No pneumatosis	Tolerates no NG		
Persistent thrombocytopenia					
Penumatosis intestinalis					
Fixed bowel loop on serial radiographs					
Blood in stool					
Increasing NG/OG output					

CHAPTER 24

Malrotation and Volvulus

Tina Shapiro and Jeannette A. Diana-Zerpa

DESCRIPTION

Malrotation is an asymptomatic anatomic variant that occurs as a result of failure to complete normal rotation and fixation of the bowel (Beasley, Hutson, & Auldist, 1996). Malrotation becomes a surgical emergency and a potentially life-threatening situation when the midgut twists or kinks, causing an intestinal obstruction known as volvulus (Kenner, Brueggemeyer, & Gunderson, 1993; Scipien, Barnard, Chard, Howe, & Phillips, 1986). Midgut volvulus may lead to widespread intestinal ischemia and progress rapidly to necrosis of the bowel, perforation, shock, and death if surgical intervention is not initiated emergently. This condition is one of the most serious surgical emergencies seen in the neonate or infant (Smith, 1986).

The incidence of malrotation is difficult to estimate because only 50% of children with complications of the anomaly present with symptoms during the neonatal period (Rowe, O'Neill, Grosfeld, Fonkalsrud, & Coran, 1995). Many of these children remain asymptomatic until adult life when the diagnosis is made. Malrotation occurs twice as often in boys as in girls (Lister, 1990). Most patients with malrotation and midgut volvulus are infants. Thirty percent of these infants present during the first week of life, and 50% to 60% present within the first month of life (Kluth & Lambrecht, 1994).

EMBRYOLOGY

To comprehend the pathophysiology of malrotation and volvulus effectively, one must understand normal embryologic development of the intestinal tract, including normal rotation and fixation of the bowel (Nixon & O'Donnell, 1992). During embryologic life, two important events occur related to intestinal development. These two events, rotation of the duodenojejunal loop and rotation of the cecocolic loop, take place simultaneously but are described here as two separate events (Rowe et al., 1995).

At about the fourth week of embryonic life, the gut begins to change from a straight line structure to an elongated tube herniating into the umbilical cord (Raffensperger, 1990). The upper portion of this elongated structure, the duodenojejunal loop, later develops into duodenum and jejunum. The lower portion, known as the cecocolic loop, later becomes the terminal ileum, cecum and colon (Smith, 1986). The superior mesenteric artery, which provides the blood supply to this portion of the bowel, is the main pivotal point.

During this time, the duodenojejunal loop lies above the superior mesenteric artery (SMA). The loop begins to rotate 90 degrees counterclockwise to the right of the SMA, then another 90 degrees to beneath the SMA. Finally, the loop rotates 90 degrees to the left of the SMA and upward, completing a 270-degree rotation (Figure 24–1). As a result of this rotation, the duodenojejunal junction now lies in the left upper quadrant in an area to be marked by the ligament of Treitz (Rowe et al., 1995).

The cecocolic loop originates beneath the SMA and begins rotation counterclockwise also in 90-degree intervals. The first rotation places this loop to the left of the SMA. Next, the loop rotates 90 degrees above the artery. The last 90-degree rotation of the cecocolic loop is a downward movement to the right of the SMA (Figure 24–2). This completes a 270-degree rotation, making it possible for the cecum to become fixed in the right lower quadrant (Rowe et al., 1995).

Acknowledgments: We thank Marc Diana, Kara McGee, Elizabeth Ruiz, Dr. Malvin Weinberger, and Carlos Zerpa for their generous contributions in helping us complete this chapter.

Duodenojejunal loop

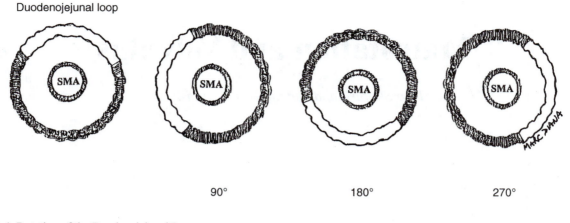

90°   180°   270°

Figure 24–1 Rotation of the Duodenojejunal Loop

With normal rotation completed, the intestines return from the umbilical cord to the abdominal cavity, where fixation begins from the tenth week of gestational life and continues postnatally (Pillitteri, 1987). The normal fixation of the mesentery of the midgut is best illustrated in Figure 24–3.

As illustrated in Figure 24–3, the broad-based mesentery is maintained in position after normal rotation and fixation occur by the ligament of Treitz (Figure 24–3A) and the ileocecal junction (Figure 24–3B). The duodenum becomes securely fixed to the retroperitoneum as the C loop. In addition, the ascending and descending colon are attached retroperitoneally. The bowel is now stabilized by the broad-based mesentery, preventing any twisting or kinking of the intestines from occurring.

The process of rotation and fixation is complex in nature and has been broken down in this text as a series of events. In reality, intestinal rotation is a spectrum with a multitude of stages occurring almost simultaneously (Smith, 1986).

PATHOPHYSIOLOGY OF MALROTATION

Malrotation is a term that describes a number of different rotational errors. The most common of these anomalies occurs with an incomplete rotation of 180 degrees instead of the normal 270-degree rotation. When the previously described normal 270-degree rotation of the bowel is interrupted or deviated, the duodenum lies behind the superior mesenteric artery or fails to cross the midline. The cecum does not reach the right iliac fossa but lies anterior to the duodenum, and adhesions form running from the cecum across the duodenum to the right lateral wall of the abdomen (Figure 24–4). These adhesions, called Ladd's bands, may obstruct the duodenum (Marlow & Redding, 1988).

PATHOPHYSIOLOGY OF MIDGUT VOLVULUS

Midgut volvulus occurs as a complication of the malrotation. Because the intestines are not fixed normally and do not

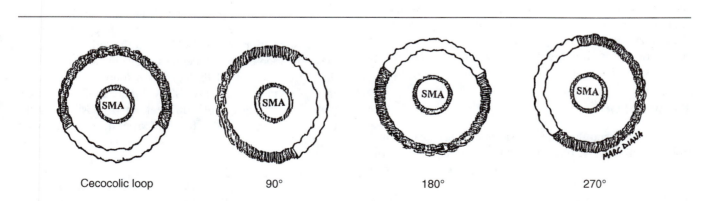

Cecocolic loop   90°   180°   270°

Figure 24–2 Rotation of the Cecocolic Loop

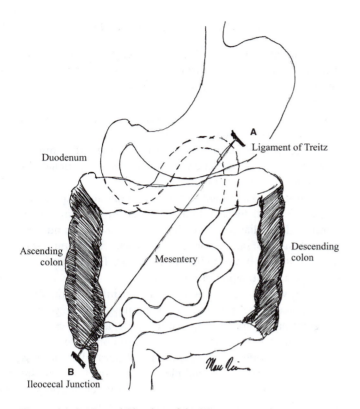

Figure 24–3 Normal Fixation of the Mesentery

may consist of gastric contents but quickly becomes bilious. A well neonate with bilious vomiting should be treated as having a midgut volvulus until proven otherwise. Bilious vomiting indicates high intestinal obstruction. As a result of vomiting, pancreatic gastric secretions and bile are lost, resulting in rapid electrolyte imbalance and dehydration (Kenner et al., 1993).

Initial examination of the abdomen may be normal in 50% of infants, but the clinical picture deteriorates rapidly (Holland, Price, & Lilly, 1993). The infant appears pale and in acute distress with abdominal pain, distention, and grunting respirations. Passage of bloody stools is a late sign and indicative of a gravely ill infant (Holland et al., 1993).

DIFFERENTIAL DIAGNOSIS

The differential diagnosis for midgut volvulus includes sepsis, duodenal atresia, duodenal stenosis, and jejunoileal atresia (Kenner et al., 1993). The possibility of pyloric stenosis may be considered with a healthy infant who suddenly begins to vomit. However, this diagnosis is quickly ruled out when the vomitus becomes bilious. The infant should then be evaluated emergently for malrotation with midgut volvulus.

have a broad-based mesentery, there is a high incidence for twisting of the midgut on its narrow pedicle. Volvulus usually involves a 360-degree or more turn of the intestines on the narrow stalk containing the superior mesenteric vessels. The entire arterial and venous blood supply is contained in this pedicle or stalk. The twisting causes vascular obstruction, and complete necrosis of the midgut develops rapidly (Rowe et al., 1995). Unless immediate diagnosis and surgical treatment are initiated, the necrosis may quickly lead to shock and death (Figure 24–5).

CLINICAL PRESENTATION

Malrotation may present as a chronic problem with asymptomatic periods combined with episodes of abdominal pain and vomiting. The bands across the duodenum may lead to varying degrees of obstruction manifested as recurrent episodes of vomiting. Often children are not diagnosed with malrotation until well into their teens, when chronic symptoms warrant a gastrointestinal workup. Malrotation with midgut volvulus, however, presents with acutely intense symptoms. The typical clinical picture is that of a healthy infant who suddenly begins to vomit. At first, the vomiting

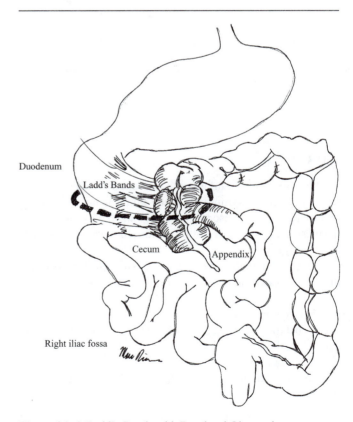

Figure 24–4 Ladd's Bands with Duodenal Obstruction

HISTORY AND PHYSICAL EXAMINATION

The infant or child with malrotation generally appears well. The history obtained from the parents usually describes an infant or child with chronic gastrointestinal upset or sporadic episodes of vomiting.

On physical examination, the infant or child is alert and hydrated. The abdomen is rarely distended because the stomach is decompressed by occasional episodes of vomiting (Raffensperger, 1990). The vomiting is due to duodenal obstruction by Ladd's bands.

The history of an infant with midgut volvulus is quite different. Usually, these infants are seen in the emergency room, at the pediatrician's office, or in the newborn nursery with a history of sudden onset of vomiting. The vomiting is formula at first, but soon becomes bilious. The parents may also report constipation or loose stools.

The physical examination reveals an infant in distress. The infant may be crying intensely, pulling up the legs, having grunting respirations, appear lethargic, and may be pale. Once the midgut becomes ischemic, the abdominal examination reveals evidence of distention and marked tenderness (Beasley et al., 1996). Rectal bleeding or sloughed mucosal tissue per rectum may occur as a result of vascular compromise of the intestines. This is an ominous sign.

The abdomen becomes more tender as the ischemia involves the serosal surface of the bowel and as sequestration of fluid in the abdomen results in peritoneal irritation (Rescorla & Grosfeld, 1991). On rectal examination, stool is usually absent, but if present, is guaiac positive or shows gross blood.

LABORATORY WORK

The following laboratory values should be obtained when evaluating an infant for midgut volvulus:

- complete blood count (CBC)
- type and screen or type and cross-match for packed red blood cells
- electrolytes

Electrolyte imbalance is expected in a child diagnosed with volvulus. A low hemoglobin and hematocrit may be noted as well because of pooling of blood in the intestine. The correction of metabolic abnormalities and any necessary transfusions begin immediately.

RADIOLOGIC DIAGNOSIS

An immediate radiologic evaluation is essential if the infant or child shows clinical signs of acute or chronic intesti-

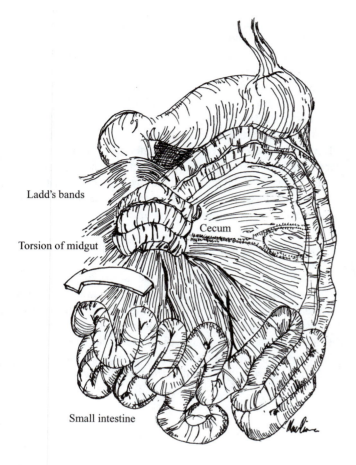

Ladd's bands

Torsion of midgut

Cecum

Small intestine

Figure 24–5 Midgut Volvulus

WORKUP

The workup for an infant with malrotation differs according to severity of symptoms. If the infant is not acutely ill, malrotation may be discovered during an elective upper gastrointestinal (UGI) series to rule out pyloric stenosis or gastroesophageal reflux.

However, if midgut volvulus is suspected, the work-up must be initiated rapidly. The workup should include

- history and physical examination
- Stat laboratory values with placement of intravenous (IV) access
- IV hydration
- Stat flat and upright plain radiographic films of the abdomen
- Stat UGI series

nal obstruction. Initially, flat and upright plain abdominal radiographic films are sufficient. Plain abdominal radiographic findings may include any of the following: a normal or nonspecific gas pattern, duodenal obstruction, gastric distention with mild duodenal dilation, or generalized distention of small bowel loops (Ford, Senac, Srikanth, & Weitzman, 1992).

Infants with clinical findings suggestive of impending bowel necrosis such as bloody emesis and stools, abdominal tenderness, dehydration, and lethargy, in addition to plain films revealing duodenal obstruction, require immediate operation. No further radiologic studies are necessary (Smith, 1986).

If the diagnosis is in doubt and compromised bowel is not evident, a contrast study may be helpful. A UGI series is usually preferred rather than a barium enema (BE) (Seashore & Touloukian, 1994). A UGI series evaluates the position of the ligament of Treitz, which is normally located to the left of the spine, thereby providing a broad base for the mesentery (see Figure 24–3). A barium enema evaluates the position of the cecum and colon. (Kluth & Lambrecht, 1994). Infants with a floppy or mobile cecum, which does not appear in the right iliac fossa on BE, do not necessarily have malrotation.

Findings on UGI in the child with malrotation include

- abnormal position of the ligament of Treitz, which is normally located on the left side of the spine
- partial obstruction of the duodenum, with a spiral or corkscrew appearance
- proximal jejunum in the right abdomen (Kluth & Lambrecht, 1994)

When volvulus is present, the barium column is noted to end with a peculiar beaking effect (Figure 24–6). The beaking appearance is pathognomonic of a volvulus and is caused by twisting of the bowel into a sharp point resembling the beak of a bird (Kenner et al., 1993). Distally, if visualized, the mucosal folds of the jejunum may be thickened as a result of mucosal edema (Rowe et al., 1995).

Ultrasonography, a noninvasive study, may also be valuable in the diagnosis of malrotation. An abnormal relationship of the superior mesenteric vein (SMV) to the SMA is diagnostic of malrotation. As the SMV wraps around the SMA, a whirlpool sign is formed, evident on color Doppler ultrasonography. The ultrasonogram is diagnostic of midgut volvulus when the whirlpool sign has a clockwise direction (Shinanuki et al., 1996).

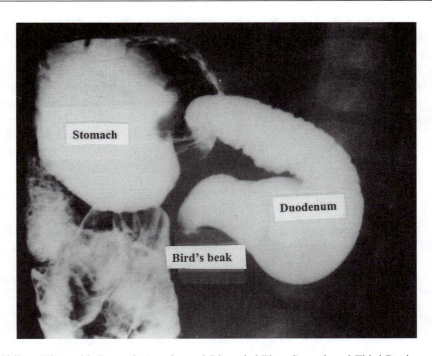

Figure 24–6 Lateral Oblique View with Stomach Anterior and Distended First, Second, and Third Portions of the Duodenum. Note the abrupt narrowing or "beaking" effect.

TREATMENT AND OPERATIVE CONSIDERATIONS

Children with symptomatic malrotation undergo immediate surgery to avoid bowel necrosis. In the asymptomatic patient, elective surgery may be indicated to avoid the risk of volvulus. Parents should be provided with precautionary instructions to return immediately to the hospital if the infant becomes symptomatic. Nearly 75% of all cases of malrotation are complicated by volvulus (Kenner et al., 1993). Therefore, some pediatric surgeons choose to operate on all children diagnosed with malrotation, regardless of symptoms.

The treatment of malrotation, based on the description by Ladd (1936), includes

- laparotomy, with reduction of midgut volvulus, if present
- division of peritoneal bands obstructing the duodenum (Figure 24–7)

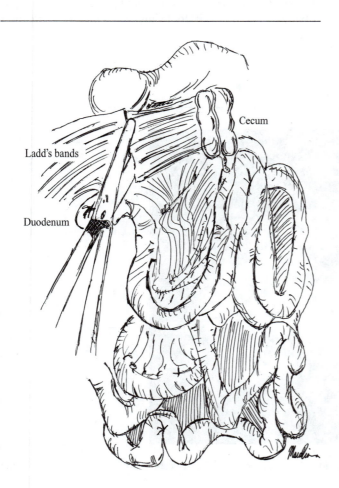

Figure 24–7 Division of Ladd's Bands

- placement of the small and large bowel in a state of nonrotation or wide disassociation of the duodenojejunal junction and cecum (Figure 24–8)
- appendectomy

A diagnostic and therapeutic dilemma for the surgeon is the patient with vague abdominal complaints and an intestinal contrast study that indicates an intestinal rotational abnormality (Mazziotti, Strasberg, & Langer, 1997). A laparoscopic approach to these children with suspected malrotation or volvulus may be useful. The advantage of this procedure in a child with chronic abdominal symptoms is that laparoscopy may diagnose and allow correction of the intestinal obstruction with possibly a lessened morbidity (Mazziotti et al., 1997).

SURGICAL PROCEDURE

After fluid resuscitation, the patient is emergently taken to the operating room. Laparotomy is performed through a supraumbilical transverse incision. Volvulus occurs in a clockwise manner. Therefore, the bowel is detorsed in a counterclockwise direction (Rescorla & Grosfeld, 1991). After detorsion, the bowel is evaluated for viability. If the bowel turns pink and appears viable, a Ladd's procedure is performed. This involves releasing all duodenal and duodenojejunal bands. The entire cecum and ascending colon are mobilized and moved to the left side of the abdomen. This procedure relieves the existing obstruction and also minimizes the chance of a recurrent volvulus by spreading out the base of the mesentery (Figure 24–9). The main goal of the Ladd's procedure is preservation of maximal length of intestine. In addition, because of the abnormal position of the appendix in the left lower abdomen after the Ladd's procedure, most surgeons remove the appendix.

If no question of viability of the intestine exists, the Ladd's procedure is carried out as described previously. However, if the viability of the bowel is questioned, three events are possibly encountered:

1. A short segment of bowel is necrotic and the remaining intestine seems healthy. The necrotic bowel is resected and an anastomosis is performed, preserving maximal length of intestines as the goal.
2. A short portion of intestine is obviously necrotic, but after resection, varying lengths of proximal and distal bowel appear compromised. In this case, both ends of bowel may be brought to the skin as stomas. After 24 to 48 hours, reexploration and resection of further necrotic intestine is performed if the stoma ends still appear necrotic.
3. A large segment of the small bowel seems questionable, or regions of both necrotic and viable intestine

ther compromise the bowel and result in short-gut syndrome (Smith, 1986).

Particular care must be given to the parents of the infant at this time, especially before emergency surgery. All procedures should be explained to the parents by the surgeon, with reinforcement of explanations by the pediatric surgical nurse. Social services may be contacted to provide additional family support during this crisis.

POSTOPERATIVE NURSING MANAGEMENT

Postoperative care of the infant with midgut volvulus is similar to that of any infant undergoing intestinal surgery. Principles of fluid and electrolyte management, bowel decompression, and pain relief are instituted. Fluid and electrolyte balance must be carefully monitored. Adequate urine output of 1 ml/kg of body weight per hour is measured by weighing the infant's diapers on a gram scale.

A nasogastric tube (NG) is inserted, placed to low suction, and left intact until bowel function returns. NG output is monitored and recorded every 4 hours. The tube is kept patent by flushing with 5 to 10 ml of normal saline every 2 hours. Skin breakdown from NG pressure on the nares is

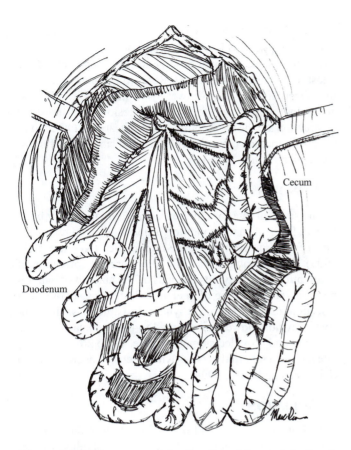

Figure 24–8 Placement of the Small and Large Intestine in Nonrotation

are noted. The bowel is then put back into the peritoneal cavity without resection. A second operation is performed 24 hours later, the bowel reassessed, and if necrotic bowel is present, resection is done (Rowe et al., 1995).

PREOPERATIVE NURSING MANAGEMENT

Once the diagnosis of malrotation is made, antibiotic or cleansing preparation of the bowel is not necessary. The correction of metabolic abnormalities must immediately begin. IV fluids are administered to correct hypovolemia. All preparations must be initiated quickly when volvulus is considered because bowel necrosis can develop rapidly and involve the whole small bowel and half of the large intestine (Rowe et al., 1995).

The child receives broad-spectrum IV antibiotics because bacteria may be translocated through the necrotic bowel wall. A nasogastric tube is inserted and placed to suction to decompress the gastrointestinal tract. Delaying the surgery for complete resuscitation is avoided because this may fur-

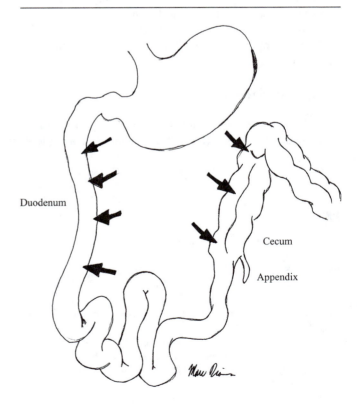

Figure 24–9 Spreading the Mesentery with Disassociation of the Cecum and Duodenum

avoided by applying a clear, adhesive dressing on the infant's cheek to secure the NG tube. Abdominal girth is measured and bowel sounds are auscultated every 2 to 4 hours.

Postoperative pain relief is achieved by administering IV morphine every 2 hours as necessary. The infant's vital signs are monitored continuously by cardiorespiratory and oxygen saturation monitors while receiving morphine. Tylenol suppositories may also be administered for pain or fever.

Parents of the infant should be informed about all aspects of their infant's care. Encouraging early handling of the infant after surgery is beneficial to both parent and infant. Rocking and holding are nonpharmacologic comfort measures to be used along with analgesics.

As soon as bowel function returns, feedings are started. Appropriate formula and amounts are ordered depending on the extent of the surgery. Feedings are usually advanced as tolerated. If a large portion of necrotic bowel was removed leaving an infant with short-gut syndrome, a gastrostomy feeding tube (GT) is placed at the time of operation. Initial feedings through the GT usually are started with very dilute elemental formula in small amounts. The volume and then the concentration are gradually increased until full-strength formula can be tolerated. This feeding progression is a tedious process, with many interruptions and delays in progression. The delays are usually frustrating to the parents. In addition, parenteral nutrition may be necessary in the case of short-gut syndrome until the intestine has had an opportunity to recover and grow (Kenner et al., 1993).

Refer to Appendix 24–A for a caremap for pre- and postoperative care.

COMPLICATIONS

Early postoperative complications include wound infection, pneumonia, sepsis (rare), anastomotic leak, and bleeding (Spigland, Brandt, & Yazbeck, 1990). A serious postoperative complication is short-bowel syndrome, which occurs as a result of the removal of large necrotic segments of the intestine (Kenner et al., 1993). Refer to Chapter 23 for further discussion of short-bowel syndrome. As in all intra-abdominal surgery, postoperative adhesions and intestinal obstruction are the most common complications. Other complications include recurrent volvulus and small bowel intussusception (Smith, 1986).

PROGNOSIS

The survival rate for children with malrotation may be as high as 92% when the condition is uncomplicated by infarction of the bowel or associated anomalies (Kenner et al., 1993). The outcome for a child after surgical correction of malrotation with volvulus depends on the amount of gangrenous bowel at the time of operation. Extensive small bowel resection results in short-gut syndrome. Children with extensive nonviable bowel are returned to the neonatal intensive care unit and provided supportive care. Up to 20% mortality rate has been reported in cases with extensive necrotic bowel (Kluth & Lambrecht, 1994).

CONCLUSION

Malrotation is the result of an aberration in the complex embryologic development of the GI tract. Volvulus is a life-threatening complication of malrotation. Astute nursing assessment to identify infants who are not tolerating feedings is critical in the early identification of malrotation and volvulus. In general, infants with malrotation have a good prognosis. The prognosis for children with volvulus is variable, depending on the amount, if any, of damage to the intestine. Ongoing nursing care includes support and education to the family.

REFERENCES

Beasley, S.W., Hutson, J.M., & Auldist, A.W. (1996). *Essential pediatric surgery*. London: Arnold.

Ford, E.G., Senac, M.O., Srikanth, M.S., & Weitzman, J.J. (1992). Malrotation of the intestine in children. *Annals of Surgery, 215*(2), 172–178.

Holland, R.M., Price, F.N., & Lilly, J.R. (1993). Pediatric surgery. In G.B. Merenstein & S.L. Gardner (Eds.), *Handbook of neonatal intensive care* (p. 478). St. Louis, MO: Mosby.

Kenner, C., Brueggemeyer, A., & Gunderson, L.P. (1993). *Comprehensive neonatal nursing*. Philadelphia: W.B. Saunders Company.

Kluth, D., & Lambrecht, W. (1994). Disorders of intestinal rotation. In N.V. Freeman, D.M. Burge, M. Griffiths, & P.S.J. Malone (Eds.), *Surgery of the newborn* (pp. 201–209). Edinburgh: Churchill Livingstone.

Ladd, W.E. (1936). Surgical diseases of the alimentary tract in infants. *New England Journal of Medicine, 215,* 705–708.

Lister, J. (1990). Neonatal surgery. In J. Lister & I.M. Ihring (Eds.), *Malrotation and volvulus of the intestine* (pp. 442–452). Oxford: Butterworth-Heinemann.

Marlow, D.R., & Redding, B.A. (Eds.). (1988). *Textbook of pediatric nursing*. Philadelphia: W.B. Saunders Company.

Mazziotti, M.V., Strasberg, S.M., & Langer, J.C. (1997). Intestinal rotation abnormalities without volvulus: The role of laparoscopy. *Journal of the American College of Surgeons, 185,* 172–176.

Nixon, H., & O'Donnell, B. (Eds.) (1992). *Essentials of pediatric surgery*. Oxford: Butterworth-Heinemann.

Pillitteri, A. (1987). *Child health nursing*. Boston: Little, Brown and Company.

Raffensperger, J.G. (Ed.). (1990). *Swenson's pediatric surgery*. Norwalk, CT: Appleton & Lange.

Rescorla, F.J., & Grosfeld, J.L. (1991). Common problems in pediatric surgery. In J.L. Grosfeld (Ed.), *Malrotation with midgut volvulus* (pp. 84–91). St. Louis, MO: Mosby.

Rowe, M.I., O'Neill, J.A., Jr., Grosfeld, J.L., Fonkalsrud, E.W., & Coran, A.G. (1995). *Essentials of pediatric surgery.* St. Louis, MO: Mosby.

Scipien, G.M., Barnard, M.U., Chard, M.A., Howe, J., & Phillips, P.J. (Eds.). (1986). *Comprehensive pediatric nursing.* New York: McGraw-Hill.

Seashore, J.H., & Touloukian, R.J. (1994). Midgut volvulus: An ever-present threat. *Archives of Pediatric and Adolescent Medicine, 148,* 43–46.

Shinanuki, Y., Aihara, T., Takano, H., Moritano, T., Oguma, E., Kuroki, H., Shibata, A., Nozawa, K., Ohkawara, K., Hirata, A., & Imaizumi, S. (1996). Clockwise whirlpool sign at color doppler US: An objective and definitive sign of midgut volvulus. *Radiology, 199*(1), 261–264.

Smith, E.I. (1986). Malrotation of the intestine. In K.J. Welch, J.G. Randolph, M.M. Ravitch, J.A. O'Neill, Jr., & M.I. Rowe (Eds.), *Pediatric surgery* (pp. 882–895). Chicago: Year Book Medical Publishers.

Spigland, N., Brandt, M.L., & Yazbeck, S. (1990). Malrotation presenting beyond the neonatal period. *Journal of Pediatric Surgery, 25*(11), 1139–1142.

Appendix 24–A

Caremap for Volvulus/Malrotation (Symptomatic)

	Preoperative	Operating Room	Postoperative Day 1	Postoperative Day 2	Postoperative Day 3	Postoperative Day 4
Monitor/assess	VS q4h Consent for surgery Social work screening		VS q2–4h Monitor urine output (1 ml/kg/hr) D/C dressing, Steri-strips dry & intact Assess incision Measure abdominal girth q4h Second look surgery if necessary			
Meds	Ancef 50 mg/kg/IV Preop meds per anesthesia		Tylenol 10–15 mg/kg/dose PRN for T>101F or pain Morphine IV 0.1 mg/kg/dose q2h PRN pain Ancef 50 mg/kg/IV (depending on surgical findings)			
Activity			OOB in parents' arms Ambulate ad lib			
Diet	NPO		NPO	NPO until bowel function returns Start TPN if delay in PO feeding is expected	Begin elemental diet when bowel function returns	
Tests	CBC Type and screen Electrolytes UGI		CBC Electrolytes			CBC Electrolytes if patient still NPO
Consults	Anesthesia		Nutrition		GI for short-gut syndrome	

	Preoperative	Operating Room	Postoperative Day 1	Postoperative Day 2	Postoperative Day 3	Postoperative Day 4
Treatments	IV fluid bolus LR 20 ml/kg over 1 hr IV maintenance fluids Transfusion if necessary Electrolyte replacement if necessary		OOB Ambulate ad lib Flush NGT with 5–10 ml NS q4h & PRN		Decrease IV rate when tolerating PO feedings	
Lines/drains	Peripheral IV NGT to low intermittent suction	Broviac if necessary GT if necessary	Replace NGT losses ml/ml q4h		DC NGT when bowel function returns	Heplock IV if tolerating PO feedings
Patient/family teaching	Explanation of diagnosis with need for emergency surgery		Explanation of all tubes, lines, meds, and treat- ments			
Discharge planning			Depends on extent of surgery			
Outcomes	Electrolytes corrected? Yes __ No __ Orientation to unit initiated? Yes __ No __ Family version of path shared? Yes __ No __ Child life assessment completed? Yes __ No __ Discharge needs assessed? Yes __ No __		Abdominal dressing dry and intact? Yes __ No __	Abdominal dressing removed? Yes __ No __ Incision clean and dry? Yes __ No __	NGT D/C'd? Yes __ No __	Feedings started? Yes __ No __

CHAPTER 25

Hypertrophic Pyloric Stenosis

Joanna Joyce Morganelli

Hypertrophic pyloric stenosis (HPS) is a common surgical disorder in infancy that produces nonbilious emesis as its hallmark symptom (Rowe, O'Neill, Grosfeld, Fonkalsrud, & Coran, 1995). Classically the disease presents itself at approximately 2 to 3 weeks of age with nonbilious vomiting that may be described as forceful or projectile. In patients with HPS, the emesis is clear without a green or straw-colored appearance. This emesis usually appears as stale, curdled milk. It may also have a coffee-ground appearance that is associated with bleeding from a proximal gastritis (Dudgeon, 1993). The projectile nature of the vomiting is described as being forcefully ejected from 1 to 4 feet from the child. The emesis is more projectile when the infant is in a sidelying position. The vomiting occurs within 30 to 60 minutes of feeding. Most infants with HPS experience vomiting in small amounts at about 2 weeks of life because of partial obstruction, and as the disease progresses, nearly complete obstruction develops by the second to fourth week of life (Rowe et al., 1995).

PATHOPHYSIOLOGY

HPS is defined as an acquired condition in which the circumferential muscle of the pyloric sphincter becomes thickened, resulting in elongation and obliteration of the pyloric channel. This process produces a high-grade, gastric outlet obstruction, with compensatory dilation, hypertrophy, and hyperperistalsis of the stomach (Magnuson & Schwartz, 1997). HPS has been reviewed and its clinical features and pathology discussed by many. In the nineteenth century Dr. Hirschsprung described two cases of HPS that established it as a discrete clinical entity. The first successful surgical treatment of HPS was performed by Dr. Lobker in 1898, using a gastrojejunostomy. In 1911, Dr. Ramstedt developed and

described the pyloromyotomy that remains the standard surgical procedure today for treatment of HPS (Dudgeon, 1993).

EMBRYOLOGY

The cause of HPS has long been debated. In Ireland in 1987, sonographic studies were obtained on 1,400 newborns to determine whether HPS is acquired rather than congenital. These studies confirmed that pyloric muscle hypertrophy visualized on ultrasonography is not present in the early newborn period of infants who later developed infantile HPS. This suggests that HPS is an acquired disease (Rollins, Shields, Quinn, & Wooldridge, 1989).

Multiple theories of etiology include immature or degenerated pyloric neural elements, variations of infant feeding regimens, and excess production of gastrin in either mother or infant (Dudgeon, 1993; Rowe et al., 1995). Other hypotheses include a theory of dyscoordination between gastric peristaltic activity and pyloric relaxation, causing inappropriate pyloric contraction in the face of elevated intragastric pressures. This results in work-related hypertrophy of the pyloric muscle, initiating a cycle of increasing pyloric obstruction and gastric contractions (Magnuson & Schwartz, 1997). Recent theories of abnormalities in the enteric nervous system and abnormalities in the distribution of neuropeptides and neurotransmitters have also been reviewed (Magnuson & Schwartz, 1997). Hypotheses exist exploring involvement of a reduction in the neuronal nitric oxide synthase in the hypertrophic circular layer of the pylorus, suggesting that nitric oxide is a potent inhibitory neurotransmitter that induces relaxation of smooth muscle. Therefore, absence of the enzyme producing nitric oxide implies that the gastric outlet obstruction of HPS might be related to a defect of pyloric relaxation (Vanderwinden et al., 1996).

INCIDENCE

The incidence of HPS ranges from 0.1% to 1% in the general population. HPS has a significant male predominance of 4:1. Its incidence varies with ethnic origin, being more predominant in Caucasians and encountered less often in infants of Asian or Indian descent (Magnuson & Schwartz, 1997; Rowe et al., 1995).

The development of HPS also appears to involve the variable transmission of an inheritable trait between generations, with the transmission of the trait more common from mothers than from fathers (Magnuson & Schwartz, 1997).

PRESENTATION

HPS most commonly is seen in full-term male infants, at approximately 3 to 6 weeks of age. Initial symptoms may begin as early as 2 to 3 weeks of life. Parents describe an infant previously well, who starts with episodes of vomiting. Initially, the infant may intermittently regurgitate after a feeding. However, as the pyloric obstruction increases, the vomiting occurs with every feeding. This emesis is described as progressive, projectile, and nonbilious. Commonly the infant appears ravenous and eager to eat immediately after the previous episode of emesis (Dudgeon, 1993). Some infants may appear well on presentation, depending on where they are in the course of their illness. However, infants who are symptomatic for several days before diagnosis may have weight loss, slight jaundice, and significant dehydration, and appear quite ill. On clinical examination, palpation of the hypertrophied pylorus is diagnostic.

DIFFERENTIAL DIAGNOSIS

Many differential diagnoses are considered in the initial examination of an infant who is vomiting, including feeding intolerance, milk allergy, overfeeding, and gastroesophageal reflux. Other disease entities such as pylorospasm, gastroesophageal reflux, primary gastric atony, salt-wasting adrenogenital syndrome, central nervous system lesions with increased intracranial pressures, gastric antral web, pyloric atresia, pyloric duplication cyst, ectopic pyloric pancreas, and pancreatic adenomas may also be considered in the differential diagnosis (Dudgeon, 1993). It is the persistent, forceful, and progressive nature of the nonbilious emesis, the abrupt onset of the disease in a previously healthy infant, and the degree of illness that the child presents with that usually lead to the consideration of hypertrophic pyloric stenosis as the leading diagnosis.

PHYSICAL EXAMINATION

On physical examination the infant may or may not appear acutely ill and dehydrated. Other clinical manifestations include projectile vomiting, weight loss, and persistent hunger despite the recent emesis. Palpation of a small oval mass, olive-like in nature, in the midepigastrium usually is diagnostic of pyloric stenosis. Most clinicians believe that if this "olive-like" mass may unequivocally be palpated in the midepigastrium, no further diagnostic studies are indicated. However, palpation of this mass is not always possible. It should be attempted when the infant is not crying and the abdominal muscles are relaxed. Having the stomach empty during palpation such as after an episode of emesis or nasogastric decompression is helpful on clinical examination. The practitioner should elevate or gently bend the infant's knees or move the infant's lower extremities while the infant is sucking on a pacifier or bottle. This technique promotes increased abdominal muscle relaxation (Rowe et el., 1995). Palpation begins just over the spine and above the umbilicus. Two or three fingers are pressed lightly into the deeper tissues in a sweeping motion superiorly to inferiorly. The pyloric olive is found to be smooth, hard, and oblong, usually about 1 to 2 cm long. Another technique that aids in the diagnosis of HPS is observing feeding.

Peristaltic waves that move across the infant's abdomen from left to right just before emesis may be observed. This provides an opportunity to assess the forcefulness and character of the emesis.

SERUM LABORATORY WORK

Serum laboratory work in an infant with HPS may demonstrate hypochloremia and hypocalcemia with a metabolic alkalosis, hypoglycemia, and an elevated unconjugated hyperbilirubinemia (Magnuson & Schwartz, 1997). Persistent vomiting results in loss of fluid and hydrochloric acid from the stomach. The gastric mucosa that produces hydrochloric acid is lost through vomitus, but the bicarbonate continues to enter the blood and is not buffered by the hydrogen equivalent. This causes a metabolic alkalosis. The hypokalemia results from the distal renal tubules responding to the renin-aldosterone system. This process promotes the excretion of potassium and hydrogen in exchange for sodium. This continues to exacerbate the metabolic alkalosis by producing hypokalemia and increasing distal bicarbonate reabsorption associated with hydrogen ion secretion. The hyperbilirubinemia is associated with a decrease in hepatic glucuronyltransferase activity (Siegel, Carpenter, & Gaudio, 1994).

RADIOLOGY

HPS can be clinically diagnosed easily by a skilled clinician. In most cases radiologic confirmation of HPS is not required. However, both contrast studies and ultrasonography can aid in the diagnosis of HPS. Contrast studies such as an upper gastrointestinal series are favored by some surgeons who believe they are more cost-effective than ultrasonography because they may demonstrate many other disease entities (Hulka, Campbell, Harrison, & Campbell, 1997a). Upper gastrointestinal contrast studies can diagnose gastroesophageal reflux, pylorospasm, and delayed gastric emptying. An upper gastrointestinal tract study is diagnostic of HPS by demonstrating an elongated and narrowed pyloric channel, an enlarged stomach, and minimal transit of contrast through the pylorus. This is commonly referred to as the "string sign," defining one narrow channel, or a "railroad track sign," defining two narrow channels. Other characteristic findings on upper gastrointestinal studies include visualization of the "shoulders" of the hypertrophied pylorus bulging into the gastric lumen (Rowe et al., 1995). Refer to Figure 25–1 for a visual description of these characteristic findings.

Some criticize the use of upper gastrointestinal studies compared with ultrasonographic studies in diagnosing HPS because upper gastrointestinal contrast studies expose an infant to ionizing radiation. There is also the risk of aspiration of gastrointestinal contents and barium if the infant undergoes surgery with general anesthesia (Dudgeon, 1993). In 1977, ultrasonography was used in making the diagnosis of HPS, and today it is favored by many as a reliable, inexpensive, noninvasive diagnostic study in evaluation of HPS (Rollins et al., 1989). The abdominal ultrasonogram measures the length and diameter of the pyloric muscle. An overall diameter of 17 mm or more, muscular wall thickness of 4 mm or more, and a channel length of 17 mm or more confirms the diagnosis of HPS with ultrasonography. In infants who are less than 30 days of age, smaller measurements are

used as the criteria for the diagnosis of HPS (Magnuson & Schwartz, 1997).

Godbole, Sprigg, Dickson, and Lin (1996) compared ultrasonography with clinical examination in diagnosing HPS. Their findings indicated that ultrasonographic study was useful in cases in which the clinical examination was negative. However, it was not necessary if an experienced clinician was able to palpate the hypertrophied pylorus (Godbole et al., 1996).

RECOMMENDED THERAPY

Recommended therapy for HPS is surgical intervention. Preoperative preparation of the infant with HPS is critical because most of these infants experience significant electrolyte abnormalities that place them at risk when undergoing a surgical procedure with general anesthesia. Surgical correction of HPS is not an emergency. A child can be stabilized and managed easily by having nothing by mouth and rehydrated with intravenous solutions. The infant who has no signs of dehydration, normal glucose and electrolytes, and excellent urine output can proceed to surgery as soon as possible. However, the infant who is significantly dehydrated with electrolyte imbalances and a metabolic alkalosis needs aggressive preoperative fluid resuscitation. This may require 24 to 48 hours. The infant should have normal serum chloride, potassium, and bicarbonate levels, as well as normal vital signs and good urine output, suggesting adequate fluid

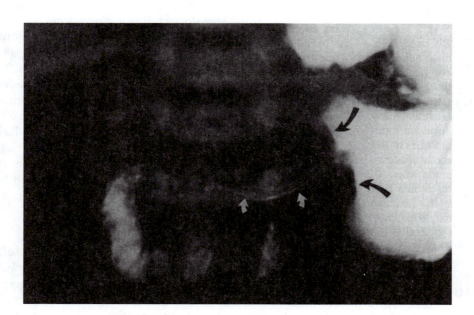

Figure 25–1 Upper Gastrointestinal Tract Contrast Study Findings in HPS, Displaying the "String Sign" of a Stenotic Channel Lumen (*white arrows*) and the Bulging Shoulders of the Hypertrophic Pyloric Muscle (*black arrows*)

repletion, before proceeding to surgery (Magnuson & Schwartz, 1997).

OPERATIVE CONSIDERATIONS/SURGICAL PROCEDURE

The surgical treatment most commonly used in infants with HPS is the Rammstedt pyloromyotomy (Greason, Thompson, Downey, & Sasso, 1995). The most common surgical approach used when performing a pyloromyotomy is to enter the peritoneal cavity through a transverse incision in the right upper quadrant over the rectus muscle at or above the liver edge (Garcia & Randolph, 1990; Rowe et al., 1995). The pyloromyotomy is commenced where the pylorus is thickest and its fibers most easily split. A longitudinal incision is made down to the mucosa, splitting the hypertrophied muscle (Magnuson & Schwartz, 1997). Refer to the illustration shown in Figure 25–2, which demonstrates the operative technique of pyloromyotomy.

During the pyloromyotomy extreme care is taken to avoid gastric mucosal tears because duodenal perforations are a potential complication in infants with HPS (Hulka, Harrison, Campbell, & Campbell, 1997b; Poon, Zhang, Cartmill, & Cass, 1996). If a gastric mucosal tear is recognized, it can be repaired without associated morbidity or compromise to the pyloromytomy. However, if a mucosal tear is not recognized during the surgery, it can be associated postoperatively with complications such as peritonitis. This increases the infant's overall risk of morbidity (Magnuson & Schwartz, 1997). Postoperatively, the nasogastric tube is removed as soon as the infant awakens from anesthesia unless the duodenal mucosa was perforated. In this case the nasogastric tube should

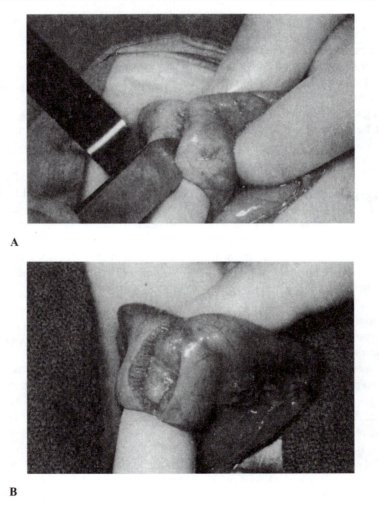

A

B

Figure 25–2 Operative Technique of Pyloromyotomy. A, The pyloric muscle is split longitudinally with the blunt end of a scalpel handle. B, Completed myotomy allows the submucosal layer to bulge out to the level of the serosa.

remain for an additional 24 to 48 hours to ensure gastric decompression (Rowe et al., 1995).

Another surgical option used recently in infants with HPS is laparoscopic pyloromyotomy. Greason et al. (1995) reported on a case series of 11 infants with HPS comparing open pyloromyotomy with the laparoscopic approach. The findings indicated laparoscopic surgery to be equally safe and effective with superior cosmetic results. Surgical times or postoperative time until feedings were initiated were not significantly different. Although these authors recognized that the open pyloromyotomy is the most consistently successful operation ever described, they are supportive of the idea that laparoscopic pyloromyotomy is an excellent alternative procedure in the management of HPS (Greason et al., 1995).

Complications associated with pyloromyotomy are rare. Children treated for HPS using a standard surgical procedure by an experienced pediatric surgeon, with expert anesthesia, and appropriate preoperative resuscitation have minimal risk of mortality (Magnuson & Schwartz, 1997). However, rare postoperative complications can occur. These include duodenal perforation, wound infections, and postoperative vomiting. Most infants experience some postoperative vomiting. This is not considered a true complication unless it exceeds 48 hours (Hulka et al., 1997b). If persistent vomiting continues for greater than 2 weeks and a contrast study has been performed to rule out a gastric leak or fluid collection obstructing the gastric outlet, a presumptive diagnosis of incomplete myotomy should be considered (Magnuson & Schwartz, 1997).

DEVELOPMENTAL CONSIDERATIONS

Developmental concerns foremost in the nurse's mind in caring for the infant and parents of the infant with HPS include caring for a newborn infant and his or her family, with the added psychological stresses of a hospitalization and impending surgery. Infants are first seen with HPS anywhere from 2 to 4 weeks of age; that is just enough time for parents to begin to establish some routine with their newborn child at home. They are recovering from the birth process and now are confronted with multiple new issues and adjustments. These might include sleep deprivation, fatigue, learning to breastfeed, sibling rivalry, and possibly entertaining family and friends who are admiring their infant. This family is already stressed to some degree. A social service consultation may be indicated and supportive for many of these families.

Many parents may feel that they have caused their infant to be sick in some way, possibly by overfeeding their infant, by giving the wrong formula, or by not choosing to breastfeed. Other parents may feel guilt knowing there is a hereditary link to HPS. Nevertheless, this family and infant need intense support and encouragement. These parents may

have an extremely high anxiety level. Therefore, information may need to be reinforced repeatedly. Specific data should be shared with them to help decrease their anxieties, for example, the prognosis in infants with pyloric stenosis and how long the procedure takes and what they can expect perioperatively.

Separation, interrupted bonding, and not feeding a hungry infant are concerns that many parents experience preoperatively. In some cases the infant may still be allowed to feed small amounts of dextrose water or breast milk until a few hours before surgery. This may help to console the infant. Mothers who breastfeed should be encouraged to pump, save their breast milk, and have skin-to-skin contact with their infant because this may be very consoling. Parents should be advised of the time anticipated before the child will proceed to surgery. Parental education should also involve the need to correct the infant's dehydration and electrolyte abnormalities before surgery. Postoperatively, parents need to be educated that many infants will continue to intermittently vomit for a few feedings, and may continue to do so for a few days. This is normal and expected. If this is not reinforced, parents may have heightened anxiety that the pyloromyotomy did not cure their infant.

SPECIAL SERVICES/REFERRALS/DISCHARGE NEEDS

Once the child is ready to be discharged, follow-up appointments should be arranged with the infant's primary care provider and pediatric surgeon. A discharge summary and operative note are forwarded to the infant's primary care provider. The family should be educated to recognize specific signs and symptoms of infection. Parents should be instructed to call for fever, persistent emesis, abdominal pain demonstrated by persistent crying, tenderness to touch, the infant pulling the legs up, lethargy, decreased urine or stool output, wound drainage or redness, and any other concern or question that arises.

PREOPERATIVE AND POSTOPERATIVE NURSING CONSIDERATIONS

Preoperative nursing considerations in caring for the child with HPS include obtaining an accurate nursing assessment of the infant and family on admission. Family supports, family dynamics, and recent stresses should be discussed. Admission time is crucial for the nurse to establish a therapeutic relationship with the family and to assess and educate the parents. Other key assessments should include the onset of the symptoms in the infant and a description of the vomiting. Vital signs and accurate intake and output should be recorded, including last wet diaper and stool pattern, weight before illness, and current weight. The patient should have blood chemistry studies done, including sodium, potassium, chloride, carbon dioxide, glucose, blood, urea and nitrogen, and creatinine levels. Bilirubin levels may also need to be evaluated. Other preoperative laboratory tests, such as prothrombin time, partial thromboplastin time, and complete blood count with platelets, are sometimes assessed as well. If the patient is extremely ill and dehydrated, specific tests may be ordered to assess the infant's acid base balance, such as arterial blood gases, since these children can have metabolic alkalosis develop. Invasive procedures during admission include starting intravenous fluids and drawing blood, and may include placing a nasogastric tube.

Routine postoperative care includes frequent assessments of the infant's vital signs and pain, assessments of the infant's dressing for bleeding or drainage, and accurate assessment of intake and output. If the infant is having difficulty advancing on feedings and the abdomen is full and distended, abdominal girth measurements can be used. Refer to the critical pathway in Appendix 25–A for a multidisciplinary approach to managing the child with pyloric stenosis.

An example of a current feeding regimen for postoperative pyloromyotomies is to primarily maintain a "nothing by mouth" status for 6 hours postoperatively. Then sugar water solution is fed, 30 ml every 2 hours for two feedings; then half-strength formula, 30 ml every 2 hours for two feedings; then full-strength formula, 45 ml every 2 hours for two feedings; then formula, 60 ml every 3 hours for two feedings; then formula ad lib every 4 hours. If the infant is breastfed, breast milk is substituted for formula and the above regimen is followed. To help the breastfed infant successfully resume breastfeeding, consider allowing the infant to go directly to the breast. Two effective means of quantifying the volume of breast milk consumed by the breastfeeding infant are the utilization of a supplemental nursing system and the utilization of a breastfeeding scale. A supplemental nursing system allows the clinician to offer an approximate volume of breast milk to be administered at the mother's breast while the infant nurses. A breastfeeding scale is also helpful by accurately assessing the infant's pre- and postbreastfeeding weight, thus allowing a fairly accurate cal-

culation of volume intake. Postoperative vomiting is common during the initiation of feedings. If vomiting occurs with feedings, the feeding is held for 2 hours and then the regimen is reinitiated. Intravenous fluids may be infused and tapered accordingly as the infant tolerates the feeding regimen (Adzick et al., 1998).

Georgeson, Corbin, Griffen, and Breaux (1993) retrospectively reviewed feeding regimens of 223 infants who underwent pyloromyotomy for HPS. They concluded that delaying feedings overnight or advancing feedings slowly every 4 hours did decrease the incidence and amount of postoperative vomiting. However, the authors were supportive of initiation of feedings 6 hours postoperatively and advancing feedings every 2 hours. They suspected that the latter feeding regimen increased the incidence of postoperative vomiting. However, it did not delay the eventual tolerance for ad lib feedings. This feeding regimen was not associated with any increased incidence of postoperative complications, and it lessened the overall hospital stay and decreased hospital charges.

Once the infant tolerates the feeding regimen and appears well, the infant can be prepared for discharge. The nurse should review anticipated pain management, signs and symptoms of infection, the current feeding regimen, plans for progression, and adequate urine and stool outputs. The nurse should remind the parents that intermittent emesis is normal postoperatively. If persistent emesis occurs with every feeding, the parents should be instructed to call their primary care provider and the pediatric surgeon. The infant and family should follow up with their primary care provider within a few days from discharge and the pediatric surgical team within 1 to 2 weeks after discharge.

CONCLUSION

Infants diagnosed with HPS have an excellent prognosis. Nursing care focuses on the management of fluid and electrolytes and on education and support to the parents. Although some vomiting does occur postoperatively, most infants achieve normal feeding patterns and good weight gain by their first postoperative visit. Parents can then begin to focus on the normal growth and development of their infant.

REFERENCES

Adzick, N.S., Wilson, J.M., Caty, M.G., Fishman, S.J., Saenz, N.C., Jennings, R.W., Buchmiller, T.L., & DiFiore, J.W. (1998). *Department of surgery's house officer's manual* (10th ed.). Boston: Children's Hospital.

Dudgeon, D.L. (1993). Lesions of the stomach. In K. Ashcraft & T. Holder (Eds.), *Pediatric surgery* (pp. 289–304). Philadelphia: W.B. Saunders Company.

Garcia, G.F., & Randolph, J.G. (1990). Pyloric stenosis: Diagnosis and management. *Pediatrics in Review, 11*(10), 292–295.

Georgeson, K.E., Corbin, T.J., Griffen, J.W., & Breaux, C.W. (1993). An analysis of feeding regimens after pyloromyotomy for hypertrophic pyloric stenosis. *Journal of Pediatric Surgery, 28*(11),1478–1480.

Godbole, P., Sprigg, A., Dickson, J.A.S., & Lin, P.C. (1996). Ultrasound compared with clinical examination in infantile hypertrophic pyloric stenosis. *Archives of Disease in Childhood, 75*, 335–337.

Greason, K.L., Thompson, W.R., Downey, E.C., & Sasso, B.L. (1995). Laparoscopic pyloromyotomy for infantile hypertrophic pyloric stenosis: Report of 11 cases. *Journal of Pediatric Surgery, 30*(11), 1171–1574.

Hulka, F., Campbell, J.R., Harrison, M.W., & Campbell, T.J. (1997a). Cost-effectiveness in diagnosing infantile hypertrophic pyloric stenosis. *Journal of Pediatric Surgery, 32*(11), 1604–1608.

Hulka, F., Harrison, M.W., Campbell, T.J., & Campbell, J.R. (1997b). Complications of pyloromyotomy for infantile hypertrophic pyloric stenosis. *The American Journal of Surgery, 173*, 450–452.

Magnuson, D.K., & Schwartz, M.Z. (1997). Acquired abnormalities of the stomach and duodenum. In K.T. Oldham, P.M. Colombani, & R.P. Foglia (Eds.), *Surgery of infants and children* (pp. 1152–1156). Philadelphia: Lippincott-Raven Publishers.

Poon, T., Zhang, A., Cartmill, T., & Cass, D. (1996). Changing patterns of diagnosis and treatment of infantile hypertrophic pyloric stenosis: A clinical audit of 303 patients. *Journal of Pediatric Surgery, 31*(12), 1611–1615.

Rollins, M.C., Shields, M.D., Quinn, R., & Wooldridge, M. (1989). Pyloric stenosis: Congenital or acquired? *Archives of Disease in Childhood, 64,* 138–139.

Rowe, M., O'Neill, J., Grosfeld, J., Fonkalsrud, E., & Coran, A. (1995). *Essentials of pediatric surgery* (pp. 481–485). St. Louis, MO: Mosby.

Siegel, N., Carpenter, T., & Gaudio, K. (1994). The pathophysiology of body fluids. In F. Oski, C. DeAngelis, R. Feigin, J. McMillan, & J. Warshaw (Eds.), *Principles and practice of pediatrics* (p. 74). Philadelphia: Lippincott-Raven Publishers.

Vanderwinden, J., Liu, H., Menu, R., Conreur, J.L., De Laet, M.H., & Vanderhaeghen, J.J. (1996). The pathology of infantile hypertrophic pyloric stenosis after healing. *Journal of Pediatric Surgery, 32*(11), 1530–1537.

Appendix 25–A

Critical Pathway for Pyloric Stenosis

	Preoperative	*Operating Room*	*POD 1*	*POD 2*
Treatments	1. IV Placement 2. D51/4 w/10KCL/ 500 @ maint. after electrolytes evaluated 3. May need additional fluid 1– 1½ maint. or NS boluses, 20 ml/kg PRN. 4. Nasogastric tube to low wall suction, PRN	1. Comfort measures	1. IV @ maint. 2. NPO X 6 hr postop. 3. Initiate PO feeds 6 hr postop. Begin with 30 ml D5w Q2 X2, then 1/2 str form. or breast milk 30 ml Q2 X2, then full-strength form. or B.M. 45 ml Q2 X2, then FS form. or B.M. 60 ml Q3 X2, then ad lib feeds Q 4 hr. 4. Decrease IV or heploc as tolerates feedings	1. Cont. feeding regimen, until reaches goal 2. Discharge home if reaches feeding goals
Medications	1. Preoperative antibiotics on call to OR	1. Intraoperative antibiotics	1. Postoperative antibiotics and acetaminophen PRN	1. Acetaminophen q4h and PRN
Assessment/ monitoring	1. Admission nursing assessment 2. Vital signs q4h and PRN 3. Check nasogastric tube output q4h 4. Accurate input and output 5. Admission weight	1. Continuous anesthesia and nursing assessment 2. Vital signs and O_2 saturation 3. Check wound for signs & symptoms of bleeding 4. Assess dressing clean, dry & intact	1. Vital signs q4h and PRN, with continuous O_2 saturation 2. Assess NGT if in place q4h, keep to low wall suction 3. Check dressing clean, dry, & intact 4. Strict input and output 5. Discharge weight	1. Vital signs q4h and PRN 2. If NGT present, d/c as able 3. Strict input and output 4. Discharge weight
Consults	1. Social service referral 2. Anesthesia consult 3. Other consult services if indicated (if child with preexisting illnesses or concerns)		1. Continuing care team PRN for anticipated discharge needs	1. Continuing care team, PRN for anticipated discharge needs

continues

Courtesy of Johns Hopkins Hospital, Baltimore, Maryland.

Appendix 25–A continued

	Preoperative	Operating Room	POD 1	POD 2
Tests	1. Check electrolytes, glucose, BUN, creat., CBC w/plts., PT/PTT, and PRN bilirubins. Repeat labs PRN. Type and screen PRN. 2. Ultrasound or upper gastrointestinal study if indicated	1. PRN		
Education	1. Orient to unit 2. Discuss preop, intraoperative & postop care w/ family	1. Cont. to reinforce teaching regarding HPS	1. Cont. to reinforce teaching, review signs and symptoms of infection, bleeding, feeding tolerance, expect occasional emesis, abdominal tenderness, wound care, pain management and who to call if parents have concerns	1. Cont. to reinforce teaching
D/C Planning	1. Assess anticipated D/C needs	1. Continue discharge planning	1. Assess readiness of infant/parents to be D/C'd 2. Assess D/C needs 3. Follow-up call to PCP review hospital course, feeding tolerance, discharge weight and any concerns 4. Implement D/C supports PRN 5. Make F/U appt. w/ surgical team and PCP	1. Assess readiness of infant/parents to be D/C'd 2. Implement previously stated discharge plans from POD 1
Evaluation outcomes	1. Electrolytes within normal limits Yes __ No __ 2. Orientation to unit Yes __ No __ 3. HPS pre, intra, postoperative course reviewed Yes __ No __ 4. Social services screen Yes __ No __ 5. Discharge needs assessed Standard __ Complex __	1. Electrolytes within normal limits Yes __ No __ 2. Abdominal dressing clean, dry, and intact Yes __ No __	1. Tolerating advancement of feedings Yes __ No __ 2. Abdominal dressing clean, dry, and intact Yes __ No __ 3. Vital signs stable and afebrile Yes __ No __ 4. Family demonstrates comprehension of all teaching Yes __ No __ 5. Family comfortable with anticipated discharge Yes __ No __	

CHAPTER 26

Intussusception

Lynn Fagerman and Margaret Meyer

INTRODUCTION

Intussusception is the invagination or telescoping of one intestinal segment into another adjacent segment of bowel, which creates a mechanical obstruction. Although this can occur at any age, it is most common in children less than 3 years old, with the greatest incidence between 5 and 10 months of age (Sherman & Consentino, 1993). The incidence of intussusception in the United States is 1.5 to 4 cases per 1,000 live births, with males more frequently affected (Sherman & Consentino, 1993). Without prompt medical attention and accurate diagnosis, intestinal perforation and bowel death can occur, creating significant morbidity. Because of the age of the child, an explanation of symptoms and discomfort may be mistaken for a benign illness. Intussusception should be high on the list of differential diagnoses when children, especially less than 1 year of age, are seen with sudden onset of abdominal pain.

The cause of intussusception falls into one of three categories: idiopathic, lead point, or postoperative. The idiopathic type has no readily identifiable cause, although it is the most common type (Sty, Wells, Starshak, & Gregg, 1992). Lead point is so named because an identifiable change in the intestinal mucosa can be discovered, usually during surgical treatment for intussusception. Postoperative intussusception is not common but can occur after operative procedures involving the abdomen or even the chest.

PATHOPHYSIOLOGY

The most common segment of bowel involved in intussusception is the ileocecal region. When small bowel (ileum) and the attached mesentery, lymphatic tissue, and blood vessels invaginate into the large bowel (cecum), the folding over

of intestines and vessels impedes normal blood flow to the tissues (Raffensperger, 1990). This leads to further swelling, which in turn decreases blood flow further. If not recognized and treated, bowel death occurs and may involve significant portions of intestine.

Although there is no readily identifiable cause of idiopathic intussusception, it is not uncommon to obtain a history of recent upper respiratory or gastrointestinal illness. It is hypothesized that viral infection leads to hypertrophy of Peyer's patches, a type of lymphoid tissue in the intestinal wall, creating a slightly thickened segment, thereby encouraging invagination to occur (Rowe, 1995). Idiopathic intussusception is the most common form seen in infants.

Lead point intussusception is the form more commonly found in children who are older than 2 to 3 years of age (Stevenson & Ziegler, 1993). It is estimated that between 2% and 8% of all intussusceptions in infants are due to a recognizable malformation in the intestinal mucosa (Rowe, 1995). For all age groups the list of malformations includes polyps, cysts, tumors, Meckel's diverticulum, and hematomas, which can occur in Henoch-Schönlein purpura, all of which create points where invagination and subsequent telescoping of bowel can occur. Children with cystic fibrosis and the characteristic changes in the bowel secondary to thick inspissated stool and mucus are also at risk for lead point–type intussusception (Rowe, 1995).

Intussusception after surgical procedures in the abdomen or chest is thought to be due to the disordered motility that can occur after receiving general anesthesia or as a result of direct handling of intestinal tissue. Intussusception may also occur after placement of long tubes for decompression or direct feedings into the bowel (Rowe, 1995). Bowel obstruction, of which intussusception is one type, should be considered if there is an increase in nasogastric drainage 2 to 5 days postoperatively, rather than the usual decrease in such output seen in the postoperative period.

CLINICAL PRESENTATION

The typical clinical scenario is that of a usually healthy, well-nourished, and active child in later infancy who experiences a sudden onset of abdominal pain, which may also create a change in behavior. The child is seen drawing up his or her legs to the abdomen as if experiencing colicky pain and may not like being held or moved. This episode may occur in waves, with periods of rest in between. Initially, the child has no change in appetite but eventually becomes anorectic and may have vomiting that progresses to a bilious color. The child becomes increasingly more irritable and lethargic as the bowel becomes more compromised. Some children pass stools consisting of sloughed mucosa that have a dark red color with a mucoid consistency. These have been termed "currant jelly" stools, which, although a classic sign of intussusception, are also a later appearing sign and indicates damage to the intestines (Stevenson & Ziegler, 1993).

The picture of an infant who is irritable yet lethargic, with decreased appetite and vomiting, and who seems to be in pain when the body is moved creates a confusing picture for many examiners. It is not unusual for such children to be evaluated for possible pneumonia, sepsis, or meningitis first.

PHYSICAL EXAMINATION

The physical examination of the child varies depending on when in the course of the intussusception the child presents. Young children whose critical condition is less obvious to parents may be brought to medical attention late, at which time they have dehydration, lethargy, shock, or even coma. One study found only one third of patients have the classic symptoms of colicky pain, vomiting, and bloody stools (Chung et al., 1994).

As the course progresses, the abdomen changes from soft to tender and distended. Between episodes of pain, with the child relaxed, it may be possible to palpate a sausage-shaped mass in the mid to upper right abdomen. The lower right quadrant is empty. Palpation may be difficult because of the child's irritability. If the abdomen is auscultated during a crisis, hyperperistaltic rushes (borborygmi) may be heard. There are decreased or absent bowel sounds with significant ileus or peritonitis. Hematochezia (maroon-colored stool) is not always present. The rectal examination is significant if there is bloody mucus on the examiner's fingertip. Sixty percent to 90% of children have gross or occult blood on rectal examination, 20% to 50% have passed mucoid bloody stools, and the remaining have occult blood on testing (Losek & Fiete, 1991).

Vital signs are normal early in the course, but as abdominal distention and vomiting continue, with loss of fluid and bacteremia, the child becomes tachycardic, hypotensive, and may have a temperature elevation. If fever is significant, the examiner must check for an extra-abdominal source. Specifically, pneumonia should be considered. The groin should be palpated for incarcerated hernia or torsion of the testicle or ovary as other possible sources of sudden onset of abdominal pain (Stevenson & Ziegler, 1993).

LABORATORY STUDIES

Initial studies of the child should include complete blood count, electrolytes, and urinalysis. The white blood cell count is often elevated because of necrotic tissue and inflammation. Electrolyte imbalances should be expected if the child is acidotic or dehydrated from vomiting (Losek & Fiete, 1991). Urine output may be low (less than 0.5 to 1.0 ml/kg/hr), with an elevated specific gravity in the dehydrated child as well.

RADIOGRAPHS

Radiologic techniques may not only be diagnostic but therapeutic as well. After a thorough physical examination, supine and upright abdominal series may be ordered. If the intussusception is very early in the course, these may be relatively normal. With progression, a more obvious pattern of small bowel obstruction with absence of gas in the colon is found (refer to Figure 26–1). The finding of a right upper quadrant soft tissue density is helpful in predicting intussusception (refer to Figure 26–2). If these radiographic findings of bowel obstruction are seen and are consistent with the history and physical examination, an air or barium enema is attempted if no intraperitoneal air has been detected (Sty et al., 1992). If intraperitoneal air is found, this indicates that intestinal perforation has occurred, and emergency surgery is indicated.

Before the enema, intravenous access should be obtained to administer fluids, sedation, pain relief, and in some cases antibiotics. A nasogastric tube may also be placed for gastric decompression. The child should be well hydrated and stable before any radiologic reduction attempts.

The barium enema has long been considered the most reliable diagnostic technique for an ileocolic intussusception and was the accepted treatment for most children. The air enema is now being widely used and is considered safer and as effective in diagnosing and reducing an intussusception. Because of the risk of perforation a surgeon should be present during the barium enema. A noninflatable rectal tube is inserted into the rectum, and the buttocks are taped together. Contrast enters the rectosigmoid by gravity under

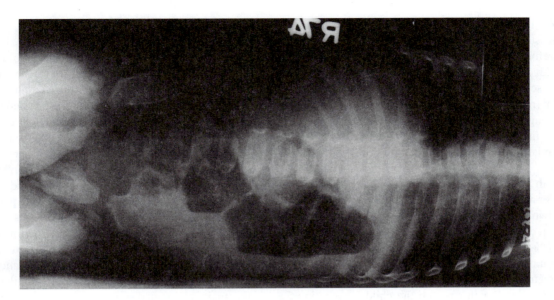

Figure 26–1 Lateral Decubitus Radiograph Showing Absence of Air in Ascending Colon

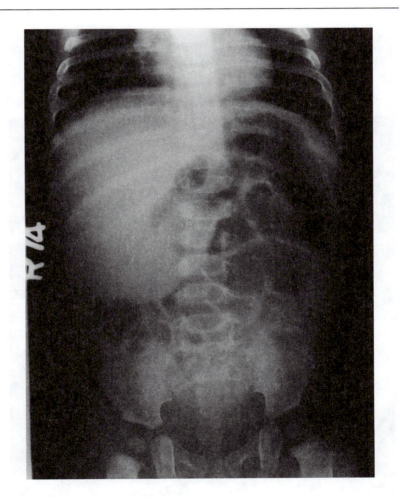

Figure 26–2 Upright Radiograph Showing Right Upper Quadrant Mass

fluoroscopic guidance. If air is used, it is delivered under constant pressure. The pressure instilled during the reduction must be carefully controlled, regardless of the material used, to avoid inadvertent perforation. Commonly, a concave filling defect is seen in the transverse colon that can be reduced to the cecum (refer to Figure 26–3). As the intussusceptum is reduced through the ileocecal valve, contrast or air should reflux freely into the small intestine; this radiographic finding is essential to document a successful reduction. If the first enema is not successful, a second or third attempt may be made with periods of waiting while the child evacuates the barium or air. Usually, the intussusception is reduced after one or two attempts (Doody, 1997). Success rates with hydrostatic reduction have been reported to range between 70% and 90% of cases (Menor, Cortina, Marco, & Olague, 1992). The most common complication after radiologic reduction is recurrence of intussusception, which occurs soon after the reduction. For this reason the child is sometimes admitted to the hospital for 24 hours of observation. Most children are able to tolerate a liquid diet and are discharged from the hospital within that period.

SURGICAL TREATMENT

Immediate surgery is indicated if barium or air reduction fails or in children who have clinical evidence of peritonitis or bowel perforation on radiographic examination. A transverse right lower quadrant incision is made and the intussusception is brought out into the wound. Gentle and continuous massage from the distal to proximal end usually results in manual reduction of the intussusception (Shorter, 1990). Resection and end-to-end anastomosis are performed if manual reduction cannot be accomplished or if the reduced bowel is gangrenous or perforated. Resection is also performed if a specific lead point is found. Often during these surgical procedures an incidental appendectomy is performed. Postoperative complications are rare except in those cases in which the child is in shock or when a significant amount of dead bowel is present. The complications are similar to those of other major abdominal surgeries, including wound infection, abscess formation, and pneumonia (see Appendix 26–A).

Recurrence rates of intussusception are lower if surgical reduction was performed, ranging between 1% and 4% in

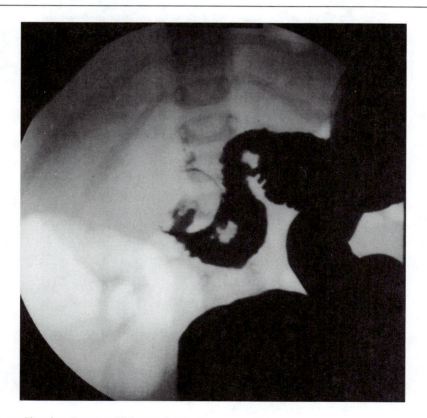

Figure 26–3 Contrast Enema Showing Concave Filling Defect in Transverse Colon

contrast to enema reduction, which averages approximately 10% recurrence. Recurrences usually develop within days after the enema procedure and longer after operative reduction (Stringer, Pablot, & Bereton, 1992). With all recurrences an underlying abnormality should be considered such as is found in lead point–type intussusception.

DEVELOPMENTAL CONSIDERATIONS

Intussusception is primarily a condition that occurs in infants and toddlers. During this time, the infant is in a period of rapid psychosocial and cognitive development. The period of infancy corresponds to Erikson's stage of basic trust versus mistrust (Erikson, 1963). Brazleton (1984) characterizes the infant as having a variety of individual differences or temperaments, ranging from quiet to active to difficult. This at times may affect how examiners interpret symptoms in the young child.

The developmental work of the infant is to acquire a sense of trust in the world by having physical and emotional needs met by competent caregivers. Once this is accomplished, the toddler strives for autonomy by adventuring out further into the world as physical and mental abilities increase (Erikson, 1963). If the treatment for intussusception involves a long hospitalization, painful procedures, and withholding of food, these developmental processes may be interrupted for a period of time.

Beginning around 6 months of age through the preschool years, the predominant fear for children is separation from their usual care provider, known more commonly as separation anxiety. During this time, it is important for the child to have consistent caregivers and to minimize separation from the primary caregiver, which is extremely stressful for young children. Allowing favorite toys or blankets to be in bed with the child or to accompany them to procedures is comforting. Children younger than 24 to 28 months are not capable of verbally expressing their fears or fully remembering fearful situations in the way that older children with developed language capabilities do (Terr, 1988). Infants and toddlers will use play to act out fears that may develop as a result of the invasive procedures (Terr, 1981). Some children have regression in behavior and skills.

INDICATIONS FOR REFERRAL

Anticipatory guidance with parents of hospitalized children can prevent long-term adverse reactions to invasive procedures and separation. Most children with intussusception requiring surgical treatment resume their healthy preoperative status fairly quickly. On postoperative follow-up the child should have resumed the former eating pattern and be gaining weight. If the child lost a significant amount of

bowel when a resection was performed, special nutritional supplementation may be required for a time. These cases, although rare in occurrence, often benefit from monitoring by a visiting nurse agency until the family is comfortable with any special care needs.

RESEARCH

The cause of intussusception remains vague, even for those children with lead point–type intussusception. For example, most children who have upper respiratory viruses, gastrointestinal illnesses, or even a Meckel's diverticulum do not have intussusception develop. Research and epidemiologic studies should continue to search for those commonalities in children with intussusception, which may help primary care providers to provide anticipatory guidance to families with young children.

NURSING CONSIDERATIONS

Nursing care of the child with intussusception includes strict attention to maintaining intravenous fluids, nasogastric decompression of the stomach at low intermittent suction, and frequent assessment of hydration status by observation of strict intake and output records. Vital signs are also monitored closely, both before and after treatment of the intussusception, being mindful of the changes seen in young children with fluid volume deficit or shock. Age-appropriate pain assessment tools should be used to aid in the decision making regarding administration of ordered pain medications. Nonpharmacologic pain relief techniques are useful as adjunctive therapy, as well as possibly decreasing the need for frequent use of pain medications.

Attention to the psychosocial care of the child and family is an equally important role for the nurse. Separation between the child and the primary support person(s) should be minimized and may be accomplished by facilitating rooming in. The child should be allowed to keep a transitional object, such as a favorite blanket or toy at all times. Family caregivers should be encouraged to bring in the child's own pajamas, slippers, and clothes if hospitalized. Explanations should be offered to the family at their level of understanding, and new situations should be explained to decrease anxiety and promote comfort for the child. The child should be provided with play opportunities as appropriate because play is necessary to their well-being. Assigning the same nursing personnel as much as possible will provide continuity of care and decrease the number of strangers that come into contact with the child. Painful procedures should be performed in a treatment room whenever possible, thereby maintaining the concept of the child's bed or room as a safe haven.

DISCHARGE INSTRUCTIONS

After a radiologic reduction, parents should be instructed to return with the child to a medical facility again if signs such as vomiting, abdominal pain, or bloody stools return. If surgical treatment was necessary, the family should be instructed in the signs and symptoms of wound infection: fever, redness, swelling, or drainage from the incision, as well as symptoms of recurrence of the intussusception. The incidence of recurrence ranges from 5% to 7% regardless of the type of treatment undertaken (Rowe, 1995).

CONCLUSION

Intussusception is a serious mechanical bowel obstruction most commonly seen in young children less than 3 years of age. The symptoms may mimic other more frequently occurring illnesses in young children, which may hamper and delay the diagnostic process. Barium or air contrast enemas may be both diagnostic and therapeutic interventions. Intussusception must be diagnosed and treated quickly to prevent bowel ischemia and necrosis, which may lead to significant morbidity for the child.

REFERENCES

Brazelton, T.B. (1984). *Neonatal behavior assessment scale* (2nd ed.). Philadelphia: Lippincott-Raven.

Chung, J.L., Kong, M.S., Lin, J.N., Wang, K.L., Lou, C.C., & Wong, H.F. (1994). Intussusception in infants and children: Risk factors leading to surgical reduction. *Journal of Formosan Medical Association, 93*(6), 481–485.

Doody, D. (1997). Intussusception. In K.T. Oldham, P.M. Colombani, & R.P. Foglia (Eds.), *Surgery of infants and children*. Philadelphia: Lippincott-Raven.

Erikson, E.H. (1963). *Childhood and society.* New York: W.W. Norton & Company.

Losek, J.D., & Fiete, R.I. (1991). Intussusception and the diagnostic value of testing stool for occult blood. *American Journal of Emergency Medicine, 9*(1), 1–3.

Menor, F., Cortina, H., Marco, A., & Olague, R. (1992). Effectiveness of pneumatic reduction of ileocolic intussusception in children. *Gastrointestinal Radiology, 17,* 339–343.

Raffensperger, J.G. (1990). Intussusception. In *Swenson's pediatric surgery* (5th ed., pp. 224–226). Stamford, CT: Appleton & Lange.

Rowe, M.I. (1995). *Essentials in pediatric surgery* (pp. 542–544). St. Louis, MO: Mosby.

Sherman, J.O., & Consentino, C.M. (1993). Intussusception. In K.M. Ashcraft & T.M. Holder (Eds.), *Pediatric surgery* (2nd ed.). Philadelphia: W.B. Saunders Company.

Shorter, N.A. (1990). Intussusception. In P.F. Nora (Ed.), *Operative surgery*. Philadelphia: W.B. Saunders Company.

Stevenson, R., & Ziegler, MZ. (1993). Abdominal pain unrelated to trauma. *Pediatrics in Review, 14*(8), 302–311.

Stringer, M.D., Pablot, S.M., & Bereton, R.J. (1992). Intussusception. *British Journal of Surgery, 79,* 867–876.

Sty, J., Wells, R., Starshak, R., & Gregg, D. (1992). *Diagnostic imaging of infants and children* (Vol. 1). Gaithersburg, MD: Aspen Publishers.

Terr, L. (1981). Forbidden games: Post-traumatic child's play. *Journal of the American Academy of Child Psychiatry, 20,* 740–759.

Terr, L. (1988). What happens to the early memories of trauma? A study of 20 children under age five at the time of documented traumatic events. *American Journal of Child and Adolescent Psychiatry, 27,* 96–104.

Appendix 26–A

Caremap for Intussusception

	ED/Clinic	Radiology	OR	POD 1	POD 2
Treatments	NPO IVF (bolus fluid) Weight	NPO IVF	NPO IVF Reduction of intussusception	NGT output IVF CR monitor	Advance to DAT Hep cap IV
Medications		Broad-spectrum antibiotics Sedation	Continue broad-spectrum antibiotics then dc antibiotics postoperatively	Broad-spectrum antibiotics x 7 days with bowel compromise Pain medication	Broad-spectrum antibiotics dc'd if bowel is viable Pain medication
Assess and monitor	Strict I & O Lab tests Vital signs Pain intensity Abdominal distention Stools for frequency and blood Hydration status	Strict I & O Radiographs Vital signs Pain intensity Abdominal distention Hydration status	Strict I & O Vital signs Bowel viability and perfusion Hydration status	Strict I & O Urine/NGT output Vital signs Pain intensity Abdomen: auscultate, palpate, percuss, observe Stools/flatus Hydration status Wound: signs and symptoms of infection	Abdomen: auscultate, palpate, percuss, observe Stools/flatus Hydration status Wound
Consults	MSW PRN Radiology	Anesthesia	Anesthesia		
Tests	CBC, electrolytes	Barium/air enema			
Education	Radiology procedure Disease process Recurrence rate	Operative procedure and complications Recurrence rate		Postoperative course	Signs and symptoms of recurrence Wound care Signs and symptoms of wound infection
Discharge planning		Signs and symptoms of recurrence Follow-up visit			Pain control Nutrition Follow-up visit

continues

Appendix 26–A continued

	ED/Clinic	Radiology	OR	POD 1	POD 2
Outcomes					Temp <38° for 12 hrs Yes __ No __ ↓ abd pain Yes __ No __ 1 stool c̄ no blood Yes __ No __ Reg diet and no vomiting Yes __ No __ Parents state s/s of recurrence of intussusception Yes __ No __

CHAPTER 27

Appendicitis

Luanne Pelosi

INTRODUCTION

Abdominal pain is a common complaint in the pediatric population and usually presents a diagnostic dilemma. The most common cause of abdominal pain is acute gastroenteritis, although more serious causes must be excluded. Acute appendicitis is the most common condition requiring emergency surgery in childhood and adolescence, with approximately 60,000 children undergoing appendectomies each year (Ashcraft & Holder, 1993). The diagnosis of appendicitis should be included in the differential diagnosis in all age groups but is most common during late childhood and early adulthood, usually occurring between 8 and 18 years of age. The incidence of appendicitis is greater in males than in females (Ashcraft & Holder, 1993).

PATHOPHYSIOLOGY

Appendicitis is the result of obstruction of the lumen of the vermiform appendix. The lumen is usually obstructed by a fecalith, a small hardened ball of feces, or less commonly hyperplasia of submucosal follicles occurring after a viral infection. Pinworm infestation and carcinoid tumor are rare causes of obstruction. This obstruction of the lumen results in edema, venous engorgement, and increased intraluminal pressure. Ultimately, bacteria invade through the wall of the appendix and, along with arterial infarction, this leads to gangrene and perforation (Lawrence, 1993).

BACTERIOLOGY

The organism most commonly found when an appendix becomes gangrenous or perforated is the aerobic organism, *Escherichia coli*, a gram-negative rod. As symptoms progress, multiple organisms including *Klebsiella, Strepto-*

coccus, and *Pseudomonas* are found. The most common anaerobic pathogen is *Bacteroides fragilis*, a gram-negative organism (Mosdell, 1994).

CLASSIFICATION

The stages of appendicitis have five classifications. The stage is determined during appendectomy and microscopic evaluation of the pathological specimen. See Exhibit 27–1 for a description of the various stages.

HISTORY

A careful history and thorough physical examination are paramount in the diagnosis of appendicitis. It is important to obtain this history from both the primary caregiver and the child. The classic presentation of appendicitis begins with a gradual onset of diffuse periumbilical pain. This is usually followed by loss of appetite, then nausea and vomiting. In time, the pain localizes to the right lower quadrant and increases in intensity. Many patients describe a change in bowel habits, usually diarrhea, that is related to pelvic inflammation. However, the amount of diarrhea is less volume than expected with gastroenteritis. Fevers of 38° to 39° C are common; however, some children do not have fever. Temperatures greater than 39° C with associated peritoneal signs usually suggest perforation (Rowe, 1995).

An unusual location of the appendix results in varied symptoms and creates tremendous diagnostic confusion. Flank pain can be caused by a retrocecal appendix, or urinary symptoms may occur when the appendix tip meets the bladder. Regardless of the location of the appendix, the first site of pain with appendicitis is usually periumbilical referred pain. When the pain shifts, it localizes on the site of the appendix.

Exhibit 27–1 Stages of Appendicitis

Acute/simple—The appendix shows mild hyperemia and edema; serosal exudate is not evident.

Suppurative—The appendix is edematous, vessels are congested, and fibrin exudate forms. The peritoneal fluid may be clear or turbid.

Gangrenous—In addition to the findings of suppurative appendicitis, purple or black areas of gangrene appear in the appendix wall. There may be microperforations present on microscopic examination, and the peritoneal fluid is increased and cloudy.

Perforated—There is visible perforation of the appendix wall, and the peritoneal fluid may be purulent and odorous.

Abscess—Abscess formation occurs adjacent to the perforated appendix and contains fetid pus. The abscess location can be pelvic, retrocecal, or subcecal.

PHYSICAL EXAMINATION

A child with appendicitis quite often appears ill, frightened, and apprehensive. Many children are found lying on their side with their knees drawn up and flexed. It is important to perform a complete physical examination, including neck, throat, and chest examination because other conditions such as streptococcus pharyngitis and a right middle lobe pneumonia can mimic appendicitis symptoms.

A cardinal sign of appendicitis is point tenderness. This is a defined area of maximum tenderness in the right lower quadrant. This occurs at McBurney's point, which is one third of the distance along the line from the right anterior iliac spine to the umbilicus (Lawrence, 1992).

On examination the child exhibits right lower quadrant tenderness with palpation, coughing, and shaking. As peritoneal irritation progresses, voluntary guarding (stiffening of the rectus muscle) and rebound tenderness, in which pain occurs with release of pressure, occur. The inflamed appendix causes irritation of the psoas muscle. Pain with passive hip extension or flexion is a positive psoas sign. If the inflamed appendix should lie on the obturator internus muscle, pain may be elicited on passive internal rotation of the flexed thigh. This is the obturator sign. A positive Rovsing's sign also suggests appendicitis (Bates, 1991). The child has pain in the right lower quadrant during palpation of the left lower quadrant. Auscultation generally demonstrates diminished bowel sounds, but an obviously silent abdomen suggests peritonitis (Bates, 1991).

A rectal examination may also elicit tenderness of the right vault or a pelvic abscess. It can also rule out constipation and fecal impaction as a cause of abdominal pain. A rectal examination aids in diagnosing a pelvic mass. Teenage girls who are sexually active need a thorough pelvic examination to rule out bacterial infections.

LABORATORY FINDINGS

Laboratory tests are not always helpful in the diagnosis of appendicitis. The white blood count is usually elevated between 10,000 and 15,000 but at times may not be elevated. The smear may show a left shift with increased polymorphics and bands. This increases the probability of a bacterial infection rather than a viral infection. A urinalysis is also important because elevated white blood cells, hematuria, and nitrates may be consistent with a urinary tract infection, which may mimic appendicitis symptoms (Lawrence, 1993).

RADIOGRAPHIC FINDINGS

Several radiologic tests aid in the diagnosis of appendicitis. These include abdominal and chest radiographs, abdominal ultrasonography, computed tomography scan, and barium enema. Abdominal radiographic films are often nonspecific unless a calcified fecalith is visualized. This occurs in a small percentage of patients (Friedland, 1997). Other abdominal radiographic findings include mild distention of loops of small bowel and obliteration of the right psoas muscle shadow. Ultrasonography identifies an acutely inflamed appendix by visualizing a noncompressible, tubular structure at the point of maximal tenderness. If the appendix diameter is greater than 6 mm and evidence of free fluid is noted, appendicitis is confirmed (Lawrence, 1993). Ultrasonography can also be used in cases to rule out pelvic inflammatory disease or ovarian torsion or cysts in females. When the diagnosis is still unclear, an abdominal computed tomography scan should be obtained (Friedland, 1997). Barium enemas are rarely used in this era. Historically, if the lumen of the appendix does not fill with barium, or partially fills, indicating perforation, appendicitis is confirmed. A chest radiographic film is needed to rule out right middle or lower lobe pneumonia when abdominal pain and respiratory signs and symptoms are involved.

DIFFERENTIAL DIAGNOSIS

Gastroenteritis is the most common cause of abdominal pain in children and can often be mistaken for appendicitis (Mones, 1991). Children with gastroenteritis have abdominal pain that coincides with or occurs after vomiting. In appendicitis abdominal pain occurs before vomiting. Diarrhea in gastroenteritis is usually high volume and frequent; diarrhea is low volume and irritative in appendicitis.

Fever, leukocytosis, and dysuria are common in patients with urinary tract infections and appendicitis.

Careful examination, including evaluation of flank pain and urinalysis results that reveal positive nitrates and 10,000 to 20,000 white blood cells, may indicate urinary tract infection.

Constipation is a common cause of abdominal pain in the school-age child and adolescent and can be accompanied by fever, vomiting, and leukocytosis. Usually right lower quadrant pain experienced as a result of constipation persists but fails to progress. Fecal masses can sometimes be palpated in smaller children. Stool in the rectal vault can be noted on rectal examination. Abdominal radiographs can confirm constipation.

Pelvic inflammatory disease (PID) mimics appendicitis. Adolescents with PID have pain in both lower quadrants and fever. Cervical and adnexal tenderness is noted on rectal examination in patients with PID. A pelvic examination may reveal cervical discharge and positive cultures.

Pneumonia of the right middle or lower lobe causes referred pain to the abdomen. Respiratory symptoms and associated radiographic findings can confirm appendicitis or pneumonia.

Intussusception is a common cause of abdominal pain in children less than 3 years of age. The symptoms are usually intermittent severe colicky pain, abdominal mass in the right lower quadrant, and bloody stools. Radiologic intervention is diagnostic and often therapeutic (see Chapter 26).

Mesenteric adenitis is a condition that is most likely due to viral infection and causes mild abdominal symptoms. Inflammation of the lymph nodes clustered in the mesentery of the terminal ileum are noted. This can be diagnosed by ultrasonography or is frequently confirmed during surgery.

Other conditions that mimic appendicitis in childhood include ovarian cyst, midmonthly cycle ovulation (mittelschmerz), inflammatory bowel disease, Meckel's diverticulum, cholecystitis, pancreatitis, and sickle cell disease pain during crisis (Zitelli, 1992).

TREATMENT

The child with suspected appendicitis should be observed closely, including vital signs and temperature. Intravenous hydration should be administered while maintaining NPO status. Serial abdominal examinations should be performed and monitored along with follow-up diagnostic studies. Children with viral gastroenteritis usually improve with intravenous fluid hydration. The child with appendicitis usually does not improve, aiding in the confirmation of appendicitis.

Preoperative antibiotics should be administered to all patients with presumed appendicitis. Clinical experience demonstrates that prophylactic and perioperative antibiotics reduce the infectious complications of appendicitis (Soderquist-Elinder, 1995). Usually a second-generation cephalosporin, such as cefoxitin or cefazolin (Kefzol), given perioperatively covers most gram-positive and gram-negative organisms in the patient with acute appendicitis. The length of administration of the antibiotic varies, but commonly 24 hours of coverage is the standard of practice (Lawrence, 1993).

OPERATIVE PROCEDURE

For simple appendicitis, a transverse right lower quadrant incision is made. The abdominal muscle and peritoneum are opened. The cecum is identified. The inflamed appendix is identified, isolated, clamped, divided, and tied. A purse-string suture is placed in the cecal wall, and the base of the appendix is crushed and tied. The appendix is excised and the appendiceal stump is inverted into the cecal wall. The purse-string suture is tied. The area is irrigated with sterile saline. The muscle layers are closed, and the skin layer is closed in a running subcuticular fashion (Rowe, 1995). Adhesive strips are applied and a sterile dry dressing covers the incision.

In the patient with perforated appendicitis, an appendectomy is performed as previously described through a right lower quadrant incision. Peritoneal cultures are obtained if the fluid is cloudy to test antibiotic sensitivity to the organism. Antibiotics may be changed on the basis of the sensitivity of the organisms that have grown. This practice varies in some institutions because recent studies have shown that obtaining cultures at the time of opening the peritoneum resulted in no appropriate adjustment of the patient's antibiotic regimen (Mosdell, 1994). The abdominal cavity is then irrigated with sterile saline or saline with cephalothin (4 gm/L). If the appendix is perforated, it is important to look for the fecalith, which may be free in the peritoneal cavity (Rowe, 1995).

Intraperitoneal drains placed in the pelvis and pericolic gutter to provide intra-abdominal abscess drainage demonstrate low infectious complications (Lund & Murphy, 1994). Wounds are then closed primarily. Drains are inserted in cases with a localized abscess cavity (Blewett & Krummel, 1995). Few institutions continue the use of delayed primary closure of wounds, in which the wound is left opened and packed with wet-to-dry dressings. As healing and granulation occur the skin is later closed. This usually necessitates delayed hospital discharge, frequent dressing changes, discomfort for the child, and less than satisfying cosmetic results (Blewett & Krummel, 1995).

LAPAROSCOPIC APPENDECTOMY

Recently, the use of laparoscopic appendectomy for acute appendicitis has been met with enthusiasm. This technique also requires general anesthesia. The procedure begins with insufflation of the peritoneal cavity with carbon dioxide through a Veress needle inserted through the umbilicus. A 10-mm port and a 5-mm port are inserted at the umbilicus and at the hypogastrium along the midline. An additional 5-

mm cannula is inserted in the epigastrium between the umbilicus and the xiphoid. Appendectomy is then performed.

A recent study demonstrates no significant difference in operative time or use of narcotics when laparoscopic appendectomy was compared with open appendectomy. Increased intraoperative costs were reported with laparoscopic appendectomy: $4,600 laparoscopic versus $1,700 open (Williams, 1996).

APPENDICEAL ABSCESS

Patients who have a perforated appendix and a walled-off abscess are managed conservatively with computed tomography–guided or ultrasonography-guided percutaneous drainage of the abscess. Parenteral antibiotics are administered until the fever defervesces. Normal diet is resumed when abdominal pain resolves and appetite returns. Drains are removed after output decreases. An interval appendectomy is planned in 6 to 8 weeks when the inflammatory process has subsided (Jamieson, Chait, & Filler, 1997).

POSTOPERATIVE MANAGEMENT

In the immediate postoperative period, the child undergoing an appendectomy receives intravenous hydration and antibiotics until the fever defervesces, usually 24 hours. Clear fluids are begun when bowel function returns and advanced to a regular diet as tolerated. Pain medication is administered as needed. Ambulation is encouraged in the first few hours after surgery. A dry, sterile dressing covers the right lower quadrant incision and should be observed for any excess drainage. Minimal serosanguineous drainage is normal. Discharge usually occurs within 48 hours of surgery when the child is tolerating a regular diet, afebrile, and receiving effective pain control with oral medications (Borkowski, 1994). The patient with a gangrenous or perforated appendix requires more aggressive postoperative management. Vital signs should be monitored every 4 hours along with temperature. Aggressive postoperative fluid rehydration should be provided at maintenance or maintenance and one half to maintain adequate urine output. Refer to Appendix 27–A for a pathway to guide the pre- and postoperative care of the child with uncomplicated appendectomy.

Antibiotic coverage choices vary by surgeon preference but continue for the chosen length of time (5, 7, or 10 days) or until the patient is afebrile. Broad-spectrum antibiotics are recommended for perforated appendix with aerobic and anaerobic organisms. Antibiotic choices and length of treatment continue to be a controversial subject and vary among institutions. The "gold standard" of treatment includes ampicillin, gentamicin, and clindamycin for 10 days with a reported infectious complication rate of 4.8% (Lund & Murphy, 1994). Keller, McBride, and Vane (1996) suggests

the length of antibiotic treatment be dependent on improvement in the patient's clinical status. The use of single-drug therapy is proving to be as effective as multiple-drug treatment. Piperacillin/tazobactam (Zosyn) is active against resistant gram-negative bacteria, beta-lactam–producing staphylococci, and anaerobic organisms (Polk, 1993). The use of single-agent antibiotics in the treatment of perforated appendicitis decreases the length of stay and costs by allowing home antibiotics to be given by means of a peripherally inserted central venous catheter (Stovroff, 1994). Prospective studies, which encourage decreased length of stay and better use of health care dollars, need to continue in this time of managed care to ensure continued quality outcomes for children.

Fevers are expected in the first few days postoperatively as a result of fluid shifts and because of the extent of the peritonitis from the perforation. A prolonged ileus is expected after surgery because of the extent of the peritonitis. Many children require nasogastric tube decompression for the first few days. When bowel function resumes, the nasogastric tube is discontinued and a clear liquid diet is begun. Diet is advanced slowly to regular as the child tolerates.

Pulmonary toilet, including incentive spirometry, coughing, deep breathing, and ambulation, is encouraged. Children who have significant peritonitis may have a sympathetic pleural effusion develop in the base of either lung. This is another potential source of fever and requires continued antibiotics and aggressive pulmonary toilet. Wound inspection, whether it be a closed or open wound with or without drains, is important. The site should be observed for erythema, warmth, purulent drainage, and increased tenderness.

Intravenous pain medication, morphine or ketorolac tromethamine (Toradol), is used during the first few days after surgery. Then transition to oral pain medication occurs with tolerance of fluids.

The patient can be discharged home if he or she is afebrile for at least 24 hours, has a white blood cell count less than 12,000, is tolerating a regular diet and oral pain medication, has normal bowel movements, and is ambulating without difficulty.

DISCHARGE INSTRUCTIONS

Families are instructed to notify the surgeon or primary care provider if the child has a fever greater than 38.5° C, emesis, diarrhea, new-onset abdominal pain, or anorexia. They are to notify the surgeon if erythema, warmth, increased tenderness, or purulent drainage is noted around the incision. Children are allowed to bathe 3 to 7 days after surgery. They can usually return to school within 1 week. Physical education, recess, and sports should be limited for 4 weeks after surgery because of healing of the abdominal muscles.

COMPLICATIONS

Intra-abdominal abscess is considered in the patient after treatment for a perforated appendicitis with fever, abdominal pain, irritability, leukocytosis, anorexia, and emesis. A rectal examination may elicit tenderness or a mass, and focal tenderness on palpation may be helpful to diagnose an abscess. An abdominal computed tomography scan or ultrasonography can confirm the presence, size, and location of the fluid collection. If the abscess is accessible, a percutaneous or transrectal drain is inserted into the collection under fluoroscopy, and antibiotic coverage is started (Jamieson et al., 1997).

A wound infection can occur a few days after surgery and manifest with erythema, warmth, purulent drainage, and increased tenderness. If the wound is open and pus is noted, cultures should be obtained and the wound should be irrigated and then packed to allow slow granulation and closure. Antibiotics are usually reinstitued or changed depending on what the cultures and sensitivities are.

A side effect of administering broad-spectrum antibiotics is *Clostridium difficile* colitis. Patients have profuse, liquid, foul-smelling diarrhea, abdominal pain, and fever. This occurs because broad-spectrum antibiotics disrupt the normal colonic flora, allowing *C. difficile*, a spore-forming anaerobe, to colonize the colon causing mucosal inflammation and subsequent diarrhea (Infection Control, 1996). If *C. difficile* toxin is positive, the treatment is oral metronidazole (Flagyl) for 7 days and rehydration. Symptoms resolve within 24 to 48 hours of treatment.

Adhesions are bands of scar tissue between or around organs. Adhesions form as aging scar tissue shrinks. After any abdominal surgery, adhesions may occur in the abdominal cavity and can cause an intestinal obstruction. All patients should be aware of the signs and symptoms of intestinal obstruction, which include bilious emesis and severe abdominal pain (Lawrence, 1992).

RESEARCH

Diagnosis and management of appendicitis varies from surgeon to surgeon. As the health care arena continues to change, costs, length of stay, and patient outcomes are closely monitored. Quality improvement is the key to the direction of further research. The development of clinical practice guidelines that standardize management plans are on the forefront. Nurses actively participate in the development and ongoing evaluation of patient outcomes of children with acute appendicitis.

CONCLUSION

Children undergoing appendectomies account for a large percentage of pediatric surgical patients. The management of these children may seem routine to some but continues to change. It is the experienced nurse who will continue to provide excellent care, providing not only the technical skills backed by strong clinical knowledge but also the emotional support to the family and child undergoing this surgery.

REFERENCES

Ashcraft, K.W., & Holder T.M. (1993). *Pediatric surgery* (2nd ed.). New York: W.B. Saunders Company.

Bates, B. (1991). *A guide to physical examination and history taking* (5th ed.). Philadelphia: Lippincott-Raven.

Blewett, C.J., & Krummel, T.M. (1995). Perforated appendicitis: Past and future controversies. *Seminars in Pediatric Surgery, 4*(4), 234–238.

Borkowski, S. (1994). Common pediatric surgical problems. *Nursing Clinics of North America, 29,* 560–562.

Friedland, J.A. (1997). CT appearance of acute appendicitis in children. *American Journal of Radiology, 168,* 439–441.

Infection Control Newsletter. (1996). *Children's Hospital, 4* (5).

Jamieson, D.H., Chait, P.G., & Filler, R. (1997). Interventional drainage of appendiceal abscesses in children. *American Journal of Radiology, 169,* 1619–1622.

Keller, M.S., McBride, W.J., & Vance, D.W. (1996). Management of complicated appendicitis: A rational approach based on clinical course. *Archives of Surgery, 131,* 261–264.

Lawrence, P.F. (1992). *Essentials of surgery* (2nd ed.). Baltimore: Williams & Wilkins.

Lawrence, P.F. (1993). *Essential surgical specialities*. Baltimore: Williams & Wilkins.

Lund, D., & Murphy, E. (1994). Management of perforated appendicitis in children. A decade of aggressive treatment. *Journal of Pediatric Surgery, 29,* 1130–1134.

Mones, R.L. (1991, August). Acute abdomen in children. Appendicitis and beyond. *Emergency Medicine,* 179–186.

Mosdell, D.M. (1994). Peritoneal cultures and antibiotic therapy in pediatric perforated appendicitis. *The American Journal of Surgery, 167,* 313–316.

Polk, H.C. (1993). Prospective randomized study of piperacillin/tazobactam therapy of surgical intra-abdominal infection. *The American Surgeon, 59,* 598–605.

Rowe, M.I. (1995). *Essentials of pediatric surgery*. St. Louis, MO: Mosby.

Soderquist-Elinder, C. (1995). Prophylactic antibiotics in uncomplicated appendicitis during childhood. *The European Journal of Pediatric Surgery, 5,* 282–285.

Stovroff, M. (1994). PIC lines save money and hasten discharge in the care of children with perforated appendicitis. *Journal of Pediatric Surgery, 29,* 245–247.

Williams, M.D. (1996). Laparoscopic versus open appendectomy. *Southern Medical Journal, 69*(7), 668–674.

Zitelli, B.J. (1992). *Atlas of pediatric physical diagnosis* (5th ed.). Philadelphia: Lippincott-Raven.

Appendix 27–A

Caremap for Appendicitis

	Preop/Day of Surgery	POD 1	POD 2/Discharge
Assessment and monitoring	Vital signs with temp q4h Serial abdominal examinations I & O	— Assess bowel sounds — Pain assessment Assess dressing	— — — —
Treatments	10–15 ml/kg fluid bolus Intravenous fluids @ maintenance Nasogastric tube if indicated	— DC NGT when bowel sounds return Pulmonary toilet Ambulate	Heplock IV — —
Tests	Abdominal radiograph Abdominal ultrasound CT scan if indicated CBC with diff, lytes, bun, creat, LFTs, amylase, lipase	Repeat CBC if elevated	
Medications	Perioperative antibiotics Pain medication as ordered IV	Postoperative antibiotics Change to PO pain when tolerating PO	Antibiotics dc'd —
Diet	NPO	Clear when bowel function, advanced to regular as tolerated	—
Education	Preop teaching as appropriate for age and clinical status	Postop/discharge planning	— Assess learning Follow-up appointments scheduled
Outcomes/evaluations	Parents oriented to ward	—	Afebrile for 24h Tolerating reg diet Pain managed with oral medication Incision without evidence of infection

CHAPTER 28

Splenectomy, Cholecystectomy, and Meckel's Diverticulum

Susan E. Olsen and Marilyn Miller Stoops

Advances in pediatric surgery offer new approaches in the management of children requiring splenectomy, cholecystectomy, or a diverticulectomy and excision of Meckel's diverticulum. This chapter provides an overview of the indications for each of these surgical procedures, including the laparoscopic approach, and nursing care of children who undergo splenectomy, cholecystectomy, and excision of Meckel's diverticulum.

SPLENECTOMY

Embryology and Pathophysiology of the Spleen

Embryologic development of the spleen begins during the fifth week of gestation. It is lobulated at first and assumes its characteristic shape early in the fetal period (Moore & Persaud, 1993). The splenic artery comes from the celiac artery and is the largest branch of the celiac trunk. It is located posterior to the omental bursa and anterior to the left kidney. The spleen consists of a capsule, connective tissue framework, and parenchyma. It functions as the hematopoietic center until late fetal life and retains this potential for blood cell formation into adult life (Moore & Persaud, 1993). It is the largest of the secondary lymphoid organs, with mononuclear phagocytes to filter and cleanse the blood and lymphocytes for immune response to blood-borne microorganisms. It also serves as a blood reservoir (McCancre & Huether, 1990). Because asplenic children are at great risk of developing overwhelming sepsis, splenectomies are performed only when absolutely necessary. There has been a recent trend toward partial splenectomy to retain the phagocytic properties of the remaining spleen.

Indications for Splenectomy

Splenectomies are largely performed on an elective basis and, rarely, emergently. One reason for emergency pediatric splenectomy is idiopathic thrombocytopenic purpura (ITP) with major bleeding in the central nervous system. Acute ITP is a disease of children that often follows a viral infection. Acute ITP lasts a few weeks to 1 or 2 months and has no residual effects. Chronic ITP affects adolescents and adults, begins insidiously, and lasts longer. Corticosteroid treatment is usually effective, but occasionally splenectomy is the treatment of choice (Zamir et al., 1996). More than 80% of children affected with ITP respond to corticosteroid treatment within a few days to several weeks of treatment (Ben-Yehuda, Gillis, & Eldor, 1990). The spleen has been proven to be a major organ for platelet destruction and a site for antiplatelet antibody production (Bussel, 1990). Splenectomy has long been used as an effective therapeutic modality with complete remission achieved in 75% to 90% of patients undergoing splenectomy (Ben-Yehuda et al., 1990; Chirletti et al., 1992). The indications for splenectomy in ITP include lack of response to medical treatment, a drop in platelet count while attempting to taper the corticosteroids, or severe side effects of steroid therapy (Ben-Yehuda et al., 1990).

Children who sustain a splenic injury undergo splenectomy if the injury is too severe for splenic salvage. If a trauma-related emergency splenectomy is indicated, it would typically be a traditional open splenectomy as opposed to a laparoscopic procedure. The incidence of mortality from septicemia is increased 50-fold in children who have had splenectomy after trauma (Peter, 1997).

339

The most common indications for elective splenectomy are hereditary spherocytosis and sickle cell anemia. Spherocytosis is the presence of spherocytes in the blood. Spherocytes are completely hemoglobinated erythrocytes in the blood that are abnormally fragile and break down, leading to jaundice and splenomegaly. Sickle cell disease is a hereditary, genetically determined hemolytic anemia, largely occurring in the African-American population in which the erythrocytes are sickle shaped and become clumped in the vascular system, causing arthralgia, attacks of abdominal pain, and splenomegaly (Ein, 1993; Peter, 1997). Among the other indications for splenectomy are Gaucher's disease, idiopathic hypersplenism, thalassemia, preleukemia, Evan's syndrome, and Wiskott-Aldrich syndrome (Janu, Rogers, & Lobe, 1996).

Gaucher's disease is a genetically acquired illness that results in massive accumulation of glycocerebroside in the reticuloendothelial system, bone marrow, and the central nervous system. Massive splenomegaly and hepatomegaly develop because of deposition of lipids in these organs. Holcomb and Greene (1993) note that, until recently, total splenectomy has been recommended to manage hypersplenism-associated anemia and thrombocytopenia. Recently, because the risk of postsplenectomy sepsis is so great, partial splenectomy has been used in the treatment of children with hypersplenism. Partial splenectomy for type I Gaucher's disease, which is the most common, has been found to be successful, whereas its use for type III Gaucher's disease, the rarest form of disease, remains in question (Holcomb & Greene, 1993). Type I Gaucher's disease is characterized by hepatosplenomegaly in almost all patients. Children with this form usually are seen in mid to late childhood and may have a normal life expectancy. Type III Gaucher's disease results in progressive neurologic decline early in life (Holcomb & Greene, 1993).

Elective splenectomy may be indicated for the child with a chronic form of leukemia such as juvenile myelogenous leukemia. These children become so physically compromised with extremely large spleens and livers that splenectomy is performed as a palliative procedure to help keep the child mobile and as comfortable as possible for as long as possible.

Splenectomy is sometimes indicated in the patient with Hodgkin's disease. There is a staging system for Hodgkin's disease that ranges from stage I to stage IV. This system is fairly reliable because the disease almost always has one focus and then spreads by a pattern through the lymphatics. If the disease has progressed to stage III, which includes involvement of lymph nodes on both sides of the diaphragm, localized involvement of an extralymphatic organ or site, and/or involvement of the spleen, splenectomy may be indicated. Included in the staging laparotomy are splenectomy, wedge and needle biopsy of both lobes of the liver, and biopsy of seven node groups (Shorter & Filston, 1993).

In the past, staging for Hodgkin's disease was necessary because the diagnostic testing was less sophisticated or able to identify the extent of the disease. Recent advances in imaging have radically decreased the use of this procedure in many institutions. Pediatric hematologists are more likely to rely on imaging studies than surgical intervention at present.

Preoperative Preparation

In the case of elective surgery, a polyvalent vaccine against streptococcal pneumococcus and *Haemophilus influenzae* should be administered 10 days to 2 weeks before surgery (Peter, 1997).

Preoperative preparation for laparoscopic surgery and open surgery is the same because there is always the possibility that a laparoscopic approach may need to be abandoned in favor of an open approach. The child begins a clear liquid diet 24 hours before the surgery. Some institutions recommend giving a Phospho-Soda enema the evening before surgery to decrease the chance of injuring the colon with the laparoscopic equipment. Prophylactic antibiotics are administered intravenously immediately before the procedure.

Operative Procedure

Laparoscopic Surgery

Surgeons have been performing laparoscopic splenectomies in children since 1992 (Tulman, Holcomb, Karamanoukian, & Reynhout, 1993). The increased frequency of these procedures has resulted in the development of new instruments and techniques that make the technical aspects more reliable and easier to perform (Schleef, Morcate, Steinau, Ott, & Willital, 1997).

First, a Foley catheter and nasogastric tube are placed for bladder and gastric decompression. Then, a 1-cm incision is made through the umbilicus, a Veress needle is passed, and pneumoperitoneum or air is introduced into the peritoneal cavity to 12 mm Hg. Next, a 10-mm laparoscope is inserted, and then three or four small 5-mm ports are inserted at various points in the abdomen. The patient is put in a steep Trendelenburg position with the left side elevated. The vessels supplying the spleen are stapled and cut, as are the ligaments. A Lap Sac (Cook Urological, Spencer, IN) is then introduced, and the spleen is placed in the sac with the use of four instruments. The splenic tissue is morselized or cut into strips and suctioned out of the sac to a point where the sac can be removed. The splenic bed and pancreas are examined to be sure there is no bleeding. The trocars are then removed and the sites sutured in the standard way. Finally, the Foley catheter and nasogastric tube are removed (Smith et al., 1994).

Schleef et al. (1997) have found that using a loop of umbilical band as an atraumatic way of grasping and manipulating the spleen is an improvement over grasping the spleen with forceps, which can cause damage to the capsule and intracapsular bleeding. A new instrument called a harmonic scalpel facilitates the division of blood vessels and coagulation, thus reducing blood loss (Janu et al., 1996).

Open Surgery

Open splenectomy requires either a midline or left subcostal incision (Figure 28–1). The spleen is exposed by moving or mobilizing the intestines and the vessels are tied off and cut (Figure 28–2A, B) (Ashcraft, 1994). The spleen is removed (Figure 28–2C) and the abdomen is explored for any accessory spleens. Accessory spleens are small nodules of splenic tissue that are most commonly found around the splenic hilum or the tail of the pancreas (Ein, 1993). They resemble lymph nodes but may be as large as 10 cm (Ein, 1993). Accessory spleens must be removed at the time of surgery if the surgery is necessary for any reason other than trauma (Ein, 1993). Accessory spleens function in the same manner as the spleen that has been removed and may cause future complications for the patient. If the accessory spleens are not excised during the initial procedure, further surgery is required. After removal of the spleen and any accessory spleens, the abdomen is closed.

Postoperative Care

Postlaparoscopic patients tolerate fluids a few hours postoperatively and resume eating solid foods the following day.

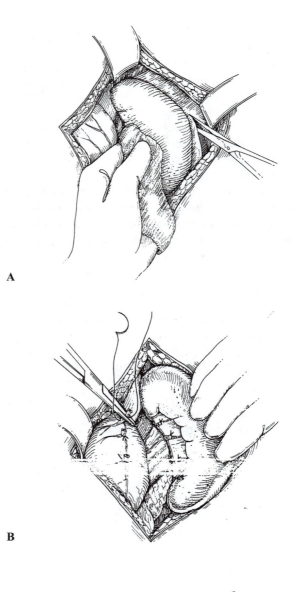

A

B

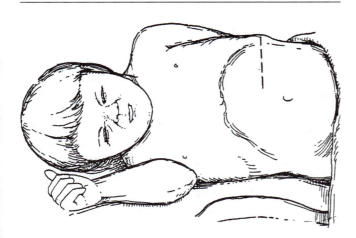

Figure 28–1 Left Subcostal Incision Made in Open Splenectomy

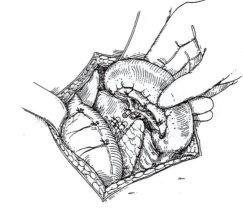

C

Figure 28–2 Open Splenectomy. A, Exposure of spleen. B, Vessels tied off and cut. C, Removal of spleen.

Discharge from the hospital is on day 2 or 3 with an antibiotic, usually penicillin, and analgesics.

After open surgery, the Foley catheter is removed on postoperative day 1. The nasogastric tube remains in place for approximately 48 hours. Clear liquids are given after removal of the nasogastric tube, and the diet is advanced to full liquids and regular diet as tolerated. The average hospital stay is 4 days. Refer to Appendix 28–A for specific details about nursing care.

Exhibit 28–1 shows advantages and disadvantages of laparoscopic splenectomy compared with traditional open splenectomy. Figure 28–3 illustrates the time involved to perform open versus laparoscopic splenectomy, and Figure 28–4 shows the hospital costs associated with each procedure.

Preventing Postsplenectomy Sepsis

The spleen serves an important phagocytic function because of its special type of anatomy and circulation. The spleen removes particulate matter, colloid, and bacteria from the circulation (Ein, 1993). *Streptococcus pneumoniae* is the most frequent bacteremia in infants and children older than 1 year of age (Ein, 1993). Prevention of overwhelming postsplenectomy infection known as OPSI caused by *S. pneumoniae* (lancet-shaped, gram-positive diplococci) is

achieved by administering pneumococcal vaccine about 2 weeks or more before the surgery (Ein, 1993). The vaccine is composed of 23 pneumococcal serotypes (Peter, 1997). There have been 84 pneumococcal serotypes identified thus far. The vaccine dose (0.5 ml) contains 25 mg of each polysaccharide antigen and is given either subcutaneously or intramuscularly. The effectiveness of this vaccine in preventing pneumonia has been demonstrated in healthy young adults and children who are predisposed. Vaccinated children who have undergone splenectomy experience significantly less pneumococcal disease than the unvaccinated children. Children 2 years and older should be vaccinated. The vaccine has limited immunogenicity in children younger than 2 years of age. Common side effects of the vaccine include erythema and pain at the infection site. Uncommon side effects include fever, myalgia, and severe local reactions. Anaphylaxis has rarely been reported (Peter, 1997).

Pneumococcus is the responsible organism in more than 50% of cases of OPSI. Other microorganisms causing OPSI include meningococcus, *Escherichia coli*, *Haemophilus influenzae*, *Staphylococcus*, and *Streptococcus* (Ein, 1993; Peter, 1997). Immunization with polyvalent capsular polysaccharide antigens of pneumococci (and possibly *H. influenzae* and meningococci) may be given at least several weeks before anticipated splenectomy because asplenic individuals have a diminished response to such immunization (Ein, 1993). If the child has received the entire three doses of *Haemophilus influenzae* type B vaccine, it is not necessary to revaccinate. If the child has not received the entire three doses, the immunizations should be completed before or after splenectomy.

The risk of OPSI is greatest in infancy and slowly declines as the child reaches adulthood. Approximately 80% of OPSI occurs within 2 years after splenectomy (Ein, 1993). The more serious the underlying splenic disease, the greater the risk for serious infection developing. Asplenic children have a morbidity rate of 1.5% to 80%, depending on the reason for which the spleen was removed (Ein, 1993). OPSI after splenectomy for trauma has the lowest rate and thalassemia has the highest rate, with all other diseases between these two extremes (Ein, 1993). The mortality rate in asplenic patients averages about 3% but can be as high as 11% (Ein, 1993).

The Committee on Infectious Diseases of the American Academy of Pediatrics (Peter, 1994, 1997) emphasizes that vaccination does not guarantee protection from fulminant pneumococcal disease and death (case fatality rates are 50% to 80%). The onset of OPSI may be sudden with fever, nausea, vomiting, and confusion being the initial symptoms. Left untreated the illness may progress to seizures, shock, disseminated intravascular coagulation, coma, and death within hours in 50% to 75% of affected children (Ein, 1993). Therefore, asplenic patients with unexplained fever greater than 38.5° C or other manifestations of sepsis should receive

---

Exhibit 28–1 Advantages and Disadvantages of Laparoscopic Splenectomy in Children

---

Advantages of Laparoscopic Approach
- smaller incisions, less painful than upper abdominal incisions[a]
- need for less pain medication postoperatively[a,b]
- fewer respiratory complications[a]
- improved return of respiratory function[a]
- reduced or absent postoperative ileus[a,b]
- shorter hospital stay[a,b]
- faster return to unrestricted activities[b]
- small scars cosmetically more preferable[b]
- reduced operative exposure to bodily fluid[b]

Disadvantages of Laparoscopic Approach
- increased operative time[a,b]
- more expensive cost of equipment[b]
- may not be possible if splenomegaly is in advanced stage[a]
- may require conversion to open procedure[b]
- possible complaints of shoulder pain[b]

[a] Smith et al., 1994. [b] Janu, Rogers, & Lobe, 1996.

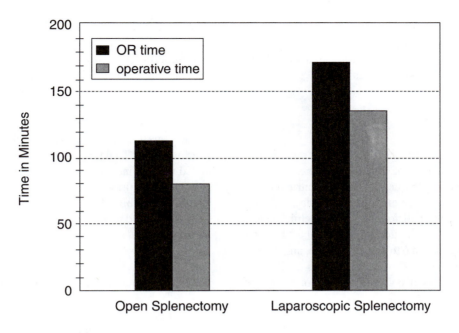

Figure 28–3 Open versus Laparoscopic Splenectomy. A comparison of operating room (OR) and operative time.

prompt medical attention, including treatment for suspected bacteremia, the initial signs and symptoms of which may be subtle. Antimicrobials selected for therapy should be effective against *S. pneumoniae*, *Neisseria meningitidis*, and beta-lactamase–producing *H. influenzae* type b (Peter, 1997).

In addition to vaccination, many experts recommend daily antimicrobial prophylaxis with oral penicillin G or V. Children less than 5 years of age receive 125 mg twice daily and older than 5 years of age 250 mg twice daily. This prophylaxis may be continued through childhood and into adulthood, depending on the practitioner. Antimicrobial prophylaxis may be particularly useful in children less than 2 years old because they are not likely to respond to the vaccine.

Surgeons vary significantly in their practice about sending children back to school and resuming full activities. Some believe that resuming normal activities is best accomplished

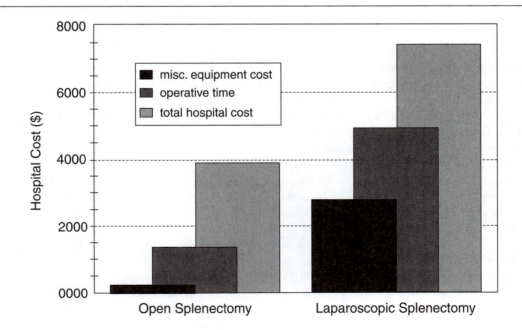

Figure 28–4 Open versus Laparoscopic Splenectomy. A comparison of hospital cost.

as soon as the child feels up to them. Others are more conservative in their beliefs and insist on a 4-week postoperative hiatus. School can be resumed anywhere from a week to 10 days after the surgery in most instances.

CHOLECYSTECTOMY

Another common pediatric problem is inflammation of the gallbladder and formation of stones. Gallstones are being diagnosed with increasing frequency in the pediatric population. In children, the incidence of gallstones varies with age. The reported incidence of gallstones is 7.7% in children less than 1 year of age, 2.7% in children between the ages of 1 and 5 years, 8.5% in children 6 to 10 years of age, and 43% in children 11 to 21 years of age (Friesen & Roberts, 1989). The symptoms of cholelithiasis also vary depending on the age of the child.

Embryology

The liver, gallbladder, and biliary duct system are formed from an outgrowth of the caudal portion of the foregut during the fourth week of gestation. This liver bud or hepatic diverticulum divides into a larger cranial portion, which becomes the liver. The smaller caudal portion becomes the gallbladder, with its stalk forming the cystic duct (Moore & Persaud, 1993). Congenital anomalies of the gallbladder itself are of significance to the surgeon who may be attempting to identify anatomy during a cholecystectomy or other surgical procedure (Shaffer, 1996).

Nonhemolytic Cholelithiasis

The conditions that predispose a child to cholelithiasis depend on the age of the child at presentation (see Figure 28–5). Nonhemolytic cholelithiasis refers to the formation of gallstones in the absence of a hemolytic disorder. The use of long-term total parenteral nutrition (TPN) has been implicated as a significant contributing factor to the increasing incidence of cholelithiasis in the pediatric population. The cause of this process is not well understood, but it is thought that the lack of enteral feedings reduces the effectiveness of gallbladder contractions, thus reducing the flow of bile from the gallbladder and resulting in biliary stasis. In addition, some of the actual components of the TPN may contribute to cholelithiasis. One study found that 13% of pediatric patients requiring TPN for longer than 30 days had cholelithiasis develop (King, Ginn-Pease, Lloyd, Hoffman, & Hohenbrink, 1987). Other nonhemolytic factors contributing to the development of cholelithiasis include obesity, history of ileal resection, cystic fibrosis, oral contraceptive use, and pregnancy (Flake, 1997) (see Figure 28–5).

Hemolytic Cholelithiasis

Hemolytic cholelithiasis is the most common cause of gallstones at urban academic medical centers where there is a large population of children with sickle cell disease (Holcomb & Pietsch, 1998). More than 50% of children with sickle cell disease have evidence of cholelithiasis by the age of 18 years (Lachman, Lazerson, Starshak, Vaughters, & Werlin, 1979). Thalassemia and spherocytosis are also associated with an increased incidence of gallstones. The bile of patients with these disorders contains a large amount of unconjugated bilirubin. This can lead to the formation of gallbladder sludge, thus increasing the risk for cholelithiasis (Rescorla, 1997).

Biliary Dyskinesia and Acute Acalculous Cholecystitis

Other indications for cholecystectomy include biliary dyskinesia and acute acalculous cholecystitis. Biliary dyskinesia occurs when the gallbladder has poor contractility and emptying, perhaps with cholesterol crystals present within the bile in the gallbladder. This may be an early stage of the formation of cholesterol gallstones (Rescorla, 1997). These children present with a history of chronic abdominal pain but are otherwise healthy and have normal laboratory and radiologic studies. A nuclear medicine study using an injection of cholecystokinin (CCK) is performed if biliary dyskinesia is suspected. CCK induces contraction and emptying of the gallbladder and relaxation of the sphincter of Oddi. During this examination, an ejection fraction is mathematically calculated by measuring the initial and residual amounts of a radioactive bile marker in the gallbladder (Krishnamurthy, Bobba, & Kingston, 1981). An ejection fraction of less than 35% is considered abnormal (Rescorla, 1997). Exact time of the onset and relief of pain and its relation to the emptying of the gallbladder are important in establishing the diagnosis. Pain occurring outside the gallbladder-emptying phase could be nonbiliary in origin (Krishnamurthy & Krishnamurthy, 1997). Cholecystectomy is the treatment of choice for cases of documented biliary dyskinesia.

In the pediatric population, acute acalculous cholecystitis (ACC) generally occurs after episodes of sepsis or other severe infections. In ACC, the gallbladder becomes acutely inflamed. In contrast to the children with biliary dyskinesia, patients with ACC have fever, vomiting, and right upper quadrant pain. They may also have abnormal liver function tests and white blood cell counts (Tsakayannis, Kozakewich, & Lillehei, 1996). On ultrasonographic examination, the wall of the gallbladder is markedly thickened and contains debris. Cholecystectomy is the treatment of choice if the gallbladder becomes progressively distended or if the patient's clinical status deteriorates (Flake, 1997).

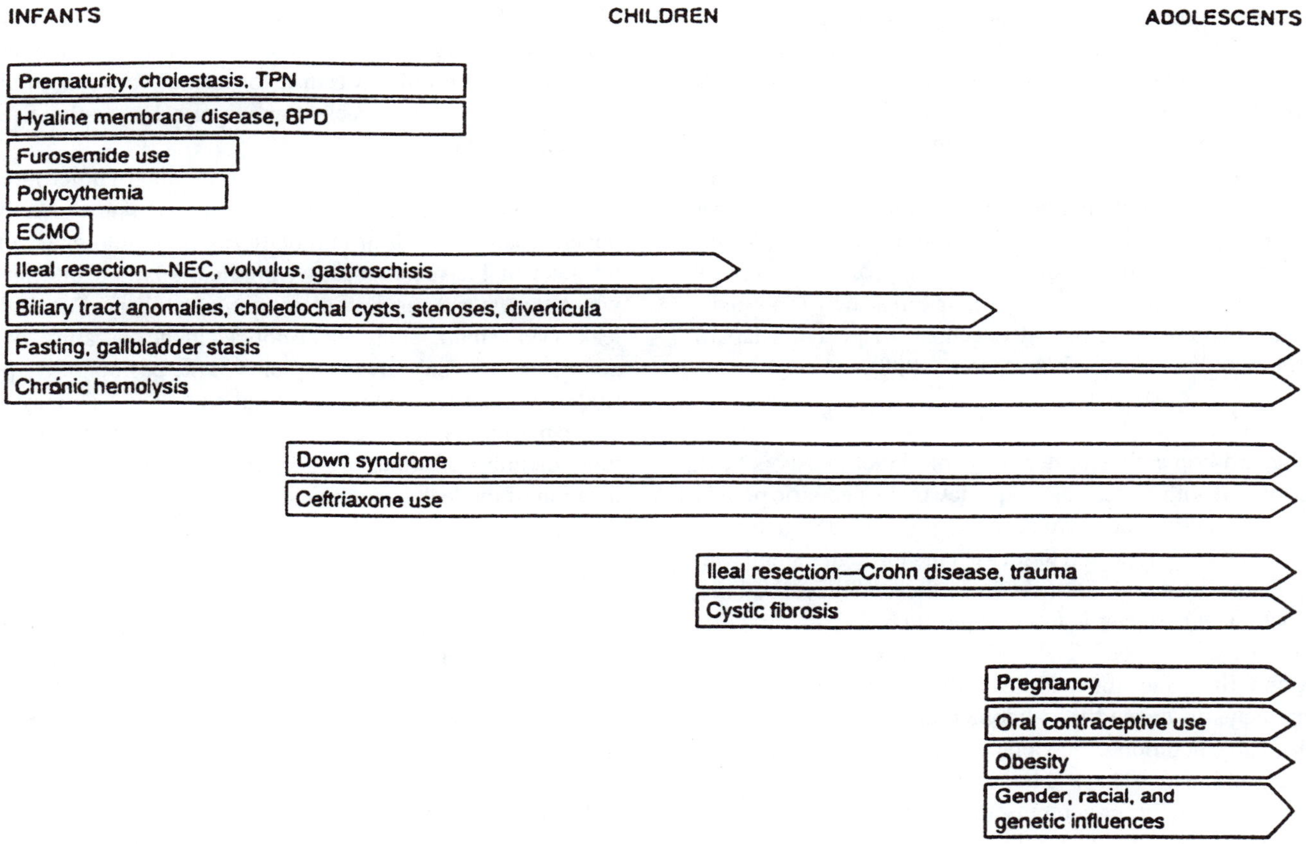

INFANTS   **CHILDREN**   **ADOLESCENTS**

Prematurity, cholestasis, TPN

Hyaline membrane disease, BPD

Furosemide use

Polycythemia

ECMO

Ileal resection—NEC, volvulus, gastroschisis

Biliary tract anomalies, choledochal cysts, stenoses, diverticula

Fasting, gallbladder stasis

Chronic hemolysis

Down syndrome

Ceftriaxone use

Ileal resection—Crohn disease, trauma

Cystic fibrosis

Pregnancy

Oral contraceptive use

Obesity

Gender, racial, and genetic influences

Figure 28–5 Predisposition to Cholelithiasis at Different Stages of Development

Clinical Presentation

Symptoms of gallstones vary, depending on the age of the patient. Occasionally, gallstones are found incidentally during an evaluation for another clinical problem. In infants, the presence of gallstones may result in fever and direct hyperbilirubinemia along with other abnormal liver function tests. Children tend to be initially seen with fever, abdominal pain, and an elevated white blood cell count. Older children complain of right upper quadrant or epigastric pain. This pain may radiate to the right scapula or shoulder, and the patient may experience nausea and vomiting. The pain and nausea may or may not occur in relation to meals or the ingestion of fatty foods. On physical examination, pain may be elicited as the patient deep breathes while the examiner palpates the abdomen in the region of the gallbladder. This is referred to as Murphy's sign and is an indication of possible gallbladder disease. Differential diagnoses include other causes of upper abdominal or epigastric pain and other conditions that may result in jaundice or abnormal liver function tests.

The diagnostic studies that are performed depend on the age of the child, the presence of risk factors for gallstones developing, and the presenting symptoms. Studies may include liver function tests, a complete blood count, abdominal radiographs or ultrasonography, and perhaps a nuclear medicine study. If the radiologic studies do not indicate a gallbladder disorder but one is still suspected, an endoscopic retrograde cholangiopancreatography (ERCP) can be performed to evaluate the pancreas and common bile duct. During this procedure, an endoscope is passed through the esophagus into the duodenum. A catheter is then passed through the endoscope into the pancreatic duct and bile ducts. Contrast medium is injected through this catheter into the ducts, and the biliary tract is evaluated for an obstruction or other abnormality. If stones are found, the physician may decide to remove them during this procedure.

Management

Nonsurgical

The management of gallstones depends on the age of the child and the symptoms that are present. In infants, gallstones sometimes spontaneously resolve without any intervention (Jacir, Anderson, Eichelberger, & Guzzetta, 1986). If the infant is asymptomatic, the physician may closely observe the patient for a period of time. If the child is older than 2 years of age and presents with pain or abnormal diagnostic studies, cholecystectomy is the treatment of choice. Even if the older child is asymptomatic, some would advocate elective cholecystectomy to prevent any future problems such as cholecystitis (Shaffer, 1996). Nonsurgical treatments, such as lithotripsy and oral dissolution therapy, are rarely used in children because of limited pediatric research trials using these techniques and the advancement of pediatric laparoscopic surgery (Holcomb & Pietsch, 1998).

Surgical

Laparoscopic cholecystectomy for cholelithiasis is being performed with increasing frequency in the pediatric population. When using the laparoscopic approach, all visualization of the operative field and tissues occurs through a small camera inserted through an incision in the umbilicus. A Foley catheter and nasogastric tube are placed before the first incision in the umbilicus. The abdomen is insufflated through the umbilical incision with an infusion of carbon dioxide. This helps to distend the abdomen and improve visualization. Three additional incisions are made at various locations in the abdomen. These three incisions serve as port sites through which the surgeon inserts other instruments, such as grasping forceps and dissecting forceps, to perform the procedure. During the procedure, a cholangiogram may be performed. A cholangiogram is performed by injecting radiopaque dye directly into the bile ducts. This helps the surgeon better identify the common bile duct and any structural abnormalities that may exist. Once the cystic duct, common bile duct, and other structures are identified, the gallbladder is removed through the umbilical incision. The instruments are removed from the other port sites in the abdomen with the laparoscope still in place to observe for any bleeding from the areas of the incisions. The laparoscope is then removed, the abdomen desufflated, and the incisions are closed with absorbable, subcuticular sutures. Wound closure strips or transparent tape and gauze are placed over each incision. The laparoscopic procedure may be contraindicated in a patient who has had previous abdominal surgery. In such a case, an open cholecystectomy can be performed through a traditional right upper quadrant incision (Monson, 1993).

Recent studies have compared laparoscopic and traditional operative or open cholecystectomy procedures in pediatrics. Kim, Wesson, Superina, and Filler (1995) compared both of these procedures evaluating cost, length of stay, and use of parenteral analgesics postoperatively. The average cost per patient, duration of hospitalization, and use of parenteral analgesics were all significantly less in the patients who underwent laparoscopic cholecystectomy. Another study has documented similar findings (Holcomb,

Sharp, Neblett, Morgan, & Pietsch, 1994). In addition, laparoscopic surgery has a much better cosmetic result, and the children are able to return to normal activities much sooner, often within 1 week after surgery (Holcomb, Olsen, & Sharp, 1991).

Complications after laparoscopic or open cholecystectomy include wound infections, bleeding, and postoperative pneumonia as a result of immobility or poor pulmonary toilet. One of the most serious complications is a bile leak, which occurs as a result of disruption of a biliary duct. If the leak is very small, it may not be noticed in the operating room and the patient may have symptoms in the postoperative period, including fever and abdominal pain. The leak may result in peritonitis. If the leak does not seal itself within a short time, diagnostic studies are performed to identify the exact location of the leak and surgical repair may be necessary.

Nursing Considerations

The exact content of preoperative teaching for the patient and family depends on whether the procedure is performed on an urgent or elective basis. All teaching should include the routine information about surgery, as well as reinforcing specific details regarding the recovery time and expected length of stay postoperatively. If the procedure is scheduled to be performed laparoscopically, the family and patient should be aware that the procedure might be converted to an open cholecystectomy if indicated.

There are several conditions in which special preoperative circumstances exist. If the child has an acutely inflamed gallbladder, surgery may be delayed until the patient has received several days of antibiotics and the inflammation is decreased. If pain medication is required, morphine sulfate is avoided because it increases spasm of the sphincter of Oddi. When the sphincter of Oddi spasms, it obstructs the normal flow of bile into the intestine, resulting in an increase in pain. If the child has sickle cell anemia, the patient should be admitted the day before surgery for hydration and a possible blood transfusion to ensure a hemoglobin level of 10 to 12 preoperatively (Al-Salem & Nourallah, 1997). Other hemolytic disorders also may require some preoperative blood work.

For most elective procedures, the patient arrives at the hospital the day of surgery and is admitted postoperatively. After recovering in the postanesthesia care unit, the child is transferred to the surgical floor. Nursing interventions for these patients are similar to those of any postoperative patient, consisting of assessment of vital signs, managing pain, recording intake and output, and wound assessment. If the procedure was performed laparoscopically, the child should be offered clear liquids the night of surgery. If the liquids are tolerated, the child is quickly advanced to a regular diet. The child is usually discharged the day after surgery if afebrile, tolerating a regular diet, and pain can be managed with oral narcotics and is otherwise doing well.

In addition to incisional pain, the child may complain of shoulder pain after laparoscopic surgery. This is referred pain from the diaphragm caused by reabsorption of residual carbon dioxide used for insufflating the abdomen during the operative procedure (George, Hammes, & Schwarz, 1995). This excess carbon dioxide can irritate the diaphragm. The patient should be encouraged to cough and deep breathe, and the patient should be positioned with the head of the bed only slightly elevated. If the procedure was performed open, the patient may require more pain medication and will have a longer recovery time. Because of this, these patients are usually discharged 3 to 5 days after the procedure. Patients with sickle cell anemia may also have a longer hospitalization and recovery time because of potential pulmonary complications, as well as the risk for developing a sickle cell crisis.

On discharge, the nurse should provide the family and patient with information regarding pain medication, wound care, and activity. Narcotics are rarely needed past the first 4 to 5 postoperative days. The child can then transition to over-the-counter medications. Wound care, whether the surgery was performed laparoscopically or open, consists of keeping the sites dry, usually for less than 1 week, depending on the kind of dressing that was applied by the surgeon intraoperatively. The child can return to regular activity within a couple of weeks if the surgery was performed laparoscopically and in 4 to 6 weeks if an open procedure was performed. Patients should be advised that if they experience any pain as they begin to increase their activity, that specific activity should be stopped and they should wait several days before attempting that activity again. Parents should be educated on the signs and symptoms of infection and encouraged to call the surgeon's office with any additional questions after discharge. Follow-up with the surgeon should be arranged approximately 2 weeks postoperatively. If the child is doing well at that time, he or she will only need to see the surgeon again if additional concerns arise.

MECKEL'S DIVERTICULUM

Embryology and Pathophysiology of Meckel's Diverticulum

Meckel's diverticulum is defined as a persistence in the omphalomesenteric duct or stalk of the yolk sac. The yolk sac develops on approximately day 10 in the inner mass of the embryo and expands to become both the primitive gut and the cavity of the chorion (which gives rise to the placenta). It does this by creating a passageway known as the omphalomesenteric duct. After supplying nourishment to the embryo, the yolk sac usually disappears around the seventh week of pregnancy. If the stalk of the yolk sac or omphalo-

mesenteric duct persists, it becomes a protuberant sac somewhere between 30 and 90 cm from the ileocecal valve in the distal ileum, the Meckel's diverticulum (also called diverticulum ilei verum). Meckel, a German anatomist and embryologist, is credited with this discovery in 1812. Meckel's diverticulum occurs in 2% of the population and is usually asymptomatic. It is one of the most common anomalies of the digestive tract (Moore & Persaud, 1993). Although only 15% of diverticuli contain gastric mucosa, 95% of those that present with bleeding contain some gastric mucosa (Grosthwaite & Leather, 1997).

Meckel's diverticulum is clinically significant in two instances: when it produces symptoms and when it is found incidentally at the time of a laparotomy. Half of the patients who present with symptoms do so by 2 years of age (Foglia, 1993).

Clinical Presentation

The three most common presentations of a symptomatic Meckel's diverticulum are lower gastrointestinal bleeding, intestinal obstruction, and abdominal pain (Foglia, 1993). Meckel's diverticula are most commonly manifested in children by painless lower gastrointestinal bleeding and in adults as an inflammatory process or obstruction (Digiacomo & Cottone, 1993).

Bleeding is present in 25% to 56% of children with symptomatic lesions (Vane, West, & Grosfeld, 1987). Bleeding can be slight, with dark, tarry stools or it may be massive with a more reddish stool. There may be copious bright red blood per rectum with no stool. It may also have a mucoid-like currant jelly appearance because Meckel's diverticulum can be the lead point of an intussusception. Except in the case of intussusception, the bleeding is almost always painless and stops spontaneously. Excessive bleeding can lead to anemia with the necessity of a blood transfusion (Foglia, 1993).

The child should be assessed for signs of hemodynamic instability because rectal bleeding is the most common presenting symptom. Frequently, though, the bleeding is slight and may not cause changes in the child's hemodynamic picture.

The second symptom, intestinal obstruction, occurs in about one third of all patients and is a frequent finding in younger patients. Besides acting as the lead point in an intussusception, Meckel's diverticulum can become the cause of a volvulus, a twisting of the bowel, or the cause of an internal hernia (Digiacomo & Cottone, 1993; Foglia, 1993).

Differential Diagnosis

One quarter of patients report abdominal pain or inflammation as the presenting symptom (Soltero & Bill, 1976).

The pain may be confused with acute appendicitis. One third of patients with Meckel's diverticulum have a perforation (Foglia, 1993). This occurs when there is gastric mucosa in the Meckel's diverticulum and peptic ulceration develops, leading to perforation (Gandy, Byrne, & Lees, 1997).

Workup

The "gold standard" for diagnosing Meckel's diverticulum is the "Meckel's scan" or scintigraphy (Foglia, 1993) (Figure 28–6). A scintigraph is a picture produced by an imaging device that shows the distribution and intensity of radioactivity in various tissues and organs after the administration of a radiopharmaceutical. Technetium (Tc) pertechnetate, an isotope, is readily absorbed by gastric mucosa and will appear anywhere gastric mucosa exists in the body. Because a symptomatic Meckel's diverticulum contains gastric mucosa in most instances, this scan accurately confirms diagnosis in 80% to 90% of cases. Defects that include less than 1 cm of gastric mucosa in the diverticulum are beyond the resolution of the camera. Some institutions premedicate with an H_2 blocker such as cimetidine. Cimetidine lengthens the amount of time the radioisotope remains in the area of interest by slowing the isotope's removal, thereby aiding in the diagnosis (Foglia, 1993). Meckel's diverticulum can occur anywhere in the abdomen but is most often found in the right lower quadrant (Jewett, Duszynski, & Allen, 1970).

The diagnostic Meckel's scan should be explained to the family. The excretion of isotope from the kidneys and bowel within 24 hours of administration should also be discussed.

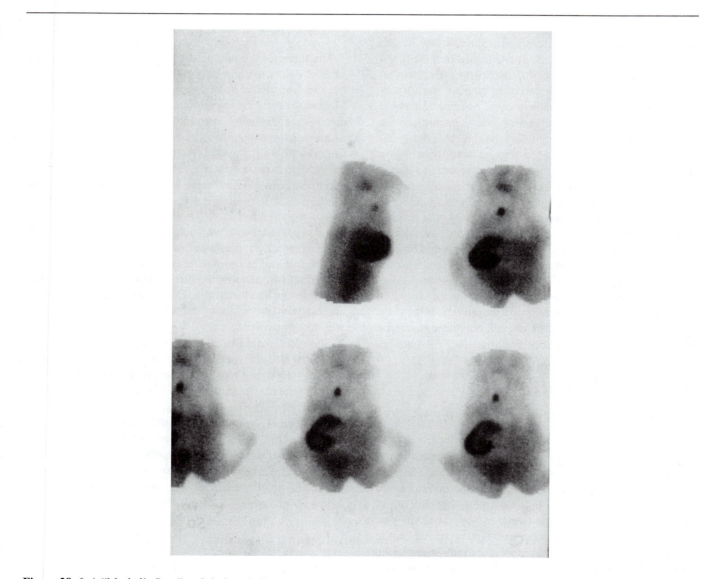

Figure 28–6 A "Meckel's Scan" or Scintigraph Showing the Location of Meckel's Diverticulum (i.e., Ectopic Site of Isotope)

The nurse should explain why there are no long-term aftereffects from this small dosage to either the child or the family members. If the child is too young to be cooperative, it may be necessary to administer conscious sedation for the duration of the scan. Rarely, the bleeding has been so great as to cause the child to be self-sedated throughout the procedure. The child becomes weak and lethargic from the blood loss. Close monitoring is necessary.

The Meckel's scan takes approximately 30 minutes to complete. As the isotope circulates, it quickly reaches the kidneys, bladder, stomach, and ectopic gastric mucosa. Between 10% and 20% of it is absorbed into the soft tissues. Tc-pertechnetate has a half-life of 6 hours and is fully excreted from the body in 24 hours.

The differential diagnosis of the patient with a positive scan includes ectopic gastric mucosa located elsewhere and a false-positive study (Sfakianakis & Conway, 1981). Duplication cysts and Barrett's esophagus are two areas where gastric mucosa will be found and that absorb a radiopharmaceutical. A duplication cyst, otherwise known as an alimentary tract duplication, can occur anywhere from the mouth to the anus and, in addition to being lined with normal gastrointestinal mucosa, has smooth muscle walls like those in the intestines. Barrett's esophagus is a disorder of the lower esophagus resulting from gastroesophageal reflux of acid from the stomach and causes a benign ulcerlike lesion in the area.

False-positive studies can be caused by bleeding of the mucosa as in intussusception, bowel obstruction, ulcers, arteriovenous malformations, and urinary tract anomalies (Fries, Mortensson, & Robertson, 1984). An intestinal duplication is the second most common cause of a false-positive scan.

If the initial scan is negative and there is a strong suspicion of a Meckel's diverticulum, the scan should be repeated. It is possible that the bladder, which rapidly fills with the isotope, may block the diverticulum from view. Further, a patient with a bowel obstruction is not usually diagnosed preoperatively with Meckel's diverticulum as the cause. Finally, if the intussusception containing a Meckel's diverticulum is reduced by a barium enema, the diagnosis may not be made at this time (Foglia, 1993).

Goyal and Bellah (1993) reported a 24-day-old male infant who presented with symptoms of bowel obstruction and was diagnosed preoperatively by sonography. Because sonography is an excellent method of diagnosing many different disorders involving the bowel, it may be helpful in diagnosing Meckel's diverticulum, too.

In cases in which there is a high index of suspicion of Meckel's diverticulum but the scan is negative, the patient will undergo an exploratory laparotomy. It is at this time the cause of the complete bowel obstruction will often be found to be a Meckel's diverticulum (Foglia, 1993). The laparo-

scopic approach for diagnosis and excision of Meckel's diverticulum in children is described in the literature (Grosthwaite & Leather, 1997; Huang & Lin, 1993; Swaniker, Soldes, & Hirschi, 1999; Teitelbaum, Polley, & Obeid, 1994). This approach may be indicated instead of scintigraphic scanning in the assessment of the anemic pediatric patient with lower gastrointestinal bleeding and suspected Meckel's diverticulum (Swaniker et al., 1998).

Treatment of Meckel's Diverticulum

Patients who have painless bleeding usually stop bleeding spontaneously, and the scan and surgery can be performed electively (Figure 28–7). Patients who have active bleeding require fluid resuscitation provided as a blood transfusion and stabilization before going to the operating room. Bleeding should not recur after excision of a Meckel's diverticulum (Foglia, 1993).

Considerable controversy exists over the value of performing a diverticulectomy if a Meckel's diverticulum is found incidentally at the time of laparotomy. Most surgeons believe that it is best to leave the Meckel's diverticulum alone and not excise it. Mackey and Dineen (1983) reported 32 cases of incidental Meckel's diverticula left in situ without subsequent complications. Leijonmarck, Bonman-Sandelin, Frisell, and Raf (1986) reported 28 additional cases of incidental Meckel's diverticula left in situ without complications during a mean follow-up of 7.8 years. They also reported a 6% reoperation rate for incidental Meckel's diverticula that were removed.

Operative Procedure

The patient must be hemodynamically stable at the time of surgery. If necessary, a blood transfusion should be administered. Clear fluids should be provided up to 2 hours before surgery if this is an elective diverticulectomy. A bowel preparation is usually not necessary but may be routine in some institutions. The incision in the abdomen is made at the location of the diverticulum, in the right lower quadrant, as noted on the Meckel's scan. The diverticulum is divided at the junction of the small intestine and closed with sutures or possibly staples if the child is older and larger. It is important not to narrow the lumen of the intestine when suturing or stapling because such narrowing may cause an intestinal obstruction postoperatively (Cullen & Kelly, 1996).

If the patient has an intussusception, this should first be reduced and the diverticulum removed afterward. If a narrowing of the bowel and gangrene exist, it may be necessary to resect that portion of the bowel and anastomose or sew the ends of the bowel together. Occasionally, it may be necessary to give the patient a temporary stoma to allow for healing of the anastomosed bowel. If the obstruction has been

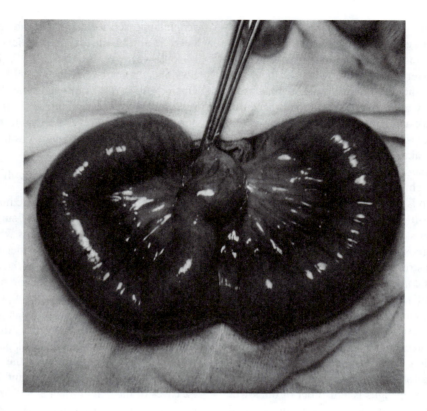

Figure 28–7 Intraoperative View of Meckel's Diverticulum with Mild Bleeding and Anemia

caused by a volvulus or twisting of the bowel or by an internal hernia (caused by a remnant of the omphalomesenteric duct), the treatment consists of reduction of the volvulus or hernia and removal of the duct (Cullen & Kelly, 1996).

Major complications occur as a result of the preceding presentations in conjunction with Meckel's diverticulum. Infection is the most common postoperative complication (Vane et al., 1987). As with any child who undergoes bowel surgery, the development of adhesions is a potential complication.

The risk of long-term complications like strictures, adhesions, or subsequent bowel obstruction developing (20 years after the surgery) is between 2% and 6%. Men have a greater chance of suffering long-term complications than do women (Cullen & Kelly, 1996). Possible complications such as postoperative bleeding and/or intestinal obstruction should be discussed with the family.

Nursing Considerations

Nursing care for children undergoing diverticulectomy is similar to the care of children with splenectomy or cholecystectomy. Preoperative teaching focuses on the surgery, de-

tails about expected length of stay, and the recovery time. Children remain NPO until bowel sounds return. Then the diet is advanced from clear liquids to regular as tolerated. Patients are usually discharged in 3 to 4 days if they meet the following criteria: no fever, ambulating, no infection, and eating a regular diet. School-age children are ready to return to school in 1 week and to full activities in 3 weeks. Information about signs of infection should be reinforced and information about pain medication provided. Follow-up should be planned with the surgical team in approximately 2 weeks.

CONCLUSION

Nurses caring for pediatric patients are frequently responsible for children who undergo splenectomy, cholecystectomy, and excision of a Meckel's diverticulum. The surgeries are generally well tolerated, requiring short hospital stays, ranging from 1 to 5 days and result in minimal morbidity. An understanding of the conditions necessitating these surgeries, the evaluation required, the operative procedure, and the nursing interventions is essential to providing quality care.

REFERENCES

Al-Salem, A.H., & Nourallah, H. (1997). Sequential endoscopic/laparoscopic management of cholelithiasis and choledocholithiasis in children who have sickle cell disease. *Journal of Pediatric Surgery, 21,* 1432–1435.

Ashcraft, K.W. (1994). *Atlas of pediatric surgery.* Philadelphia: W.B. Saunders Company.

Ben-Yehuda, D., Gillis, S., & Eldor, A. (1990). Clinical and therapeutic experience in 712 Israeli patients with idiopathic thrombocytopenic purpura. *Acta Hematologica, 91,* 1–6.

Bussel, J.B. (1990). Autoimmune thrombocytopenic purpura. *Hematology Oncology Clinics of North America, 4,* 179–191.

Chirletti, P., Cardi, M., Barillary, P., Vitale, A., Sammartino, P., Bolognese, A., Caiazzo, R., Ricci, M., Muttillo, I.A., & Stipa, V. (1992). Surgical treatment of immune thrombocytopenic purpura. *World Journal of Surgery, 16,* 1001–1005.

Cullen, J. J., & Kelly, K.A. (1996). Current management of Meckel's diverticulum. *Advances in Surgery, 29,* 207–214.

Digiacomo, J.C., & Cottone, F.J. (1993). Surgical treatment of Meckel's diverticulum. *Southern Medical Journal, 86,* 671–675.

Ein, S.H. (1993). Splenic lesions. In K.W. Ashcraft & T.M. Holder (Eds.), *Pediatric surgery* (pp. 535–545). Philadelphia: W.B. Saunders Company.

Flake, A.W. (1997). Disorders of the gallbladder and biliary tract. In K.T. Oldham, P.M. Colombani, & R.P. Foglia (Eds.), *Surgery of infants and children: Scientific principles and practice* (pp. 1405–1414). Philadelphia: Lippincott-Raven Publishers.

Foglia, R.P. (1993). Meckel's diverticulum. In K.W. Ashcraft (Ed.), *Pediatric surgery* (2nd ed., pp. 435–439). Philadelphia: W.B Saunders Company.

Fries, M., Mortensson, W., & Robertson, B. (1984). Technetium pertechnetate scintigraphy to detect ectopic gastric mucosa in Meckel's diverticulum. *Acta Radiologica: Diagnosis, 25,* 417–422.

Friesen, C.A., & Roberts, C.C. (1989). Cholelithiasis: Clinical characteristics in children. *Clinical Pediatrics, 28,* 294–298.

Gandy, J., Byrne, P., & Lees, G. (1997). Neonatal Meckel's diverticular inflammation with perforation. *Journal of Pediatric Surgery, 32,* 750–751.

George, C., Hammes, M., & Schwarz, D. (1995). Laparoscopic Swenson pull-through procedure for congenital megacolon. *AORN Journal, 62,* 727–736.

Goyal, M.K., & Bellah, R.D. (1993). Neonatal small bowel obstruction due to Meckel diverticulitis: Diagnosis by ultrasonography. *Journal of Ultrasound Medicine 12*(2), 119–122.

Grosthwaite, G.L., & Leather, A.J.M. (1997). Laparoscopy: The ultimate diagnostic tool for a bleeding Meckel's diverticulum. *Australia & New Zealand Journal of Surgery, 67,* 223–224.

Holcomb, G.W., & Greene, H.L. (1993). Fatal hemorrhage caused by disease progression after partial splenectomy for type III Gaucher's disease. *Journal of Pediatric Surgery, 28,* 1572–1574.

Holcomb, G.W., III, Olsen, D.O., & Sharp, K.W. (1991). Laparoscopic cholecystectomy in the pediatric patient. *Journal of Pediatric Surgery, 26,* 1186–1190.

Holcomb, G.W., III, & Pietsch, J.B. (1998). Gallbladder disease and hepatic infections. In J.A. O'Neill, Jr., M.I. Rowe, J.L. Grosfeld, E.W. Fonkalsrud, & A.G. Coran (Eds.), *Pediatric surgery* (5th ed., pp. 1495–1503). St. Louis, MO: Mosby.

Holcomb, G.W., III, Sharp, K.W., Neblett, W.W., III, Morgan, W.M., III, & Pietsch, J.B. (1994). Laparoscopic cholecystectomy in infants and children: Modifications and cost analysis. *Journal of Pediatric Surgery, 29,* 900–904.

Huang, C.S., & Lin, L.H. (1993). Laparoscopic Meckel's diverticulectomy in infants: Report of three cases. *Journal of Pediatric Surgery, 28*(11), 1486–1489.

Jacir, N.N., Anderson, K.D., Eichelberger, M., & Guzzetta, P.C. (1986). Cholelithiasis in infancy: Resolution of gallstones in three of four infants. *Journal of Pediatric Surgery, 21,* 567–569.

Janu, P.G., Rogers, D.A., & Lobe, T.E. (1996). A comparison of laparoscopic and traditional open splenectomy in childhood. *Journal of Pediatric Surgery, 31,* 109–114.

Jewett, T.C., Jr., Duszynski, D.O., & Allen, J.E. (1970). The visualization of Meckel's diverticulum with 99mTc-pertechnetate. *Surgery, 68,* 567–570.

Kim, P.C.W., Wesson, D., Superina, R., & Filler, R. (1995). Laparoscopic cholecystectomy versus open cholecystectomy in children: Which is better? *Journal of Pediatric Surgery, 30,* 971–973.

King, D.E., Ginn-Pease, M.E., Lloyd, T.V., Hoffman, J., & Hohenbrink, K. (1987). Parenteral nutrition with associated cholelithiasis: Another iatrogenic disease of infants and children. *Journal of Pediatric Surgery, 22,* 593–596.

Krishnamurthy, G.T., Bobba, V.R., & Kingston, E. (1981). Radionuclide ejection fraction: A technique for quantitative analysis of motor function of the human gallbladder. *Gastroenterology, 80,* 482–490.

Krishnamurthy, S., & Krishnamurthy, G.T. (1997). Biliary dyskinesia: Role of sphincter of Oddi, gallbladder, and cholecystokinin. *Journal of Nuclear Medicine, 38,* 1824–1830.

Lachman, B.S., Lazerson, J., Starshak, R.J., Vaughters, F.M., & Werlin, S.L. (1979). The prevalence of cholelithiasis in sickle cell disease as diagnosed by ultrasound and cholecystography. *Pediatrics, 64,* 601–603.

Leijonmarck, C.E., Bonman-Sandelin K., Frisell, J., & Raf, L. (1986). Meckel's diverticulum in the adult. *British Journal of Surgery 73,* 146–14.

Mackey, W.C., & Dineen, P.A. (1983). A fifty year experience with Meckel's diverticulum. *Surgery Gynecological Obstetrics, 156,* 56–64.

McCancre, K., & Huether, S. (1990). *Pathophysiology, the biological basis for disease in adults and children.* St. Louis, MO: Mosby.

Monson, J.R.T. (1993). Advanced techniques in abdominal surgery. *British Medical Journal, 307,* 1346–1350.

Moore, K.L., & Persaud, T.V.N. (1993). *The developing human: Clinically oriented embryology.* Philadelphia: W.B. Saunders Company.

Peter, G. (Ed.). (1994). *Red Book: Report of the Committee on Infectious Diseases* (23rd ed.). Elk Grove Village, IL: American Academy of Pediatrics.

Peter, G. (Ed.). (1997). *Red Book: Report of the Committee on Infectious Diseases* (24th ed.). Elk Grove Village, IL: American Academy of Pediatrics.

Rescorla, F.J. (1997). Cholelithiasis, cholecystitis, and common bile duct stone. *Current Opinion in Pediatrics, 9,* 276–282.

Schleef, J., Morcate, J.J., Steinau, G., Ott, B., & Willital, G.H. (1997). Technical aspects of laparoscopic splenectomy in children. *Journal of Pediatric Surgery, 32,* 615–617.

Sfakianakis, G.N., & Conway, J.J. (1981). Detection of ectopic gastric mucosa in Meckel's diverticulum and in other aberrations by scintigraphy:

II. Indications and methods—A 10-year experience. *Journal of Nuclear Medicine, 22,* 732–738.

Shaffer, E.A. (1996). Gallbladder disease. In W.A. Walker, P.R. Durie, J.R. Hamilton, J.A. Walker-Smith, & J.B. Watkins (Eds.), *Pediatric gastrointestinal disease: Pathophysiology, diagnosis, management* (5th ed., pp. 1399–1419). St. Louis, MO: Mosby.

Shorter, N.A., & Filston, H.C. (1993). Lymphomas. In K.W. Ashcraft & T.M. Holder (Eds.), *Pediatric surgery* (pp. 863–874). Philadelphia: W.B. Saunders Company.

Smith, B.M., Schropp, K.P., Lobe, T.E., Rogers, D.A., Presbury, G.J., Wilimas, J.A., & Wong, W.C. (1994). Laparoscopic splenectomy in childhood. *Journal of Pediatric Surgery, 28,* 975–977.

Soltero, M.J., & Bill, A.H. (1976). The natural history of Meckel's diverticulum and its relation to incidental removal. A study of 202 cases of diseased Meckel's diverticulum found in King County, Washington, over a fifteen year period. *American Journal of Surgery, 132,* 168–173.

Swaniker, F., Soldes, O., & Hisrchi, R. (1999). The utility of technetium 99m pertechnetate scintigraphy in the evaluation of patients with Meckel's diverticulum. *Journal of Pediatric Surgery, 34*(5), 760–764.

Teitelbaum, D.H., Polley, T.Z., & Obeid, F. (1994). Laparoscopic diagnosis and excision of Meckel's diverticulum. *Journal of Pediatric Surgery, 29*(4), 495–497.

Tsakayannis, D.E., Kozakewich, H.P.W., & Lillehei, C.W. (1996). Acalculous cholecystitis in children. *Journal of Pediatric Surgery, 31,* 127–131.

Tulman, S., Holcomb, G.W., III, Karamanoukian, H.L., & Reynhout, J. (1993). Pediatric laparoscopic splenectomy. *Journal of Pediatric Surgery, 28,* 689–692.

Vane, D.W., West, K.W., & Grosfeld, J.L. (1987). Vitelline duct anomalies: Experience with 217 childhood cases. *Archives of Surgery, 122,* 542–547.

Zamir, O., Szold, A., Matzner, Y., Ben-Yehuda, D., Seror, D., Deutsch, I., & Freund, H.R. (1996). Laparoscopic splenectomy for immune thrombocytopenic purpura. *Journal of Laparoendoscopic Surgery, 6*(5), 301–304.

Appendix 28–A

Caremap for Splenectomy

	Preop	OR	POD 1	POD 2	Day 3	Day 4 / Day 5
Monitoring/ assessment	VS q4h Strict I & O		Incisional dressing D & I NG output 4qh Social work screening			D/C dressing
Treatments	Bowel prep. consisting of golytely 100 ml every 10 min to 1/2 hr until effluent is clear		Irrigate NG with 10 ml NS q4h Replace NG output ml/ml with D_5 45 NS & 20 mEq KCl/L			
Line drains		Foley catheter Nasogastric tube for decompression IV	Foley catheter removed Nasogastric tube removed, if laparoscopic procedure	DC IV if laparoscopic Nasogastric tube removed if open procedure	DC IV if open	
Medications	Polyvalent vaccine 10 days to 2 wk before splenectomy Corticosteroids if indicated (as in ITP)		Laparoscopic patients: All ages: Tylenol with codeine; Tylenol suppositories Open patients: Under 6 months: Tylenol suppositories 6 months to 6 years: Morphine sulfate suppositories 6 years and over: PCA (IV morphine)	Same as day 1	Tylenol with codeine for both	Tylenol if laparoscopic Tylenol with codeine if open
Activity	Ambulatory		OOB to chair—open Ambulate— laparoscopic	Ambulate both		

continues

Appendix 28–A continued

	Preop	OR	POD 1	POD 2	Day 3	Day 4 / Day 5
Diet	Clear liquids 24 hr preop NPO after midnight	NPO if open or laparoscopic	NPO if open Clear liquids if laparoscopic	Clear liquids if NG tube removed Full liquids to solid if laparoscopic	Full liquids advance as tolerated if open	
Tests	CBC with diff. Chem7 Type and screen or type and crossmatch Platelets ready PRBCs ready					
Consults/referral						Follow-up ID specialist
Patient teaching	Preop movie for age 4 and older Family teaching explain operation postop, NG tube and Foley, pain medication					
Discharge planning				Laparoscopic procedure by day 2 to 2 1/2		Open procedure
Evaluation of outcomes				Afebrile x 24 hours Incision(s) clean and dry Tolerating regular diet Parents state s/s of infection, return to activity/school; administration of pain meds Parents given prescription of PCN G or PCN VK Follow-up appointment		

PART VI

Nursing Care of Children with Complex Surgical Conditions

CHAPTER 29

Biliary Atresia and Choledochal Cysts

Laura M. Flanigan

INTRODUCTION

The liver is the largest organ in the body and the site of varied and complex physiologic tasks. Included are vascular, metabolic, and storage functions, as well as detoxification and excretion of drugs and chemical alteration and excretion of hormones. A vital excretory function of the liver is formation of bile, which then flows into the intestinal tract through a system of ducts. Bile salts are required for the digestion and absorption of fat. The extrahepatic biliary system is crucial as a means of excreting bilirubin, the end product of hemoglobin degradation (Guyton, 1991).

Neonatal cholestasis is a common presentation of jaundice that implies an absence or impairment of bile flow from the hepatocyte to the duodenum. Causes of neonatal cholestasis vary from anatomic abnormalities, metabolic disorders, hepatitis, chromosomal abnormalities, and miscellaneous causes. This chapter discusses the diagnosis and treatment of two anatomic abnormalities—biliary atresia and choledochal cyst. Appendixes 29–A and 29–B provide critical pathways for biliary atresia and choledochal cyst, respectively.

BILIARY ATRESIA

Description

Biliary atresia (BA) is an obstructive condition of the liver and bile ducts that presents in early infancy and results in obliteration of the extrahepatic biliary tree. Although the term atresia implies congenital absence of the biliary tree, this condition is a dynamic one. There is an ongoing, inflammatory process of bile duct epithelium that scleroses and obliterates the normal ductal system. The cause is unknown, but once fibrosis obliterates the bile ducts, bile can no longer be transported from the liver to the gastrointestinal tract. This results in profound cholestasis, jaundice, and progressive cirrhosis, ultimately leading to liver failure. Biliary atresia is the most common cause of chronic cholestasis in infants and children (Balistreri et al., 1996).

No causal relationship exists between the cholestatic jaundice of biliary atresia and the physiologic jaundice of the newborn that begins at 3 to 5 days of life and generally resolves by 2 weeks. The incidence of BA is approximately 1 in 15,000 live births. It is rarely seen in premature infants and more females than males are affected. Polysplenia and intestinal malrotation are present in 15% to 20% of patients (Altman, Lilly, Greenfeld, Weinberg, vanLeeuwan, & Flanigan, 1997). Biliary atresia is the most common cause of death from liver disease in children (Ohi & Ibrahim, 1992). If untreated, biliary atresia results in progressive liver failure with the usual life expectancy of less than 2 years (Adelman, 1985).

Clinical Presentation

Most infants with BA have an uneventful perinatal course. Initially, the infant appears to be well and thrives despite the presence of asymptomatic jaundice that becomes apparent at 2 to 3 weeks of age (Wyllie & Hyams, 1993). Stools, which initially have a normal appearance, gradually become acholic (pale or clay colored). Urine becomes dark in appearance because the kidneys filter some excess bilirubin. In addition to being markedly icteric, the infant's liver is enlarged and firm. The gradual onset of the symptoms may go unnoticed by the parents and are often first appreciated by the primary health care provider at a regular visit at 4 to 8 weeks of life.

Differential Diagnosis and Workup

The presence of jaundice after 2 weeks of age is unlikely to be physiologic. Any jaundiced infant older than 2 weeks of age should be evaluated. Successful outcome in the treatment of BA is strongly influenced by the age at surgical intervention, which makes prompt diagnosis imperative. The likelihood of the surgical drainage procedure (Kasai procedure) being successful is markedly reduced in infants older than 10 weeks of age (Altman et al., 1997). No single test result is diagnostic of biliary atresia but certain tests may eliminate other conditions that are seen in early infancy with jaundice.

Laboratory Studies

Serum Bilirubin

An elevated bilirubin may result from obstructive, metabolic, or infectious causes that result in cholestasis. The hyperbilirubinemia of physiologic jaundice is indirect (unconjugated), appearing at about 2 days of age and generally resolving by the second week of life. The jaundice of BA is characterized by direct (conjugated) hyperbilirubinemia, with the total bilirubin being elevated to 4 to 8 mg/dl or greater with the direct level being 15% to 20% of the total. This is indicative of an obstructive process.

Liver Function

Liver enzymes are usually modestly elevated, indicative of hepatocellular injury (Table 29–1). This is not specific to biliary atresia. At the onset, prothrombin time and partial thromboplastin time are usually normal because the synthetic functions of the liver are still intact (Altman, 1991).

Other

Hepatitis serologic findings, "TORCH" titers, and alpha$_1$-antitrypsin studies are obtained to rule out some of the infectious and metabolic causes of jaundice. The hematocrit, hemoglobin, and white blood count are generally normal.

Radiologic Studies

Ultrasonography

An abdominal sonogram is a safe, noninvasive study that documents the presence and size of the gallbladder. In biliary atresia, the gallbladder is not visualized or is small (<1.5 cm) and noncontractile. A fasting infant with a gallbladder greater than 1.5 cm, which contracts with feeding, is unlikely to have biliary atresia (Karrer, Lilly, & Hall, 1993).

Hepato-Iminodiacetic Acid Scan

The hepatobiliary scan using technetium-99 iminodiacetic acid (HIDA) detects bile flow from the liver through the bil-iary tree and into the gastrointestinal tract. The isotope is quickly concentrated by the liver and normally excretion begins immediately. It can be detected in the gallbladder within 5 minutes and in the small bowel by 30 minutes. If isotope activity is not detected in the small bowel within a few hours, a delayed scan is obtained in 24 hours. In infants with biliary obstruction, no excretion into the bowel is detectable. Children with severe intrahepatic cholestasis, without extrahepatic biliary obstruction, may also demonstrate impaired excretion. Patients are prepared for the scan by receiving oral phenobarbital (5 to 10 mg/kg/day) for 3 to 5 days before the study. The choleretic effect of the phenobarbital encourages bile flow in patients with cholestasis. This study helps to identify patients whose lack of bile excretion is due to parenchymal disease rather than extrahepatic ductal obstruction (Madj, Reba, & Altman, 1981).

Percutaneous Liver Biopsy

The percutaneous liver biopsy is performed with local anesthesia and sedation. Intramuscular vitamin K is administered before the biopsy to enhance clotting. The potential risk of bleeding after a percutaneous liver biopsy necessitates close observation and monitoring of the infant's hemodynamic status for 6 hours. The histologic findings consistent with a diagnosis of biliary atresia are bile duct proliferation, cholestasis (which may be mild, moderate, or severe), and portal tract fibrosis (Ohi & Ibrahim, 1992).

Exploratory Laparotomy and Intraoperative Cholangiogram

The workup to this point cannot provide a secure diagnosis of BA. No test or combination of tests is absolutely diagnostic. Other causes of jaundice may be eliminated and findings may provide evidence to support, but not make, the diagnosis. Diagnosis is confirmed with surgical exploration to identify the anatomy of the extrahepatic bile ducts. With the patient under general anesthesia, a right upper quadrant incision is made. In BA the liver is firm and the surface appears greenish brown, coarse, and irregular. A generous liver specimen is obtained to confirm the findings of the previous percutaneous biopsy. If inspection of the extrahepatic biliary tree reveals complete fibrosis, the diagnosis of biliary atresia is confirmed. If the gallbladder has an obvious lumen, it is aspirated. If the contents are bilious, a cholangiogram is performed by instilling a small amount of radiopaque contrast. If the entire biliary tree, from the liver to the duodenum, can be visualized on the radiographic film, the diagnosis of BA is eliminated and the procedure terminated (Altman, 1991).

In BA there are anatomic variations of the diseased extrahepatic ducts. In approximately 25% of patients, the distal common duct is patent to the duodenum. In 75% the entire extrahepatic biliary tree is atretic. If the gallbladder is obviously fibrotic, a cholangiogram is deferred. Dissection in the

Table 29–1 Liver Function Tests

Test	Description
Albumin	Serum protein produced by the liver, decreased in chronic disease due to impaired synthesis, which contributes to formation of ascites
Alkaline phosphatase	Enzyme produced by liver, bone, and intestine; elevated in liver disease indicating biliary obstruction
ALT (SGPT)	Enzyme present in liver cells, elevated with hepatocellular injury (i.e., hepatitis, obstruction, cirrhosis)
AST (SGOT)	Enzyme present in cells of heart, muscle, liver; increases with hepatocellular injury
GGT (GGPT)	Enzyme found in many tissues but a sensitive test for both hepatocellular and obstructive liver disease
LDH	Enzyme found in many tissues; relatively insensitive to liver injury
PT (Protime)	Measure of phase II clotting; prolonged in liver decompensation
PPT (Partial thromboplastin time)	Measure of phase I clotting; prolonged in liver decompensation

portal area of the liver is then undertaken to identify the anatomy of the fibrotic biliary tree (Kasai, Kimura, & Asakura, 1968). If the diagnosis is confirmed by inability to visualize the complete biliary tree, the procedure converts from exploratory to therapeutic.

Surgery

Without surgical treatment to establish bile flow, BA is uniformly fatal. In 1968, following his earlier work in Japan, Kasai published the first report in the U.S. literature on the hepatic portoenterostomy (Kasai et al., 1968). The results were extremely encouraging, and the procedure gained gradual acceptance as the definitive procedure for BA in the 1970s (Altman & Lilly, 1975).

The hepatoportoenterostomy or Kasai procedure involves excision of the fibrotic biliary tract and anastomosis of a 45-cm Roux-en-Y limb of the jejunum to the periductal tissue at the porta hepatis (Figure 29–1). The procedure is based on Kasai's observations that the fibrous tissue at the porta contains microscopically patent biliary channels that communicate with the intrahepatic duct system (Kasai et al., 1968). This newly created conduit provides a channel for bile flow from liver to intestine. Although there are three common variants of BA (Figure 29–2), all require complete excision

of the extrahepatic biliary tree and creation of the Kasai hepatoportoenterostomy. Many modifications of the conduit, including exteriorization of the jejunal limb with cutaneous diversion of bile drainage and creation of an antireflux valve in the jejunal limb (Karrer et al., 1993), have been proposed with the intent of reducing the incidence of ascending bacterial cholangitis. None of the modifications intended to reduce the incidence of cholangitis affect outcome (Altman et al., 1997).

The goal of the Kasai procedure is to establish bile flow from the liver. The first appearance of bile in the stool may be scant, streaky, and intermittent and usually occurs by the end of the first postoperative week. When adequate bile flow is achieved, the pigmented appearance of the stool becomes normal.

Complications

The most common complication of the Kasai procedure is bacterial cholangitis. Initially, the bile flow from the liver may be sluggish. Infection results from the bile stasis and bacterial contamination from the intestinal conduit. All patients should receive intravenous antibiotics in the immediate postoperative period and continue oral prophylaxis for 12 to 24 months. Cholangitis is most likely within the first 2

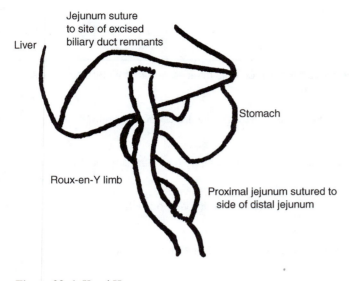

Figure 29–1 Kasai Hepatoportoenterostomy

years after surgery, although it may also occur later (McEvoy & Suchy, 1996). After a Kasai procedure, any patient with fever and leukocytosis and a rising bilirubin with no obvious other causes is presumed to have cholangitis and is treated with intravenous antibiotics and steroids. With each attack comes the risk of permanent liver damage with complete shutdown of bile flow. Institution of early treatment may prevent irreversible liver damage (Karrer et al., 1993).

Outcome

Kasai's hepatoportoenterostomy has revolutionized the outlook for infants with BA. Early recognition; prompt, effi-

cient workup; and timely referral for surgical correction are critical to achieving the best outcome. Without biliary drainage, there is no possibility of altering the inexorable course of the disease. When surgery is carried out before the infant reaches 70 days, there is a significantly greater chance of achieving bile flow. Another factor influencing outcome is the diameter of microscopic biliary ductules at the porta where the fibrous biliary tree has been resected. Patients with larger ductal lumens have a significantly better chance of long-term survival (Altman et al., 1997).

Bile drainage can be achieved in about 90% of patients who undergo a Kasai procedure at less than 10 weeks of age (Altman et al., 1997; Karrer et al., 1993). Approximately 30% to 40% of patients become jaundice free and liver functions return to normal, resulting in an optimistic long-term outcome. Another 30% to 40% of patients will have evidence of hepatic damage but with medical and nutritional support will continue to grow and develop. The fibrotic liver may eventually decompensate, often precipitated by some physiologically stressful event. In nearly another 30% of patients, even with bile drainage having been achieved, the process causing BA continues uninterrupted, with progressive biliary cirrhosis leading to early liver failure (Altman, 1991; Karrer et al., 1993).

Portal hypertension is another potential problem after portoenterostomy, even with adequate bile flow. The portal vein carries blood and its newly acquired nutrients from the viscus into the liver. A scarred liver impedes this flow, increasing the portal venous pressure. Portal hypertension ultimately results in hypersplenism, ascites, and esophageal and gastric varices. Hemorrhagic bleeding from esophageal varices may be sudden, repeated, and life threatening. Varices are managed by endoscopic sclerosing or banding (Karrer et al., 1993).

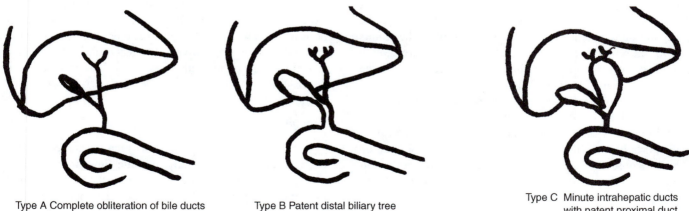

Type A Complete obliteration of bile ducts   Type B Patent distal biliary tree   Type C Minute intrahepatic ducts
                                                                                                   with patent proximal duct
                                                                                                   and gallbladder

Figure 29–2 Most Common Types of Biliary Atresia

At present, the treatment for end-stage liver disease or severe portal hypertension is hepatic transplantation. Patients with BA comprise most of the pediatric recipients undergoing liver transplantation (Whitington & Balistreri, 1991). It has been suggested that transplantation replace the Kasai procedure as the treatment of choice (Azarow, Phillips, & Sandler, 1997). However, there is evidence in a large series that median survival after achieving biliary drainage with the Kasai procedure is 15 years. Some children may never need transplantation, whereas others survive with their native liver many years before needing transplantation. With the limited supply of organs available to infants, decreased survival in infant recipients, and the problems associated with long-term immunosuppression along with the likelihood that the portoenterostomy will extend pretransplant survival, the Kasai procedure and liver transplantation should be considered complementary therapies (Altman et al., 1997).

The advent of successful outcomes using living, related, and reduced sized orthotopic liver grafts has made it possible to plan liver transplants for infants after a failed Kasai procedure. Transplantation may then take place before patients reach end-stage liver disease. For additional information on liver transplantation refer to Chapter 31.

Developmental Considerations

When the Kasai procedure is successful in establishing biliary drainage and liver function returns to normal, there is a negligible impact on development. If the course of hepatic fibrosis is not interrupted by the portoenterostomy, delays in growth and development are inevitable. Fat, carbohydrate, and protein metabolism normally occur in the liver, and this process is increasingly impaired as hepatic fibrosis progresses. A critical indication of impaired hepatic function is an infant's failure to maintain his or her own curve on the growth chart for height, weight, and head circumference. As the child's nutritional status worsens, the ability to achieve expected developmental milestones becomes markedly impaired. Increasing abdominal girth, secondary to hepatosplenomegaly, and ascites make being placed in the prone position difficult, which interferes with development of head control. As nutrition worsens, the child develops muscle wasting and decreased strength and energy to perform normal, age-appropriate activities.

Susceptibility to infection may require isolating a child from his or her peer group and interfere with normal social development. Interventions designed to stimulate physical and social development should be encouraged. As children become sicker and require intermittent hospitalization, physical and occupational therapy and child life can ensure that appropriate interventions and activities are available. Parents and the health care team should participate in and reinforce planned developmental activities.

Referrals

Several parent support groups may be helpful to parents as they struggle to cope with their child's diagnosis. For example, the Biliary Atresia and Liver Transplant Network Inc. (BALT) and Children's Liver Association for Support Services (CLASS) provide support networks for families of children with BA and chronic liver disease, both before and after transplantation. Refer to Appendix A for additional information.

Referrals to home care agencies should be made as appropriate. If the biliary conduit is exteriorized, the family is referred to a home health agency for additional support and teaching until parents are comfortable caring for the ostomy. If the liver disease becomes progressive, parents may find themselves facing increasingly complex care issues at home. Equipment and home nursing support may be required for nasogastric feedings, total parenteral nutrition, central line care, and pain management.

CHOLEDOCHAL CYST

Description

Choledochal cyst is a malformation of the biliary system manifested by localized dilation of all or some portion of the intrahepatic and extrahepatic biliary tree. The first description appeared in the literature in the seventeenth century (Douglas, 1852). In 1959 the entity was classified into three anatomic groups by Alonso-Lej, and since then two variants have been added (Caroli, 1968; Flanigan, 1975). The most common presentation is type I, cystic dilation of the common bile duct that represents more than 75% of cases. The other four classifications describe a spectrum of complex pathologic anomalies in the biliary tree that together make up the remaining less than 25%. Type II represents a diverticulum of the common bile duct and type III an intraduodenal dilation of the common bile duct (also called choledochocele). In type IV there is intrahepatic and extrahepatic cystic dilation. If intrahepatic cysts are present with a normal extrahepatic biliary tree, it is classified as type V, also called Caroli's disease.

The origin of choledochal cyst formation is unclear, although many mechanisms have been proposed. It is likely that a number of factors lead to their formation and that the cysts actually represent a spectrum of anomalies in the pancreaticobiliary system. The common features, in addition to cystic dilation of the bile duct, include (1) anomalous junction of the pancreatic and common bile duct; (2) distal bile duct stenosis; (3) intrahepatic ductal dilation; (4) abnormal histologic findings of the common bile duct; and (5) hepatic histologic findings from normal to cirrhotic (Altman, 1992). The bile duct stenosis results in cholestasis leading to cholangitis. The liver injury that results may range from mild periportal infiltrates to marked biliary cirrhosis and subsequent portal hypertension (Lazar & Altman, 1999). Adenocarcinoma resulting from long-term inflammation of the bile ducts has also been reported (Howard, 1991). Surgical intervention is necessary to relieve the chronic obstruction.

Choledochal cyst is considered a rare entity, with a worldwide incidence reported anywhere between 1 in 13,000 to 1 in 1,000,000 (Wyllie & Hyams, 1993). It is much more frequently seen in the Japanese, with an incidence of 1 in 1,000 but only 1 in 15,000 in the United States (Howard, 1991). In all races, the female to male incidence is about 4:1.

Clinical Presentation

Choledochal cyst can be diagnosed at any age, but approximately 25% are diagnosed by 1 year and 60% by age 10. Clinical presentation in early infancy, less than 6 months of age, may include signs of complete extrahepatic biliary obstruction: jaundice, hepatomegaly, and acholic stools. These symptoms make it indistinguishable from biliary atresia (Rowe, O'Neill, Grosfeld, Fonkalsrud, & Coran, 1995). Increased use of ultrasonography as a screening technique has led to prenatal diagnosis in a number of cases (Holland & Lilly, 1992). Older infants or children present with subtle episodic but recurrent abdominal pain. The accompanying minimal jaundice may go unnoticed (Altman, 1992). Approximately 15% of patients actually present with what is referred to as the classic triad: intermittent pain, jaundice, and abdominal mass. Pancreatitis and cholangitis occur secondary to the bile stasis caused by the obstructive nature of the cyst (Lazar & Altman, 1999). Untreated choledochal cyst may result in chronic liver failure or biliary carcinoma (Karrer et al., 1993).

Diagnosis

The initial workup depends on the nature, severity, and duration of the symptoms. Laboratory findings are nonspecific. The main finding is conjugated hyperbilirubinemia, which is generally more pronounced in the infant. Other laboratory abnormalities include elevated alkaline phosphatase, transaminases, and gamma glutamyl transpeptidase. An abdominal ultrasonography and computed axial tomography scan establish the diagnosis of choledochal cyst. Both studies clearly define the dimensions of the cyst and the extent of involvement. In patients in whom symptoms are intermittent and marked cystic enlargement is not present, a DISIDA (technetium-99m) scan should be obtained with follow-up scanning to define extrahepatic anatomy and the pattern of bile excretion. Endoscopic retrograde cholangiopancreatography (ERCP) is also used to diagnose a choledochal cyst. This invasive study increases the risk of cholangitis (Altman & Hicks, 1996). Recently, magnetic

resonance cholangiopancreatography (MRCP) has replaced endoscopic retrograde cholangiopancreatography because it provides the same information noninvasively.

Recommended Therapy

Definitive treatment for choledochal cyst is surgical. Internal drainage by cystenterostomy, once considered the procedure of choice, has been abandoned. However, patients treated with this method had a high incidence of anastomotic obstruction leading to bile stasis, cholangitis, biliary cirrhosis, and possible malignancy in the retained cyst wall (Flanigan, 1977).

Total cyst removal with reconstruction using a Roux-en-Y jejunostomy with anastomosis of the normal, proximal bile ducts to a limb of jejunum is now the preferred treatment in most cases (Altman & Hicks, 1996). Anastomosis of the mucosa of the proximal bile duct to the mucosa of a jejunal loop is important to avoid postoperative stricture. If inflammation around the cyst makes resection hazardous, the entire mucosal lining may be removed, leaving the outer wall in place. In type V, in which the cystic structure is inside the liver, a lobectomy may be indicated. If the disease affects both lobes, transplant is the only treatment (Lazar & Altman, 1999).

Outcome

Early postoperative complications are generally minor. The most common late complications are cholangitis, obstructive jaundice, pancreatitis, and complications of portal hypertension such as bleeding esophageal varices (Karrer et al., 1993). The long-term results after biliary reconstruction are favorable in patients who have surgery before the onset of advanced liver disease (Lazar & Altman, 1999). If biliary cirrhosis develops because of delayed diagnosis or postsurgical complications, the child may have the hallmarks of chronic liver disease such as malnutrition, hepatosplenomegaly, ascites, and susceptibility to infection.

Developmental Considerations

Prompt diagnosis and treatment alleviate impact on a child's growth and development. Infants usually undergo surgery before chronic liver disease has any effect on growth and development. In older children, symptoms such as recurrent episodes of severe abdominal pain and a child's ability to eat normally, go to school, and play may be severely impacted.

Referrals

Most children recover with no long-term sequelae. Families with children who have chronic liver disease may find that contact with families in similar circumstances is helpful.

The Children's Liver Association for Support Services (CLASS) is a support group for families of children with chronic liver disease.

NURSING CARE OF THE CHILD WITH BILIARY ATRESIA AND CHOLEDOCHAL CYSTS

Preoperative

Families have a wide variety of understanding about the diagnosis of BA and choledochal cysts, the treatment, and possible outcomes. Most are overwhelmed and frightened by the news that their young infant or child has a serious condition and needs an urgent, major surgical procedure. Some have limited knowledge about the diagnosis and its life-threatening implications, whereas others are well informed. Often parents come with lists of questions and information obtained from an Internet search.

Nursing assessment of the family's level of functioning will make it possible to provide the appropriate level of teaching and support. The nurse needs to repeat and reinforce the information about diagnosis, prognosis, surgical procedure, and the perioperative course.

If the patient with BA is close to 70 days of age when referred to the pediatric surgeon, the situation must be treated with urgency to enhance the chances of a favorable outcome (Altman et al., 1997).

Patients are admitted to the hospital the morning of surgery. Bowel preparation is not necessary. Additional blood work is usually unnecessary. If transfusion is anticipated, a specimen for typing and cross-match is obtained. Information regarding giving donor-designated blood should be made available prior to surgery. Results of laboratory work obtained outside the hospital should be documented. Intramuscular vitamin K may be administered before surgery.

Nursing mothers should be informed that breastfeeding will be interrupted for a few days. Mothers should be provided with information and assistance in pumping and storing breast milk while their infant is unable to feed orally.

Because the diagnosis of BA cannot always be confirmed before exploration, it is important to communicate with the family from the operating room. This may be done by a call or visit from a member of the surgical team.

Postoperative

Care after a Kasai procedure or total cyst removal is similar to that for any infant or child who has had abdominal surgery with intravenous hydration, antibiotics, and narcotic. The first antibiotic dose is given before surgery. When the patient is tolerating feedings, an oral antibiotic at a prophylactic dose is begun. Adequate postoperative pain management requires continuous narcotic infusion. This may be pro-

vided quite safely even in infants and young children with appropriate dosing and frequent assessment. The addition of rectal acetaminophen may potentiate the effect of the opioid in treating postoperative pain. Reduction of the narcotic dose can result in fewer adverse effects (Tobias, 1996).

The Kasai procedure or cyst removal requires a generous right upper quadrant incision. The right incision is covered with a small dressing that allows assessment of the wound. A soft drain is brought out through a stab wound several centimeters below the incision and dressed separately. This keeps ascitic fluid, serum, or bile from collecting within the abdomen. The drain is advanced several centimeters per day until it is removed, usually by the fifth postoperative day. The dressing is changed as needed, using sterile technique.

The patient remains NPO and has a nasogastric tube to low suction for decompression of the stomach and gastrointestinal tract. A tube that is not in the stomach will not drain properly. If there is no drainage initially or anytime in the early postoperative period or the patient becomes distended, patency and position of the tube are assessed. Five to 10 ml of normal saline instilled gently may clear an obstructed tube. If suction is too strong, it may pull gastric mucosa into the suction holes and prevent proper drainage from occurring. If a sump type tube is used, it may be necessary to instill a few milliliters of air in the sump lumen to clear it. The tube should then be repositioned as needed and secured. Return of bowel function is indicated by reduction of nasogastric drainage or passage of flatus or stool. This generally occurs 2 to 3 days postoperatively. Presence of bowel sounds alone does not provide assurance that bowel function is sufficient to allow removal of the tube. If the infant does not become distended within 6 to 8 hours after tube removal, small feedings of 15 ml of water, glucose water, or electrolyte solution are initiated. If this is tolerated for several feedings, the infant advances to expressed breast milk or formula, gradually advancing the volume. Unrestricted breast or formula feeding can generally be resumed without problem about 24 hours after feedings are initiated. Intravenous fluids should be reduced as oral volume increases. In older infants and children clear liquids may be offered and the diet advanced as tolerated.

The appearance of bile in the stool indicates that the portoenterostomy has been successful in providing a conduit from the liver to the gastrointestinal tract. The first stools may have been in the colon preoperatively and still be clay colored. The first appearance of bile is usually green plugs. Because of the severe intrahepatic cholestasis, bile flow is sporadic initially. It is important to warn parents of this so they are not alarmed by the passage of acholic stools. The flow of bile from the liver increases gradually until the stools are normally pigmented. Within a few days of initiating feedings, patients begin ursodeoxycholic acid (Actigol), 12 to 20 mg/day in two divided doses. This is a choleretic agent that promotes bile flow. Ursodeoxycholic acid is continued for a minimum of 1 to 2 years if there is good return of liver function. Patients with continued evidence of cirrhosis may remain on Actigol indefinitely.

Some infants with BA have an externalized conduit that should be fitted with an appropriate ostomy device. The family should be instructed to measure the output and feed the bile into the distal stoma using a small catheter. This provides the infant's gastrointestinal tract with bile salts to absorb fats. Discharge planning includes arranging delivery of appropriate supplies. The possibility of bleeding from the stoma should varices develop must be discussed. Closure of the ostomy is performed in several months whether good bile flow has been established or not.

Because the fat, carbohydrate, and protein metabolism that occurs in the liver is impaired and because of the reduced presence of bile acids in the intestine of patients with biliary atresia, nutrition is always an important consideration. Postoperatively, patients are fed breast milk or formula containing medium-chained triglycerides as the source of fat, such as Pregestimil and Alimentum. These formulas do not require bile acids for digestion. Absorption of the fat-soluble vitamins A, D, E, and K is usually compromised. These are available as a single preparation and should be started when the patient is tolerating oral feedings. Serum vitamin E levels can be monitored in 4 to 8 weeks. It is sometimes necessary to increase the dose to get adequate levels because of impaired absorption (Hendricks & Walker, 1990).

Even with evidence of biliary drainage and resolution of jaundice, improvement in liver function parameters cannot be expected for 4 to 6 weeks. Obtaining studies before that time creates unnecessary anxiety for the family and is not predictive of outcome. It will be several months before it can be established whether liver functions will return to normal.

Postoperative support for these families is critical. If biliary drainage does not occur promptly, anxiety is heightened. The reality that, even in the face of successful biliary drainage, the likelihood of this being a chronic illness is beginning to be understood. Introduction of information on support groups for families of infants with BA and liver disease is appropriate at this time. Families are discharged from the hospital not knowing whether the Kasai procedure will be successful in interrupting the course of the disease. Whether the child's liver will recover sufficiently or they will face the problems of chronic liver failure, ultimately requiring transplantation for survival, is still to be determined.

CHRONIC LIVER DISEASE

When the degree of hepatic fibrosis is significant or continues to worsen, despite a portoenterostomy, the family must begin to deal with the sequelae of biliary cirrhosis. The patient and family benefit from continued nursing support when the child is managed at home or during those periods when hospitalization might be required.

Maintaining the child's nutritional status at a level where growth and development continue to occur at an acceptable rate is critically important. Fat digestion and metabolism present the greatest problems, but initially most babies will gain weight on breast milk or medium-chain triglyceride oil formulas. Early introduction of solids that are higher in carbohydrate and have greater caloric density may be helpful. The addition of a carbohydrate supplement, such as Polycose, to both formula and solids will boost caloric intake. As the disease progresses, hepatosplenomegaly and ascites may compress the stomach so that small, frequent feedings become necessary. This is a difficult time for families as they begin to see their child fail.

During the later stages of disease, nasogastric feedings are needed to supplement oral intake or become the primary source of nutrition. Admission to the hospital is usually required for parents to learn to pass the tube, secure it, and administer the feedings safely. Nighttime continuous feeding with oral feeding during the daytime allows maximum freedom. If enteral feeding is unsuccessful, total parenteral nutrition is used but has the potential for further adverse effects on the liver. Optimizing the child's nutritional status improves chances of becoming a successful liver transplant recipient. Failure to thrive even with nutritional support measures is indication for transplantation in these infants (Whitington & Balistreri, 1991).

Many infants have pruritus develop because of increased serum concentrations of bile salts. This leads to deposits in the epidermis causing itching that can become severe. The child's nails should be kept short to prevent damage to the skin. Cloth mitts should be applied to prevent scratching so that hands do not need to be restrained. Cholestyramine may be administered to bind bile salts in the intestine and promote their excretion. However, this also reduces the bile salts available to aid in fat digestion. If bile is not present in the gastrointestinal tract, as evidenced by acholic stools, cholestyramine will not be effective (Wyllie & Hyams, 1993). Antihistamines may also be used. Severe, uncontrolled pruritus is considered an indication for transplantation.

Generalized edema and increasing ascites result from decreasing serum albumin levels and the presence of portal hypertension. This may become severe, resulting in discomfort and respiratory distress. Spironolactone (Aldactone) or furosemide (Lasix) may be used to control this problem (Wyllie & Hyams, 1993). Serum electrolytes should be monitored carefully after diuretics are initiated to detect abnormalities. Keeping the head elevated may also increase the child's comfort level.

RESEARCH

Further research is required to identify the cause of BA. Genetic, ischemic, and infectious causes have been proposed as causes of the process that causes the sclerotic obliteration of the biliary tract. Most recently, an autoimmune basis has been proposed on the basis of the presence of the inflammatory mediator, intercellular adhesion molecule-1, found in the ductal epithelium of six patients with biliary atresia (Dillon, Belchis, Minnick, & Tracey, 1994).

CONCLUSION

There are many causes of jaundice in early infancy; however, only in the case of BA does early intervention have such a critical influence on outcome. Studies have shown that early diagnosis and surgical treatment by 10 weeks of age will result in a far greater likelihood of success. Since the advent of the Kasai hepatoportoenterostomy, more than 30% of patients have stable, normal liver function. Another 30% have gained enough improvement in liver function to reach normal growth and development milestones for months or years. Only one third of patients do not appear to gain any benefit and require early rescue with liver transplantation to survive.

Infants presenting with choledochal cysts may have symptoms similar to those of BA but may be distinguished with ultrasound or CT scan. Older infants and children generally present with episodic abdominal pain due to cholangitis or pancreatitis. Total excision of the cyst and Roux-en-Y drainage procedure are the preferred treatment in all age groups.

REFERENCES

Adelman, S. (1985). Prognosis of uncorrected biliary atresia. *Journal of Pediatric Surgery, 20,* 529–534.

Alonso-Lej, F., Rever, W., & Pessagano, D. (1959). Congenital choledochal cyst with a report of 2 and an analysis of 94 cases. *International Abstracts of Surgery, 108,* 1–30.

Altman, R.P. (1991). Infantile obstructive jaundice. In M. Schiller (Ed.), *Pediatric surgery of the liver, pancreas and spleen* (pp. 59–75). Philadelphia: W.B. Saunders.

Altman, R.P. (1992). Choledochal cyst. *Seminars in Pediatric Surgery, 1*(2), 130–133.

Altman, R.P., & Hicks, B. (1996). Choledochal cyst. In D. Carter, R. Russell, H. Pitt, & H. Bismuth (Eds.), *Hepatobiliary and pancreatic surgery* (pp. 362–368). London: Chapman & Hall.

Altman, R.P., & Lilly, J.R. (1975). Technical details in the surgical correction of extrahepatic biliary atresia. *Surgery, Gynecology & Obstetrics, 10,* 952.

Altman, R.P., Lilly, J.R., Greenfeld, J., Weinberg, A., vanLeeuwen, K., & Flanigan, L. (1997). A multivariate risk factor analysis of the portoenterostomy (Kasai) for biliary atresia: A twenty five year experience from two centers. *Annals of Surgery, 226,* 348–355.

Azarow, K., Phillips, M., & Sandler, A. (1997). Should all patients undergo a portoenterostomy. *Journal of Pediatric Surgery, 32,* 168–174.

Balistreri, W., Grand, R., Hoofnagle, J., Suchy, F., Rykman, F., Perlmutter, D., & Sokol, R. (1996). Biliary atresia: Current concepts and research directions. *Hepatology, 23,* 1682–1692.

Caroli, J. (1968). Disease of intrahepatic bile ducts. *Israel Journal of Medical Science, 4,* 21–25.

Dillon, P., Belchis, D., Minnick, K., & Tracey, T. (1994). Differential expression of the major histocompatibility complex antigens and ICAM-1 on bile duct epithelial cells in biliary atresia. *Tohoku Journal of Experimental Medicine, 181,* 33–40.

Douglas, A.H. (1852). Case of dilatation of the hepatic bile duct. *Monthly Journal of Medical Science, 14,* 97.

Flanigan, D.P. (1975). Biliary cysts. *Annals of Surgery, 182,* 635–643.

Flanigan, D.P. (1977). Biliary carcinoma associated with biliary cysts. *Cancer, 40,* 880–883.

Guyton, A.C. (1991). *Textbook of medical physiology* (8th ed.). Philadelphia: W.B. Saunders.

Hendricks, K., & Walker, W.A. (1990). *Manual of pediatric nutrition* (2nd ed.). Toronto: B.C. Decker.

Holland, R., & Lilly, J.R. (1992). Surgical jaundice in infants: Other than biliary atresia. *Seminars in Pediatric Surgery, 1*(2), 126–129.

Howard, E.R. (1991). Choledochal cysts. In E.R. Howard (Ed.), *Surgery of liver disease in children.* Oxford: Butterworth-Heinemann.

Kasai, M., Kimura, S., & Asakura, Y. (1968). Surgical treatment of biliary atresia. *Journal of Pediatric Surgery, 3,* 665–675.

Karrer, F., Lilly, J.R., & Hall, R.J. (1993). Biliary tract disorders and portal hypertension. In K.W. Ashcraft & T.M. Holder (Eds.), *Pediatric surgery* (2nd ed., pp. 448–485). Philadelphia: W.B. Saunders Company.

Lazar, E., & Altman, R.P. (1999). Surgical disease of the biliary tract. Manuscript submitted for publication.

Madj, M., Reba, R., & Altman, R.P. (1981). Effect of phenobarbital on 99mTc-IDA scintigraphy in the evaluation of neonatal jaundice. *Seminars in Nuclear Medicine, 11,* 194–204.

McEvoy, C., & Suchy, F. (1996). Biliary tract disease in children. *Pediatric Clinics of North America, 43,* 75–98.

Ohi, R., & Ibrahim, M. (1992). Biliary atresia. *Seminars in Pediatric Surgery, 1,* 115–124.

Rowe, M., O'Neill, J. Jr., Grosfeld, J., Fonkalsrud, E., & Coran, A. (1995). Choledochal cyst. In *Essentials of pediatric surgery.* St. Louis, MO: Mosby.

Tobias, J. (1996). Postoperative pain management. In J. Deshpande & J. Tobias (Eds.), *Pediatric pain handbook* (p. 55). St. Louis, MO: Mosby.

Whitington, P.F., & Balistreri, W.F. (1991). Liver transplantation in pediatrics: Indications, contraindications, and pre-transplant management. *Journal of Pediatrics, 118,* 169–177.

Wyllie, R., & Hyams, J. (1993). Abnormalities of the bile duct. In R. Wyllie & J. Hyams (Eds.), *Pediatric gastrointestinal disease* (pp. 917–921). Philadelphia: W.B. Saunders Company.

Appendix 29–A

Critical Pathway for Biliary Atresia

Day/Date	Preop	OR Day	POD 1	POD 2	POD 3	POD 4	POD 5	POD 6
Consults/ Assessment	Laboratory Liver function Hepatitis screen TORCH titers Alpha₁- antitrypsin Radiologic HIDA scan Abdominal ultrasonog- raphy Percutaneous liver biopsy	Exploratory laparotomy Liver biopsy Cholangio- gram Preop weight Vital signs C-R monitor or pulse oximetry (while on IV narcotics) Strict I & O Assess pain, wound, abdominal distention	Weight		Vital signs Strict I & O Pain, wound, drainage ? return of bowel function (NG drainage, flatus or stool)	Observation of stool color		Notify pediatrician of discharge
				Assess fluid balance				
Treatments		Kasai procedure (portoenter- ostomy)			Change drain dressing PRN			dc drain site dsg if dry
Medications	Phenobarbital 5–10 mg/kg/ day × 3 days before scan	IV antibiotics IV narcotic/ continuous	Add rectal acetamino- phen to pain management regimen		Continue IV antibiotics Reduce IV narcotic dose Continue rectal acetamino- phen	Narcotics PRN	Start oral antibiotics, vitamins, & Actigol dc narcotics Acetaminophen PRN PO/PR	Discharge on oral antibiotics, vitamins, & Actigol Acetaminophen PRN PO/PR for discomfort
Lines/Drains		IV fluids 1½ maintenance NG tube to suction Penrose drain/ abdominal wound		Decrease IV to maintenance Advance drain 1–1.5 cm/day	IV at mainte- nance NG to gravity Advance drain	Remove NG if no distention & evidence of bowel function	IV at 1/2 main- tenance if PO >hep cap Drain out	dc IV Both if drain site dry

Day/Date	Preop	OR Day	POD 1	POD 2	POD 3	POD 4	POD 5	POD 6
Diet	Formula or breast	Formula or breast until 6 hours preop Clears until 2 hours preop then NPO	NPO	NPO	NPO>clear	Clear>advance as tolerated	Feed ad lib	
Activity	Normal infant	Provide safe environment	Assist family in holding baby safely & comfortably	Infant stimulation activities/props				
Family Teaching	Diagnosis specific & standard preop teaching	Orientation to environment Reinforce teaching re periop course Provide lactating mother with teaching & facilities	Provide opportunity & teaching for families to be involved in care as desired				Teach med administration, wound assessment S & S cholangitis	Reassess parental knowledge and ability Written home care instructions
Discharge Planning		Begin assessment of home care needs	Begin discharge planning				Home health referral PRN	Discharge Return appt. Telephone number for problems, questions

Appendix 29–B

Critical Pathway for Choledochal Cyst

Day/Date	Preop	OR Day	POD 1	POD 2	POD 3	POD 4	POD 5	POD 6
Consults/ Assessment	Laboratory Liver function Hepatitis screen TORCH titers Alpha$_1$-antitrypsin Radiologic Abdominal ultrasonography ERCP/MRCP	Preop weight Vital signs C-R monitor or pulse oximetry (while on IV narcotics) Strict I & O Assess pain, wound, abdominal distention	Weight	Assess fluid balance	Vital signs strict I & O Pain, wound, drainage ? return of bowel function (NG drainage, flatus, or stool) Change drain dressing PRN			Notify pediatrician of discharge dc drain site dsg if dry
Treatments		Cyst excision Roux-en-Y jejunostomy						
Medications		IV antibiotic IV narcotic/ continuous	Add rectal acetaminophen to pain management regimen		Continue IV antibiotics Reduce IV narcotic dose Continue rectal acetaminophen	Narcotics PRN	Start oral antibiotics dc narcotics Acetaminophen PRN PO/PR	Discharge on oral antibiotics Acetaminophen PRN PO/PR for discomfort
Lines/Drains		IV fluids 1½ maintenance NG tube to suction Penrose drain/ abdominal wound		Decrease IV to maintenance Advance drain 1–1.5 cm/day	IV at maintenance NG to gravity Advance drain	Remove NG if no distention & evidence of bowel function	IV at 1/2 maintenance if PO >hep cap Drain out	dc IV

Day/Date	Preop	OR Day	POD 1	POD 2	POD 3	POD 4	POD 5	POD 6
Diet	Regular for age	Infant: formula or breast until 6 hours preop Child: regular until 8 hours preop All, clears until 2 hours preop then NPO	NPO	NPO	NPO > clear	Clear > regular for age	Feed ad lib	
Activity	Normal	Provide safe environment	Assist family in holding or positioning safely & comfortably	Age-appropriate stimulation, activities/props		Normal		Bathe if drain site dry
Family Teaching	Diagnosis specific & standard preop teaching	Orientation to environment Reinforce teaching re: periop course Provide lactating mother with teaching & facilities	Provide opportunity & teaching for families to be involved in care as desired				Medication administration Wound assessment S & S cholangitis	Assess parental knowledge & ability Written instructions
Discharge Planning		Begin assessment of home care needs	Begin discharge planning				Home health referral PRN	Discharge Return appt. Telephone number for problems or questions

CHAPTER 30

Solid Tumors

Barbara S. Ehrenreich and Laura San Miguel

"Within Western industrialized nations, the proportion of all cancers occurring in the pediatric age range is approximately 2%" (Robison, 1997). Cancer in childhood, however, is the second leading cause of childhood mortality and the most common cause of death from disease in the United States in children from age 1 to age 15 (Leonard, Alyono, Fischel, Nesbit, Nguyen, & McClain, 1985; Robison, 1997; Young & Miller, 1975). Demographically, the incidence for cancer in children less than 15 years of age is greater in males than females and in whites than blacks (Gurney, Severson, Davis, & Robinson, 1995). The incidence is greater in the early years from birth to 3 years of age, with a steady decline until adolescence when the rate begins to increase again (Gurney et al., 1995).

In the past, resection was the only treatment of solid tumors. It has now become an integral part of a combined program of treatment, along with chemotherapy, radiation, and even immunotherapy. Each modality plays a specific role at a specific point, with each role being dependent on the one before and after it for success.

Malignant solid tumors account for most cases of cancer in children, with central nervous system (CNS) tumors being the most common. The most common extracranial solid tumors are neuroblastoma, non-Hodgkin's lymphoma, Wilms' tumor, Hodgkin's disease, rhabdomyosarcoma, and Ewing's sarcoma in that order of occurrence (Gurney et al., 1995).

This chapter focuses on the cause, demographics, sites of origin, signs and symptoms, tests and procedures performed for diagnosis, staging, and treatment of extracranial solid tumors, including neuroblastoma, Wilms' tumor, hepatoblastoma, and rhabdomyosarcoma. In addition, the preoperative and postoperative management of children is reviewed.

NEUROBLASTOMA

Neuroblastoma is the third most common malignancy and the most common extracranial tumor of childhood (Adams et al., 1993; Robison, 1997). For incidence, see Table 30–1.

Neuroblastoma is one of the small round blue cell tumors of childhood (which include Ewing's sarcoma, rhabdomyosarcomas, lymphomas, desmoplastic round cell tumor, and primitive neuroectodermal tumors). Neuroblastoma arises from the neural crest progenitor cells that normally give rise to the sympathetic nervous system. These cells ultimately become the sympathetic ganglia and adrenal medulla, as well as other sites (Brodeur & Castleberry, 1997). The outcome for infants and children with neuroblastoma varies widely on the basis of age and stage of disease at diagnosis and tumor biology. Generally, the lower the stage the better the outcome. Despite recent advances in treatment, however, advanced stage and older age at diagnosis are still poor prognostic indicators.

Etiology

The cause of neuroblastoma is unknown, but a subset of patients with neuroblastoma do exhibit an autosomal dominant predisposition to having this disease develop (Brodeur & Castleberry, 1997). In addition, there have been a number of reports of familial occurrence, and it has been suggested that genetic abnormalities occur in approximately 80% of tumors (Caty & Shamberger, 1993).

Neuroblastoma has also been associated with neurofibromatosis type 1 and aganglionosis of the colon (Hirschsprung's disease). These findings suggest that neuro-

Table 30–1 Incidence of Neuroblastoma, Wilms' Tumor, Hepatic Tumors, and Rhabdomyosarcoma

Tumor Type	Incidence in Children < 15 Yr	Notes
Neuroblastoma	7.3% of malignancies 754 cases/yr M:F 1.02:1 W:B 1.31:1	Third most common malignancy Most common extracranial tumor of childhood 36% cases diagnosed <1 yr 79% cases diagnosed <4 yr 97% cases diagnosed ≤10 yr
Wilms' tumor	6% of malignancies 640 cases/yr M:F 0.78:1 W:B 0.88:1	Second most common extracranial tumor of childhood
Primary hepatic tumors	1.1% of malignancies 1.4 cases/million children M:F 1.5:1	Rare in children 70% of all hepatic tumors are malignant Median age at diagnosis for hepatocellular carcinoma is 10 years, most cases present in adolescence Hepatoblastoma usually occurs in infancy with most cases <3 yr of age
Rhabdomyosarcoma	10–12% of malignancies 354 cases/yr M:F 1.44:1 W:B 1.15:1	Most common soft tissue sarcoma Two incidences of peak occurrence, with two thirds of cases in children ≤6 yr and second peak mid adolescent years

blastoma may be part of a syndrome involving the maldevelopment of the neural crest (Gaisie, Oh, & Young, 1979; Knudson & Amromin, 1966; Knudson & Meadows, 1976). Further, neuroblastoma has also been associated with Beckwith-Wiedemann syndrome and Van Waardenburg's syndrome (Grosfeld, 1986). The relative uniform incidence of neuroblastoma worldwide suggests that industrial or other environmental exposures associated with developed countries have not had a significant impact on the incidence of this disease (Brodeur & Brodeur, 1991).

Sites of Origin

The location of primary tumors at the time of diagnosis varies according to age. Most tumors occur within the abdomen (65%) at any age. The primary site in the adrenal gland accounts for 40% of all children but only 25% of infants. Also, cervical and thoracic tumors are more commonly seen in infants, 7% and 58%, respectively. Pelvic tumors are more commonly seen in children, whereas 12% of tumors have no known primary site (Castleberry, Shuster, Smith, & Members Institutions of the Pediatric Oncology Group, 1994; Nemes & Donahue, 1994).

Clinical Presentation

The signs and symptoms of neuroblastoma reflect the location of the primary tumor and the extent of regional or metastatic disease (Robison, 1997). Some tumors may be discovered incidentally when a child seeks medical attention for other reasons. Most children with neuroblastoma, however, are often not diagnosed until the disease has progressed, resulting in an ill appearance. Table 30–2 reviews the presenting signs and symptoms for neuroblastoma by anatomic site.

Paraneoplastic Syndromes

Several paraneoplastic syndromes have been associated with neuroblastoma whether it is localized or has metastasized. About 1% to 5% of patients with neuroblastoma experience hypertension. Excessive catecholamine secretion results from lateral displacement of the kidney by the adrenal gland or paraspinal primary tumor causing hypertension (Brodeur & Brodeur, 1991; Lanzkowsky, 1995). This excessive catecholamine production can also result in intermittent attacks of sweating, flushing, pallor, headaches, and palpitations.

Table 30–2 Presenting Signs and Symptoms for Neuroblastoma by Site

Site	Signs and Symptoms
Generalized	Anorexia, irritability, fatigue, diarrhea, and hypertension
Orbital	Proptosis, periorbital ecchymosis
Superior stellate or cervical ganglion	Horner's syndrome, neurologic findings
Thoracic	Dysphagia, respiratory symptoms of infection, dyspnea, respiratory compromise especially if tumor is displacing the trachea
Abdominal	Rapid increase in abdominal girth,[a] hard and fixed mass
Adrenal	Difficult to palpate when small
Pelvic	Bladder and bowel compromise, a result of neuronal compression or mass effect
Paraspinal	Severe pain, weakness, or hypotonia of the extremities, scoliosis or paraplegia, depending on the location of the mass
Cortical bone	Pain, limping, refusal to ambulate
Bone marrow	Asymptomatic or anemia, thrombocytopenia, leukopenia, or pancytopenia
Skin nodules	Characteristic of stage IV-S disease and seen in children under age 1

[a] These tumors often occur with a rapid increase in abdominal girth, which is suggestive of malignancy compared with benign processes, which are more indicative of gradual abdominal distention.

Another syndrome associated with neuroblastoma is opsoclonus and myoclonus. This consists of rapid involuntary chaotic conjugate eye movements and motor incoordination manifested as frequent, irregular, jerking movements of muscles of the limbs and trunk (Lanzkowsky, 1995). This syndrome is generally associated with a more favorable outcome, and although the mechanism is unclear, it generally resolves after the tumor is removed (Koh et al., 1994).

Vasoactive intestinal peptides (VIP) produce watery diarrhea syndrome, which results from the secretion of vasoactive peptides of the tumor. This can be seen in patients diagnosed with frank neuroblastoma but more frequently in lower grade tumors such as ganglioneuromas or ganglioneuroblastomas. This syndrome presents as intractable watery diarrhea, resulting in failure to thrive, abdominal distention, and hypokalemia (El Shafie, Samuel, Klippel, Robinson, & Cullen, 1983).

Workup

Screening for neuroblastoma can be divided into several study groupings: radiologic findings, urinary catecholamine metabolism, serum values, and pathologic and histologic characteristics of the tumor (see Figure 30–1 and Table 30–3).

The histology of the tumor is important in determining the tumor type and in directing the choice of therapy. Tissue is obtained for biologic variables, including tumor histology, cellular deoxyribonucleic acid (DNA) content or chromosome number, N-*myc* copy number, and deletion of the short arm of chromosome 1 (1p deletion) (Cohn et al., 1988). Tumor histology by Shimada classification is characterized as favorable or unfavorable. Those tumors with favorable histology are usually of a lower stage and have a good prognosis. Those with unfavorable histology are generally stage 3 or 4 and are aggressive tumors with a poorer outcome. DNA content is determined by flow cytometry. Tumors that have few cytogenetic rearrangements and are hyperdiploid or near-triploid are generally found in patients under the age of 1 with localized disease and a good prognosis (Brodeur, 1990). Tumors that are near-diploid or near-tetraploid karyotype with no consistent cytologic rearrangement are generally found in older patients with more advanced stages of disease that progress slowly but are frequently fatal (Brodeur, 1990). Tumors that are characterized as near-diploid or tetraploid karyotype with

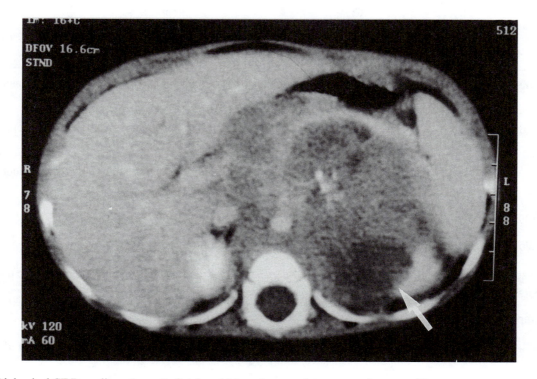

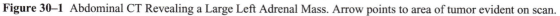

Figure 30–1 Abdominal CT Revealing a Large Left Adrenal Mass. Arrow points to area of tumor evident on scan.

chromosomal deletions and/or N-*myc* amplification are generally found in older patients with advanced stages of disease that progress rapidly (Brodeur, 1990).

N-*myc* copy number has been shown to be an independent predictor of survival in patients with neuroblastoma. N-*myc* amplification contributes to the aggressiveness of neuroblastoma cells and to their malignant phenotype (Seeger et al., 1985). Amplification of N-*myc* is found predominantly in patients with advanced stages of disease (Robison, 1997). Tumors with one to three copies of N-*myc* are in the lower stages of disease or stage IVS. Tumors with 3 to 10 copies of N-*myc* may not suppress the capability of the tumor to regress (Nakagawara et al., 1962). Tumors with greater than 10 copies of N-*myc* have more advanced and progressive stages of disease.

Spontaneous Regression

In selected patients it has been noted that neuroblastomas are able to regress or mature spontaneously. Actual overall incidence of regression is probably 5% to 10% and is most often seen in infants (Brodeur et al., 1992).

Staging

Neuroblastomas are staged to predict survival and determine the intensity of treatment required. A variety of staging systems exist, each with its own strengths and weaknesses. In 1988 an International Neuroblastoma Staging System (INSS) was established in an attempt to provide uniformity in staging (Table 30–4).

Treatment

Treatment for neuroblastoma depends on degree of risk. Low-risk tumors do not require chemotherapy or radiation. Resection of the primary lesion is followed by observation. High-risk tumors require a multimodality approach and still have overall survival rates of only 10% to 30% (LaQuaglia, 1997). Chemotherapy, radiation therapy, and surgery are all recommended treatment for high-risk disease.

Chemotherapy/Radiation

Chemotherapy is the mainstay of treatment for advanced neuroblastoma. A variety of single agents, including cyclo-

Table 30–3 Diagnostic Evaluation for Suspected Neuroblastoma

Examination or Test	Rationale
History and physical examination	Assess general condition and underlying problems; assess size of primary tumor, areas of metastatic disease
Complete blood count	Anemia and/or thrombocytopenia may result from bone marrow replacement
Serum ferritin	Levels on the upper limit of normal or higher are indicative of advanced disease
Lactic dehydrogenase (LDH)	Elevated levels are indicative of malignancy
Neuron-specific enolase (NSE)	Tumor marker for neuroblastoma
Bone marrow aspirations times four sites, bone marrow biopsies times two sites	Assess for bone marrow involvement and metastatic disease, a single positive site is indicative of disease
Chest radiograph	Assessment for metastatic disease
CT scan or MRI scan of the primary site	Evaluation of tumor size, invasiveness, enlargement of regional nodes
CT scan or MRI of possible metastatic sites	Metastatic disease can be found in the head and neck, abdomen, liver, or chest; evaluation of tumor size and invasiveness
Meta-iodobenzylguanidine scintigraphy (MIBG)	Assesses primary tumor and sites of distant metastasis (that may not be identified on other scans)
Bone scan	Assesses sites of bone and bone marrow involvement
Urinary catecholamines [homovanillic acid (HVA) and vanillylmandelic acid (VMA)]	90% to 95% of tumors produce catecholamines; 24-hour urine levels measuring VMA and HVA are performed and elevation confirms the diagnosis

phosphamide, doxorubicin, platinum, vincristine, and doxorubicin (Adriamycin), produce responses. Pairs and combinations of these drugs are more effective than single-dose agents.

Radiation has a limited role in the overall management of patients with neuroblastoma because of the high frequency of metastatic disease. Indications for use include (1) as an adjunct therapy to primary and bulky sites of disease; (2) for unresectable tumors after chemotherapy and surgery; (3) treatment of microscopic disease after chemotherapy and surgery; and (4) palliation in unresectable masses that cause pain or organ dysfunction like bony metastases. Radiation should generally be administered after surgery because it makes excision of the tumor more difficult.

Surgical Management

Before treatment all patients with advanced stages of disease require placement of a central venous access device for the administration of chemotherapy, antibiotics, blood products, total parenteral nutrition, and other intravenous needs. Patients with low-risk disease usually undergo complete resection of the tumor and surrounding lymph nodes at the time of diagnosis (Figure 30–2). These patients may require no further therapy other than observation. Patients with more advanced stages of disease (stage 3 and 4) require a different approach. Initial surgery should be confined to acquisition of diagnostic tissue and staging. Increased complication rates are reported when the operation is performed at the time of

Table 30–4 Comparison of Staging Systems for Neuroblastoma

Children's Cancer Study Group (CCSG) System	Pediatric Oncology Group (POG) System	International Neuroblastoma Staging System (INSS)
Stage I Tumor confined to the organ or structure of origin	*Stage A* Complete gross resection of primary tumor, with or without microscopic residual disease; intracavitary lymph nodes not adhered to primary tumor and histologically free of tumor; nodes adhered to the surface of or within primary tumor possibly positive	*Stage 1* Localized tumor to the area of origin; complete gross excision, with or without microscopic residual disease; identifiable ipsilateral and contralateral lymph nodes negative microscopically
Stage II Tumor extending in continuity beyond the organ or structure of origin, but not crossing the midline; regional lymph nodes on the ipsilateral side possibly involved	*Stage B* Grossly unresected primary tumor; nodes and nodules the same as in stage A	*Stage 2A* Unilateral tumor with incomplete gross excision; identifiable ipsilateral and contralateral lymph nodes negative microscopically *Stage 2B* Unilateral tumor with complete or incomplete gross excision; with positive ipsilateral regional lymph nodes; identifiable contralateral lymph nodes negative microscopically
Stage III Tumor extending in continuity beyond the midline; regional lymph nodes possibly involved bilaterally	*Stage C* Complete or incomplete resection of primary tumor; intracavitary nodes not adhered to primary tumor histologically positive for tumor; liver and in stage A	*Stage 3* Tumor infiltrating across the midline with or without regional lymph node involvement; or unilateral tumor with contralateral regional lymph node involvement; or midline tumor with bilateral lymph node involvement
Stage IV Remote disease involving the skeleton, bone marrow, soft tissue, and distant lymph node groups (see Stage IV-S)	*Stage D* Dissemination of disease beyond intracavitary nodes (i.e., extracavitary nodes, liver, skin, bone marrow, bone, etc.)	*Stage 4* Dissemination of tumor to distant lymph nodes, bone, bone marrow, liver, or other organs (except as defined in stage 4S)
Stage IV-S As defined in stage I or II, except for the presence of remote disease confined to the liver, skin, or marrow (without bone metastases)	*Stage DS* Infants <1 year of age with stage IV-S disease (see CCSG)	*Stage 4S* Localized primary tumor as defined for stage 1 or 2 with dissemination limited to liver, skin, or bone marrow

diagnosis before chemotherapy in high-risk neuroblastoma (DeCou et al., 1995; Shamberger, Allarde-Segundo, Kozakewich, & Grier, 1991). Resection is attempted after several cycles of high-dose chemotherapy. Survival is not decreased with delayed surgery (DeCou et al., 1995; Shamberger et al., 1991).

Bone Marrow Transplantation

Another therapy offered to children with neuroblastoma is autologous bone marrow transplantation (BMT) (Graham-Pole, 1991; Graham-Pole et al., 1991). BMT in children with neuroblastoma is used in children with high-risk, stage 4 dis-

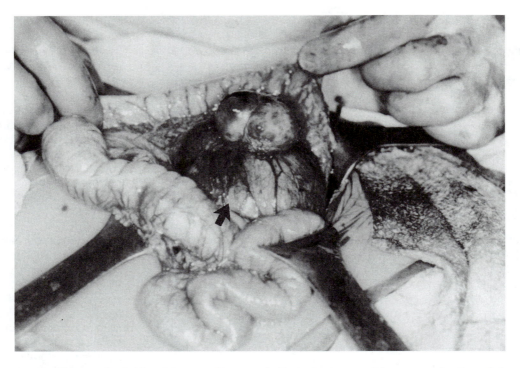

Figure 30–2 Intraoperative Photograph of a Neuroblastoma. The arrow indicates the tumor as it is seen growing through the mesentery of the bowel.

ease. This therapy is used less frequently today because of the high mortality rate and relapse in children (Brodeuer & Castleberry, 1997). Outcome after autologous transplantation ranges from 8% to 34% survival at 2 years after diagnosis. Allogeneic transplantation has worse results (Matthay et al., 1994). Thus, the role of BMT has not been fully defined in the treatment of neuroblastoma.

Prognosis

The most important variables in determining the prognosis for a child with neuroblastoma include the age of the patient at diagnosis, stage of disease, the site of the primary tumor, and the histologic findings of the tumor. On the basis of the INSS criteria for neuroblastoma, the 3-year survival rate is as follows: (1) stage 1 patients have a 97% 3-year survival rate; (2) stage 2A and 2B patients have a 87% and 86% 3-year survival rate, respectively; (3) stage 3 patients have a 62% 3-year survival rate; (4) stage 4 patients have less than a 40% 3-year survival rate; and (5) stage 4S patients have a 75% 3-year disease-free survival rate. The relapse rate is greater as the stage of the tumor increases. Stage 4S tumors are the exception, with a 75% relapse-free rate (LaQuaglia, 1997).

Future Directions

Immunotherapy is used in the treatment of various forms of cancer. Antigen-specific immunity is a strong natural defense system within the body, and it is a key target within the system to find microscopic disease. Chemotherapy, resection, and radiation are the treatments of choice for newly discovered malignancies. These, however, severely immunocompromise the patient and have a dose-limiting factor. Immunotherapy is not overly immunosuppressive, and toxicity is low so it can be used in conjunction with other modalities to achieve maximal treatment efficacy. However, immunotherapy is highly experimental and is available at a limited number of centers. There are no data that immunotherapy alone is effective.

Several types of immunotherapy are used in the treatment of neuroblastoma. They include nonradiolabeled (which works with the complement system and antibody-dependent cell-mediated toxicity) and radiolabeled (which delivers a dose of radioactivity to the tumor site) monoclonal antibodies.

Other innovative strategies include (1) vaccines that stimulate the body to create antibodies against the tumor; (2) interferon, which stimulates the natural killer cell activity to destroy tumor cells; (3) retinoic acid, which causes neuro-blastoma cells to differentiate and mature; (4) deferoxamine (Desferal), which helps by starving the tumor cells of iron; and (5) gene therapy, which is thought to target neuroblastoma cells and eradicate them.

WILMS' TUMOR

Wilms' tumor, also known as nephroblastoma, is the most common primary malignant renal tumor of childhood and is the paradigm for multimodal treatment of a pediatric malignant solid tumor (Green et al., 1996). The tumor presents at an earlier age in males, with a mean age of 41.5 months for unilateral tumors compared with 46.9 months for females. The mean age for patients with bilateral disease is 29.5 months for males and 32.6 months for females (Breslow et al., 1991). Wilms' tumor is rare in children younger than 6 months of age and in children older than 10 (for incidence, see Table 30–1).

Wilms' tumor is a malignant embryoma of the kidney that arises from metanephric blastema. Individual tumors not only contain metanephric cells but may also have cartilage, skeletal muscle, and squamous epithelium (Green et al., 1997). The classic tumor is an encapsulated or pseudo-encapsulated intrarenal mass arising from the periphery of the renal cortex. They are globular or spherical with a soft gray-tan appearance. They appear to occupy an entire pole of the kidney, and calcification is not often present.

Wilms' tumor is considered a prototype for the success of cancer chemotherapy because the survival rates have improved from less than 30% to almost 90% since the advent of modern chemotherapy (Brodeur & Brodeur, 1991).

Etiology

Evidence suggests the presence of an autosomal dominant pattern of inheritance and the predisposition of Wilms' tumor developing (Brodeur & Brodeur, 1991). Two chromosomal abnormalities have been associated with the development of Wilms' tumor. The first is the aniridia association, sometimes associated with genitourinary anomalies, such as cryptorchidism and hypospadias, and mental retardation. The second is the Beckwith-Wiedemann syndrome, which includes macroglossia, omphalocele, and visceromegaly (Brodeur & Brodeur, 1991; Beckwith, 1969). Hemihypertrophy occurs as an isolated abnormality or in association with Beckwith-Wiedemann syndrome (Green et al., 1997).

Clinical Presentation

Most children with Wilms' tumor present with an incidentally discovered abdominal mass in an otherwise healthy child. It is most often discovered by a family member or caregiver. The tumor may reach an enormous size before a diagnosis is made. The "classic" findings are abdominal pain, gross hematuria, and fever (Green et al., 1997).

A subset of patients have rapid abdominal enlargement associated with anemia, hypertension, gross hematuria, and sometimes fever. This is attributed to intratumoral hemorrhage and may be associated with spontaneous rupture (Green et al., 1997; LaQuaglia, 1997). Hypertension is noted in about 25% of cases as a result of an increase in renin activity (Steinbrecher & Malone, 1995).

On physical examination of the male a varicocele may be evident as a result of obstruction of the spermatic vein, which may be associated with the presence of tumor thrombus in the renal vein or inferior vena cava. Persistence of the varicocele when the child is supine suggests venous obstruction (Green et al., 1997).

Workup

The chief differential diagnosis is in distinguishing Wilms' tumor from neuroblastoma and to a lesser degree hepatoblastoma. It should be easy to differentiate because most neuroblastomas arise from the adrenal gland and Wilms' tumor is intrarenal. Initial imaging studies are restricted to those necessary to establish the presence of an intrarenal mass (Figure 30–3). Additional important data include the presence and function of the opposite kidney, whether the opposite kidney has tumor involvement, and the presence and extent of intravascular tumor thrombus (Green et al., 1997) (see Table 30–5).

Staging

Staging depends on whether the primary tumor is confined to the renal capsule; the presence or absence of abdominal lymph node involvement; rupture of the tumor before or during surgery; and hematogenous dissemination to distant sites such as liver, lung, bone, or brain (Brodeur & Brodeur, 1991). Exhibit 30–1 reviews staging.

Surgical Management

The standard of care in the United States for low-risk Wilms' tumor is initial resection. Exceptions to this rule include extensive intracaval tumors that require cardiopulmonary bypass for extraction, obviously unresectable tumors with documented invasion of contiguous structures, and possibly bilateral tumors, especially if it is unclear which side is more heavily involved (LaQuaglia, 1997).

Resection usually requires a radical nephroureterectomy (see Figure 30–4). Questions have arisen as to whether patients with stage 1 unilateral disease should undergo a radical nephrectomy or parenchymal sparing procedure if feasible

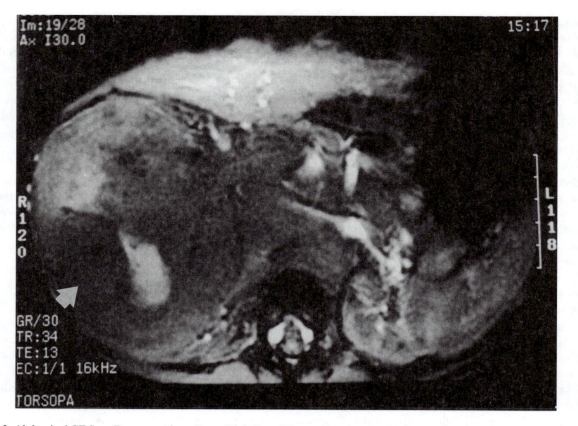

Figure 30–3 Abdominal CT Scan Demonstrating a Large Right Renal Tumor Crossing the Midline (see arrow). Abdominal aorta is displaced anteriorly by tumor.

(Cozzi et al., 1996; Ritchey, 1996; Urban et al., 1995). A nephron-sparing procedure could reduce the risk of subsequent renal morbidity. In addition, it is useful in patients with solitary kidneys or renal insufficiency. However, this approach remains controversial and additional trials are needed to evaluate the risks and benefits of this approach.

The resection of Wilms' tumor begins with a thorough abdominal exploration using a transabdominal approach. Strict attention is paid to the local tumor extent or tumor rupture and status of the regional periaortic, interaortocaval, paracaval, and perirenal lymph nodes. The liver is carefully palpated for metastasis (LaQuaglia, 1997). Direct visualization and palpation of the contralateral kidney are also performed before resection. A study by Kessler et al. (1996) suggests that contralateral exploration in radiologically demonstrated unilateral involvement should be abandoned to reduce the high incidence of postoperative intestinal obstruction. However, at this time contralateral exploration is still considered standard therapy. This is supported by reports of contralateral involvement not recognized on imaging stud-

ies. The frequency of contralateral kidney involvement with Wilms' tumor ranges from 4% to 7% (Green et al., 1997).

Patients with extensive intracaval tumors, unresectable tumors with documented invasion of contiguous structures, and bilateral tumors with an unclear picture of which kidney is more heavily involved benefit from preoperative chemotherapy and/or radiation (Crombleholme, Jacir, Rosenfield, Lew, & Harris, 1994; Lee, Saing, Leung, Mok, & Cheng, 1994; McLorie, Khoury, Weitzman, & Greenberg, 1996; Shaul, Srikanth, Ortega, & Mahour, 1992). By initiating preoperative chemotherapy treatment (after tumor biopsy), tumor burden is reduced. This reduces the risk of tumor rupture and patient morbidity and mortality.

Pathology

Tumors are histologically characterized as favorable or unfavorable. Tumors with quantitative (blastemal, epithelial, and stromal predominant) deviations of triphasic nephroblastoma have favorable histologic findings (Lanzkowky,

1995). Tumors with anaplastic features occur in approximately 5% of patients and are associated with increased rates of relapse and death (Ritchey, Haase, & Shochat, 1993a).

Treatment

After the stage of disease is determined by the surgeon and pathologist, a treatment plan is determined. In general, all patients receive postoperative chemotherapy. The exception to this rule consists of stage 1 favorable histologic findings in patients who are younger than 24 months of age at diagnosis and have tumors less than 250 g in weight at resection (Green et al., 1997; Larsen et al., 1990). There also should be no vascular invasion beyond the renal hilar plane and absence of capsular invasion (LaQuaglia, 1997).

Chemotherapy/Radiation Therapy

Chemotherapy for Wilms' tumor involves several agents, including actinomycin-D, vincristine, doxorubicin, and cy-clophosphamide. The doses, frequencies, and types of the drugs given are based on the stage of disease and histologic findings.

Radiation therapy, when applicable, is initiated when the patient is stable postoperatively; is free of ileus, atelectasis, or diarrhea; has an absolute neutrophil count of greater than $100/mm^3$; and has a hemoglobin of at least 10 g/dl. Radiation therapy is not given postoperatively to patients with stage 1 favorable histologic findings and stage 2 favorable histologic findings who receive actinomycin-D and vincristine (Green et al., 1997; Ritchey et al., 1993a).

Patients with stage 3 disease receive whole abdomen external beam radiation therapy in daily fractionated doses. The entire kidney bed and areas of gross residual disease are targeted. Patients with stage 4 disease receive radiation therapy to the primary tumor in the same doses as those with stage 3 disease. Pulmonary metastases are treated with whole thoracic external beam radiation in fractions. Patients with unresectable liver metastases also receive radiation. Lo-

Table 30–5 Diagnostic Evaluation for Suspected Wilms' Tumor

Examination or Test	Rationale
History and physical examination	Assess general condition and underlying problems Assess size of primary tumor, areas of metastatic disease
Complete blood count	Bone marrow replacement is associated with anemia and thrombocytopenia, helps to differentiate from neuroblastoma because Wilms' tumor does not generally metastasize to the bone marrow
Liver function tests	Elevation indicates presence of malignancy and possible site of metastasis
Renal function tests	Assess kidney function secondary to presence of disease; help to determine ability to tolerate chemotherapy
Urinalysis	Assess for presence of blood and renal function secondary to disease
Abdominal ultrasound/Doppler ultrasound	Determines whether mass is cystic or solid, may identify organ of origin; Doppler study is done to identify intracaval extension, liver metastasis, or enlarged retroperitoneal lymph nodes; inferior vena cava thrombosis occurs with a 7% frequency
CT scan	To further evaluate nature and extent of mass, important in detecting liver metastasis and localizing intra-abdominal tumors; may identify tumors in the opposite kidney
Chest radiograph	Assesses for pulmonary metastasis
Chest CT scan[a]	Assesses for pulmonary metastasis

[a] If the chest CT scan is positive and the chest radiograph is negative, a biopsy is required to verify diagnosis.
[b] Bone marrow aspirates and biopsies and urine catecholamines may be done to differentiate Wilms' tumor from neuroblastoma.

Exhibit 30–1 National Wilms' Tumor Study Group Staging System for Wilms' Tumor

---

Stage I

The tumor, limited to the kidney, was completely excised. The renal capsule has an intact outer surface. The tumor was not ruptured or sampled for biopsy before its removal (fine-needle aspiration biopsy is excluded from this restriction). The vessels of the renal sinus are not involved. No evidence of tumor at or beyond the margins of resection is visible.

Stage II

The tumor extended beyond the kidney, but was completely excised. One may see regional extension of tumor (i.e., penetration of the renal capsule or extensive invasion of the renal sinus). The blood vessels outside the renal parenchyma, including those of the renal sinus, may contain tumor. Biopsy was performed (except fine-needle aspiration), or tumor spillage before or during surgery was confined to the flank and did not involve the peritoneal surface. No evidence of tumor at or beyond the margins of resection is present.

Stage III

Residual nonhematogenous tumor is present, confined to the abdomen. Any one of the following may occur: (1) lymph nodes within the abdomen or pelvis are found to be involved by tumor (renal hilar, paraaortic, or beyond; lymph node involvement in the thorax or other extraabdominal sites is a criterion for stage IV); (2) the tumor has penetrated the peritoneal surface; (3) tumor implants are found on the peritoneal surface; (4) gross or microscopic tumor remains postoperatively (e.g., tumor cells are found at the margin of surgical resection on microscopic examination); (5) the tumor is not completely resectable because of local infiltration into vital structures; or (6) tumor spillage not confined to the flank occurred either before or during surgery.

Stage IV

Hematogenous metastases (lung, liver, bone, brain, etc.) or lymph node metastases outside the abdominopelvic region are present.

Stage V

Bilateral renal involvement is present at diagnosis. An attempt should be made to stage each side according to the foregoing criteria on the basis of the extent of disease before biopsy or treatment.

---

calized liver lesions receive focal radiation. Bulky nodal, brain, and skeletal metastases receive radiation with focal boosts as needed (Green et al., 1997).

Prognosis

The overall prognosis for children diagnosed with Wilms' tumor is excellent. Children with stage 1 and 2 disease have a 95% to 97% 4-year survival rate. Children with stage 3 disease have a 91% 4-year survival rate. Children with stage 4 and bilateral disease have a 78% 4-year survival rate.

The prognosis for children who have relapsed with favorable histologic findings with Wilms' tumor depends on their initial stage, the site of recurrence, the time from initial diagnosis to recurrence and their previous therapy (Green et al., 1997). Favorable prognostic factors include no prior treatment with doxorubicin, relapse more than 12 months after diagnosis, and subdiaphragmatic relapse in a patient who has not received abdominal irradiation (Grundy et al., 1989). These children should be treated aggressively because they have shown a good response to further therapy.

Children who have recurrences often have pulmonary metastases. The role of surgery in these cases is for biopsy or excision of the lesion. For recurrent abdominal tumors, an attempt is made to reduce the tumor burden before the use of chemotherapeutic agents not previously used.

Children who have a recurrence after receiving doxorubicin or who have an abdominal recurrence after previous irradiation have a poor prognosis. The use of autologous bone marrow transplant has been investigated, as well as several phase 1 and 2 studies that involve drug combinations.

HEPATIC TUMORS

Historically, children with liver tumors were uniformly considered to have a poor prognosis. However, over the last decade with advances in diagnostic imaging studies, chemotherapy and surgical techniques outcomes have improved.

Frequently, liver tumors are the result of metastatic disease, most commonly from neuroblastoma or Wilms' tumor (see Table 30–1 for incidence). The two most common liver tumors in children are hepatoblastoma and hepatocellular carcinoma (HCC). Hepatoblastoma is the most common pediatric hepatic malignancy, and HCC is the second most common. Hepatoblastomas usually occur in infancy and most are diagnosed before age 3. HCC has two age peaks, one before age 4 and another between 12 and 15 years (Shochat, 1992). Table 30–6 reviews distinctive features of hepatic tumors.

Hepatoblastoma

Hepatoblastoma is the most frequently occurring liver tumor in children, accounting for more than 25% of pediatric

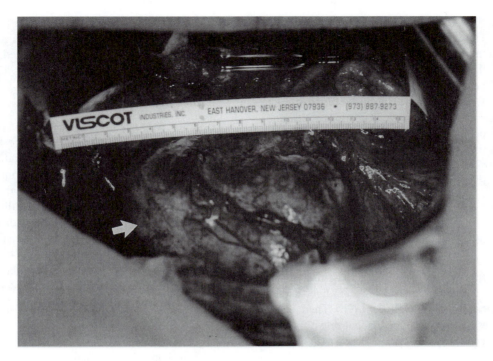

Figure 30–4 Intraoperative Photograph of a Large Right Renal Wilms' Tumor. Arrow indicates tumor.

Table 30–6 Useful, Distinctive Features of Hepatic Tumors

Feature	Hepatoblastoma	Hepatocellular Carcinoma	Fibrolamellar Variant of HCC
Usual age at presentation	0–3 yr	5–18 yr	10–20 yr
Associated congenital anomalies	Dysmorphic features: hemihypertrophy, Beckwith-Wiedemann	Metabolic	None
Usual site of origin	Right lobe	Right lobe-multifocal	Right lobe
Abnormal liver function tests	15–30%	30–50%	Rare
Jaundice	5%	25%	Absent
Elevated alpha-fetoprotein	80–90%	50%	10%
Positive hepatitis B serology	Absent	Present in some	Absent
Abnormal B_{12}-binding protein	Absent	Absent	Present
Distinctive radiographic appearance	None	None	None
Pathology	Fetal and/or embryonal cells ± mesenchymal component	Large pleomorphic tumor cells and tumor giant cells	Eosinophilic hepatocytes with dense fibrous stroma

hepatic tumors and nearly 50% of those that are malignant (Stocker, 1994). Hepatoblastoma is an embryonal tumor composed of immature hepatic epithelial tissue in various stages of differentiation. It is most often unifocal, and the right lobe of the liver is most commonly affected (Weinberg & Finegold, 1983). Microscopic vascular spread may be found beyond the encapsulated tumor. The gross appearance is that of a lobulated, bulging, tan mass, often punctuated by geographic areas of necrosis and surrounded by a pseudo-capsule (Greenberg & Filler, 1997). The tumor has no association with cirrhosis.

Etiology

Hepatoblastoma is associated with the congenital anomalies Beckwith-Wiedemann syndrome and hemihypertrophy. It has also been reported in sibling pairs and children with diaphragmatic or umbilical hernias, Meckel's diverticulum, and renal anomalies (Bowman & Riely, 1996). There is also a synchronous association between hepatoblastoma and Wilms' tumor (Greenberg & Filler, 1997; Bowman & Riely, 1996).

Hepatoblastoma has been reported in association with maternal use of both oral contraceptives and gonadotropins and in fetal alcohol syndrome. High frequency of maternal exposure to metals, petroleum products, and paints and of paternal exposure to metals has been noted, although the significance is unclear (Greenberg & Filler, 1997).

Clinical Presentation

Children with hepatoblastoma have an asymptomatic abdominal mass. Approximately 10% are found on routine physical examination, which is remarkable for hepatomegaly or a right upper quadrant midline mass. Other associated symptoms include pain, irritability, minor gastrointestinal disturbances, vomiting, fever, and pallor, although these are usually associated with advanced disease. Significant weight loss and failure to thrive are unusual. Jaundice occurs in only 5% of patients. Rarely, patients may have isosexual precocious puberty (including genital enlargement and pubic hair resulting from androgen release of tumor, usually in males) or severe osteoporosis (Bowman & Riely, 1996).

Workup

The workup for hepatoblastoma involves physical assessment, laboratory, and radiological studies (see Table 30–7 and Figure 30–5).

Table 30–7 Diagnostic Evaluation for Hepatoblastoma/Hepatocellular Carcinoma[a]

Examination or Test	Rationale
Physical examination and history	Assess general condition and underlying problems Assess size of primary tumor, areas of metastatic disease
Complete blood count	Mild anemia and thrombocytosis are often seen
Liver function tests	Nonspecifically elevated
High serum cholesterol	High levels are associated with a poor prognosis
Alpha-fetoprotein (AFP)	Occurs in 84%–91% of cases; is often extreme; useful marker to monitor disease reduction
Abdominal radiograph	Identifies presence of a right upper quadrant mass
Abdominal ultrasound	Distinguishes between space-occupying lesions and diffuse hepatomegaly
Abdominal CT scan or MRI	Most sensitive for diagnostic discrimination and to assess operability; also identifies nodal disease
Chest CT scan	Assesses for pulmonary metastasis; evident in 10%–20% of patients

[a] The radiologic evaluation is the same for both diseases. Preoperative differentiation is difficult.

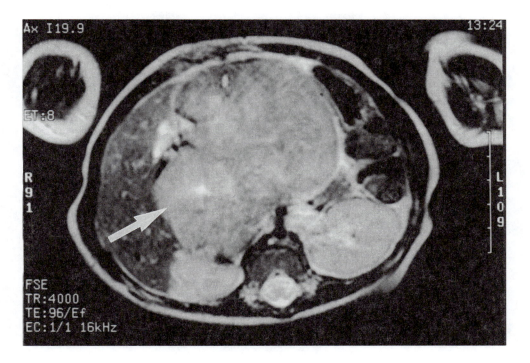

Figure 30–5 Abdominal CT Scan Demonstrating a Large Lesion in the Left Lobe of the Liver (see arrow)

Staging

Staging is based on operative findings, nodal involvement, and metastasis (Evans et al., 1982; LaQuaglia, 1997) (see Table 30–8).

Chemotherapy/Radiation Therapy

Several chemotherapeutic agents are used to treat hepatoblastoma in an effort to reduce tumor burden preoperatively. These agents include cisplatin, vincristine, 5-fluorouracil (5-FU), doxorubicin, and carboplatin. It is recommended that all hepatoblastoma patients with inoperable tumors undergo initial treatment with vincristine, cisplatin, and 5-FU (LaQuaglia, 1997). Children with bilobar disease without extrahepatic involvement who do not respond to chemotherapy are candidates for liver transplantation (Caty & Shamberger, 1993). The role of radiation therapy is not clearly defined.

Surgical Management

Historical data indicate that cure of malignant liver tumors in children is not possible without complete resection of the primary hepatic tumor. However, less than half of the patients have resectable disease. Unresectable disease includes those tumors that occupy both lobes of the liver, involve the portal vein, and extend extrahepatically. Fortunately, hepatoblastomas are highly chemosensitive, so initial surgical management should be directed toward obtaining diagnostic material if total resection is not feasible. Once the tumor burden has been reduced, a successful resection can be performed, reducing the morbidity and mortality in these patients (see Figure 30–6) (Reynolds, Douglass, Finegold, Cantor, & Glicksman, 1992).

Prognosis

Survival of children with hepatoblastoma is related to the histologic findings of the tumor and completeness of the surgical resection. The 3-year survival rate for patients who initially are seen with resectable tumors is 90%. Children who

Table 30–8 Clinical Groupings of Malignant Hepatic Tumors

Designation	Criteria
Group I	Complete resection of tumor by wedge resection lobectomy, or by extended lobectomy as initial treatment
Group IIA	Tumors rendered completely resectable by initial irradiation or chemotherapy
Group IIB	Residual disease confined to one lobe
Group III	Disease involving both lobes of the liver
Group IIIB	Regional node involvement
Group IV	Distant metastases, irrespective of the extent of liver involvement

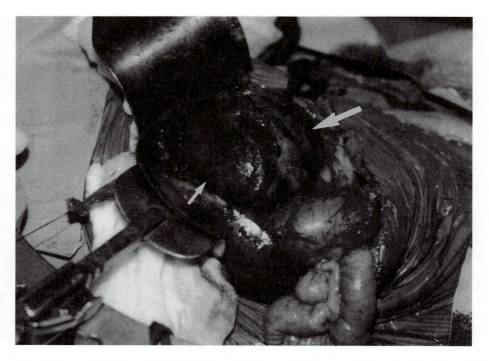

Figure 30–6 Intraoperative Photograph of a Large Right Lobe Hepatoblastoma. Small arrow indicates healthy liver. The larger arrow identifies the tumor.

have unresectable primary tumors have an estimated 65% 3-year survival rate, and children who have metastatic disease at diagnosis do poorly, with a 10% to 20% 3-year survival rate (Bowman & Riely, 1996). In addition, those children who have anaplastic hepatoblastoma have a poor prognosis (von Schweinitz, Hecker, Schmidt-Von-Arndt, & Harms, 1997).

Hepatocellular Carcinoma

HCC in childhood is similar in gross and microscopic features to its adult counterpart, except for the lack of underlying cirrhosis in most pediatric cases (Merten & Gold, 1994). However, approximately one third of patients have cirrhosis as a result of metabolic abnormalities, glycogen storage disease, malnutrition, biliary atresia, or giant cell hepatitis (Bowman & Riely, 1996). It has also been associated with the hepatitis B virus infection.

HCC tumor cells are larger than normal hepatocytes and have pleomorphic nuclei and prominent nucleoli (Weinberg & Finegold, 1983). There are two major histologic subtypes, classic and fibrolamellar. The tumor is often bile stained, and intratumoral calcification occurs infrequently (Bowman & Riely, 1996; Greenberg & Filler, 1997). These tumors are

often multicentric and may involve both the right and left lobes simultaneously (Merten & Gold, 1994).

Clinical Presentation

Unlike hepatoblastoma, the presenting signs and symptoms of HCC are not incidental. Children frequently have a distended abdomen and a mass in the right upper quadrant. Pain is common even in the absence of a palpable mass. Nausea, vomiting, anorexia, significant weight loss, and fever are likely at the time of diagnosis. Jaundice is evident in 25% of cases. Small numbers of patients may present acutely with tumor rupture.

Workup

The radiologic evaluation is the same as in hepatoblastoma. The computed tomographic appearance of both tumors is similar. The most common sites of metastasis are the lungs and lymph nodes. As a result, preoperative differentiation between hepatoblastoma and HCC is difficult (see Table 30–7).

Staging

The staging system is the same as for hepatoblastoma (see Exhibit 30–1). The prognosis for each stage in HCC is equivalent to hepatoblastoma. However, patients with HCC usually are initially seen with advanced disease.

Treatment

Complete resection is a prerequisite for cure in HCC. It is the only effective treatment and only possible in one third of cases. The fibrolamellar variant has a higher resection rate at 48% to 60% and, thus, has a better prognosis. Relapse after resection is common for both types (LaQuaglia, 1997).

Chemotherapy has no effect on these tumors. Radiation has been used, but, even in combination with chemotherapy, the treatment has not been curative.

As with hepatoblastoma, liver transplantation is an additional therapy when there is no evidence of metastatic disease. Some children who have undergone transplantation have had their metastases eradicated by preoperative chemotherapy or surgery (Greenberg & Filler, 1997).

Prognosis

Overall survival in the pediatric age group for HCC is less than 20%. Children who have undergone liver transplantation have an overall 2-year survival of only 20% to 30% (Greenberg & Filler, 1997).

Rhabdomyosarcoma

Malignant tumors derived from primitive mesenchymal cells are called sarcomas. Mesenchymal cells mature into skeletal or smooth muscle, fat, fibrous tissue, bone, and/or cartilage. Sarcomas are divided into categories according to the mature cell type they resemble. For example, tumors that arise from the fat tissue are called liposarcomas. Sarcomas are highly aggressive tumors and tend to be locally invasive with a high propensity for local recurrence. Rhabdomyosarcoma is the most common soft tissue sarcoma in childhood, accounting for approximately 50% of all sarcomas (Pappo, 1996). It arises from tissue resembling striated muscle tissue, which contains rhabdomyoblasts, or primitive muscle cells (Pack & Eberhart, 1985). Some sarcomas are called undifferentiated because they come from cells that are primitive and do not resemble any specific mature tissue type.

Soft tissue sarcomas rank fifth among all reported tumors (Pappo, 1996) and rhabdomyosarcoma accounts for 10% to 12% of all malignant solid tumors in children (Lanzkowsky, 1995). For incidence statistics, see Table 30–1.

There are four histopathologic subtypes of rhabdomyosarcoma: embryonal, alveolar, botryoid, and pleomorphic. Embryonal is the most common type in children, accounting for 53% of cases (Figure 30–7). Usual primary sites of embryonal types are the head and neck, orbit, and genitourinary tract. Alveolar sites include extremities, trunk, and perineum. Botryoid sites include the bile ducts and submucosal locations such as the bladder, vagina, and nasopharynx. The pleomorphic subtype is uncommon in infants and children, but when it occurs, the extremities and trunk are the usual locations (Lanzkowsky, 1995; Rowe, O'Neill, Grosfeld, Fonkalsrud, & Coran, 1995).

Etiology

The cause of rhabdomyosarcoma is unknown although there is some association with neurofibromatosis, the Li-Fraumeni syndrome (LFS), and Beckwith-Wiedemann syndrome (Wexler & Helman, 1997; Lanzkowsky, 1995).

Sites of Origin

Rhabdomyosarcoma is found virtually everywhere in the body and like neuroblastoma, it is a small round blue cell tumor of childhood. The most common sites for rhabdomyosarcoma are the head and neck, accounting for 35% of cases, followed by genitourinary tract (22%), extremities (18%), and other sites (25%) (Figure 30–7).

Clinical Presentation

Rhabdomyosarcoma generally is seen as a mass and/or a disturbance in bodily function resulting from the presence of the tumor. Presenting signs and symptoms depend on the tumor site and the presence of metastasis. Table 30–9 details the signs and symptoms of rhabdomyosarcoma by anatomic locations.

Workup

Management of rhabdomyosarcoma depends on the tumor site and the extent of the disease. A thorough workup to evaluate the primary tumor site and the presence and extent of metastases is necessary. A computed tomographic scan of the primary tumor site should be obtained to evaluate the tumor size and invasiveness, regional lymph node involvement, and other complicating features. Figure 30–8 demonstrates computed tomography scans of an extremity rhabdomyosarcoma. Table 30–10 reviews the standard workup. Additional examinations may be warranted for some tumor sites. For suspected rhabdomyosarcoma of the parameningeal and head and neck regions ophthalmologic examination, cerebrospinal fluid cytologic studies, and an ear, nose, and throat examination with the patient under anesthesia provide further information (Lanzkowsky, 1995). After the initial workup is complete, incisional biopsy of the primary tumor site and any metastatic regional lymph nodes is performed to provide tissue for pathologic examination and biologic markers. Specific surgical management is discussed later, but if the tumor is small, noninvasive, and accessible, resection of the tumor with an attempt to obtain clear margins is performed after a complete workup.

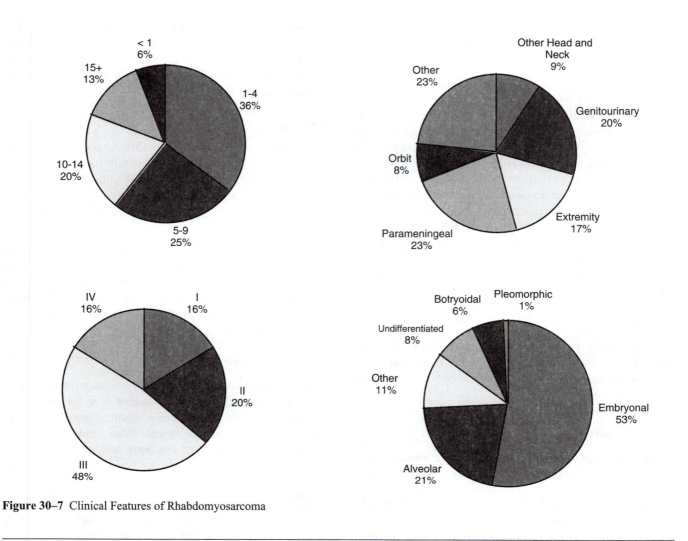

Figure 30–7 Clinical Features of Rhabdomyosarcoma

Staging

Careful staging is important to both the treatment and prognosis of rhabdomyosarcoma. The current Intergroup Rhabdomyosarcoma Study IV (IRS-IV) trial incorporates a tumor, node, metastases (TNM) classification system. It is a preoperative staging system that evaluates tumor size, invasiveness, lymph node involvement, and primary site (Table 30–11). The combination of the clinical staging, TNM evaluation, and results of tissue pathologic and histopathologic studies provides the information needed to initiate treatment.

Treatment

Multimodality therapy, including surgery, chemotherapy, and radiation therapy, is paramount to achieving and maintaining remission for patients with rhabdomyosarcoma. The role of each modality depends on the stage and classification of the tumor at presentation and the responsiveness to therapy. The results of the IRS-III study indicate that therapy

should be risk directed and based primarily on tumor site and extent of disease (Crist et al., 1995).

Surgical Management. Before the advent of chemotherapy and radiation therapy, surgery was the mainstay of treatment for patients with rhabdomyosarcoma. Survival rates have risen to 50% or greater with the addition of chemotherapy. At this point, the role of surgery became somewhat unclear. If tumors responded well to chemotherapy, was resection in fact indicated? And what is the impact of resection on survival? Given present-day survival rates, however, it would be unethical to randomize a patient with a resectable, nonmetastatic tumor to a nonsurgical arm of treatment (LaQuaglia, 1997). The goals of surgery are as follows:

1. Complete resection of the tumor, if it can be performed without mutilating or debilitating consequences
2. Procurement of tissue before the initiation of other therapies for tumor biology and histopathologic study

3. Debulking of the tumor before chemotherapy and radiation
4. Evaluation of response to therapy or excision of residual tumor
5. Placement of a central venous catheter for the administration of chemotherapy

Surgical management varies with the site of disease (Table 30–12). Resection is the most rapid method to eradicate tumor and is the treatment of choice if it can be done without significant cosmetic or functional deficit. Figure 30–9 demonstrates an extremity rhabdomyosarcoma before resection. Reexcision is performed if surgical margins are positive for disease or if the existence of a neoplasm was unknown at the time of the initial excision. Some tumors are not amenable to surgical resection (e.g., parameningeal) but are responsive to chemotherapy. For these tumors, the role of surgery is biopsy of the tumor to confirm the diagnosis and to obtain tissue for biologic studies. Incisional biopsy is generally performed but computed tomography–guided needle biopsy is also an option.

If the tumor is large and gross total resection is not possible, debulking of the tumor may reduce tumor burden before the initiation of chemotherapy and/or radiation therapy.

Table 30–9 Presenting Signs and Symptoms of Rhabdomyosarcoma

Site	Signs and Symptoms
Vaginal	Discharge or bleeding from vaginal introitus, prolapse of polypoid mass with possible hemorrhage; with advanced disease there may be urethral compression and constipation
Uterus	Prolapse of polyp through the cervix, abdominal pain, abdominal distention
Bladder	Urinary frequency, urinary obstruction, frequent UTIs, hematuria, dysuria, dribbling, acute urinary retention, abdominal mass, hydrocephalus, and renal deterioration (secondary to urethral obstruction)
Prostate	Pelvic mass, constipation, hematuria
Paratesticular	Unilateral, firm, slightly mobile mass palpable above and separate from the testes, usually painless, sometimes associated with a hydrocele, which may obscure the tumor presence and delay diagnosis
Extremity	Presence of a mass, may be painless or painful, associated limp, overlying skin changes, pathologic fracture (local bony invasion)
Nasopharyngeal	Local pain, sinusitis, epistaxis, dysphagia, airway obstruction
Middle ear	Pain, history of chronic otitis, aural discharge, polypoid mass in the external canal, Bell's palsy
Orbit	Eyelid swelling, proptosis, headache, decreased visual acuity, conjunctival mass, visual disturbances, extraocular muscle imbalance
Facial lesion	Painful swelling associated with trismus, skin discoloration or cellulitis over the mass
Laryngeal	Pertussis-like cough, hoarseness
Chest wall/paraspinal	Chest pain, mass, pleural effusion with occasional shortness of breath
Retroperitoneum	Abdominal pain, abdominal mass, compression of surrounding organs and subsequent symptoms
Perianal/perineum	Subcutaneous mass, verrucous superficial tumor, constipation, dysuria
Bile duct tumors	Pain, fever, jaundice

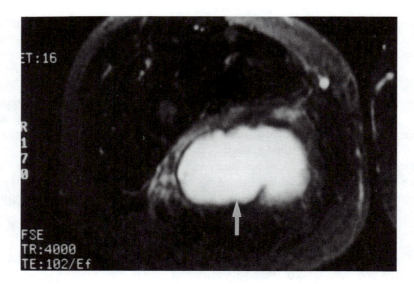

Figure 30–8 MRI Scan of the Upper Leg Demonstrating a Large Tumor (Rhabdomyosarcoma) in the Thigh

Table 30–10 Diagnostic Evaluation for Suspected Rhabdomyosarcoma[a]

Examination or Test	Rationale
History and physical examination	Search for lymph nodes, size of primary mass, general condition, underlying conditions
Complete blood count	Bone marrow replacement associated with anemia or thrombocytopenia; bone marrow toxicity is the major side effect of chemotherapy
Electrolytes, renal and hepatic function tests, creatinine clearance	Renal toxicity associated with cisplatin and other alkylators; genitourinary tumors may obstruct ureters; hepatic toxicity with dactinomycin
Four-site bone marrow aspirations, two-site bone biopsies	Bone marrow metastases reported in up to 6% of patients at diagnosis (29% of stage 4 patients have marrow involvement); bone marrow assessment before chemotherapy
Bone scan	Possibility of bone and bone marrow metastases
CT of the primary site	Evaluation of tumor size, invasiveness, enlargement of regional nodes and complicating ureteral, biliary, bowel, or airway patency
CT of possible metastatic sites	CT scanning of the lungs and liver should be done to rule out parenchymal metastases. CT scanning is superior to MR imaging in assessing the degree of bone destruction in paraspinal, extremity, and head and neck (base of skull) lesions.
MR imaging	MR imaging is done for the same rationale as CT scanning. It may give more detailed information regarding the extent of viable tumor (T2 weighted imaging) and the presence of hepatic metastases. It is also the most useful tool for evaluation of the epidural space in paraspinal or base of skull primaries.
Gallium scanning	Both the primary tumor and metastatic deposits may be identified by gallium scanning

[a] The same workup is applicable to other high-grade sarcomas.

Table 30–11 TNM Staging of Rhabdomyosarcoma: TNM Pretreatment Staging Classification for IRS-IV[a]

Stage	Sites	T Invasiveness	T Size	N	M
1	Orbit Head and Neck[b] Genitourinary[c]	T1 or T2	a or b	N0 N1 or Nx	M0
2	Bladder/prostate Extremity Cranial parameningeal Other[d]	T1 or T2	a	N0 or Nx	M0
3	Bladder/prostate Extremity Cranial parameningeal Other[d]	T1 or T2 T1 or T2	a b	N1 N0 N1 or Nx	M0 M0
4	All	T1 or T2	a or b	N0 or N1	M1

[a] T (tumor): T1, confined to anatomic site of origin; T2, extension; a, ≤5 cm in diameter; b, >5 cm in diameter. N (regional nodes): N0, not clinically involved; N1, clinically involved; Nx, clinical status unknown. M (metastases): M0, no distant metastases; M1, distant metastasis present.
[b] Excluding parameningeal.
[c] Nonbladder/nonprostate.
[d] Includes trunk, retroperitoneal, and so on.

Second look surgery is also performed after other therapies have been initiated to evaluate responsiveness to therapy (and potentially limit further therapy) or for excision of residual tumor. Hays et al. (1990) found that for patients with selected tumor sites (clinical groups III and IV) excision of residual tumor mass after intensive chemotherapy and radiotherapy may favorably influence patient outcome. Debilitating or disfiguring surgery is only performed if residual disease is found after all other modes of therapy have been exhausted. LaQuaglia (1997) recommends that "amputation of extremity rhabdomyosarcoma does not enhance cure and should only be performed when lesions are bulky, invade bone or neurovascular structures, or are recurrent."

Chemotherapy. Multiagent chemotherapy is used for the treatment of rhabdomyosarcoma. Dosing, use of specific agents, and length of therapy depend on the stage at diagnosis. Effective agents in rhabdomyosarcoma include actinomycin-D, doxorubicin, cisplatin, cyclophosphamide, etoposide (VP-16), ifosfamide, melphalan, and vincristine. Chemotherapy is used for the eradication of microscopic disease after resection, reduction of tumor size before resection of initially unresectable tumors, or cytoreduction before autologous bone marrow rescue. It is also used for the treatment of recurrent disease.

Radiation Therapy. Radiation therapy plays an essential role in the treatment of rhabdomyosarcoma. It is particularly useful for tumors in areas that are difficult to resect (i.e.,

head, neck, pelvis). Rhabdomyosarcoma is only moderately sensitive to radiation. Therefore, high doses are required to obtain cell kill. An IRS-IV-P study confirmed that hyperfractionated radiation (HF XRT) in children with rhabdomyosarcoma was both feasible and tolerable. Hyperfractionated techniques allow the delivery of high doses to maximize tumor kill, while minimizing morbidity. At present, a prospective randomized trial is under way to test the efficacy of HF XRT compared with conventional radiation (Donaldson et al., 1994). The use of radiation therapy is based on stage at diagnosis. Dose does not depend on age, although dose modifications have been made for young children.

Complications of Treatment

Complications of treatment range from the devastating hematopoietic side effects of chemotherapy and radiation therapy to surgical scarring, tissue loss, and secondary neoplasms. For the purposes of this chapter, only the complications related to surgical management will be reviewed. Surgical complications occur intraoperatively or postoperatively. Intraoperative complications could include blood loss; damage to surrounding vessels, nerves, or organs; and reactions to anesthesia. Potential postoperative complications include, but are not limited to, fluid and electrolyte imbalance, pneumonia, prolonged ileus, and wound infection. Assessments to recognize and methods to minimize these complications are addressed later in the chapter.

Table 30–12 The Role of Surgery for Primary Sites of Rhabdomyosarcoma in Children

Primary Site	Role of Surgery
Head and neck	
Superficial (scalp, temporal region, facial structures, neck)	Wide excision with normal margins of tissue provided no significant cosmetic and/or functional deficits occur.
Parameningeal (paranasal sinuses, nasopharynx, middle ear, pterygo-palatine fossa)	Rarely amenable to local excision; incisional biopsy for diagnosis; routine cervical lymph node sampling is unnecessary unless nodes are clinically suspicious.
Orbit and eyelid	Incisional biopsy only, orbital exenteration only for recurrent disease.
Genitourinary tract	
Paratesticular	Radical orchiectomy and resection of entire spermatic cord (inguinal approach to avoid scrotal contamination). For stage I, group I patients with no evidence of lymph node involvement, no retroperitoneal lymph node dissection is recommended; stages II–IV, groups II–IV, RPLN sampling is recommended to evaluate ipsilateral high infrarenal and low infrarenal nodes and bilateral iliac nodes.
Vulvar, vaginal	Respond well to chemotherapy; incisional biopsy for diagnosis, limited local excision after chemotherapy.
Uterine	Transvaginal biopsy for polypoid cases, D&C for intrauterine infiltrative tumors; radical resection is limited to patients with gross residual disease after initial resection, chemotherapy and radiation or for those patients with progression despite therapy.
Bladder/prostate	Endoscopic, perineal, or suprapubic diagnostic biopsy; complete resection only if preservation of bladder and urethra assured.
Bladder dome	Partial cystectomy (ureteral reimplantation and bladder augmentation may be necessary), total cystectomy, anterior pelvic exenteration only if no local control is obtained after combination chemotherapy and radiation therapy.
Extremities	Complete surgical resection if limb function will not be greatly impaired (independent of whether microscopically clear margins can be obtained or not); biopsy of axillary, inguinal lymph nodes in upper and lower extremities; if immediate regional nodes are positive, more distal nodes should be explored; with an unplanned excision with positive margins, re-excision of the primary site to achieve tumor-free margins.
Trunk	Aggressive surgical management recommended with chest wall, diaphragmatic and pulmonary resection; wide local resection of chest wall tumors includes removal of the entire soft tissue mass and a block of uninvolved tissue extending at least 1 rib above and below the lesion.
Retroperitoneum	Incisional biopsy for diagnosis, debulking before or after other therapies.

Prognosis

The prognosis for patients diagnosed with rhabdomyosarcoma has greatly improved over the years. At present, predictors of outcome include primary tumor site, histologic findings, age at diagnosis, tumor invasion, metastases, and regional lymph node involvement (LaQuaglia et al., 1994). Favorable tumor sites include orbital, paratesticular, and vaginal primary tumors and unfavorable sites include the parameningeal head and neck, extremities, retroperitoneum,

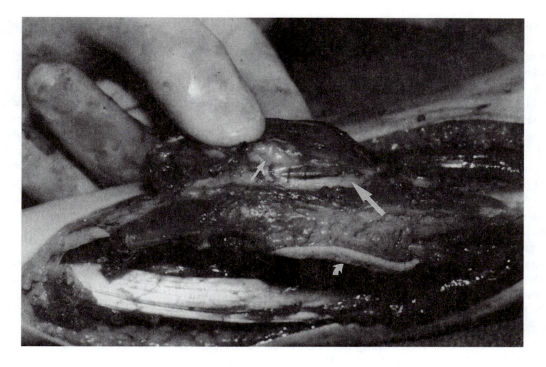

Figure 30–9 Intraoperative Photograph of an Upper Extremity Rhabdomyosarcoma. Curved arrow indicates skin. The long arrow points to the tumor. The short arrow indicates the ulnar nerve, which was sacrificed for complete tumor resection.

and trunk. Extent of disease is an important variable, with noninvasive, small, nonmetastatic tumors with no regional lymph node involvement having a more favorable outcome. Embryonal types have a better prognosis than alveolar, anaplastic, or monomorphous round cell types. There is a higher incidence of advanced disease and alveolar disease in children older than 7 years, making the prognosis better for children between 1 and 7 years (Lanzkowsky, 1995).

Future Directions

Research efforts are now focused on patients with metastatic disease at presentation and gross residual tumor after conventional therapy. Hyperfractionated versus conventional radiotherapy is being evaluated in the IRS-IV study. Autologous bone marrow transplant or stem cell rescue after myeloablative chemotherapy and radiation is being investigated, as are surgical approaches that combine interstitial brachytherapy and intraoperative radiation with resection. Understanding more about cell lines and genetics will assist in tailoring treatment protocols to patient risk factors, which will potentially reduce toxicities of treatment. Maintaining current outcomes while minimizing short-term and long-term side effects of therapy is essential in the treatment of rhabdomyosarcoma.

OPERATIVE CONSIDERATIONS

The preoperative and postoperative considerations are similar for neuroblastoma, Wilms' tumor, hepatic tumors, and rhabdomyosarcoma based on the site of the primary tumor. The caremaps in Appendixes 30–A, 30–B, and 30–C review the nursing care for thoracic, extremity, and abdominal/pelvic tumors. The abdominal/pelvic caremap reflects the nursing care for patients undergoing exploratory laparotomy. Laparoscopy for biopsy is not addressed because it is covered in Chapter 28.

PREOPERATIVE MANAGEMENT OF THE PEDIATRIC PATIENT WITH A SOLID TUMOR

Most pediatric surgery involving solid tumors is performed with patients arriving at the hospital on the morning of surgery. In general, patients are no longer being admitted to the hospital preoperatively. This is not only cost-effective but, more importantly, has an anxiety-reducing effect for both the patient and the family. Reasons for admission before surgery might include bowel preparation for low abdominal or pelvic tumors, intravenous hydration for sickle cell patients, or handling of a difficult social situation.

Surgical management of patients with solid tumors varies according to tumor type, size, extent, and patient condition. Preoperative nursing management, however, is virtually the same, regardless of tumor type. Preoperative testing is performed within 7 days and not less than 24 hours before surgery (see Table 30–13). In settings where pediatric nurse practitioners (PNPs) are present, the PNP plays a key role in the coordination of the preoperative process. She or he performs the history and physical examination, orders blood work, carries out preoperative teaching, and answers questions accordingly. If a PNP is not in the setting, the responsibilities fall to surgical residents and RNs. Preoperative education is essential because it provides information about both the preoperative and postoperative expectations. Age-appropriate language and demonstrations of the operative procedure using diagrams, photographs, and educational dolls better prepare the child and ideally alleviate some of the fear and anxiety that surround operative procedures (Figures 30–10 to 30–12). Reviewing the postoperative process, including the sites and sounds of the postanesthesia recovery room, potential drain and tube presence, and expectations regarding activity, diet, wound care, and discharge, also alleviates anxiety. For the adolescent and young adult population it is essential to stress their role in the recovery process. Body image is extremely important to adolescents, and they may be more concerned with the idea of a Foley catheter than the prospect of a life-threatening operation. Speaking to patients directly and taking the time to listen and address their specific fears will ultimately affect the outcome in a positive manner.

POSTOPERATIVE MANAGEMENT

The immediate postoperative care for children recovering from tumor resection is in a pediatric intensive care unit (PICU). The PICU stay is on average 2 to 4 days, depending on the child's recovery. The remainder of the hospital stay is generally on a pediatric inpatient unit. Nursing care plays a key role for these patients during the recovery process, especially in minimizing and recognizing complications.

Fluid and Electrolyte Management

Patients receive aggressive hydration intraoperatively. Mobilization of third space fluid occurs approximately 48 hours postoperatively. As a result, patients are hydrated at maintenance postoperatively and a negative fluid balance is expected until days 3 to 5 postoperatively.

Pulmonary Toilet

To minimize pneumonia as a postoperative complication, pulmonary toilet is emphasized with age-appropriate interventions (e.g., incentive spirometer for older children and adolescents, bubble blowing and pinwheel use for younger children). Frequent position change and ambulation are also

Table 30–13 Preoperative Management for Pediatric Patients with Solid Tumors

Evaluation	Rationale
Complete history and physical examination	Baseline preoperative evaluation, review of systems, and triage of any problems
Preoperative education	Preparation of patient and family with verbal and written information, demonstration of incentive spirometer use, review of pulmonary toilet
Blood work	Baseline evaluation or based on patient condition and prior treatment; platelet count must be >100,000 for major resections, absolute neutrophil count must be ≥1,000
Anesthesia evaluation	Obtained by anesthesiologist as a baseline evaluation, provides education for patients and families
Surgical consent	Obtained by the surgeon, risks and benefits of the procedure are fully explained
Other testing (ECHO, CXR, ultrasound, CT, MRI, renal scan)	History driven and based on prior treatment

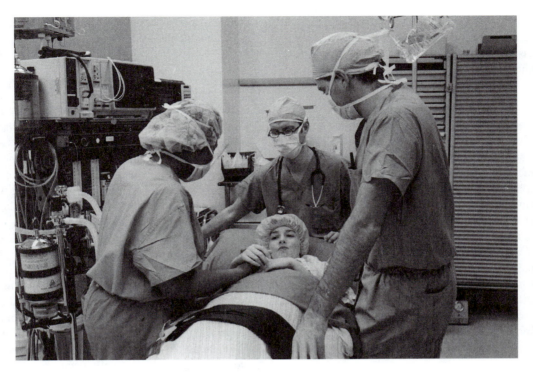

Figure 30–10 The Operating Room and Staff before Induction of Anesthesia

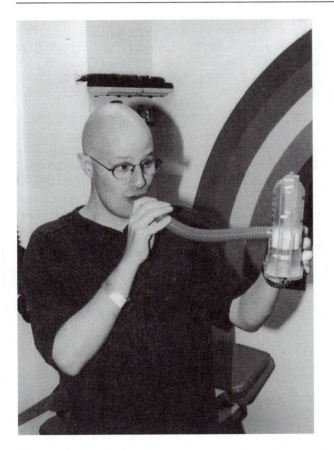

Figure 30–11 A Patient Demonstrating the Use of an Incentive Spirometer Preoperatively

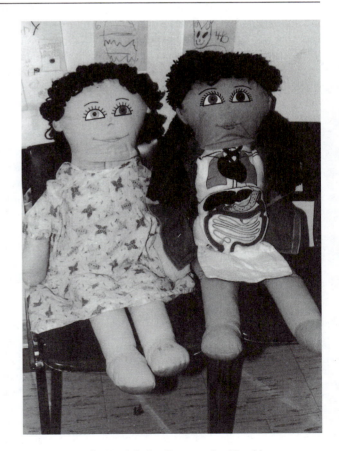

Figure 30–12 Dolls Used during Preoperative Teaching

essential as soon as allowed by the surgeon. Coughing and deep breathing are encouraged, with instructions on how to splint the incision with a pillow to minimize discomfort. Chest physiotherapy may be warranted for thoracic cases.

Pain Control

Aggressive pain management is paramount in the immediate postoperative period. Epidural catheters and patient-controlled analgesia are the standard of care. Incisional pain lasts approximately 72 hours postoperatively. The pain most patients complain of after the first 72 hours is generally muscular. Ambulation and use of the muscles affected generally provide relief. Because narcotics are ineffective for muscular pain, it is important to distinguish the difference, if possible, and explain to the patients the importance of ambulation and use of the muscles. The patient should be weaned from narcotics as quickly as possible to minimize the paralytic effect on the bowel. Pain medication is initially given intravenously or through an epidural catheter and is then tapered by replacing it with oral analgesics.

Diet

Resumption of a regular diet depends on the specific operation performed. For nonabdominal procedures, patients are started on clear liquids the evening of surgery or the next morning and are advanced as tolerated. For abdominal surgery, normal peristalsis is necessary before the introduction of liquids or solids. Nasogastric tubes are in place and removed once the secretions have minimized and with the onset of normal peristalsis. If a patient begins vomiting and the nasogastric tube is still in place, it should be irrigated to ensure patency. If the output from a nasogastric tube increases significantly and the drainage is bilious, the tube may be in the duodenum and should be pulled back slightly so it is in the stomach.

After abdominal or pelvic surgery, patients are monitored for decreased or absent bowel sounds, increasing abdominal girth, vomiting, absence of stools or disappearance of flatus, and abdominal pain because these may be signs of intestinal obstruction. Signs of perforation or peritonitis include absence of bowel sounds, tachycardia, pallor, increasing temperature, rapid shallow respirations, splinting, and sudden relief of abdominal pain followed by increasing diffuse abdominal pain. The pediatric surgeon should be notified immediately.

Prolonged ileus is a potential postoperative complication. It is important to rule out other reasons for the ileus, such as electrolyte imbalance or excess narcotic use. Bowel function usually resumes 3 to 5 days postoperatively but may be longer after extensive retroperitoneal tumor dissection or if fecal contamination has occurred. Patients with a prolonged ileus are kept NPO, and the use of hyperalimentation is es-

sential. Any patient who will be kept NPO for 7 days or more needs intravenous nutritional support.

Wound Care

Depending on the surgeon's preference, either internal, absorbable sutures are used, with adhesive strips over the incision, or internal, absorbable sutures with staples are used to close the incision. Staples or external sutures are used if the incision is large or in an area of tension or mobility. Staples and/or external sutures are removed approximately 7 to 10 days postoperatively if the wound is healing well and adhesive strips are placed over the incision. Dressings are in place for 48 to 72 hours, and the first dressing change or removal is performed by the surgical service. Once the dressing is removed, the incision is left open to air and kept clean and dry. If sutures or staples are present, a light gauze dressing is used to minimize catching on the patient's clothing. If staples or external sutures are not used, showering is allowed 48 to 72 hours postoperatively. If staples or external sutures are present, showering is at the discretion of the surgeon.

Erythema, wound drainage, or fever may be signs of wound infection. This usually occurs 5 to 7 days postoperatively. Opening the wound and draining any pus or fluid are the treatment for a wound infection. If cellulitis is present, the use of intravenous antibiotics may be warranted. Some bruising at the incision site may occur, and expansion of the incision may represent the presence of an underlying hematoma.

Drains

Drain use depends on the specific operation performed. For chest cases, generally at least one chest tube is in place. Removal of the chest tube is based on chest radiographic findings, drainage from the tube, and patient condition. Accurate measurement of output from the chest tube is paramount because it helps to determine the timing for removal of the drain. Other drains that may be in place postoperatively include nasogastric tubes, Reliavac, Jackson-Pratt and Penrose drains, and Foley catheters.

Discharge Home

On discharge from the hospital, patients are given a follow-up appointment with the surgeon. In addition, instructions regarding wound management, medications, signs and symptoms to report, and how to get in touch with the surgeon are provided.

Follow-Up Visits

The follow-up visit consists of an interval history, wound check, follow-up scans if needed (e.g., chest radiographic film), and review of return to or restrictions on full physical activity. Complete wound healing takes 6 to 8 weeks, and patients are generally instructed to limit activities for 2 weeks, at which time the patient may resume light physical activity. It is important to note, and to convey to the patient and family, that the area of healed incision is never as strong as the area was before the operation, but maximum strength will occur 6 to 8 weeks after the surgery. Swimming is at the discretion of the surgeon. Patients are encouraged to return to school but may have limitations in regard to physical education classes.

CONCLUSION

The care of the pediatric patient diagnosed with a solid tumor is complex. The role of surgery may be as simple as placement of a central line or as involved as a complicated tumor resection. Regardless of the complexity of the role, surgical nurses will find themselves caring for pediatric oncology patients. Understanding the disease process, expected outcomes, and potential complications prepares them to provide holistic and comprehensive care.

REFERENCES

Adams, G.A., Shochat, S.J., Smith, E.I., Shuster, J.J., Joshi, V.V., Altshuler, G., Hayes, F.A., Nitschke, R., McWilliams, N., & Castleberry, R.P. (1993). Thoracic neuroblastoma: A Pediatric Oncology Group study. *Journal of Pediatric Surgery, 28*, 372–377.

Beckwith, J.B. (1969). Macroglossia, omphalocele, adrenal cytomegaly, gigantism and hyperplastic visceromegaly. *Birth Defects, 5*, 188.

Bowman, L.C., & Riely, C.A. (1996). Management of pediatric liver tumors. *Surgical Oncology Clinics of North America, 5*(2), 451–459.

Breslow, N., Sharples, K., Beckwith, J.B., Takashima, J., Kelalis, P.P., Green, D.M., & D'Angio, G.J. (1991). Prognostic factors in nonmetastatic, favorable histology Wilms' tumor. Results of the third national Wilms' tumor study. *Cancer, 68*(11), 2345–2353.

Brodeur, G.M. (1990). Neuroblastoma: Clinical significance of genetic abnormalities. *Cancer Surveys, 9*(4), 673–688.

Brodeur, G.M., Azar, C., Brother, M., Hiemstra, J., Kaufman, B., Marshall, H., Moley, J., Nakagawara, A., Saylors, R., Scavarda, N., Schneider, S., Wasson, J., White, P., Seeger, R., Look, T., & Castleberry, R. (1992). Neuroblastoma. *Cancer, 70*(6), 1685–1694.

Brodeur, A.E., & Brodeur, G.M. (1991). Abdominal masses in children: Neuroblastoma, Wilms' tumor, and other considerations. *Pediatrics in Review, 12*(7), 197–206.

Brodeur, G.M., & Castleberry, R.P. (1997). Neuroblastoma. In P.A. Pizzo & D.G. Poplack (Eds.), *Principles and practice of pediatric oncology* (ed. 3, pp. 761–797). Philadelphia: Lippincott-Raven Publishers.

Castleberry, R.P., Shuster, J.J., Smith, E.I., & Members Institutions of the Pediatric Oncology Group. (1994). The Pediatric Oncology Group experience with the international staging system criteria for neuroblastoma. *Journal of Clinical Oncology, 12*(11), 2378–2381.

Caty, M.G., & Shamberger, R.C. (1993). Abdominal tumors in infancy and childhood. *Pediatric Surgery, 40*(6), 1253–1271.

Cohn, S.L., Salwen, H., Herst, C.V., Maurer, H.S., Nieder, M.L., Morgan, E.R., & Rosen, S.T. (1988). Single copies of the N-*myc* oncogene in neuroblastomas from children presenting with the syndrome of opsoclonus-myoclonus. *Cancer, 62*(4), 723–726.

Cozzi, F., Schiavetti, A., Bonanni, M., Cozzi, D.A., Matrunola, M., & Castello, M.A. (1996). Enucleative surgery for stage 1 nephroblastoma with a normal contralateral kidney. *Journal of Urology, 156*, 1788–1793.

Crist, W., Gehan, E.A., Ragab, A.H., Dickman, P.S., Donaldson, S.S., Fryer, C., Hammond, D., Hays, D.M., Herrmann, J., Heyn, R., Jones, P.M., Lawrence, W., Newton, W., Ortega, J., Raney, R.B., Ruymann, F.B., Tefft, M., Webber, B., Wiener, E., Wharam, M., Vietti, T.J., & Maurer, H.M. (1995). The third intergroup rhabdomyosarcoma study. *Journal of Clinical Oncology, 13*(3), 610–630.

Crombleholme, T.M., Jacir, N.N., Rosenfield, C.G., Lew, S., & Harris, B.

(1994). Preoperative chemotherapy in the management of intracaval extension of Wilms' tumor. *Journal of Pediatric Surgery, 29*(2), 229–231.

DeCou, J.M., Bowman, L.C., Rao, B.N., Santana, V.M., Furman, W.L., Luo, X., Lobe, T.E., & Kumar, M. (1995). Infants with metastatic neuroblastoma have improved survival with resection of the primary tumor. *Journal of Pediatric Surgery, 30*(7), 937–941.

Donaldson, S.S., Asmar, L., Breneman, J., Fryer, C., Glicksman, A.S., Laurie, F., Wharam, M., & Gehan, E.A. (1994). Hyperfractionated radiation in children with rhabdomyosarcoma—Results of an intergroup rhabdomyosarcoma pilot study. *International Journal of Radiation Oncology and Biological Physics, 32*(4), 903–911.

El Shafie, M., Samuel, D., Klippel, C.H., Robinson, M.G., & Cullen, B.J. (1983). Intractable diarrhea in children with VIP-secreting ganglioneuroblastomas. *Journal of Pediatric Surgery, 18*(1), 34–36.

Evans, A.E., Land, V.J., Newton, W.A., Randolph, J.G., Sather, H.N., & Tefft, M. (1982). Combination chemotherapy in the treatment of children with malignant hepatoma. *Cancer, 50*, 821.

Federici, S., Galli, G., Ceccarelli, P.L., Rosito, P., Sciutti, R., & Domini, R. (1994). Wilms' tumor involving the inferior vena cava: Preoperative evaluation and management. *Medical and Pediatric Oncology, 22*, 39–44.

Gaisie, G., Oh, K.S., & Young, L.W. (1979). Coexistent neuroblastoma and Hirschsprung's disease: Another manifestation of the neurocristopathy? *Pediatric Radiology, 8*, 161.

Graham-Pole, J. (1991). Autologous marrow transplants in pediatric tumors. In R.E. Champlian & R.P. Gale (Eds.), *New strategies in marrow transplantation* (p. 413). New York: John Wiley & Sons.

Graham-Pole, J., Casper, J., Elfenbein, G., Gee, A., Gross, S., Janssen, W., Kock, P., Marcus, R., Pick, T., Shuster, J., et al. (1991). High-dose chemotherapy supported by bone marrow infusions for advanced neuroblastoma: A Pediatric Oncology Group study. *Journal of Clinical Oncology, 9*, 152.

Green, D.M., Coppes, M.J., Breslow, N.E., Grundy, P.E., Ritchey, M.L., Beckwith, J.B., Thomas, P.R.M., & D'Angio, G.J. (1997). Wilms tumor. In P.A. Pizzo & D.G. Poplack (Eds.), *Principles and practice of pediatric oncology* (3rd ed., pp. 733–759). Philadelphia: Lippincott-Raven Publishers.

Green, D.M., D'Angio, G.J., Beckwith, J.B., Breslow, N.E., Grundy, P.E., Ritchey, M.L., & Thomas, P.R.M. (1996). Wilms tumor. *CA: A Cancer Journal for Clinicians, 46*, 46–63.

Greenberg, M., & Filler, R.M. (1997). Hepatic tumors. In P.A. Pizzo & D.G. Poplack (Eds.), *Principles and practice of pediatric oncology* (3rd ed., pp. 717–732). Philadelphia: Lippincott-Raven Publishers.

Grosfeld, J.L. (1986). Neuroblastoma in infancy and childhood. In D.M.

Hayes (Eds.), *Pediatric surgical oncology* (p. 63). New York: Grune & Stratton.

Grundy, P., Breslow, N., Green, D.M., Sharples, K., Evans, A., & D'Angio, G.J. (1989). Prognostic factors of children with recurrent Wilms' tumor: Results from the second and third National Wilms Tumor Study. *Journal of Clinical Oncology, 7*, 638.

Gurney, J.G., Severson, R.K., Davis, S., & Robinson, L.L. (1995). Incidence of cancer in children in the United States. *Cancer, 76*, 2186–2195.

Hays, D.M., Raney, R.B., Crist, W.M., Lawrence, W.W. Jr., Ragab, A., Wharam, M.D., Webber, B., Mehan, E., Johnston, J., & Maurer, H.M. (1990). Secondary surgical procedures to evaluate primary tumor status in patients with chemotherapy-responsive stage III and IV sarcomas: A report from the intergroup rhabdomyosarcoma study. *Journal of Pediatric Surgery, 25*(10), 1100–1105.

Kessler, O., Franco, I., Jayabose, S., Reda, E., Levitt, S., & Brock, W. (1996). Is contralateral exploration of the kidney necessary in patients with Wilms' tumor? *Journal of Urology, 156*, 693–695.

Knudson, A.G.J., & Amromin, G.D. (1966). Neuroblastoma and ganglioneuroma in a child with multiple neurofibromatosis: Implications for the mutational origin of neuroblastoma. *Cancer, 19*, 1032.

Knudson, A.G.J., & Meadows, A.T. (1976). Developmental genetics of neuroblastoma. *Journal of the National Cancer Institute, 57*, 675.

Koh, P.S., Raffensperger, J.G., Berry, S., Larsen, M.B., Johnstone, H.S., Chou, P., Luck, S.R., Hammer, M., & Cohn, S.L. (1994). Long-term outcome in children with opsoclonus-myoclonus and ataxia and coincident neuroblastoma. *Journal of Pediatrics, 125*(5), 712–716.

LaQuaglia, M.P. (1997). Childhood tumors. In L.J. Greenfield, M.W. Mulholland, K.T. Oldham, G.B. Zelenock, & K.D. Lillemore (Eds.), *Surgery: Scientific principles and practice* (pp. 2118–2140). Philadelphia: Lippincott-Raven Publishers.

LaQuaglia, M.P., Heller, G., Ghavimi, F., Casper, E.S., Vlamis, V., Hajdu, S., & Brennan, M.F. (1994). The effect of age at diagnosis on outcome in rhabdomyosarcoma. *Cancer, 73*(1), 109–117.

Lanzkowsky, P. (Ed.). (1995). *Manual of pediatric hematology and oncology* (pp. 419–475). New York: Churchill Livingstone.

Larsen, E., Perez-Atayde, A.R., Green, D.M., Retik, A., Clavell, L.A., & Sallan, S.E. (1990). Surgery only for the treatment of patients with stage 1 (Cassidy) Wilms' tumor. *Cancer, 66*, 264.

Lee, A.C.W., Saing, H., Leung, M.P., Mok, C.K., & Cheng, M.Y. (1994). Wilms' tumor with intracardiac extension: Chemotherapy before surgery. *Pediatric Hematology and Oncology, 11*, 535–540.

Leonard, A.S., Alyono, D., Fischel, R.J., Nesbit, M.E., Nguyen, D.H., & McClain, K.L. (1985). Role of the surgeon in the treatment of children's cancer. *Surgical Clinics of North America, 65*, 1387.

Matthay, K.K., Seeger, R.C., Reynolds, C.P., Stram, D.O., O'Leary, M.C., Harris, R.E., Selch, M., Atkinson, J.B., Haase, G.M., & Ramsay, N.K. (1994). Allogeneic versus autologous purged bone marrow transplantation for neuroblastoma: A report from the children's cancer group. *Journal of Clinical Oncology, 12*(11), 2382–2389.

McLorie, G.A., Khoury, A.E., Weitzman, S.S., & Greenberg, M.L. (1996). Preoperative chemotherapy in management of Wilms' tumor [editorial]. *Urology, 47*, 792–793

Merten, D.F., & Gold, S.H. (1994). Radiologic staging of thoracoabdominal tumors in childhood. *Radiological Clinics of North America, 32*(1), 133–149.

Nakagawara, A., Sasazuki, T., Akiyama, H., Kawakami, K., Kuwano, A., Yokoyama, T., & Kume, K. (1962). N-*myc* oncogene and stage IV-S neuroblastoma (preliminary observations on ten cases). *Cancer, 65*(9), 1960–1967.

Nemes, J., & Donahue, M.C. (1994). Solid tumors in childhood. *Pediatric Surgical Nursing, 29*(4), 585–598.

Ni, Y., Chang, M., Hsu, H., Chen, C.C., Chen, W.J., & Lee, C.Y. (1991). Hepatocellular carcinoma in childhood: Clinical manifestations and prognosis. *Cancer, 68*, 1737.

Pack, G.T., & Eberhart, W.F. (1985). Rhabdomyosarcoma of skeletal muscle: Report of 100 cases. *Surgery, 32*, 1023.

Pappo, A.S. (1996). Rhabdomyosarcoma and other soft tissue sarcomas in children. *Current Opinion in Oncology, 8*, 311–316.

Reynolds, M., Douglass, E.C., Finegold, M., Cantor, A., & Glicksman, A. (1992). Chemotherapy can convert unresectable hepatoblastoma. *Journal of Pediatric Surgery, 27*, 8, 1080–1084.

Ritchey, M.L. (1996). Primary nephrectomy for Wilms' tumor: Approach of the national Wilms' tumor study group [editorial]. *Urology, 47*(6), 787–791.

Ritchey, M.L., Haase, G.M., & Shochat, S. (1993a). Current management of Wilms' tumor. *Seminars in Surgical Oncology, 9*, 502–509.

Ritchey, M.L., Kelalis, P.P., Etzioni, R., Breslow, N., Shochat, S., & Haase, G.M. (1993b). Small bowel obstruction after nephrectomy for Wilms' tumor: A report of the national Wilms' tumor study-3. *Annals of Surgery, 218*(5), 654–659.

Robison, L.L. (1997). General principles of the epidemiology of childhood cancer. In P.A. Pizzo & D.G. Poplack (Eds.), *Principles and practice of pediatric oncology* (3rd ed., pp. 1–10). Philadelphia: Lippincott-Raven Publishers.

Rowe, M.I., O'Neill, J.A., Grosfeld, J.L., Fonkalsrud, E.W., & Coran, A.G. (1995). *Essentials of pediatric surgery* (pp. 249–285). St. Louis, MO: Mosby.

Seeger, R.C., Brodeur, G.M., Sather, H., Dalton, A., Siegel, S.E., Wong, K.Y., & Hammond, D. (1985). Association of multiple copies of the N *myc* oncogene with rapid progression of neuroblastomas. *New England Journal of Medicine, 313*(18), 1111–1116.

Shamberger, R.C., Allarde-Segundo, A., Kozakewich, H.P., & Grier, H.E. (1991). Surgical management of stage III and IV neuroblastoma: Resection before or after chemotherapy? *Journal of Pediatric Surgery, 26*, 1113–1117.

Shaul, D.B., Srikanth, M.M., Ortega, J.A., & Mahour, G.H. (1992). Treatment of bilateral Wilms' tumor: Comparison of initial biopsy and chemotherapy to initial surgical resection in the preservation of renal mass and function. *Journal of Pediatric Oncology, 27*(8), 1009–1015.

Shochat, S.J. (1992). Update on solid tumor management in childhood. *Surgical Clinics of North America, 72*(6), 1417–1428.

Steinbrecher, H.A., & Malone, P.S.J. (1995). Wilms' tumor and hypertension: Incidence and outcome. *British Journal of Urology, 76*, 241–243.

Stocker, J.T. (1994). Hepatoblastoma. *Seminars in Diagnostic Pathology, 11*(2), 136–143.

Urban, C.E., Lackner, H., Schwinger, W., Klos, I., Hollwarth, M., Sauer, H., Ring, E., Gadner, H., & Zoubek, A. (1995). Partial nephrectomy in well-responding stage 1 Wilms' tumor: Report of three cases. *Pediatric Hematology and Oncology, 12*, 143–152.

von Schweinitz, D., Hecker, H., Schmidt-Von-Arndt, G., & Harms, D. (1997). Prognostic factors and staging systems in childhood hepatoblastoma. *International Journal of Cancer, 74*, 593–599.

Weinberg, A.G., & Finegold, M.J. (1983). Primary hepatic tumors of childhood. *Human Pathology, 14*(6), 512–537.

Wexler, L.H., & Helman, L.J. (1997). Rhabdomyosarcoma and the undifferentiated sarcomas. In P.A. Pizzo & D.G. Poplack (Eds.), *Principles and practice of pediatric oncology* (3rd ed., pp. 799–829). Philadelphia: Lippincott-Raven Publishers.

Young, J.L., & Miller, R.W. (1975). Incidence of malignant tumors in U.S. children. *Journal of Pediatrics, 86*, 254.

Appendix 30–A

Caremap for Thoracic Solid Tumors

	Preoperative	OR	POD 1	POD 2	POD 3	POD 4
Monitoring/ assessment	Pediatric preadmission testing Social worker contacted Child life assessment	Patient may be in the PACU or on an inpatient unit, vital signs (frequency depends on location) Strict I & O Monitor chest tube output Incision/chest tube dressings clean, dry and intact	Vital signs q4h Strict I & O Dressing C/D/I Chest tube drainage recorded	Vital signs q4h Strict I & O Dressing C/D/I Chest tube drainage recorded	Vital signs q4h Strict I & O Assess old chest tube site and incision	Vital signs as per routine Assess incision, assess chest tube site
Treatments	None	Chest physiotherapy pulmonary toilet with incentive spirometer use 10 times per hour while awake	Chest PT Incentive spirometer	Chest tube removal (depends on presence or absence of air leak and drainage) Incisional dressing changed Chest tube dressing changed with removal	Chest tube removed if not done on day 2 Chest tube site dressing changed Incisional dressing removed and site left open to air Continue incentive spirometer	Continue incentive spirometer Chest tube site dressing changed
Lines/drains	Central catheter or peripheral IV access	IV fluid at maintenance until tolerating PO Chest tube to suction regulated by column of water in the Pleurovac	IV fluid to KVO if tolerating PO Chest tube to water seal	IV fluid at KVO (secondary to narcotics) Chest tube to water seal or removal	IV heplock or peripheral IV removed	None

continues

Appendix 30–A continued

	Preoperative	OR	POD 1	POD 2	POD 3	POD 4
Medications	None	Cefazolin (20 mg/kg) IV x 1 on call to OR (max 1 g) and q8h times 24 hr postop Narcotics for pain control (PCA vs epidural)	Stop cefazolin after 24 hr Pain medication (IV narcotics)	IV narcotics	Taper IV narcotics and switch to PO narcotics or acetaminophen PRN	PO narcotics or acetaminophen
Activity	Ad lib	OOB to chair	OOB to chair OOB ambulating when chest tube to water seal	OOB ambulating Full activity, no heavy lifting	Full activity Encourage frequent ambulation and frequent position changes, no heavy lifting	Activity ad lib, no heavy lifting
Diet	Regular per routine	Clears, advance as tolerated	Regular	Regular	Regular	Regular
Tests	Blood work: CBC, T&C, coag profile, screening profile CT chest within 1 month of planned surgery	CXR in PACU	CXR before and after chest tube to water seal Daily CXR while chest tube in place CBC, lytes	CXR	CXR if chest tube removed day 3, otherwise none	None
Consults/referrals	Anesthesia evaluation Pain service for possible epidural	Pain service evaluation	VNS referral (if necessary)	None	None	None
Patient teaching	Pre and postoperative process reviewed Instructions given re: incentive spirometer, bubble blowing, pinwheel use	Reinforce pulmonary toilet	Wound management Pulmonary toilet	Incision/chest tube site care reviewed	Incision, chest tube site care reviewed May shower—no tub bathing for 2 wk	Incision/chest tube site care reviewed

	Preoperative	OR	POD 1	POD 2	POD 3	POD 4
Discharge planning	Evaluation of home environment and ability of patient to return home postoperatively	None	VNS referral (if necessary)	Begin discharge teaching regarding incision/chest tube site care, bathing, activity, care of central line	Follow-up appointment scheduled	Discharge home with emergency contact numbers, instructions re: medications, & signs and symptoms to report
Evaluation of outcomes	Bloodwork WNL: Yes___ No___ / Preop chart complete? / Consent/surgeons' note / Anesthesia evaluation and orders / History and physical / Education	Dressing Clean/dry/intact Yes___ No___ / Pain well controlled Yes___ No___ / Chest tube to suction Yes___ No___ / Chest tube drainage assessed Yes___ No___ / Chest x-ray reviewed Yes___ No___ / Tolerating diet Yes___ No___ / Tolerating activity Yes___ No___	Dressing C/D/I Yes___ No___ / Pain well controlled Yes___ No___ / Chest tube to water seal Yes___ No___ / Chest tube drainage Yes___ No___ / Chest x-ray reviewed Yes___ No___ / Tolerating diet Yes___ No___ / Tolerating activity Yes___ No___	Dressing C/D/I Yes___ No___ / Pain well controlled Yes___ No___ / Chest tube removed Yes___ No___ / Chest x-ray reviewed Yes___ No___ / Tolerating diet Yes___ No___ / Tolerating activity Yes___ No___	Dressing C/D/I Yes___ No___ / Incision site assessed Yes___ No___ / Pain well controlled Yes___ No___ / Tolerating full PO Yes___ No___ / Tolerating activity Yes___ No___ / Understands discharge instructions Yes___ No___	Dressing C/D/I Yes___ No___ / Incision site assessed Yes___ No___ / Pain well controlled Yes___ No___ / Tolerating full PO Yes___ No___ / Tolerating activity Yes___ No___ / Understands discharge instructions Yes___ No___

Appendix 30–B

Caremap for Extremity Solid Tumors

	Preoperative	OR	POD 1	POD 2	POD 3	POD 4	POD 5	POD 6
Monitoring/ assessment	Pediatric preadmission testing Social worker assessment Child life assessment	Frequent vital signs Strict I&O Incisional dressing clean, dry and intact Assess capillary refill, skin temperature, sensation and color, digit mobility to affected extremity Monitor JP drainage	Frequent vital signs Strict I&O Incisional dressing clean, dry and intact Assess capillary refill, skin temperature, sensation and color, digit mobility to affected extremity Monitor JP drainage	Frequent vital signs Strict I&O Incisional dressing changed Assess capillary refill, skin temperature and color, digit mobility to affected extremity Monitor JP drainage, incisional site assessed for infection	Frequent vital signs Strict I&O Incisional dressing changed Assess capillary refill, skin temperature and color, digit mobility to affected extremity Monitor JP drainage, incisional site assessed for infection	Frequent vital signs Strict I&O Incisional dressing changed Assess capillary refill, skin temperature and color, digit mobility to affected extremity Monitor JP drainage, incisional site assessed for infection	Frequent vital signs Strict I&O Incisional dressing changed Assess capillary refill, skin temperature and color, digit mobility to affected extremity Monitor JP drainage, incisional site assessed for infection	Frequent vital signs Strict I&O Incisional dressing changed Assess capillary refill, skin temperature and color, digit mobility to affected extremity Incisional site assessed for infection Assessment of old JP site for drainage
Treatments	None	Passive ROM machine as needed Passive ROM exercises	Passive ROM exercises	Passive ROM exercises Dressing change with assessment of surgical incision	Passive ROM exercises Dressing change with assessment of surgical incision	Passive ROM exercises Dressing change with assessment of surgical incision	Passive ROM exercises Dressing change with assessment of surgical incision	Passive ROM exercises Dressing change with assessment of surgical incision	None
Lines/drains	None	IV fluid at maintenance until tolerating PO	IV at maintenance until tolerating PO, then IV at KVO secondary to IV narcotics JP to self-suction	IV at maintenance until tolerating PO, then IV at KVO secondary to IV narcotics JP to self-suction	IV at maintenance until tolerating PO, then IV at KVO secondary to IV narcotics JP to self-suction	IV removed when analgesia switched to PO JP to self-suction	JP removed when output is less than 30 ml per 8 hr or at discretion of surgeon	None

	Preoperative	OR	POD 1	POD 2	POD 3	POD 4	POD 5	POD 6
Medications	None	Cefazolin (20 mg/kg) IV times 1 or call to OR and q8h for 24 hr postop Narcotics for pain control	Stop cefazolin after 24 hr [a] Continue IV narcotics	Continue IV narcotics	Initiate taper of IV narcotics to oral narcotics or acetamino-phen	Oral narcotics or acetamino-phen	PRN analgesia	PRN analgesia
Activity	Ad lib	Keep extremity elevated and immobile Passive ROM exercises	Keep extremity elevated and immobile Passive ROM exercises	Keep extremity elevated and immobile Passive ROM exercises	Keep extremity elevated and immobile Passive ROM exercises	Initiate ROM exercises as indicated by surgeon under direction of rehab	Continue ROM exercises as indicated by surgeon under direction of rehab	ROM exercises as indicated by surgeon under direction of rehab
Diet	Regular per routine	Clears, advance as tolerated	Regular diet	Regular	Regular	Regular	Regular	Regular
Tests	Bloodwork: CBC, T&C, coag profile, screening profile	None	CBC	None	None	None	None	None
Consults/ referrals	Anesthesia evaluation Pain service evaluation	Pain service evaluation	VNS referral (if indicated) Rehab service evaluation	None	None	None	None	None
Patient teaching	Pre and postop process reviewed	None	Wound care ROM exercises	Wound care ROM exercises Assessment of incision site	Wound care ROM exercises Assessment of incision site	Wound care ROM exercises Assessment of incision site	Wound care ROM exercises Assessment of incision site Extensive review of site care Review need for follow-up care at home and need for return visit	Wound care ROM exercises Assessment of incision site Extensive review of site care Review need for follow-up care at home and need for return visit Bathing guidelines

continues

Appendix 30–B continued

	Preoperative	OR	POD 1	POD 2	POD 3	POD 4	POD 5	POD 6
Discharge planning	Evaluation of home environment and ability of patient to return home	None	VNS referral if necessary Initiate availability of rehab services near home	None	None	None	Speak with home rehab specialists regarding interventions permitted and appointment date for evaluation	Discharge home with emergency contact numbers Instructions re signs and symptoms to report
Evaluation of outcomes	Blood work WNL Yes__ No__ Preop chart complete? Yes__ No__	Dressing clean, dry and intact Yes__ No__ Pain well controlled Yes__ No__ Keeping extremity elevated Yes__ No__ Assess extremity for postop complications Yes__ No__ JP to self-suction Yes__ No__ Tolerating diet Yes__ No__	Dressing clean, dry and intact Yes__ No__ Pain well controlled Yes__ No__ Keeping extremity elevated Yes__ No__ Assess extremity for postop complications Yes__ No__ JP to self-suction Yes__ No__ Tolerating diet Yes__ No__	Dressing clean, dry and intact Yes__ No__ Pain well controlled Yes__ No__ Keeping extremity elevated Yes__ No__ Assess extremity for postop complications Yes__ No__ JP to self-suction Yes__ No__ Tolerating diet Yes__ No__	Dressing clean, dry and intact Yes__ No__ Pain well controlled Yes__ No__ Keeping extremity elevated Yes__ No__ Assess extremity for postop complications Yes__ No__ JP to self-suction Yes__ No__ Tolerating diet Yes__ No__	Dressing clean, dry and intact Yes__ No__ Pain well controlled Yes__ No__ Keeping extremity elevated Yes__ No__ Assess extremity for postop complications Yes__ No__ JP to self-suction Yes__ No__ Tolerating diet Yes__ No__ JP removed Yes__ No__	Dressing clean, dry and intact Yes__ No__ Pain well controlled Yes__ No__ Keeping extremity elevated Yes__ No__ Assess extremity for postop complications Yes__ No__ JP to self-suction Yes__ No__ Tolerating diet Yes__ No__ JP removed Yes__ No__	Dressing clean, dry and intact Yes__ No__ Pain well controlled Yes__ No__ Keeping extremity elevated Yes__ No__ Assess extremity for postop complications Yes__ No__ JP to self-suction Yes__ No__ Tolerating diet Yes__ No__ JP removed Yes__ No__ Understands discharge instructions Yes__ No__

[a] Some surgeons continue the antibiotic until the drain is removed.

Appendix 30–C

Caremap for Abdominal/Pelvic Solid Tumors

	Preop	OR	POD 1	POD 2	POD 3	POD 4	POD 5	POD 6	POD 7
MONITORING AND ASSESSMENT	History and PE, including weight & height; social work; screening; child life assessment	PICU: vitals per routine; strict I/O with specific gravity, O₂ sat q2h,[a] supplemental oxygen PRN, abdominal dressing dry/intact, assess NGT, Foley, JP/Reliavac output	PICU: vitals per routine; strict I/O with specific gravity, O₂ sat PRN, supplemental oxygen PRN, abdominal dressing dry/intact, assess NGT, Foley, JP/Reliavac output, assess for peristalsis, pain assessment	(Possible transfer to general ward) Vitals q4h, strict I/O with sg, O₂ sat PRN, supplemental oxygen PRN, abdominal dressing dry/intact, assess NGT, JP/Reliavac output, assess for peristalsis, abdominal girth, daily weight, pain assessment	(Possible transfer to general ward) Vitals q4h, strict I/O with sg, O₂ sat PRN, assess incision for drainage or erythema, assess NGT output, assess for peristalsis, abdominal girth, daily weight, pain assessment	Vitals q4h, strict I/O, assess incision, assess for peristalsis, abdominal girth, daily weight, pain assessment	Vitals q4h, strict I/O, assess incision, assess for peristalsis, abdominal girth, daily weight, pain assessment	Vitals q4h, strict I/O, assess incision, assess for peristalsis, abdominal girth, daily weight, pain assessment	Vitals q4h, strict I/O, assess incision, assess for peristalsis, abdominal girth, daily weight, pain assessment
TREATMENTS	Perioperative care possible transfusion (plts, PRBCs, FFP)		Aggressive pulmonary toilet, Foley removed	Aggressive pulmonary toilet	Aggressive pulmonary toilet, removal of abdominal dressing (by surgical service), removal of JP/Reliavac	Pulmonary toilet, removal of NGT	Pulmonary toilet, staple removal (if present) and placement of Steri-Strips over incision	None	None

continues

Appendix 30–C continued

	Preop	OR	POD 1	POD 2	POD 3	POD 4	POD 5	POD 6	POD 7
LINES AND DRAINS	Peripheral/central intravenous access NGT (if needed for bowel prep)	Peripheral/central IV access, NGT, Foley catheter, possible JP or Reliavac, arterial line	IV access-hydration at maintenance, NGT to intermittent LWS, Foley removed+, possible JP or Reliavac	IV access-hydration at maintenance, NGT to gravity, JP/Reliavac	IV access-hydration at maintenance, NGT	IV access-hydration at maintenance until tolerating oral, then to KVO	IV at KVO or HL	IV HL	IV HL
TREATMENTS	1. Bowel prep Cathartic agent based on weight and age Bowel sterilizing atbx (e.g., neomycin, erythromycin) 2. Inhalers (as needed for RAD) 3. Steroids (if indicated) 4. Blood products ordered for on call to OR (platelets, PRBCs, & FFP) 5. Antibiotic ordered on call to OR	Cefotetan (20–40 mg/kg) IV on call to OR Cefotetan (20–40 mg/kg) IV q12hr x 24 hr postop IV narcotics PRN pain (PCA or epidural)	Cefotetan discontinued after 24 hr epidural/PCA narcotics	Epidural/PCA narcotics	Epidural/PCA narcotics	Begin to taper IV narcotics, switch to oral narcotics	Discontinue IV narcotics, taper oral narcotics	Continue oral narcotic taper and use acetaminophen as needed	Continue oral narcotic taper and use acetaminophen as needed
ACTIVITY	Ad lib	Bed rest	OOB to chair, HOB elevated while NGT in place	OOB ambulating	OOB ambulating	OOB ambulating	OOB ambulating	OOB ambulating	OOB ambulating

	Preop	OR	POD 1	POD 2	POD 3	POD 4	POD 5	POD 6	POD 7
DIET	1. Clear liquid diet 24–48 hr before surgery for patients requiring bowel prep 2. Regular diet for all others 3. NPO after MN before operative day (unless otherwise directed by the anesthesiologist)	NPO	NPO	NPO	NPO	Sips of clears	Clear liquid diet, if tolerating, advance to full liquid	Full liquid diet, advance as tolerated	Regular diet
TESTS	Blood work CBC Crossmatch Coagulation profile Electrolytes, renal & liver function screen scans as indicated (CT, Doppler U/S, CXR, ECHO, renal scan)	Per intra-operative routine	CBC, lytes	CBC, lytes	CBC, lytes	None unless indicated by patient condition	None	None	None
CONSULTS/REFERRALS	Anesthesia pain service Other as indicated (e.g., cardiology, endocrine)	None	None	None	Discharge planning service	Possible nutrition consult	None	None	None

continues

Appendix 30–C continued

	Preop	OR	POD 1	POD 2	POD 3	POD 4	POD 5	POD 6	POD 7
PATIENT TEACHING	Discuss pre/postop course; Review pulmonary toilet; Orientation to inpatient unit	Pulmonary toilet	Pulmonary toilet, wound care	Pulmonary toilet, wound care	Pulmonary toilet, wound care; Discharge teaching re: wound care, signs and symptoms to report, meds	Pulmonary toilet, wound care, discharge teaching	Pulmonary toilet, wound care, discharge teaching	Wound care, discharge teaching	Wound care, discharge teaching
DISCHARGE PLANNING	Evaluation of postop home care needs (e.g., PT, wound care, nutritional support)	None	Continue eval of potential home care needs	Begin discharge teaching re: wound care, signs and symptoms to assess for	Continue discharge teaching, initiate call to home care company or to discharge planning service	Discharge teaching	Discharge teaching	Discharge teaching, finalize home care needs	Discharge teaching
EVALUATION OF OUTCOMES	Lab data obtained and corrected PRN Yes__ No__; Preop chart complete Yes__ No__; Pre op atbx/blood products ordered Yes__ No__; Bowel prep initiated (if appl) Yes__ No__; Pt./family educ complete Yes__ No__	Pain well controlled Yes__ No__; Pulmonary toilet performed Yes__ No__; Dressing clean, dry, and intact Yes__ No__; Drains assessed and output recorded Yes__ No__	Pain well controlled Yes__ No__; Pulmonary toilet performed Yes__ No__; Dressing clean, dry, and intact Yes__ No__; Drains assessed and output recorded Yes__ No__; Foley removed Yes__ No__; Peristalsis present Yes__ No__	Pain well controlled Yes__ No__; Pulmonary toilet performed Yes__ No__; Dressing clean, dry and intact Yes__ No__; Drains assessed and output recorded Yes__ No__; NGT to gravity Yes__ No__; Foley removed Yes__ No__; Peristalsis present Yes__ No__	Pain well controlled Yes__ No__; Pulmonary toilet performed Yes__ No__; Dressing removed Yes__ No__; Incision assessed Yes__ No__; JP/Reliavac removed Yes__ No__; Drains assessed and output recorded Yes__ No__	Pain well controlled Yes__ No__; Pulmonary toilet performed Yes__ No__; Incision assessed Yes__ No__; JP/Reliavac removed Yes__ No__; NGT removed Yes__ No__; Peristalsis present Yes__ No__; Activity tolerated Yes__ No__	Pain well controlled Yes__ No__; Pulmonary toilet performed Yes__ No__; Incision assessed Yes__ No__; NGT removed Yes__ No__; Peristalsis present Yes__ No__; Activity tolerated Yes__ No__; Abdominal girth and weight recorded Yes__ No__	Pain well controlled Yes__ No__; Pulmonary toilet performed Yes__ No__; Incision assessed Yes__ No__; Peristalsis present Yes__ No__; Activity tolerated Yes__ No__; Abdominal girth and weight recorded Yes__ No__	Pain well controlled Yes__ No__; Pulmonary toilet performed Yes__ No__; Incision assessed Yes__ No__; Peristalsis present Yes__ No__; Activity tolerated Yes__ No__; Abdominal girth and weight recorded Yes__ No__

	Preop	OR	POD 1	POD 2	POD 3	POD 4	POD 5	POD 6	POD 7
EVALUATION OF OUTCOMES	Pt./family oriented to inpt. unit Yes __ No __		Activity tolerated Yes __ No __	Activity tolerated Yes __ No __	NGT to gravity Yes __ No __	Abdominal girth and weight recorded Yes __ No __	Discharge teaching continues Yes __ No __	Discharge teaching continued Yes __ No __	Discharge teaching completed Yes __ No __
	Child life assessment complete Yes __ No __		Discharge planning initiated Yes __ No __	Abdominal girth and weight recorded Yes __ No __	Foley removed Yes __ No __	Discharge teaching continued Yes __ No __	Diet tolerated Yes __ No __	Diet tolerated Yes __ No __	Diet tolerated Yes __ No __
	Social work screen complete Yes __ No __		Antibiotics discontinued Yes __ No __	Discharge teaching initiated Yes __ No __	Peristalsis present Yes __ No __	Diet tolerated Yes __ No __	Continue narcotic taper Yes __ No __	Continue narcotic taper Yes __ No __	Continue narcotic taper Yes __ No __
	Discharge needs assessment complete Yes __ No __				Activity tolerated Yes __ No __	Begin taper of narcotics Yes __ No __	Staples removed Yes __ No __		Staples removed Yes __ No __
					Abdominal girth and weight recorded Yes __ No __				Follow-up appointment given Yes __ No __
					Discharge teaching continued Yes __ No __				

[a] Some patients remain intubated postoperatively for 12–24 hr. In this case, respiratory care is monitored closely per the PICU routine.

[b] Unless otherwise indicated by the surgeon.

[c] Not done for retroperitoneal tumors or as directed by the surgeon.

CHAPTER 31

Pediatric Abdominal Organ Transplants

Kathleen Falkenstein, Caroline Brass, and Joanne Palmer

The management of children with abdominal organ transplants challenges the entire transplant team before, during, and after this complex surgical procedure. For nurses, postoperative management of a child who receives an abdominal organ transplant (liver, small bowel, kidney) presents special problems in the intensive care unit (ICU) and on the transplant ward. To support a successful outcome, nurses must understand the unique physiologic changes that occur and be prepared to intervene appropriately. This chapter focuses on end-stage disease, surgical procedures, associated therapies, and possible complications that occur after transplantation.

Survival for solid organ transplant in the United States has improved dramatically over the last two decades. With the introduction of new immunosuppressive drugs, such as cyclosporine (1983) and tacrolimus (1994) along with more innovative surgical techniques, patient and graft survival continue to improve. Better long-term survival along with expansion of inclusion criteria for recipients has prompted an increase in referrals for transplantation. Today more than 50,000 people are waiting for a solid organ transplant, which has resulted in longer waiting times (UNOS, 1998). In 1996 there were 3,934 liver transplants performed in the United States (UNOS, 1998). Four hundred twenty-three children less than age 16 underwent kidney transplantation in 1996. The international registry for intestinal organs reported on 180 intestinal transplants in 170 patients from 1990 to 1996. This included 38% intestinal, 46% liver/bowel, and 16% multivisceral (Grant, 1996).

RENAL TRANSPLANTATION

The first pediatric kidney transplant was performed in the early 1960s. Success of renal transplants has improved within the last three decades so that transplantation is now the treatment of choice for children with end-stage renal dis-

ease (Mauer, Nevins, & Ascher, 1992). The transplant process, including evaluation and the medical/surgical issues associated with these children, is reviewed here.

Preemptive Transplant

According to data provided by the North American Pediatric Renal Transplant Cooperative Study (NAPRTCS), the most common diagnoses leading to chronic renal failure in children include congenital obstructive uropathy, aplastic/hypoplastic/dysplastic kidneys, focal segmental glomerulosclerosis, and reflux nephropathy (Warady, Herbert, Sullivan, Alexander, & Tejani, 1997). Exhibits 31–1 and 31–2 include indications for abdominal transplants and clinical manifestations of end-stage organ disease. Various factors affect the decision regarding the best time to perform a transplant. Preemptive transplants are considered before renal replacement therapy with dialysis becomes necessary (Salvatierra et al., 1997). In some instances preemptive transplantation is not an option because the child is initially seen with an acute episode of renal failure and dialysis has to begin immediately.

Transplant Evaluation

The transplant evaluation involves a thorough medical review to identify any contraindications to the patient receiving a kidney. An integral aspect of the evaluation involves identification of the potential recipient's ABO blood type and human leukocyte antigen (HLA) tissue typing. These antigens are proteins that are present on the surface of kidney cells and other cells in the body (Bell, 1998). The antigens are divided into class I antigens, consisting of A, B, and C, and class II antigens, the DR category. The class I antigens present the major target for antibody and T cell reactions to a

Exhibit 31–1 Indications for Organ Transplant

Renal	Liver	Intestinal
Renal dysplasia	Cholestatic	Intestinal atresia
Renal hyperplasia	Biliary atresia	Gastroschisis
Glomerulonephritis	Alagille's syndrome	Mid-gut volvulus
Prune belly syndrome	Neonatal hepatitis	Necrotizing enterocolitis
Wilms' tumor	Acute fulminant failure	Crohn's disease
Obstructive uropathy	Hepatitis A, B, or C	Gardner syndrome
Acquired disease	Neonatal hemochromatosis	TPN cholestasis
Alport's syndrome	Metabolic disease	Pseudo-obstruction
Juvenile nephrophthisis	Alpha 1-antitrypsin	Congenital hepatic fibrosis
Hemolytic uremic syndrome	Wilson's disease	
Chronic pyelonephritis	Tyrosinemia	
Sickle cell nephropathy	Sclerosing cholangitis	
Polycystic kidney disease		
Oxalosis		
Congenital nephrotic syndrome		

transplanted organ. A perfect donor-recipient match is a six-antigen match based on these three sites. Parents always have at least a three-antigen match, an inherited haplotype. The HLA typing found in the transplanted kidney is the primary stimulus for the initiation of the immune response against the renal allograft (Suthanthiran & Strom, 1994). The more antigens that match the less severe the rejection. (See Exhibit 31–3 for other testing performed in the pretransplant evaluation.) Children with congenital uropathies undergo a urologic evaluation in addition to the laboratory evaluation, physical examination, and radiologic studies. Ureterovesical reflux to the allograft ureter, native kidney, or ureteral stump increases susceptibility to urinary tract infection after a renal transplant (Zaontz, Hatch, & Firlit, 1988). Children with congenital reflux may require native ureteronephrectomies or ureteral reimplantation before transplantation to decrease the risk of urinary tract infection after transplantation.

Donor Selection

Selection of an optimal kidney donor involves numerous factors. When possible, a living donor should be considered because these recipients do significantly better than those receiving a cadaver organ (Salvatierra et al., 1997). The living donor may be a parent, sibling older than 18 years of age, or other relative. Many centers are now performing living re-

Exhibit 31–2 Clinical Manifestation of Kidney, Liver, and Intestinal Disease

Renal	Liver	Intestinal
Sodium retention	Jaundice	Jaundice
Metabolic acidosis (low CO_2)	Failure to thrive	Ascites
Hyperkalemia	Ascites	Malabsorption
Hypocalcemia	Hypoglycemia	Growth stunting
Hypokalemia	Hepatomegaly	
Anemia	Hypoalbuminemia	
Congestive heart failure	Prolonged clotting studies	
Hyperglycemia	Hyperammonia	
Hyperlipidemia	Hypercholesterolemia or	
Peripheral neuropathy	hypocholesterolemia	
Renal osteodystrophy	Encephalopathy	
Growth stunting	Portal hypertension	
	Growth stunting	
	Hepatosplenomegaly	

Exhibit 31–3 Renal Recipient Evaluation

- Renal ultrasound
- Chest radiographic film
- Electrocardiogram
- Ophthalmology examination
- Dental examination
- Comprehensive panel
- PPD
- ABO
- Complete blood cell count, clotting studies
- Urinalysis and urine cultures
- Voiding cystourethrogram
- Bone age
- Echocardiogram (ECHO)
- Audiology examination
- Viral titers—cytomegalovirus (CMV), Epstein-Barr virus (EBV), varicella (VZV), toxoplasmosis
- Immunization update
- Human leukocyte antigen (HLA)

Exhibit 31–4 Renal Point System

- <11 years—4 points extra at time of listing
- 11–18 years—3 points extra at time of listing

  As of November 2, 1998, children will receive high priority if they meet the following criteria:

- 0–5 years on list >6 months receive high priority
- 6–10 years >12 months
- 11–17 years >18 months

lated and living unrelated donor transplants. This presents providers with an ethical dilemma of exposing a healthy donor to surgery with potential morbidity. Prospective living donors undergo a thorough medical and psychological evaluation before being accepted as a donor. The donor evaluation includes the standard biochemical assessment with the addition of a glomerular filtrate rate (GFR); urine tests for protein, creatinine, and culture and sensitivity; and cancer screening for donors older than 40 years of age. A computed tomography (CT) scan is obtained for prospective laparoscopic living related donors to identify the vascular anatomy. If a living donor is not identified or is found medically unacceptable, the child is placed on a waiting list for a cadaver graft. Although pediatric patients receive some priority according to their age, they may still wait several months to years for a medically suitable cadaveric organ. See Exhibit 31–4 for a delineation of the current United Network for Organ Sharing (UNOS) regulations for pediatric kidney transplantation. Whether receiving a living or cadaveric graft, the donor must be both ABO blood type and cross-match compatible. A positive T cell cross-match indicates the possibility of hyperacute rejection, a contraindication to transplantation with that donor (Suthanthiran & Strom, 1994). A positive T cell cross-match results in hyperacute rejection and graft loss within 24 hours.

Graft survival in pediatric renal transplant recipients is 91% and 76% at 1 and 5 years, respectively, for living donors. Cadaver graft survival in contrast is 78% and 59% at 1 and 5 years. Patient survival rates at 2 years are 96% for living donor recipients and 94% for cadaver donor recipients (Warady et al., 1997).

Preoperative/Intraoperative Management

On admission for transplantation the following studies should be performed: CBC, comprehensive panel, clotting studies, type and cross-match for 2 units of blood, and a final cross-match. Patients receiving hemodialysis should be dialyzed the day before surgery, whereas those receiving peritoneal dialysis continue passes until 2 hours before surgery. Immunosuppression can be initiated preoperatively or intraoperatively according to the transplant center's protocol. Management during the operative procedure focuses on maintaining adequate central venous pressure and blood pressure, which are particularly vital during reperfusion of the allograft (Jones, Matas, & Najarian, 1994). The kidney is generally placed in the retroperitoneum unless the patient is an infant or small child, in which case it is placed in the peritoneal cavity. Two vascular anastomoses connect the donor's renal artery with the recipient's iliac artery and the donor's renal vein with the recipient's iliac vein (Jones et al., 1994). After reperfusion of the kidney, the donor ureter is anastomosed to the bladder (ureteroneocystostomy).

Postoperative Management

Postoperative nursing care of the pediatric renal transplant includes a systems approach.

Fluid and Electrolyte Therapy

Maintaining renal perfusion, adequate blood pressure, and intravascular fluid volume is extremely important in the immediate postoperative period to promote diuresis of the transplanted kidney. A combination of crystalloid and colloid solutions are administered to replace insensible water losses, urine output, gastrointestinal losses, and third space distribution. During the initial 24 hours, milliliter per milliliter urine output replacement is delivered hourly with a 0.45% NaCl solution with sodium bicarbonate and potassium added as needed. Dextrose is avoided in urine replacement fluids to prevent the development of hyperglycemia. Insensible fluid losses are replaced with a dextrose solution.

Monitoring of the central venous pressure (CVP) is crucial during the early postoperative course to prevent hypovolemia, which may impair renal function, or hypervolemia with resultant pulmonary edema (Loertscher, Parfrey, & Guttmann, 1989). The CVP should be maintained in the range of 8 to 11 cm H_2O; 0.9% saline or 5% albumin should be administered at 5 to 10 ml/kg to support blood pressure and to maintain systolic measurements of at least 100 to 110 mm Hg (Alexander, 1990). Dopamine may be administered to maintain cardiac output and increase allograft perfusion (Alexander, 1990). Evaluation of the patient's clinical status, pulse oximetry, and chest radiography are important adjuncts to CVP measurements in differentiating fluid overload from hypovolemia.

Biochemical imbalances are common during the early posttransplant period. Close monitoring and correction of serum electrolytes, calcium, phosphorous, and glucose concentrations is necessary. In the immediate postoperative period serum creatinine should be monitored every 6 hours to assess renal function. Initially, urine output is replaced milliliter per milliliter. Over the next 2 days a fraction of the hourly urine output is replaced to promote a more manageable diuresis and to allow excretion of excess fluids (Mauer et al., 1992). Maintenance intravenous fluids are generally administered by the third postoperative day and adjusted according to oral intake.

Acute Renal Failure

Nonfunction of the allograft is caused by prerenal, renal, or postrenal factors. Prerenal graft nonfunction causes hypovolemia that is easily reversed by administering intravenous fluid resuscitation to maintain adequate CVP (Loertscher et al., 1989). A leading cause of postrenal allograft nonfunction is obstruction of the bladder outlet by a blood clot. The indwelling catheter should be irrigated or replaced if necessary (Keown & Stiller, 1986; Kirkman & Tilney, 1989). Once prerenal and postrenal factors have been eliminated, renal factors such as acute tubular necrosis (ATN) must be considered. This condition is usually reversible and results from excessive ischemia to the kidney either from prolonged donor hypotension or extended warm and/or cold ischemia time during the organ recovery and transplant procedure (Shapiro & Simmons, 1991). Management of ATN includes avoidance of nephrotoxic drugs, such as cyclosporine and antibiotics, and conservative fluid replacement to prevent hypervolemia. Other causes of posttransplant renal failure include acute allograft rejection, vascular complications, cyclosporine nephrotoxicity, recurrence of primary renal disease, or development of new disease (Baluarte et al., 1994). A nuclear medicine renal scan and/or Doppler ultrasonography are obtained to evaluate graft function and abnormalities after surgery.

Surgical Complications

Bleeding after transplantation may occur from the site of the vascular anastomosis or from arterial branches that are not properly ligated during surgery (Kirkman & Tilney, 1989). Postoperative bleeding is manifested by tachycardia, hypotension, falling CVP, abdominal distention, pain, and oliguria that result from diminished perfusion of the allograft (Mauer et al., 1992). Restoration of the blood volume and surgical intervention to control the source of bleeding are required to stabilize the patient and avoid jeopardizing graft function.

Early graft loss caused by vascular thrombosis is a significant problem for pediatric renal transplant recipients (Kohaut & Tejani, 1996). This has been reported in 2.6% of all pediatric renal transplantations (Harmon, Stablein, Alexander, & Tejani, 1991). Children less than 5 years of age are at highest risk for renal vascular thrombosis related to low flow states. A young child's limited cardiac activity results in diminished renal blood flow and compromises the new graft. Renal artery thrombosis is seen as a sudden onset of anuria and is generally irreversible, requiring allograft nephrectomy. A related problem, renal artery stenosis, is caused by technical problems during organ procurement or the transplant surgery. A stenosis is diagnosed by a Doppler ultrasonographic study that demonstrates decreased or turbulent flow through the renal artery (Bunchman & So, 1994). Clinical symptoms include persistent and difficult to control hypertension, with or without erythrocytosis and deteriorating renal function (Tilney, Rocha, Strom, & Kirkman, 1984). Approximately one third of these cases are successfully treated with percutaneous transluminal angioplasty (Ingelfinger & Brewer, 1992).

In contrast, renal vein thrombosis (RVT) presents with persistent gross hematuria, graft swelling, and a gradual deterioration in renal graft function. RVT is more common in living related recipients less than 6 years of age and recipients of young cadaver donor grafts, especially those with long cold storage times (Harmon et al., 1991). It may be possible to treat a partial RVT with heparin (Shapiro & Simmons, 1991).

Urologic Complications

Another source of complications after kidney transplantation is urologic problems related to technical difficulties in performing the ureteroneocystostomy (Mauer et al., 1992). Urinary extravasation occurs during the early postoperative period and develops at the ureterovesical anastomosis site. Clinical manifestations include unexplained fever, abdominal pain, decreased urine output, elevated serum creatinine, and wound drainage. Fluid from either the surgical drain or incision may be analyzed for creatinine to determine whether the leakage is urine or lymph. Ultrasonography demonstrates a large fluid collection, and a nuclear medicine renal scan differentiates a ureteral versus a bladder urinary leak (Salvatierra, 1994). Urine leaks are treated with prolonged indwelling catheter drainage for minor leakage (Shapiro & Simmons, 1991) or immediate surgical repair to avoid infection (Salvatierra, 1994).

Obstruction at the ureterovesical anastomosis may occur at any time after transplantation, also causing oliguria, and usually requires surgical correction (Zaontz et al., 1988). After removal of the surgical drain, a lymphocele may develop because of the continued drainage of lymphatic fluid from the surface of the allograft or surrounding tissues. An ultrasonogram should be obtained to document the extraperitoneal collection. Needle aspirations and/or surgery may be required for large fluid collections, which compromise allograft function (Mauer et al., 1992).

The surgical incision should be monitored for signs of infection, including erythema, warmth, swelling, and drainage. The risk of wound infection after transplant is increased for recipients with a history of chronic anemia, malnutrition, and current immunosuppressive therapy (Rubin, 1988). Prophylactic antibiotics are administered for three doses at the time of surgery to prevent infection.

Medical Complications

According to NAPRTCS data, a high incidence of kidney allograft loss in children is due to rejection, both acute and chronic.

Acute Rejection. Acute rejection can occur as early as 2 weeks after transplantation. Refer to Exhibit 31–5 for clinical manifestations of acute organ rejection. In the first 2 years after transplantation as many as 72% of cadaver graft recipients and 56% of living donor recipients experience rejection (Kohaut & Tejani, 1996). Acute rejection is diagnosed clinically by progressive increases in creatinine levels, fever, allograft swelling and associated pain, proteinuria, hematuria, and hypertension and confirmed by biopsy. The biopsy reveals glomeruli that are being invaded by lymphocytes. Induction drugs such as antithymocyte globulin (ATG), OKT3, dacliximab (Zenapax), and Simulect reduce early acute rejection and prolong graft survival, thus increasing the supply of organs. Refer to Table 31–1 for immunosuppression regimens used in abdominal organ transplants. A recent NAPRTCS report indicates that 50% of all kidney transplant recipients receive some form of induction therapy (Kohant & Tejani, 1996).

Acute rejection can occur any time after the transplantation. A viral infection and medication noncompliance are two risk factors for late acute rejection. In the presence of acute rises in creatinine, with the suspicion of infection or noncompliance, a biopsy is obtained to diagnose acute rejection. Acute rejection is treated with steroid boluses at 10 mg/kg followed by a taper of steroids and maintaining therapeutic drug levels of cyclosporine or tacrolimus. Acute rejection that is not responsive to steroid boluses requires treatment with OKT3.

Chronic Rejection. Although effective strategies are being developed for treatment of acute rejection, chronic rejection remains a most troublesome problem. It is clinically characterized by a slow and progressive increases in creatinine, often associated with hypertension and proteinuria and generally unresponsive to present immunosuppressant agents. The cause of chronic rejection is probably multifactorial, but the most significant risk factor is a history of acute rejection (Paul, 1995). There has not been a great deal of success in treating chronic rejection. An effective strategy is a change in immunosuppression and encouragement of medication compliance. As kidney function deteriorates, the child experiences symptoms of chronic renal failure that can be conservatively treated, such as by administration of phosphate binders, vitamin D therapy, recombinant erythropoietin to stimulate red blood cell production and decrease the severity of anemia, and finally, retransplant. Children are relisted for transplant when they begin to show signs of renal failure, including growth stunting, fatigue, and poor school performance. Dialysis is reinstituted when biochemical parameters and physical findings indicate progressive renal failure. These include elevated BUN (>100), creatinine (> 6–8), hyperkalemia unresponsive to sodium polystyrene sulfonate (Kayexalate), hyperphosphatemia, and hypercalcemia.

Hypertension. The cause of posttransplant hypertension is also multifactorial, including the roles of renal factors (i.e., renin release in the face of decreased renal blood flow from ATN and cyclosporine toxicity) and hemodynamics (i.e., increased vascular volume in the presence of decreased urine output sometimes seen in rejection). A frequent side effect of many immunosuppressants is hypertension (Ingelfinger & Brewer, 1992). Short-term effects of hypertension include headache, vision problems, and light-headedness. Long-term hypertension contributes to the risk of kidney damage from glomerulosclerosis. Common treatment strategies include vasodilators, cardioselective agents, and diuretics. Frequently used antihypertensive agents are calcium-channel blockers that reduce blood pressure, treat ischemic heart disease, and reduce cyclosporine nephrotoxicity by antagonizing either the direct or indirect vasoconstrictive actions of the cyclosporine (Weir, 1990).

Maintenance Immunosuppression

Immunosuppression of children who have received an abdominal organ transplant is critically important to prevent rejection. Most centers use a combination of three immunosuppressant medications and/or induction therapy. Gener-

Exhibit 31–5 Clinical Manifestations of Acute Organ Rejection

Renal	Liver	Intestines
Fever	Fever	Fever
↑BUN	↑WBCs	Increase ostomy output
↑Creatinine	↑Liver enzymes	Diarrhea
Decrease urine output	Pain over graft	Abdominal pain
Weight gain	Dark urine	Metabolic acidosis
Abdominal pain	Jaundice	Vomiting
Irritability	Irritability	Abdominal distention

Table 31–1 Immunosuppression Therapy for Children with Abdominal Organ Transplant

Treatment	Dosage
Renal transplant	
Cyclosporine microemulsion formula (Neoral)	6–12 mg/kg/day divided BID Trough levels (100–200 RIA or 150–300 TDX)
Antilymphocytic globulin (ATG)	5–10 mg/kg/dose (until CYA level >100)
Tacrolimus (FK506)	0.1–.15 mg/kg/day divided BID Trough levels (5–10 ng)
Azathioprine (Imuran)	1–1.5 mg/kg/day once a day
Mycophenolate mofetil (CellCept)	1,200 mg/kg/m²/day given BID
Solu-Medrol	5 mg/kg/day taper over 7 days to dose of 2 mg/kg/day (total not greater than 80 mg/day) Day 8–14 1.5 mg/kg/day (40 mg maximum)
Prednisolone	6–18 months .2 mg/kg/day
Liver transplant	
Cyclosporine (Neoral)	12–20 mg/kg/day given BID or TID Trough levels (1–3 mo 200–250; 6–12 mo 150–175; 1 yr–2 yr 125)
Tacrolimus (FK506)	.2–.3 mg/kg/day PO BID to maintain trough levels of 15–20 for first month (2–12 mo) (7–15 ng/ml) (>12 mo) (5 ng/ml)
Azathioprine (Imuran)	1–2 mg/kg/day given daily for 1 yr
Mycophenolate mofetil	1,200 mg/kg/m²/day given BID
Prednisolone	10 mg/kg day 1 and then wean to 2 mg/kg/day by day 5 and 1 mg/kg/day daily or BID at discharge Wean at .2 mg/kg/every other month until total dose is .2 mg/kg dose, then QOD times 2–3 months and discontinue
Small bowel transplant	
Tacrolimus	0.15 mg/kg/day IV until tolerating oral .30/mg/kg/day PO BID to maintain trough levels (15–30)
Methylprednisolone	10 mg/kg/day on day 1 1 mg/kg/day with tapering doses over 5 days, to start on POD 2
Azathioprine (Imuran)	1 mg/kg/day IV or PO

Note: Each transplant center has individualized immunosuppressant regimens. This is just an example of management from the literature review.

ally, these medications are continued throughout the patient's lifetime. Many centers attempt to reduce the dose of prednisone to alternate-day therapy or complete withdrawal. This strategy decreases the incidence of long-term side effects and promotes growth. Each of the medications acts on a different part of the cell cycle to block organ rejection. Immunosuppressive medications suppress humoral and cellular immunity. Cyclosporine/Neoral and tacrolimus block the production of interleukin-2, thus interrupting events that lead to organ rejection. Corticosteroids decrease the number of activated lymphocytes. See Table 31–1 for a list of commonly used drugs for immunosuppression therapy. Both cyclosporine and tacrolimus require careful drug monitoring to adjust the dose in the early posttransplant period. A trough level is obtained during the hospitalization and follow-up of the patient (Lake & Kilkenny, 1992; Payne, 1992). In general, there is an increased incidence of rejection of a subsequent transplant if the previous transplant was lost because of acute rejection as opposed to technical problems (Tejani, Cortes, & Stablein, 1996).

LIVER TRANSPLANTATION

The first human liver transplant was performed in Denver by Starzl in 1963. The patient survived only briefly, as did the next four recipients of liver transplants. Measurable success was not achieved until 1967, when a child with a hepatoma received a liver transplant and survived 13 months (Starzl, Swatsuki, & Van Thiel, 1982).

As recently as 1983, 20% to 50% of children who needed liver transplantation died before a child's donor liver became available; most of these patients weighed less than 10 kg (Broelsch, Edmond, & Thistlethwaite, 1988). To address the shortage of donor organs, investigators at the University of Chicago began using portions of young teens' and adult livers for small children. This procedure is known as reduced-size liver transplantation. Thereafter, from 1988 to 1990, the mortality rate for children on waiting lists for liver transplants decreased significantly to a reported national average of 7% to 10%. Living related liver transplantation (using a portion of a parent or relative's liver for a small child) became a reality in 1989. This technique along with split liver techniques (one liver being used for two children or a child and adult recipient) has continued to allow more children to be transplanted before they are in critical condition (Hayashi et al., 1998).

Liver Structure and Function

See Figure 31–1 and Exhibit 31–6 for a review of the complex structure and physiology of the liver. The body's largest organ, the liver, rests in the right upper abdominal quadrant. The porta hepatis, located centrally behind the fourth seg-

ment of the liver, is the point of entry into the liver for the portal vein, hepatic artery, nerves, and lymph vessels and the point where the bile duct emerges from the liver. The liver receives blood from two major sources: the hepatic artery and the portal vein. The hepatic artery conveys 20% of the blood supply as oxygenated blood; the portal vein supplies 80% as nutrient-filled blood from the stomach and intestines. The celiac axis carries oxygenated blood from the aorta to the hepatic artery and to the spleen and stomach. The portal vein supplies 75% of the blood supply to the liver. When recipients have an occluded or small portal vein, the liver transplant is technically difficult. Both portal and hepatic blood flow are essential for the liver allograft to function normally (Starzl, Rutman, & Corman, 1987).

Bile is produced in the liver and secreted by parenchymal cells. Bile drains into cholangioles, small terminal bile ducts (canaliculi), that merge into the right and left hepatic ducts and form the common bile hepatic duct. The common hepatic duct joins the cystic duct from the gallbladder to form the common bile duct (CBD). The CBD exits the liver at the porta hepatis and empties into the duodenum to aid in digestion of fat. These ducts are not large, and any obstruction, whether mechanical or caused by disease, can cause liver decompensation.

The liver can function despite extensive damage; approximately 85% of the liver must be damaged before liver failure occurs. Fortunately, the liver has the unique ability to regenerate after injury; a damaged liver can regenerate within 3 weeks and resume normal function within about 4 months.

Indications for Liver Transplantation and Types of Liver Transplants

The liver transplant procedure can be performed as a whole liver graft, reduced-size graft, split liver procedure, or as a living donor operation. Reduced-size grafts can be obtained using a right lobe, left lobe, or left lateral segment from either a cadaveric or living donor. Left lateral segment grafts are used in infants and small children. Older children may require a left lobe graft to provide adequate liver tissue. Recently, living related transplants have been performed on adult recipients who receive the right lobe. In a split liver procedure, the liver is divided along the falciform ligament producing two segments, a right lobe graft that is used in an adolescent or small adult and a left lobe or left lateral segment that can be used for an infant or small child.

Refer to Exhibit 31–1 for indications for liver transplant and Figure 31–2 for a schematic diagram of reduced-size allografts.

Recipient Evaluation and Donor Selection

The evaluation of potential recipients for liver transplant includes a multidisciplinary approach and a thorough physi-

Reviewing liver structure and function

The body's largest internal organ, the liver rests in the right upper abdominal quadrant. An adult's liver weighs about 3 lb (1.36 kg). A thick covering of connective tissue called Glisson's capsule surrounds the liver. The liver attaches to the anterior abdominal wall and diaphragm by the falciform ligament, which also grossly divides the liver into right and left lobes. The right lobe has three sections; the left lobe, two.

Lobules, the liver's functional units, subdivide each lobe section.

The liver contains approximately 50,000 to 100,000 lobules, hexagonal rows of hepatic cells called hepatocytes. Blood that enters from the portal vein and hepatic artery flows through lobular channels called sinusoids, which drain into the central vein. Kupffer's cells (part of the reticuloendothelial system), line the sinusoids. A crucial filtering system, these cells phagocytically destroy old and defective red blood cells and remove bacteria and foreign particles from blood.

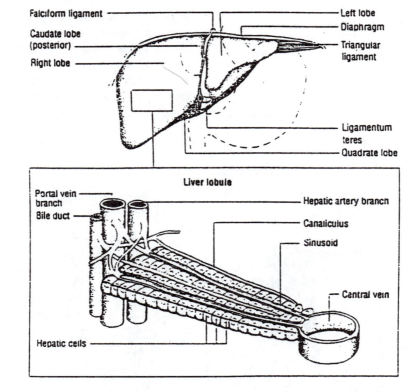

Figure 31–1 Liver Structure and Function. Figure 31–1A is a schematic diagram of the liver and Figure 31–1B indicates the venous and arterial blood flow to the hepatocytes.

cal and laboratory evaluation (Exhibit 31–7). In addition to testing performed for renal transplant recipients (see Exhibit 31–3), liver recipients undergo a liver biopsy and duplex scan of the liver. The cadaveric donor evaluation involves complete serologic studies, liver enzymes, a complete history of prior illness, substance abuse, and any adverse events during the hospitalization. Potential recipients are matched by blood group, weight, and wait time on the UNOS list (see Table 31–2 for UNOS liver transplant status criteria).

Living related donor evaluations are performed on an outpatient basis. Initially, a family conference occurs to discuss risks and benefits of the procedure with the transplant team. Issues related to postoperative recovery and return to work

are discussed. The donor evaluation includes a history and physical examination with an adult hepatologist, laboratory evaluation, volumetric CT scan, and a hepatic arteriogram to determine liver anatomy (Boone, Kelly, & Smith, 1992) (Exhibit 31–8). Occasionally, unfavorable vascular anatomy is found. At this point a different living donor is considered or the child continues to wait for an appropriate cadaver donor. The operation is scheduled after determining that all studies are normal. In the case of acute liver failure, donors can be evaluated in approximately 6 to 8 hours and donate the same day. This has become a lifesaving measure when children are in imminent danger of dying and no cadaveric organs are available (Casas, Falkenstein, Gallagher, & Dunn, 1999).

Exhibit 31–6 Functions of the Liver

A. Metabolism
   1. Carbohydrates: maintain normal glucose level (gluconeogenesis).
   2. Fats: oxidation of fatty acids for energy.
   3. Proteins: breaks down proteins, removes ammonia from blood.
B. Storage of vitamins: fat-soluble A, D, E, K, and B_{12}.
C. Detoxification and removal of drugs from blood (alter doses with liver failure).
D. Secretion of bile: needed to break down fat globules and absorb fatty acids. Failure of bile flow results in malnutrition.
E. Synthesis of plasma protein: albumin, fibrinogen (blood coagulation).
F. Kupffer cell activity: destroys old and defective RBCs and removes bacteria from blood.

Pretransplant Management and Complications

Because transplantation survival rates have continued to improve, liver transplant is the modality of choice for children with end-stage liver disease. The most common reasons to initiate transplant in children with chronic liver disease are poor growth and development, portal hypertension, and mental changes (McDiarmid, 1998).

Nutritional and Developmental Concerns

Cognitive deficits are not unusual in children with liver disease because the children have organomegaly and malabsorption, resulting in protein-calorie malnutrition and low energy levels (Stewart, Kennard, Waller, & Fixler, 1994). The brain is particularly vulnerable to the effects of protein-energy malnutrition during early life. Malnutrition during the early months of life, independent of cause, has a deleterious effect on development (Stewart et al., 1989). Recogni-

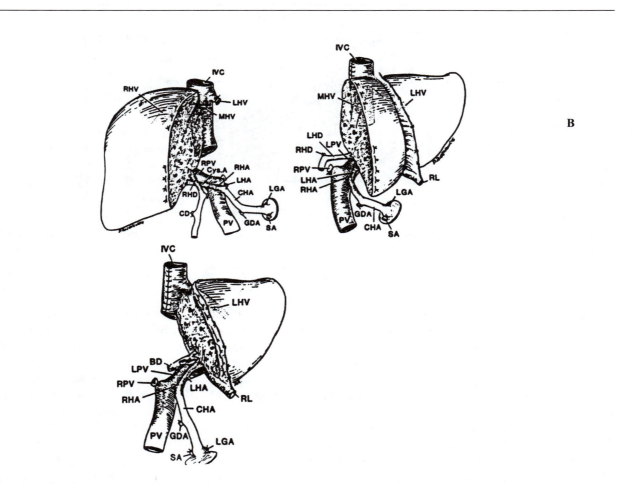

Figure 31–2 Schematic Diagrams of Reduced-size Allografts after Graft Preparation. A, Right hepatic lobe. B, Left hepatic lobe. C, Left lateral segment.

Exhibit 31–7 Liver Transplant Recipient Evaluation

- Physical examination
- Laboratory tests (chemistry, hematology, viral, ABO, HIV, hepatitis, tissue typing)
- Consults (renal, cardiology, social work, neurology, pulmonary)
- Liver biopsy

Exhibit 31–8 Living Related Donor Liver Evaluation

- History and physical examination
- Laboratory tests (same as recipient)
- Chest radiographic film, ECG
- CT scan for size and volume of liver
- Hepatic arteriogram

tion and prevention of growth failure in a transplant candidate is necessary to institute maximal nutritional support (Balistreri, Bucuvalas, & Ryckman, 1995). The treatment of nutritionally depleted patients requires the administration of adequate calories to ensure optimal anabolic use of protein sources (Moukarzel et al., 1990). (For additional information about nutrition in children with end-stage liver disease see Chapter 4).

Children who are in a better nutritional state before transplantation have better outcomes after transplantation (Moukarzel et al., 1990). When oral intake is not adequate to provide for calories and weight gain, nasogastric or gastrostomy tube feedings should be initiated (Kaufman, Murray, Wood, Shaw, & Vanderhoof, 1987).

Portal Hypertension

Children with chronic liver disease are at increased risk for esophageal varices that result from decreased blood flow to the liver and increased flow, by means of collateral circulation, to the spleen and stomach. These children require frequent evaluations because medical management is based on symptoms. Sclerotherapy is the temporizing treatment of choice for bleeding varices. Other therapies include propra-

nolol (Inderal) or portal-venous shunt (Goh & Meyers, 1994).

Encephalopathy

Children with chronic liver disease may have obvious changes in mental status related to elevated NH_3 levels. Changes in wake-sleep cycle, decreased concentration in school resulting in change in grades, frustration, and inability to perform simple fine motor skills are common. Evaluation and treatment with medications such as neomycin and lactulose and a decrease in dietary protein may help.

Infections

Children awaiting liver transplantation are at increased risk of infection because of chronic nutritional deficits and impaired liver function. Good hand washing and the avoidance of day care centers and large crowds while on the transplant list are recommended.

Surgical Procedure and Operative Management

When a liver becomes available, the recipient is brought to the hospital and preoperative blood work, including a com-

Table 31–2 UNOS System for Liver Candidates

UNOS Status	Description of Status	Special Status Considerations
Status 3	At home with stable liver function as an outpatient	
Status 2B	Requires ongoing care as an inpatient or outpatient. Outpatient criteria include malnutrition, gastrointestinal bleeding, growth failure, and peritonitis	Documentation on status 2B Form. Audit may occur.
Status 1	Requires ICU and one of the following criteria: Primary graft nonfunction Grade 3–4 encephalopathy, vasopressors, hemodialysis, mechanical ventilation, or gastrointestinal bleeding	Reevaluation of status in 7 days, reapply with completion of UNOS status 1 form, audit may occur.

prehensive panel, CBC, PT/ PTT, and type and cross-match for blood products, is obtained. A chest radiographic film, urinalysis, and physical examination are part of the preoperative evaluation.

The surgical procedure is approximately 8 to 12 hours from induction of anesthesia and line placement until final skin closure. The procedure involves a bilateral subcostal incision to visualize and mobilize all major structures (portal vein, hepatic artery, and bile ducts) of the liver before the hepatectomy. Before removing the liver, the surgeon cross-clamps the suprahepatic and infrahepatic venae cavae, portal vein, and hepatic artery. Clamping of the venae cavae can lead to acidosis, hypotension, and bleeding. The donor liver is placed in an orthotopic position, and the vascular anastomoses are performed in the following order: suprahepatic vena cava, infrahepatic vena cava (which is flushed with 5% albumin to remove any leftover preservation solution), portal vein establishing blood flow to the graft, and finally, the hepatic artery. Reperfusion of the graft occurs once portal venous blood flow is reestablished. During the reperfusion phase, the results of clamping can lead to swelling of the intestine, fluid shifts (third spacing), and renal failure. Children generally tolerate caval clamping well because of their collateral circulation (Falkenstein, 1993). Reconstruction of the biliary drainage involves a Roux-en-Y limb of the jejunum and insertion of two to three Jackson-Pratt drains. The child remains intubated and is transferred directly to the intensive care unit (Falkenstein, 1993).

The donor liver is stored in Wisconsin preservation solution and ice until it is prepared for implantation. Use of this solution has increased cold times from 8 to 24 hours. Extended preservation time permits careful inspection of the donor organ and reconstruction or back table surgery of the hepatic allograft. One of the advantages of living related donation is that the liver can be removed from the donor and almost immediately be placed in the recipient, thus decreasing cold ischemic time.

Postoperative Management

Postoperative care of the child after liver transplantation involves assessment and monitoring of the cardiovascular, pulmonary, neurologic, gastrointestinal, and immune systems; liver function; and fluid and electrolyte and nutrition (Falkenstein, 1993). Nursing care must also address the psychosocial and emotional needs of the child and family members.

Cardiovascular Monitoring

Adequate perfusion of body organs, especially the new liver, is important. Hypothermia may occur as a result of the large incision, the exposure of the bowel during surgery, and the transfusion therapy required. Hemorrhage is possible as a result of coagulopathy or bleeding from the anastomosis. To detect bleeding, one should observe for increased abdominal girth, oozing from suture lines, and large amounts of drainage from Jackson-Pratt drains. Children have an arterial line, two central lines, and peripheral lines in the upper extremities because of cross-clamping of the vena cava. Hypertension or hypotension may occur postoperatively. Hypertension in the first 24 to 48 hours is usually related to the amount of colloids and blood products given in the operating room. It also may be due to altered function of the renin-angiotensin system from decreased renal flow caused by intravenous cyclosporine. Hypotension also results from bleeding or depleted fluid volume.

Pulmonary Monitoring

Ventilatory support is usually required for the first 24 to 48 hours after liver transplantation. Children are less likely to breathe effectively on their own because of the large incision and large hepatic allograft. Gentle chest percussion and suctioning facilitated with adequate pain management should be provided.

Fluid and Electrolytes

CVP monitoring aids in evaluating the child's fluid status. A complicating factor of maintaining fluid and electrolyte balance is the shift of fluid into the vascular beds and abdomen that occurs after the portal vein and vena cava are unclamped in the operating room (Falkenstein, 1993). Children with this complication usually have a low CVP (1 to 3 cm H_2O) and low urine output, suggesting hypovolemia, although they appear edematous and weigh more than their preoperative weight. Effective diuresis is accomplished with furosemide (Lasix) or ethacrynate sodium (Edecrin). Fluids are administered at 80% of maintenance. Electrolytes are monitored every 6 hours, and fluid and electrolyte correction is made accordingly (Falkenstein, 1993). Hypocalcemia, hypokalemia, and hypomagnesia are common problems in the child immediately after liver transplantation. Intake and output (Jackson-Pratt drains, Foley catheter, nasogastric tube) should be accurately measured to monitor fluid balance. Decreased urine output (<1 ml/kg/hr) may reflect early graft dysfunction or cyclosporine-induced nephrotoxicity. As liver function improves, urine volume and concentration improve, and urine changes from an orange to a straw color.

Neurologic Evaluation

Neurologic assessments should be performed using a modified Glasgow coma scale until the child is fully awake. Central nervous system status is a crucial indicator of allograft function. Seizure activity is uncommon and usually limited to extremely ill children with multiple risk factors.

Gastrointestinal and Nutritional

A nasogastric tube is placed to keep the stomach decompressed and prevent vomiting and aspiration postoperatively. Parenteral nutrition begins on day 2 or 3 and continues until the child is receiving adequate calories either orally or by nasogastric tube. Small children have an increased metabolic rate and require increased calories by mouth or nasogastric tube for at least 6 months after transplantation.

Care on the Transplant Unit

The average stay in the intensive care unit is 3 to 5 days, at which point children are moved to the transplant unit. The most common problems after transplantation are rejection and infection. Other complications include hepatic artery thrombosis, bile leaks, bowel perforation, hypertension, and fluid retention (Falkenstein, 1993). Nursing interventions include monitoring for signs and symptoms of rejection and infection, monitoring of blood pressure, and discharge teaching.

Surgical Complications

Hepatic Artery Thrombosis

Hepatic artery thrombosis (HAT) occurs 1 to 6 days after transplantation and is usually related to mechanical problems. HAT results in graft failure, necessitating prompt detection. Signs and symptoms include irritability, fever, increasing liver enzymes, and inability of clotting studies to normalize. Doppler ultrasonography is used to confirm the diagnosis. HAT requires thrombectomy and restoration of arterial blood flow. Late artery thrombosis may result from chronic rejection and is less damaging to the graft because of collateral circulation. Bile duct complications are common in all patients with hepatic artery thrombosis because the bile duct receives flow from the hepatic artery. Retransplantation may be required at a later time (Stevens et al., 1992).

Bile Duct Stricture

Bile duct stricture may occur at any time. Children who are at an increased risk for strictures are those with chronic rejection, cytomegalovirus infections, or who required placement of a stent for a small duct during anastomosis of the bile duct (Dunn et al., 1994).

Bile Leaks

Bile leaks can develop at any time after transplantation. Leakage of bile is evidenced by a change in color of the drainage from the Jackson-Pratt drains. Diagnosis is confirmed by measuring bilirubin from the drain. If it is higher than the systemic bilirubin, a bile leak is suspected. Early diagnosis and treatment can prevent a major episode of infectious peritonitis.

Bowel Perforation

Bowel perforation is relatively uncommon and it usually occurs 5 to 7 days postoperatively. This complication results from division of adhesions during surgery. Signs and symptoms are fever, abdominal pain, distention, and irritability. Diagnosis is confirmed by a lateral decubitus radiographic film of the abdomen, assessing for free air. Surgical repair is the only treatment and should be performed immediately (Oldham, Colombani, & Foglia, 1997).

Medical Complications

The first episode of a acute rejection usually occurs 5 to 10 days after transplantation. Early signs of rejection include low-grade fever (101°F), increases in liver enzymes and bilirubin, abdominal pain over the liver graft, irritability, and ascites. Percutaneous liver biopsy confirms rejection. This procedure can safely be performed with the patient under local anesthesia with conscious sedation. Before the biopsy, prothrombin and partial thromboplastin time and a type and cross-match for 1 unit of blood should be available. After biopsy, the child should be placed on the right side for 2 to 4 hours in bed. A small infant may be held by the parent. A hemoglobin level should be obtained 4 hours after the procedure. Any decrease should be reported to the transplant team, along with any change in vital signs or irritability. Signs and symptoms of rejection are similar to those of infection but their treatments are different; therefore, careful evaluation and consideration of all differential diagnoses are vital. Bolus doses of corticosteroids used to treat rejection could enhance the process in a child with a viral infection. Initially, rejection is managed with methylprednisolone sodium succinate (Solu-Medrol). If liver enzymes continue to rise, a monoclonal antibody (OKT3) is administered.

Chronic Rejection

Chronic rejection may be the most important cause of graft loss beyond the second year after transplantation (Kerman, 1998). It is defined as progressive loss of bile ducts, along with formation of fibrosis and cirrhosis. This process begins in the first few months after transplantation or it may occur many years later. The cause is still not well understood, but early chronic rejection is associated with several episodes of early acute rejection that lead to tissue damage and scarring (Kerman, 1998). Kerman (1998) reported an increased incidence of chronic rejection in children who experience a first episode of acute rejection within 1 year after transplantation. He proposed that inconsistent immunosuppressive medication levels, secondary to malabsorption or noncompliance or related to chronic viral diseases such as Epstein-Barr virus or cytomegalovirus, contributed to chronic rejection. Bile duct complications that result in strictures are also associated with chronic rejection after liver transplantation.

Hypertension

Hypertension in the immediate postoperative period is related to several factors: stress, pain, and the administration of immunosuppressant agents. Antihypertensive agents are used to control high blood pressure. For many children these episodes are transient and resolve within 3 to 6 months (Purath, 1995). (See Table 31–3 for a list of commonly prescribed antihypertensive medications.)

INTESTINAL TRANSPLANTATION

Early attempts at human intestinal transplantation in the 1960s and 1970s, using immunosuppression agents of prednisone and azathioprine, resulted in survival rates of less than 2.5 weeks. It was not until the introduction of tacrolimus in the early 1990s that centers began to see better results (Kocoshis, 1994). There have been 55 pediatric intestinal transplants performed at the University of Pittsburgh from 1990 to 1997, with a 55% patient and 52% graft survival at 1 year. The University of Miami reported on 20 intestinal transplants: 10 liver/bowel, 3 isolated bowel, and 7 multivisceral, with 12 of 19 (70%) patients alive and 11 of 19 (60%) grafts functioning at 1 year. The experience at the University of Western Ontario from 1993 to 1997 included nine patients, with a patient and graft survival of 78% and 67%, respectively. In this group three received liver/bowel and six received isolated bowel grafts (Atkison et al., 1997).

Although total parenteral nutrition (TPN) has significantly prolonged the lives of children with intestinal failure, it is often complicated by recurrent central venous line infections and sepsis, loss of venous access, and cholestatic liver disease (Bueno et al., 1999). Approximately 70% of pediatric recipients of intestinal transplant procedures require a simultaneous liver transplant because of TPN-induced liver disease (Bueno et al., 1999). Factors associated with higher morbidity included bridging fibrosis, bilirubin >3 mg/dl, platelet count <100,000, prothrombin time >15 seconds, and combined intestinal/liver transplant. Early referral for intestinal transplant should occur before the development of liver dysfunction, taking into consideration the preceding risk factors (Bueno et al., 1999). Exhibit 31–1 reviews the diseases leading to intestinal transplantation and Exhibit 31–2 reviews signs and symptoms of intestinal failure.

Anatomy

The small intestine is a convoluted tube extending from the stomach to the large intestines. It measures approximately 7 m long (23 feet) and 4 cm (1.5 inches) in diameter. The small intestine is the site of digestion and absorption. It is divided into three sections: the first section known as the duodenum measures 25 cm in length and is arranged in the shape of the letter C. The jejunum is two fifths of the intestines and extends from the duodenum to the ileum. There is no structural line of distinction between the jejunum and ileum. The ileum extends from the remainder of the intestine and terminates by joining the large intestines at the ileocecal valve. The villi that line the intestines are fingerlike projections of mucous membrane that enhance absorption of nutrients. The crypts of Lieberkuhn are intestinal glands located in the epithelium of the mucosa that are responsible for enzymes that aid digestion (Warevich & Williams, 1980).

Recipient Selection

Children who are dependent on TPN from a variety of conditions that result in short-bowel syndrome are consid-

Table 31–3 Antihypertensive Medications

Drug	Dose	Side Effects
Captopril (Capoten)	1.5 mg/kg/day (max, 6 mg/kg/day)	Rash, proteinuria
Enalapril (Vasotec)	.15 mg/kg/day (max, .5 mg/kg/day)	Diarrhea, headache
Nifedipine (Procardia)	.25–.5 mg/kg/dose (max, 3 mg/kg/day)	Tachycardia, syncope
Propranolol (Inderal)	.5–1 mg/kg/day (max, 6 mg/kg/day)	Hypoglycemia, heart block
Hydralazine (Apresoline)	.75–3 mg/kg/day (max, 7.5 mg/kg/day)	Tachycardia, flush
Clonidine (Catapress)	.05–1 mg/kg/day	Dry mouth, dizziness

ered for small bowel transplantation. Exclusion criteria are incurable malignancy, severe cardiopulmonary insufficiency, and sepsis (Funovits, Staschak-Chicko, Kovalak, & Altieri, 1993). Whether the child receives a bowel only, liver/bowel, or multivisceral transplant depends on certain criteria. A child with short-bowel syndrome with intestinal failure with no evidence of cirrhosis but who has had problems with sepsis and line access would receive an isolated intestinal graft. A child who is TPN dependent and has evidence of cirrhosis would receive a small bowel/liver graft. Children with severe pseudo-obstruction with minimal evidence of motility in the native bowel would receive a multivisceral transplant (Atkison et al., 1997).

Recipient Evaluation

The preoperative evaluation for intestinal transplantation includes the standard biochemical assessment used for liver transplantation. Additional studies to ascertain the degree of malabsorption include mineral and trace elements, parental nutritional requirements, metabolic assessment D-Xylose tolerance test (carbohydrate absorption), fecal fat analysis (digestion), and nitrogen excretion studies. An endoscopic examination is obtained to document varices. The upper gastrointestinal radiograph, Doppler ultrasonography, and an abdominal CT are used to assess hepatic, mesenteric, and venous vasculature. Magnetic resonance imaging may be performed if there is suspicion of subclavian vein occlusion (Reyes et al., 1998).

Donor Selection

The appropriate donor is ABO compatible, of appropriate weight (no more than 20% greater than recipient), free of infection, and has normal liver function. Donor preparation requires decontamination of the intestinal tract with a combination of GoLYTELY, colistin, gentamicin, and nystatin.

Transplant Operation

The liver is included when there is TPN-induced end-stage liver disease. The intestinal graft is anastomosed on a vascular pedicle of superior mesenteric artery and superior mesenteric vein. The venous return is directed into the superior mesentery, splenic vein, or inferior vena cava or an interposition graft to the portal vein (Figure 31–3A). In children who receive both liver and small bowel grafts, the recipient vena cava is anastomosed and arterialized from the infrarenal aorta by means of conduit homograft (Figure 31–3B). In the liver/small bowel recipients, a permanent native portocaval shunt or a donor portal vein to native portal vein anastomosis is performed. Reconstruction of the gastrointestinal and biliary tracts uses a Roux-en-Y technique, and all chil-

dren have ostomies (ileostomy) and jejunostomy tubes for feedings. The ostomy is reversed when the children consume all their nutrition through the enteral route (Reyes et al., 1998).

Postoperative Phase

Care is similar to the postoperative care of liver transplant recipients with the addition of ostomy output monitoring (Beath, Kelly, & Booth, 1994).

Surgical Complications

Complications after intestinal transplant include stenosis or thrombosis of the arterial and/or vascular systems. There also may be problems with the intestinal anastomoses and bowel perforations in this group of children. Vascular problems can be assessed by observing the color and appearance of the stoma. Immediate surgical intervention prevents further complications.

Medical Complications

Rejection. Signs and symptoms are listed in Exhibit 31–5. Diagnosis is confirmed by biopsy specimens from multiple sites from the small bowel. Endoscopic changes such as ulceration, bleeding, and decreased peristalsis may be seen. Clinical signs of acute rejection include sepsis, high stomal output, abdominal distention, diffuse abdominal pain, absent bowel sounds, and a dusky stoma. Treatment depends on the severity of the rejection. Initially, the patient receives a bolus of steroids, and tacrolimus doses are increased. If the child does not respond to this therapy, OKT3 or ATG is instituted. Protocol biopsy specimens of the intestines are obtained initially biweekly, then weekly for 4 weeks while the child remains in the hospital and then monthly or as indicated. There are no biochemical markers of rejection, although it may be accompanied by increased intestinal permeability. Biopsy is the only definitive method for diagnosis of rejection (Atkison et al., 1997).

Graft vs. Host Disease (GVHD). GVHD may occur with other organ transplants, but bowel transplants have a greater incidence because of the abundance of lymphoid tissue in the intestines. GVHD results from donor T cells reacting against recipient tissue. The assumption is that donor lymphocytes settle in the recipient tissues as dormant cells that may reactivate with suboptimal immunosuppressant therapy (Abu-Elmagd, Fung, & Reyes, 1992). Pretreatment of the graft with irradiation, antilymphoid globulins, and OKT3 has been used to sterilize the donor graft before transplantation but has not successfully prevented GVHD (Funovits et al., 1993).

Infections/Translocation. The child with short-bowel syndrome on parenteral nutrition and who has an isolated

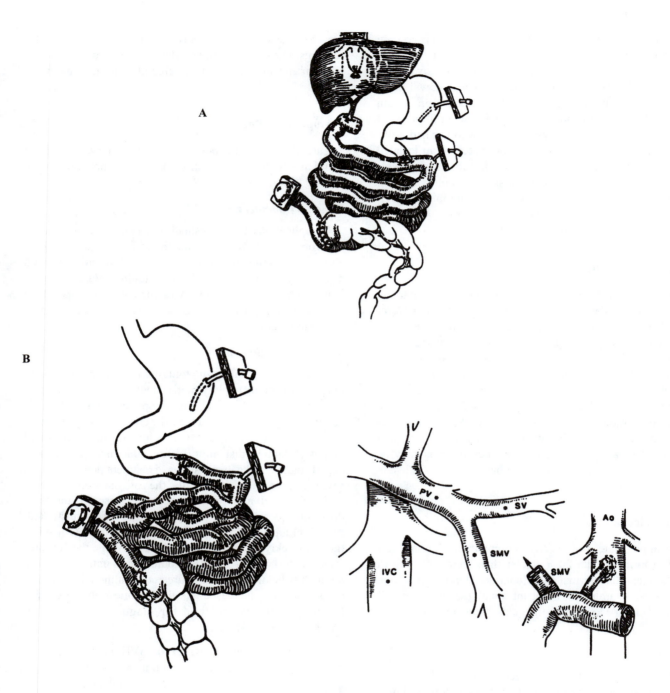

Figure 31–3 Intestinal Transplant Procedure. **A**, Liver small bowel graft. **B**, Isolated intestinal graft with arterial and venous drainage options with a conduit homograft.

bowel or liver/bowel transplantation is at increased risk for opportunistic infections because of multiple surgeries, hospitalizations, and multiple central venous catheters (Funovits et al., 1993). There is an increased incidence of intestinal overgrowth in children requiring treatment with metronida-

zole and other agents to decontaminate the bowel. Surveillance stool cultures are obtained, and particular attention is given if rejection is suspected because bacteria may translocate from the bowel lumen through the damaged mucosa to the blood (Funovits et al., 1993).

Gastrointestinal motility disorders such as reflux, esophagitis, gastric hypomotility, and pyloric spasms are more common in this group of children and usually resolve 4 to 8 weeks postoperatively. Diarrhea of unknown cause is managed with pectin, paregoric, octreotide (Sandostatin), and a low-fat diet. Surveillance stool cultures, endoscopy, and small intestinal biopsy are strongly recommended at frequent intervals to rule out the possibility of graft rejection or enteric infection as a cause of diarrhea (Funovits et al., 1993).

POSTOPERATIVE CARE OF THE PEDIATRIC ABDOMINAL TRANSPLANT RECIPIENT

Bacterial Infection

Pediatric transplant recipients are at risk for bacterial infections. Common sites are intra-abdominal abscess, central lines, Jackson-Pratt drains, and urinary catheters. Children who are immunosuppressed may not respond to bacterial infections with a fever. The combination of immunosuppression leading to infections, ongoing immunosuppression, and treatment with multiple antibiotics can lead to opportunistic infections.

Nursing assessment for signs and symptoms of infection in children with solid organ transplantation includes assessing for incisional redness, or drainage, and rhinorrhea. A fever of 38.5° C should be reported to the transplant team immediately.

Fungal Infection

Immunocompromised children are particularly vulnerable to both common and rare pathogens such as *Candida albicans*, *Aspergillus fumigatus*, and *Pneumocystis carinii* (Weil & Rovelli, 1990) because of prophylactic antibiotics administered concomitantly with immunosuppressant agents in the early postoperative period. Prophylactic antifungal agents such as clotrimazole (Mycelex) lozenges or nystatin swish and swallow are used for 4 to 6 weeks to prevent yeast infections. Amphotericin B is administered to treat systemic yeast infections (0.5 mg/kg/day given over 4 to 6 hours) for 14 to 30 days, depending on source of infection. In older children, fluconazole orally or intravenous can be used (American Academy of Pediatrics, 1997).

Viral Infection

Pediatric transplant recipients are immunologically naive related to their age at transplant. Concomitant administration of immunosuppressant medications increases the risk for primary viral infections with cytomegalovirus (CMV) and Epstein-Barr virus (EBV). Donor and recipient status for CMV should be identified, as determined by the presence of a protective mismatch titer, before transplantation. The least preferred match is a CMV (+) donor organ in a CMV (–) or (+) recipient. Serious problems occur when a CMV (+) donor organ is transplanted into a CMV (–) recipient. CMV-rich gamma globulin should be administered to provide passive immunity, or ganciclovir should be administered to treat early infection. Some centers have used both ganciclovir and acyclovir in differing protocols to reduce the effect of the CMV disease. A CMV (+) donor organ transplanted into a CMV (+) recipient raises the possibility of the recipient becoming infected with a different strain of CMV. CMV can be a pervasive disease, affecting the kidney, but also the liver, lungs, and eyes (Dickens et al., 1991). Regardless of the cause, CMV infection, which presents with fever, decreased WBC count, and gastrointestinal symptoms, requires prompt treatment (Dunn et al., 1991). If a child has an acute viral infection develop, immunosuppressive medications are tapered and the appropriate antiviral agent is begun (acyclovir, ganciclovir).

Epstein-Barr Virus

EBV is a serious complication after transplantation for pediatric recipients if the child is seronegative and receives a seropositive organ. Undiagnosed EBV leads to posttransplant lymphoproliferative disease (PTLD) (a malignancy) and death (Penn, 1998). The incidence of this disease is greatest in children who are less than 5 years of age at the time of transplant. Administration of potent immunosuppressive agents increases the incidence of this disease. Diagnosis is confirmed with biopsy of infected lymph nodes, polymerase chain reaction (PCR) DNA assay, and EBV titers. Treatment depends on the severity. If a child has a positive PCR but is asymptomatic, decreasing immunosuppressive drugs may be the only treatment. If the child is symptomatic with enlarged lymph nodes in the neck, axilla, or other places, is febrile, and has a positive PCR titer, immunosuppression should be discontinued and treatment started with ganciclovir or acyclovir. A CT scan should be obtained to identify any evidence of malignancy or tumors or dissemination to other organs. Early diagnosis of signs and symptoms such as fever, change in graft function, lymphadenopathy, and treatment may prevent mortality in this group of children. Evidence of lymphoma requires treatment with the appropriate chemotherapeutic agents (Martin, 1996).

Herpes Simplex

The herpes simplex virus will reactivate after transplant but is rarely the source of a new infection. Children who have a prior history of herpes may be started on acyclovir after transplantation for 8 to 12 weeks or longer as a prophylaxis. The mouth should be examined routinely to detect whether the infection is present.

Pneumocystis carinii

This opportunistic pathogen may cause fatal infection after transplantation. Prophylaxis with cotrimoxazole (Bactrim) given 5 mg/kg daily three times a week has been effective in preventing *P. carinii* infections (Munoz, 1996).

Varicella

Varicella (chickenpox), a common childhood illness, can be life threatening to an immunocompromised child. The pretransplant evaluation includes varicella titers. Varicella vaccine should be administered to children older than 1 year of age with negative titers. Siblings should receive the vaccine on schedule as per the American Academy of Pediatrics recommendations. Families and school nurses should be advised of children who are seronegative after transplantation and educate them concerning the importance of notifying the transplant team of any exposure. Varicella immune globulin (VZIG) should be administered within 72 hours of exposure to chickenpox. Acyclovir prophylaxis at 80/mg/kg/day for 5 days may also be used in older children. If disease does occur, intravenous or oral acyclovir is warranted. Varicella titers should be monitored 1 month after disease. Protective immunity may not occur as a result of their immunocompromised condition, and these children are at risk for a subsequent exposure. Pediatric transplant patients are also at risk for varicella zoster (shingles) developing. Acyclovir should be administered if the child has shingles develop.

Pain Management

Pain management is an integral part of postoperative care of the transplant patient. Refer to Chapter 6 for specific strategies.

Immune Response

Figure 31–4 highlights the function of the immune system (Tami, Parr, & Thompson, 1986).

Immunosuppressive Medications

Immunosuppressive medications selectively prevent rejection. Double or triple immunotherapy is required initially to prevent humoral or cellular rejection. Perhaps the most challenging and the most dynamic aspect in caring for pediatric transplant recipients remains the selection of maintenance immunosuppression because there are now so many options to choose. The goal of maintenance immunosuppres-

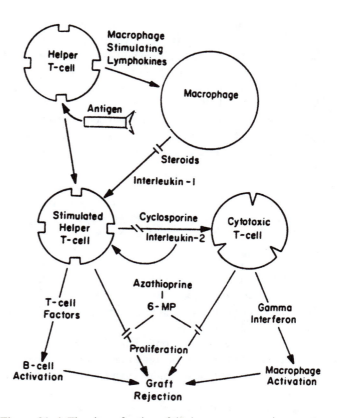

Figure 31–4 The sites of action of the immunosuppressive agents cyclosporine, azathioprine, and the corticosteroids.

sion is to maximize antirejection while minimizing potential side effects (Kahan & Ghobrial, 1994; Sollinger & Pirsch, 1995).

Corticosteroids

Corticosteroids have consistently been included in immunosuppression regimens, although the dose and continuation of steroids has evolved over the years (Hricik, Almawi, & Strom, 1994). Steroids inhibit the expression of T cells and subsequent activation, which is a predominant factor in acute transplant rejection. Steroids also play a role in preventing the immune system's recognition of the allograft antigens.

The side effects of steroids are well known and include body appearance changes (acne, cushingoid effects, obesity) and more serious considerations, including cataracts, hypertension, hyperlipidemia, glucose intolerance, and osteoporosis. Steroids slow or stunt linear growth in children. Prescribing steroids either in low-dose or alternate-day regimens reduces or eliminates the problem (Kaiser et al., 1994).

Elimination of steroids in renal transplant recipients can result in acute rejection. Steroid withdrawal in the pediatric liver transplant has been successful, with centers reporting a low rate of acute rejection (5% to 15%) requiring reinstitution of steroids (Andrews, Skimaoka, Sommerauer, Moore, & Hudgins, 1994; Dunn et al., 1994; Superina et al., 1998).

Cyclosporine

Cyclosporine was introduced in 1983 and marks the "old" versus the modern era of transplantation. Its primary action is inhibition of T-lymphocytes known to cause rejection. Cyclosporine is administered to pediatric kidney and liver recipients but rarely is it used in small bowel transplants.

Side effects of cyclosporine include nephrotoxicity, hirsutism, hypertension, gum hyperplasia, and tremors, all of which may make the child or adolescent particularly resistant to taking this medicine. Hypertension associated with cyclosporine and steroids diminishes over time and is controlled with antihypertensive medications (Exhibit 31–9).

Neoral, a microemulsion formula of cyclosporine, was developed in 1994 (Hoyer, 1994). It provides more stable absorption and longer drug exposure than cyclosporine, allowing for less variation in blood levels. The adverse effects and drug interactions are similar to the standard cyclosporine preparation with a few exceptions, including increased incidences of headaches, hypertension, hypomagnesemia, and

Exhibit 31–9 Drug Interactions with Cyclosporine and Tacrolimus

Drugs that increase absorption	
Verapamil	Reglan
Methylprednisolone	Vancomycin
Ketoconazole	Zithromax
Biaxin	Nicardipine
Cimetidine	Danazol
Erythromycin	Diltiazem
Fluconazole	

Drugs that decrease absorption	
Rifampin	Dilantin
Solu-Medrol	Phenobarbital

Nephrotoxic agents	
Bactrim	Ranitidine
Ketoconazole	Amphotericin
Aminoglycosides	Vasotec

Miscellaneous drugs (risk of ventricular arrhythmias)	
Cisapride	Erythromycin
Fluconazole	Ketoconazole
Miconazole	Itraconazole

renal tubular acidosis (Dunn, Falkenstein, Pierson, & Cooney, 1998). The side effects result from increased drug exposure. Targeting lower trough levels in children who present with symptoms of toxicity may prevent side effects (Hoyer, 1998).

Azathioprine

Azathioprine (Imuran) is a nonselective inhibitor of lymphocyte activity. Major concerns with azathioprine are the reduction of lymphocytes increasing the likelihood of infection and the long-term possibility of malignancies. The side effects include thrombocytopenia, alopecia, and hepatic dysfunction.

Mycophenolate Mofetil

Mycophenolate mofetil (CellCept) selectively inhibits the purine synthesis identified as a pathway that stimulates the immune response leading to rejection. Side effects include diarrhea and gastrointestinal upset, leukopenia, and anemia (Butani, Palmer, Polinsky, & Baluarte, 1997). When the symptoms are severe, the drug is withdrawn.

Tacrolimus

Tacrolimus works within the lymphocyte by preventing the activation of interleukin-2 present in rejection. Tacrolimus is approximately 100 times more potent than cyclosporine. Thus, smaller doses are required for the same effect. Side effects include hyperglycemia, lymphoproliferative disease (especially in children under age 5), nephrotoxicity, hypertension, hyperkalemia, neurotoxicity, and renal tubular acidosis (McDiarmid, 1998).

Monoclonal and Polyclonal Antibodies

OKT3 is a monoclonal antibody derived from mice. This drug blocks all T lymphocyte functions within hours of administration, and it clears T cell infiltrates from graft sites. OKT3 treats steroid-resistant rejection or may also be used as induction therapy, especially in children with renal dysfunction. Before administering OKT3 a chest radiographic film is obtained to evaluate for fluid overload. Premedication with methylprednisolone (Solu-Medrol), diphenhydramine (Benadryl), and acetaminophen (Tylenol) is used to decrease side effects. OKT3 is administered in a daily dose, IV push over 1 to 2 minutes for a course of 7 to 14 days. Dosing ranges from 1 mg to 5 mg, depending on the weight of the child. Side effects include pulmonary edema, fever, muscle aches, headaches, neurologic symptoms, and general flulike illness symptoms (Palmer & Slook, 1992). An increased risk of lymphoproliferative disease and CMV is associated with administration of OKT3.

Antithymocyte globulin (ATG) is a polyclonal antibody, primarily moneric IgG, from hyperimmune serum of horses immunized with human thymic lymphocytes. Its primary use is for induction therapy and treatment of acute rejection. The mechanism of action involves depletion of peripheral T and B lymphocytes. Premedication is administered with methylprednisolone (5 to 10 mg/kg), acetaminophen (10 mg/kg), and diphenhydramine (1 mg/kg) before the first dose (Payne, 1992). This "cocktail" may be needed with subsequent doses. A skin scratch test dose is imperative because of anaphylaxis. Administer 1/100 of the dose over 10 minutes, and wait 20 minutes. If no reaction occurs, give premedication and then infuse over 4 to 6 hours. Adverse reactions include fever, chills, hypotension, serum sickness, pruritus, erythema, infections, thrombocytopenia, and decrease in white blood cell count and platelets.

New Immunosuppressive Agents

Dacliximab (Zenapax), a humanized monoclonal antibody, is used to prevent early rejection. This drug acts by inhibiting interleukin-2–mediated activation of lymphocytes, a critical pathway in the cellular immune response involved in allograft rejection. While in the circulation it impairs the response of the immune system to the antigen (transplanted organ). The current dose recommended is 1 mg/kg/dose every 2 weeks for a total of five doses. It is administered over 15 minutes in 0.9% sodium chloride (Hoffman-La Roche, 1997). Minimal or no side effects are reported in clinical trials. There is a reduction in biopsy-proven rejection when used concomitantly in double and triple therapy protocols. Dacliximab increases the time to first rejection and improves patient survival while offering the safety net of using lower doses of steroids. Side effects include gastrointestinal distress, edema of the upper extremities, and tremors. Dacliximab has a longer half-life than murine antibodies, resulting in saturation of the interleukin-2 receptor for at least 3 months.

Simulect (SDZ CHI 621) is a chimeric (mouse/human) monoclonal antibody that inhibits binding of interleukin-2 receptor. It mediates effective antibody that depends on cellular cytotoxicity against CD25 cell lines. Dosing recommendations are 10 mg in children <40 kg and 20 mg in children >40 kg for two doses over 30 minutes (Novaritis Pharmaceutical, 1997). Provide the first dose within 8 hours of reperfusion of the transplanted organ and the second dose on postoperative day 4. Administer with standard double or triple therapy. Adverse reactions include diarrhea, constipation, gastritis, headache, dizziness, dyspnea, and edema.

LIVING WITH A TRANSPLANT

Postoperative care of the pediatric transplant patient requires a collaborative relationship between the primary care physician and the transplant facility.

Growth

Current strategies to improve growth in the posttransplant patient include low daily steroid dosing, alternate-day steroid dosing, and steroid withdrawal (Falkenstein & Dunn, 1998). In one study, discontinuation of corticosteroids was possible in 86% of children after liver transplantation, resulting in a significant increase in growth velocity and a low rate of acute rejection (Falkenstein & Dunn, 1998). The average follow-up period was 5 years, with no reported incidence of acute rejection. A small group of children became noncompliant with monotherapy immunosuppressant medication, which resulted in a 7% incidence of rejection. Recombinant human growth hormone prescribed in children with renal and liver disease offers a promising addition to the medical treatment of children who experience posttransplant growth delay (Bartosh et al., 1992). Other approaches focus on maximizing nutritional and metabolic contributions to promote growth.

Development

Children with chronic renal or liver disease may experience delays in sexual maturation. Adolescent girls note a delay in menarche, whereas males experience a delay in the development of secondary sex characteristics. Initial delays in menarche are ascribed to the hormonal imbalances caused by steroids (Armenti, Radmonski, & Moritz, 1995).

Diet

A well-balanced diet should be encouraged. Children who are taking steroids are encouraged to consume a diet low in sugar and salt because of fluid retention and hyperglycemia (Pipes & Trahms, 1993).

Immunizations

As a result of illness, well immunizations are often neglected. All children awaiting organ transplant should receive a full set of immunizations before transplantation on a regular or accelerated schedule. This decreases the risk of acquiring these infections after transplantation. Posttransplant, live virus vaccines, such as varicella, oral polio, and the measles, mumps and rubella vaccine, are to be avoided. Siblings should not receive the oral polio vaccine because the virus is shed for 6 weeks after immunization and may cause illness in the immunocompromised child. The IPV (Sabin) is an accepted alternative. Yearly influenza vaccine is recommended to reduce the incidence of influenza (Edvardsson et al., 1996).

Safety

Good hand washing is encouraged for the child and caregivers to decrease risk of infection. The use of sunblock, at least SPF 15, is recommended to prevent sunburn because these children are at increased risk for melanomas. Families should be provided with a Medic Alert application and the importance of a bracelet in the event of an emergency should be discussed. Exercise restrictions should be advised for 6 weeks to allow for healing. Advise that no contact sports should be played for the first year and then check with the transplant center. Encourage the use of bike helmets and car seat belts.

Screening

Children after transplantation require normal childhood hearing and vision screening because immunosuppressant medications and antibiotics make them more vulnerable to vision and hearing problems. Transplant recipients require a biannual vision test for the first year and then annually because of the risk of cataracts and pseudotumor cerebri (Lessell, 1992). An audiogram should be scheduled before discharge, 6 months after transplantation, and then yearly to assess for hearing loss related to administration of ototoxic drugs.

Dental

Good dental habits with daily brushing and flossing and biannual check-ups should be encouraged. Children who receive cyclosporine or nifedipine (Procardia) are at increased risk for developing gingival hyperplasia. Prophylactic antibiotics should be prescribed for any dental procedure, including cleaning, to prevent a *Staphylococcus aureus* infection. The American Heart Association (AHA) guidelines for SBE prophylaxis with amoxicillin or penicillin 1 hour before procedure (50 mg/kg/dose, max 3 gm) should be followed.

Follow-Up Blood Work and Evaluation

Postoperative visits include physical examination and review of systems, including weight, height, and diet. Close follow-up is essential for the first several weeks. Visits are scheduled further apart as the child stabilizes. Monitoring includes a comprehensive panel, hepatic panel (liver and intestinal transplant recipients), complete blood count, magnesium, and drug level monitoring of immunosuppressive agents. Renal transplant children will also have urinalysis and urine cultures and renin levels and a 24-hour urinalysis every 6 months.

Behavioral Issues

Children who undergo transplantation must continue immunosuppressant therapy for the remainder of their lives. Often this becomes a problem as children reach adolescence and try to "fit in" with their peers (Meyers, Thomson, & Weiland, 1996). Recipients suggest two reasons for missing medication: (1) forgetting to take their medicines or return for routine follow-up appointments and (2) avoidance of medication side effects. Several helpful strategies to improve noncompliance include simplifying the medication regimen, using weekly pill boxes to organize medications, or even investing in a watch with an alarm that gives a reminder so that medications are given on time. Appearing different from one's peers can be a devastating experience. It should be recommended that adolescents use acne creams, nutritional counseling, depilatories for unwanted hair, and proper dental care to prevent the side effects of immunosuppressant medications.

In the posttransplant phase when the children feel well, it is often difficult for the immediate and extended family to make the transition from illness to health (Jessop & Stein, 1988). In some of the pretransplant and posttransplant studies, parents have described the child with a transplant as dependent and irritable before the transplant to defiant and aggressive after the transplant (Stewart et al., 1994; Zitelli, Miller, Gartner, & Malatack 1988).

Schooling

Children with a transplant should be encouraged to attend school. Partnerships should be developed with the school nurse and classroom teacher to promote the successful return of the child with a transplant to the classroom setting. Some successful strategies to build self-esteem include encouraging them to see themselves as "normal." They must be encouraged to develop new relationships at school, participate in sports and other extracurricular activities, and dream of a future.

CONCLUSION

The goals of transplantation have changed and improved in the last decade because of innovative surgical techniques and more specific immunosuppressive agents. The support of the multidisciplinary team is essential in the immediate postoperative period and lifetime management of this acquired chronic illness. Often, parents of children who receive an organ transplantation live in constant fear of rejection and death (Hobbs & Sexton, 1995). Families may benefit from participation in support groups or chat lines. Nurses can support families to achieve a balance in normalizing their child's life and the complex management of their care.

REFERENCES

American Academy of Pediatrics. (1997). *Red book: Report of the Committee on Infectious Diseases.* Elk Grove Village, IL: Author.

Abu-Elmagd, K., Fung, J., & Reyes, J. (1992). Management of intestinal transplantation in humans. *Transplant Proceedings, 23*(3), 1992.

Alexander, S.R. (1990). Controversies in pediatric renal transplantation. *AKF Nephrology Letter, 7,* 5–21.

Andrews, W., Skimaoka, S., Sommerauer, J., Moore, P., & Hudgins, P. (1994). Steroid withdrawal after pediatric liver transplantation. *Transplant Proceedings, 26,* 159–160.

Armenti, V., Radmonski, S., & Mortiz, M. (1995). Parenthood after liver transplantation. *Liver Transplantation and Surgery, 1*(5), 84–88.

Atkison, P., Chatzipetrou, M., Tsaroucha, A., Lehmann, R., Tzakis, A., & Grant, D. (1997). Small bowel transplantation in children. *Pediatric Transplantation, 1,* 111–118.

Balistreri, W., Bucuvalas, J., & Ryckman, F. (1995). The effect of immunosuppression on growth and development. *Liver Transplantation and Surgery, 1*(5), 64–73.

Baluarte, H.J., Braas, C., Kaiser, B.A., Polinsky, M.S., Palmer, J., & Dunn, S. (1994). Postoperative management of pediatric transplant patient. In A. Tejani & R. Fine (Eds.), *Pediatric renal transplantation* (pp. 239–255). New York: John Wiley & Sons.

Bartosh, S., Kaiser, B., Rezvani, I., Polinsky, M., Schulman, S., Palmer, J.A., & Baluarte, H.J. (1992). Effects of growth hormone administration in pediatric renal allograft recipients. *Pediatric Nephrology, 6,* 68–73.

Beath, S., Kelly, D., & Booth, I. (1994). Post-operative care of children undergoing small bowel and liver transplantation. *British Journal of Intensive Care, 4,* 302–308.

Bell, J. (1998). Antigens and antibodies—The foreign language of transplantation. *Nephrology News & Issues,* January, 12–13.

Boone, P., Kelly, S., & Smith, C.D. (1992). Liver transplantation: Living related donations. *Critical Care Nursing Clinics of North America, 4,* 243.

Broelsch, C., Edmond, J., & Thistlethwaite, J. (1988). Liver transplantation with reduced size donor organs. *Transplantation, 45,* 519–524.

Bueno, J., Ohwada, S., Kocoshis, S., Mazariegos, G., Dvorchik, I. Sigurdsson, L., DiLorenzo, C., Abu-Elmagd, K., & Reyes, J. (1999). Factors impacting the survival of children with intestinal failure referred for intestinal transplantation. *Journal of Pediatric Surgery, 34*(1), 27–33.

Bunchman, T.E., & So, S.K. (1994). Diagnosis and treatment of postoperative allograft dysfunction. In A. Tejani & R. Fine (Eds.), *Pediatric renal transplantation* (pp. 257–268). New York: John Wiley & Sons.

Butani, L., Palmer, J.A., Polinsky, M., & Baluarte, H.J. (1997). Adverse effects of mycophenolate mofetil in pediatric renal transplant recipients [abstract]. *Journal of the American Society of Nephrology, 8,* 710A–711A.

Casas, A., Falkenstein, K., Gallagher, M., & Dunn, S.P. (1999). Living related transplant for acute liver failure. *Pediatric Transplantation, 3,* 1–4.

Dickens, S., Luks, L., Braandt, M., Khazal, P., Weber, A., et al. (1991). Infectious complications of pediatric liver transplantation. *Transplantation, 57,* 544–47.

Dunn, S., Falkenstein, K., Lawrence, J., Meyers, R., Vinocur, C.D., Billmire, D.F., & Weintraub, W.H. (1994). Monotherapy with cyclosporin for chronic immunosuppression in pediatric liver transplant. *Transplantation, 57,* 512–515.

Dunn, S., Mayoral, J., Gilligham, K., Loeffler, C., Brayman, K., & Kramer, M. (1991). Treatment of invasive cytomegalovirus disease in solid organ transplant patients with ganciclovir. *Transplantation, 51*(1), 98–106.

Dunn, S.P., Falkenstein, K., Pierson, A., & Cooney, G. (1998). Results of conversion from and immune to Neoral in stable pediatric liver transplant recipients after two years. *Transplant Proceedings, 30*(5), 1962–1963.

Edvardsson, V.O., Flynn, J.T., Deforest, A., Kaiser, B.A., Schulman, S.L., Bradley, A., Palmer, J., Polinsky, M.S., & Baluarte, H.J. (1996). Effective immunization against influenza in pediatric renal transplant recipients. *Clinical Transplantation, 10,* 556–560.

Falkenstein, K. (1993). Liver transplantation: Nursing care of pediatric recipients. *Med-Surg Nursing Quarterly 1*(30), 51–86.

Falkenstein, K., & Dunn, S. (1998). Growth acceleration on cyclosporine monotherapy after transplantation in children. *Transplantation Proceedings, 30*(5), 1969–1972.

Funovits, M., Staschak-Chicko, S., Kovalak, J., & Altieri, K. (1993). Transplantation of the small intestines. In M.T. Nolan & S.M. Augustine (Eds.), *Transplantation nursing* (pp. 319–345). Norwalk, CT: Appleton & Lange.

Goh, D., & Meyers, N. (1994). Portal hypertension in children. *Journal of Pediatric Surgery, 29*(5), 688–691.

Grant, D. (1996). Current results of intestinal transplantation. *Lancet, 347,* 1801–1803.

Harmon, W.E., Stablein, D., Alexander, S.R., & Tejani, A. (1991). Graft thrombosis in pediatric renal transplant recipients. *Transplantation, 51,* 406–412.

Hayashi, M., Cao, S., Concepcion, W., Monge, H., Ojogoho, O., So, S., & Esquivel, C.O. (1998). Current status of living related liver transplant. *Pediatric Transplanation, 2,* 16–25.

Hobbs, S., & Sexton, S. (1995). Cognitive development and learning in the pediatric organ transplant recipient. *Journal of Learning Disabilities, 26*(2), 28–32.

Hoffman-La Roche. (1997). Zenapax package insert. Nutley, NJ.

Hoyer, P. (1994). Cyclosporin A (Neoral) in pediatric organ transplantation. *Pediatric Transplantation, 2,* 25–39.

Hricik, D.E., Almawi, W.Y., & Strom, T.B. (1994). Trends in the use of glucocorticoids in renal transplantation. *Transplantation, 57*(7), 979–989.

Ingelfinger, J.A., & Brewer, E.D. (1992). Pediatric post transplant hypertension: A review of current standards of care. *Child Nephrology and Urology, 12,* 139–146.

Jessop, J.D., & Stein, R. (1988). Essential concepts in the care of children with chronic illness. *Pediatrics, 15,* 5–12.

Jones, J.W., Matas, A.J., & Najarian, J.S. (1994). Surgical technique. In A. Tejani & R. Fine (Eds.), *Pediatric renal transplantation* (pp. 187–200). New York: John Wiley & Sons.

Kahan, B.D., & Ghobrial, R. (1994). Immunosuppressive agents. *Surgical Clinics of North America, 74*(5), 1029–1053.

Kaiser, B.A., Polinsky, M.S., Palmer, J.A., Dunn, S., Mochon, M., & Flynn, J.T. (1994). Growth after conversion to alternate-day corticosteroids in children with renal transplants: A single-center study. *Pediatric Nephrology, 8,* 320–325.

Kaufman, S., Murray, N., Wood., P., Shaw, B., & Vanderhoof, J. (1987). Nutritional support for the infant with extrahepatic biliary atresia. *The Journal of Pediatrics,* May 679–685.

Keown, P.A., & Stiller, C.R. (1986). Kidney transplantation. *Surgical Clinics of North America, 66,* 517–539.

Kerman, R.H. (1998). Can we predict chronic rejection? *Graft Pediatric Transplantation,* 66–68.

Kirkman, R.L., & Tilney, N.L. (1989). Surgical complications in the transplant recipient. In E. Milford, B. Brenner, & J. Stein (Eds.), *Renal transplantation* (pp. 231–245). New York: Churchill Livingstone.

Kocoshis, S. (1994). Small bowel transplantation in infants and children. *Gastroenterology Clinics of North America, 23*(4), 727–742.

Kohaut, E.C., & Tejani, A. (1996). The 1994 annual report of the North American Pediatric Renal Transplant Cooperative Study. *Pediatric Nephrology, 10,* 422–434.

Lake K.D., & Kilkenny, J.M. (1992). The pharmacokinetics and pharmacodynamics of immunosuppressive agents. *Critical Care Nursing Clinics of North America, 4*(2), 205–219.

Lessell, S. (1992). Pediatric pseudo tumor cerebri (idiopathic intracranial hypertension). *Survey of Ophthalmology, 37*(3), 155–166.

Loertscher, R., Parfrey, P.S., & Guttmann, R.D. (1989). Postoperative management of the renal transplant recipient and long term complications. In E. Milford, B. Brenner, & J. Stein (Eds.), *Renal transplantation* (pp. 197–230). New York: Churchill Livingstone.

Martin S. (1996). Assessing and caring for the infant liver transplant recipient. *Critical Care Nursing, 16*(3), 734–743.

Mauer, S.M., Nevins, T.E., & Ascher, N. (1992). Renal transplantation in children. In C. Edelman (Ed.), *Pediatric kidney disease* (pp. 941–981). Boston: Little, Brown and Company.

McDiarmid, S. (1998). The use of tacrolimus in pediatric liver transplantation. *Journal of Pediatrics Gastroenterology and Nutrition, 26,* 90–102.

McNamara, E., Pike, N., Gettys, C., & Richert, B. (1996). Organ transplants. In J. Vessey & P. Jackson (Eds.), *Primary care of the child with a chronic condition* (pp. 598–622). Saint Louis, MO: Mosby.

Meyers, K.E.C., Thomson, P.D., & Weiland, H. (1996). Noncompliance in children and adolescents after renal transplantation. *Transplantation, 62*(2), 186–189.

Moukarzel, A., Najm, I., Vargas, J., McDiarmid, S., Busuttil, R., & Ament, M. (1990). Effect of nutritional status on outcome of orthotopic liver transplantation in pediatric patients. *Transplantation Proceedings, 22*(40), 1560–1563.

Munoz, S. (1996). Long-term management of the liver transplant recipient. *Medical Clinics of North America, 80*(5), 1103–1119.

Novaritis Pharmaceutical. (1997). Simulect clinical trial review. New Jersey.

Oldham, K., Colombani, P., & Foglia, R. (1997). *Surgery of infants and children.* Philadelphia: Lippincott-Raven Publishers.

Palmer, J.A., & Slook, P. (1992). Successful use of Orthoclone OKT3 for steroid-resistant acute rejection in pediatric renal allograft recipients. *American Nephrology Nurses Association Journal, 19*(4), 375–367.

Paul, L.C. (1995). Chronic renal transplant loss. *Kidney International, 47,* 1491–1499.

Payne, J.L. (1992). Immune modification and complications of immunosuppression. *Critical Care Nursing Clinics of North America, 4*(1), 43–58.

Penn, I. (1998). De novo malignancies in pediatric organ transplant recipients. *Pediatric Transplantation 2,* 56–63.

Pipes, P., & Trahms, C. (1993). *Nutrition in infancy and childhood.* St. Louis, MO: Mosby.

Purath, J. (1995). Pediatric hypertension: Assessment and management. *Pediatric Nursing, 21*(2), 173–177, 202.

Reyes, J., Bueno, J., Kocoshis, S., Green, M., Abu-Elmagd, K., Fuukawa, H., Barksdale, E.M., Strom, S., Fung, J.J., Todo, S., Irish, W., & Starzl, T.E. (1998). Current status of intestinal transplantation in children. *Journal of Pediatric Surgery, 33*(2), 243–251.

Rubin, R.H. (1988). Infection in the renal and liver transplant patient. In R. Rubin & L. Young (Eds.), *Clinical approach to infection in the compromised host* (pp. 557–621). New York: Plenum Publishing.

Salvatierra, O. (1994). Urologic complications in renal transplantation. In A. Tejani & R. Fine (Eds.), *Pediatric renal transplantation* (pp. 337–348). New York: John Wiley & Sons.

Salvatierra, O., Tanney, D., Mak, R., Alfrey, E., Lemley, K., & Mackie, V. (1997). Pediatric renal transplantation and its challenges. *Transplantation Reviews, 11,* 51–69.

Shapiro, R., & Simmons, R.L. (1991). Kidney transplantation. In L. Makowka (Ed.), *Handbook of transplantation management* (pp. 168–191). Austin, TX: R.G. Landes Company.

Sollinger, H., & Pirsch, J. (1995). *Transplantation drug pocket reference guide.* Georgetown, TX: Landis Company.

Starzl, T., Rutman, C., & Corman, J. (1987). Transplantation of the liver. In E. Schiff (Ed.), *Diseases of the liver* (6th ed.). Philadelphia: Lippincott-Raven Publishers.

Starzl, T., Swatsuki, S., & Van Thiel, T. (1982). Evaluation transplantation. *Hepatology, 2*(5), 261–265.

Stevens, L.H., Emond, J.C., Piper, J.B., Heffron, T.G., Thistlewait, J.R., Whitinton, P.F., & Broelsch, C.E. (1992). Hepatic artery thrombosis in infants. *Transplantation, 53,* 396–399.

Stewart, S., Kennard, B., Waller, D., & Fixler, D. (1994). Cognitive function in children who receive organ transplantation. *Health Psychology 13*(1), 3–13.

Stewart, S., Uauy, R., Waller, D., Kennard, B., Benser, M., & Andrews, W. (1989). Mental and motor development, social competence, and growth one year after successful pediatric liver transplantation. *The Journal of Pediatrics,* April, 574–581.

Superina, R., Zangari, A., Acal, L., DeLuca, E., Zaki, A., & Kimmel, S. (1998). Growth in children following liver transplantation. *Pediatric Transplantation, 2,* 70–75.

Suthanthiran, M., & Strom, T.B. (1994). Renal transplantation. *The New England Journal of Medicine, 331,* 365–376.

Tami, J., Parr, M., & Thompson, J. (1986). The immune system. *American Journal of Hospital Pharmacy, 43,* 2483–2493.

Tejani, A., Cortes, L., & Stablein, D.H. (1996). Clinical correlates of chronic rejection in pediatric renal transplantation: A report of the North American Renal Transplant Cooperative. *Transplantation, 61(7),* 1054–1058.

Tilney, N.L., Rocha, A., Strom, T.B., & Kirkman, R.L. (1984). Renal artery stenosis in transplant patients. *Annals of Surgery, 199,* 454–460.

UNOS Annual Report. (1998). *The U.S. scientific registry of transplant recipients and the organ procurement and transplantation network, transplant data 1988–1994.* (International standard book number 1–886651–13–2). Richmond, VA: United Network for Organ Sharing Printing Office.

Warady, B.A., Herbert, D., Sullivan, E.K., Alexander, S.R., & Tejani, A. (1997). Renal transplantation, chronic dialysis, and chronic renal insufficiency in children and adolescents. The 1995 annual report of the North American Pediatric Renal Transplant Cooperative Study. *Pediatric Nephrology, 11,* 49–64.

Warevich, R., & Williams, P. (1980). *Gray's anatomy.* Philadelphia: W.B Saunders Company.

Weil, M., & Rovelli, M. (1990). Infectious disease and transplantation. In K.M. Sigardson-Poor & L.M. Haggerty (Eds.), *Nursing care of the transplant recipient* (pp. 89–113). Philadelphia: W.B. Saunders Company.

Weir, M.R. (1990). Calcium channel blockers in organ transplantation: Important new therapeutic modalities. *Journal of American Society of Nephrology, 1,* 528–538.

Zaontz, M.R., Hatch, D.A., & Firlit, C.F. (1988). Urologic complications in pediatric renal transplantation: Management and prevention. *Journal of Urology, 140,* 1123–1128.

Zitelli, B., Miller, J., Gartner, S., & Malatack, J. (1988). Changes in life style after transplantation. *Pediatrics, 82,* 173–178.

CHAPTER 32

Nursing Care of the Cardiothoracic Transplant Patient

Jeanette M. Teets

INTRODUCTION

The areas of heart, lung, and heart-lung transplantation in the pediatric age group have made tremendous strides over the last decade. Cardiothoracic transplants are now seen as viable options for infants and children with end-stage heart and lung disease. With the use of successful immunosuppressive medications, long-term survival has dramatically improved. However, coronary artery disease and obliterative bronchiolitis continue to pose long-term complications for the cardiothoracic transplant recipient.

This chapter reviews heart, lung, and heart-lung transplants; the donor; surgical procedure; postoperative care; rejection; infection; and immunosuppression. Children are not little adults; they have special needs that need to be addressed appropriately to contribute to the success of their transplant. Topics addressed that impact the pediatric patient are immunizations, compliance, dietary issues, use of over-the-counter medications, and returning to school.

HEART TRANSPLANTATION

Pediatric cardiac transplantation is considered an acceptable option for the treatment of end-stage cardiac disease. The first reported experience with pediatric heart transplantation occurred in 1967 by Dr. Kantrowitz and associates in a 2-week-old infant with tricuspid atresia who lived for a few hours (Moodie & Stillwell, 1993). However, the first successful cardiac transplant in a pediatric patient was not performed until 1985 at Loma Linda University by Dr. Leonard Baily in an infant with hypoplastic left heart syndrome (Spray, 1995). Since the advent of cyclosporine in the mid-1980s, tremendous strides have been made in the area of immunosuppression, increasing long-term survival.

The registry of the International Society for Heart and Lung Transplantation (ISHLT) reports that the number of pediatric cardiac transplants has plateaued in the youngest populations (0 to 5 years), and the actual number of transplant procedures appears to be decreasing despite the use of expanded donor pools (Hosenpud, Bennett, Keck, Fiol, & Novick, 1997). An ever-increasing number of pediatric patients are being identified as potential cardiac transplant candidates, but the number of donors is not keeping pace with the need. This situation brings about increased waiting times on the transplant list and an increased number of deaths occurring as patients wait in intensive care units without receiving lifesaving heart transplants.

The indications for heart transplantation are congenital heart disease, cardiomyopathy, and retransplantation. The 1-year actuarial survival rate after cardiac transplantation is approximately 80% and the 5-year survival rate is approximately 63% (Hosenpud et al., 1997). Individual centers may report slightly higher percentages. Further, factors like patient selection criteria and number of transplants performed yearly have an impact on individual institution's statistics.

When a child is referred to the transplant center for an evaluation, he or she undergoes several tests and evaluations before being placed on the waiting list. The purpose of the pretransplant evaluation is to determine whether transplantation is the only option for the child and whether the child is a transplant candidate. The medical team examines the potential recipient and explains to the family what further studies are needed. Some of the studies that may be completed are a cardiac catheterization with possible drug study, echocardiogram, electrocardiogram (ECG), chest radiograph, and an exercise stress test. Neurologic evaluations are performed if central nervous system (CNS) disorders are suspected. All potential transplant candidates undergo serologic testing, which includes testing for hepatitis A, B, and C; human immunodeficiency virus (HIV); herpes simplex virus; measles, mumps, rubella; varicella zoster virus; toxoplasmosis; Epstein-Barr virus (EBV); and cytomegalovirus (CMV). Complete blood counts (CBC), liver functions tests (LFTs), thyroid function tests (TFTs), electrolytes, blood urea nitrogen (BUN), and creatinine are also evaluated. If active disease or organ dysfunction is detected through these tests, further studies may need to be completed or the patient is determined not to be a transplant candidate. The patient and family are also seen by a transplant social worker, financial counselor, and psychiatrist. Absolute contraindications to heart transplantation include major CNS abnormalities, uncontrolled infections, active malignancies, and irreversible failure of other organ systems (Gundry, 1997).

Once the child and family have completed the evaluation and it has been determined that no other options are available, the child is placed on the transplant waiting list. The child is listed according to blood type and weight. As a guideline for most children, they are listed 10% below and 30% above their weight. They are initially listed with the local organ procurement organization (OPO) and then they are placed on the national waiting list with the United Network of Organ Sharing (UNOS). According to data compiled by UNOS (1999) regarding the number of patient registrations on the national transplant waiting list as of December 31, 1997, 189 children are awaiting heart transplant in the age group under 1 year, 87 in the 1- to 5-year age group, 71 in the 6- to 11-year age group, and 72 in the 11- to 17-year age group. Heart transplants have at present two listing statuses: status 1 and status 2. Through a UNOS-directed mandate to transplant the sickest patients first, status 1 is further delineated into 1A and 1B. This is certainly a very difficult task. Therefore, criteria were outlined for each of the statuses to facilitate the set forth endeavors of identifying the sickest of recipients and providing them with a lifesaving organ. The criteria for children are different from that for the adult population, and they are also different for people with congenital heart disease. At least one of the following criteria must be met for a child to be listed as 1A: (1) requires the assistance of a mechanical assist device; (2) less than 6 months of age with congenital or acquired heart disease with pulmonary hypertension; (3) requires high-dose or multiple inotropes; and (4) life expectancy is less than 14 days without a heart transplant. These patients obviously are hospitalized in an intensive care unit while awaiting their transplant. A status of 1B meets at least one of the following criteria: (1) requires low-dose single inotrope; (2) less than 6 months of age but does not meet 1A criteria; and (3) growth failure. It is important to mention that the local region OPO has the ability to make exceptions to the status 1 criteria. Status 2 patients are those patients who do not meet status 1A and 1B criteria. These patients are typically able to wait at home.

The Donor

A pediatric heart donor is referred to the local organ procurement organization when the diagnosis of brain death is imminent. Once brain death is declared, the family is contacted for their consent regarding organ donation. The donor heart is then evaluated by echocardiogram and ECG. The heart needs to be of normal anatomic structure and the shortening fraction needs to be within the normally accepted parameters on minimum inotropic support. Maintenance of adequate intravascular volume is essential in preserving cardiac performance in brain-dead cardiac donors. Blood typing needs to be completed to match donor and recipient ABO type. The serologic status is also evaluated with particular attention to HIV and hepatitis. To be an acceptable cardiac donor active infectious and malignant issues must be absent.

Cardiac arrest in the donor before the declaration of brain death does not preclude donation. If the donor is quickly resuscitated, inotropic support can be minimized, and the cardiac function is determined to be acceptable, organ donation can take place successfully.

Donor and recipient are matched on the basis of blood ABO compatibility and recipient weight range. Once a donor and recipient have been matched and the organ accepted, the donor is managed until the heart can be harvested at the donor hospital. Oftentimes, multiple organs are being harvested from one donor. The orchestration of the organ placement and the arrival times of the procurement teams take a few hours to arrange. During this organ placement time, the donor requires constant surveillance to preserve organ function until the actual surgery takes place.

Surgical Procedure

Once an acceptable donor has been identified and accepted, the child is taken to the operating room. Under general anesthesia the patient is prepped and draped. A median sternotomy incision is performed. The patient is placed on cardiopulmonary bypass (CPB) and cooled to a nasopharyngeal temperature of 18° C. Circulatory arrest is established. The recipient's cardiectomy is performed, whereby the heart is removed. The donor heart is prepared and sewn in with suture sites at the aorta, pulmonary artery, and the right and left atrium. This procedure is called orthotopic heart transplantation. Refer to Figure 32–1 for anastomotic sites after orthotopic heart transplant.

Intracardiac lines are placed for pressure-monitoring purposes and for vascular access. Temporary ventricular pacemaker wires are inserted epicardially at the completion of the transplant surgery. It is not uncommon to need pacing in the initial postoperative phase because of denervation and possible sinus node or atrioventricular node dysfunction. The sternum is reapproximated with stainless steel wires and the incision repaired in layers.

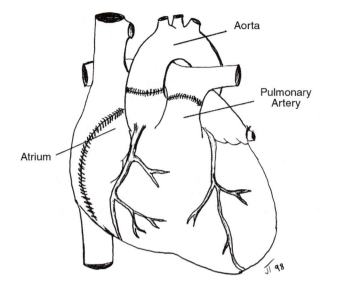

Figure 32–1 Anastomotic Sites at the Aorta, Pulmonary Artery, and Atrium after Orthotopic Heart Transplantation

Total ischemic time is the amount of time that the heart remains unperfused. It is calculated from the time that the aortic cross-clamp is placed during organ retrieval until the cross-clamp is removed at the completion of the recipient's transplant surgery. Ideally, ischemic times less than 4 hours promote the best results in the postoperative phase. However, several centers have extended their cold ischemic times to 6 and 8 hours with good results (Gundry, 1997). Ischemic times become a vital issue in light of the increased demand for lifesaving organs because transporting an organ a great distance is not possible.

Postoperative Care

The nursing care of children who have undergone an orthotopic heart transplant is not much different from the routine care that is provided to the postoperative open-heart surgery patient. The postoperative nursing care takes place in reverse-flow isolation rooms. Strict attention to good handwashing techniques by all caregivers and visitors needs reinforcement. Hemodynamic monitoring of the patient is achieved through the monitoring of intracardiac pressures, arterial blood pressure, and volume intake and output. Most of these patients receive low-dose dopamine infusion (2 to 3 mcg/kg/min) to promote renal perfusion and diuresis (Gundry, 1997). A continuous infusion of isoproterenol is used for chronotropic effects because cardiac output is largely heart rate dependent in the immediate postoperative phase and to reduce pulmonary vascular resistance.

Once hemodynamic stability is established, the patient is weaned from the ventilator. The inspired oxygen content is weaned as quickly as possible to maintain an arterial oxygen level (PaO_2) around 80 mm Hg or an arterial oxygen saturation of 90% or greater measured by means of a pulse oximeter or arterial blood gas analysis (Kshettry & Bolman, 1995). Patients are suctioned using clean technique on an as-needed basis. The overall goal is to wean patients as early as possible and liberate them from the ventilator as quickly as possible.

Invasive lines and temporary pacemaker wires are maintained according to standard hospital protocol, maintaining sterile techniques for blood drawings and dressing changes. The mediastinal chest tube is connected to a closed sterile chest tube drainage system maintained at –20 cm H_2O suction. The Foley catheter is removed as early as possible to prevent urinary tract infections. The mediastinal incision dressing is removed after 24 to 48 hours, and the incision is monitored for signs of infection.

Immunosuppressant therapy is started as soon as the patient is brought back from the operating room. The standard is a triple-drug regimen, such as intravenous cyclosporine, prednisone, and azathioprine (Imuran). Further details on dosages, levels, and weaning of the medications are discussed later in the chapter.

The potential postoperative complications that need to be monitored for are hemorrhage, decrease in cardiac output, and arrhythmias. Any complication needs to be identified quickly and managed appropriately to preserve the function of the new cardiac allograft.

Although the nurse is busy in the initial postoperative period with various tasks, he or she must keep the parents of the child well informed. Parents should be encouraged to visit soon after admission and frequently to the intensive care unit. Parents should also be encouraged to participate as much as possible in the care of their child.

Rejection

Rejection is the body's immunologic response that occurs when the body recognizes the transplant organ as foreign. Three types of rejection have been confirmed clinically and in the laboratory. They are hyperacute, acute, and chronic rejection. Hyperacute rejection, although rare, occurs immediately after the implantation of the new heart. It is the immune system's response to preformed antibodies. This form of rejection is rare yet life threatening. Hyperacute rejection is treated with retransplantation. In an attempt to avoid this situation, human leukocyte antigen (HLA) testing is performed to determine preformed antibodies, allowing prospective HLA matching for those recipients who are sensitized (Kichuk, Itescu, Michler, & Addonizio, 1997).

Acute rejection can occur at any time throughout a transplant recipient's life. However, the time that the recipient is most at risk is during the first 3 months after transplantation (Gundry, 1997). These first few months represent the time when immunosuppression is being adjusted to maintain adequate levels while preserving the function of other organ systems like the kidneys. Clinical signs of acute graft rejection include arrhythmias, an unexplained persistent high resting heart rate, increased central venous pressure (CVP), decreased cardiac output (CO), decreased ventricular compliance, presence of a third heart sound, tachypnea, diaphoresis, cool/cold extremities, and hepatosplenomegaly. Rejection should be considered as one of many possible causes of fever. Children may also exhibit signs of irritability, malaise, and changes in sleeping and feeding patterns.

The "gold standard" for diagnosing cardiac rejection is through an endomyocardial biopsy. This is an invasive procedure in which a bioptome, which is a specially designed catheter with biopsy forceps on the end, is advanced through the tricuspid valve into the apex of the right ventricle and samples of endocardium are obtained. Refer to Figure 32–2 for the jugular approach with a bioptome for endomyocardial biopsy. Microscopic examination of the specimen makes the diagnosis of rejection. No universally accepted guidelines exist for performing surveillance endomyocardial biopsies. However, most patients undergo their first biopsy within a week or two of their transplant. Then the surveillance biopsies are typically performed at 3-month intervals for the first

year and yearly thereafter. If the patient exhibits any clinical signs of rejection, there is a low threshold for performing biopsies.

In a prospective study Neuberger et al. (1997) compared the efficacy of echocardiography in diagnosing rejection in cardiac transplant recipients with endomyocardial biopsy. They found echocardiography was not as sensitive in detecting myocardial rejection (changes in left ventricular function or CVP).

After the diagnosis of rejection is made, 10 mg/kg of methylprednisolone is administered intravenously daily for a total of 3 days. The patient's regular daily dose of steroids is then adjusted accordingly. Follow-up endomyocardial biopsies are obtained within 1 to 2 weeks after treatment to ensure that the rejection is resolved.

Chronic rejection or accelerated graft atherosclerosis is a serious problem that confronts patients who have undergone a cardiac transplant. The exact cause is unknown. However, possible causes may include an antibody-mediated immune response, chronic steroid use, chronic CMV infection, and hypercholesteremia (Gundry, 1997). Typically, these lesions are diffuse in nature and the conventional methods of treating coronary artery disease (CAD) are not applicable. The ultimate treatment of posttransplant CAD is retransplantation.

LUNG TRANSPLANTATION

Pediatric lung transplantation has become an acceptable therapeutic option for children since the late 1980s. However, the number of lung transplants being performed each year by individual centers remains relatively small. The total number of pediatric lung transplants has only seen a slight increase over the years. Refer to Table 32–1 for the number of pediatric lung transplants performed from 1993 to 1997. According to the 1997 ISHLT report (Boucek et al., 1997), the leading diagnoses of children from newborn until 11 years of age who required lung transplantation included congenital alpha$_1$-antitrypsin deficiency, idiopathic pulmonary fibrosis, primary pulmonary hypertension, chronic obstructive pulmonary disease, cystic fibrosis, and retransplantation. However, cystic fibrosis was the leading diagnosis that brought 63% of the children in the 11- to 17-year age group to lung transplantation. Kurland (1996) notes that approximately 10% of pediatric lung transplant recipients also have congenital heart disease with Eisenmenger's physiology that requires surgical correction of their congenital heart disease at the time of their lung transplant surgery. Eisenmenger's syndrome exists when there is a reversal of blood flow from a left-to-right shunt to a right-to-left shunt through a pre-existing cardiac defect, such as a ventricular septal defect. The right-to-left shunting occurs as a result of elevated pulmo-

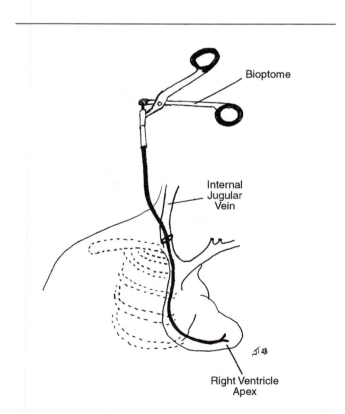

Figure 32–2 Jugular Approach with Bioptome

Table 32–1 Lung Transplant Recipients from 1993 to 1997. (UNOS, 1998)

Year	Under 1 Year of Age	1–5 Years of Age	6–10 Years of Age	11–17 Years of Age
1993	2	5	7	22
1994	5	3	6	17
1995	9	8	7	41
1996	7	3	7	32
1997	6	7	13	34

nary vascular resistance. As the right-to-left shunting increases, children exhibit cyanosis.

Patients who are referred for lung transplantation have either end-stage lung disease or pulmonary vascular disease (Shumway & Bolman, 1997). Once a child has been referred for a lung transplant, a thorough evaluation is completed. The transplant candidate needs to be evaluated by a pediatric pulmonologist who may request pulmonary function testing, a ventilation and perfusion scan, and a computed tomography (CT) scan of the thoracic cavity. Children with the diagnosis of cystic fibrosis may need an evaluation of their sinuses. Their cardiac function should also be evaluated by a pediatric cardiologist to rule out any anatomic issues such as a patent foramen ovale that will need to be repaired at the time of the lung transplant surgery along with evaluation of right ventricular pressure and function (Shumway & Bolman, 1997). A social work evaluation along with an assessment by a psychiatrist/psychologist is completed. If necessary, financial counseling should be offered to the patient and family during the evaluation process. Blood work is completed to assess blood type, serologic status especially for HIV, hepatitis, CMV, and EBV; LFTs; TFTs; CBC; electrolytes; BUN; and creatinine. During the pretransplant evaluation, if active infectious issues or organ dysfunction is detected, further studies may be necessary or the patient may be determined not to be a transplant candidate.

After the evaluation is completed and the transplant team decides that the best option for the patient is to receive a lung transplant, he or she is placed on the local OPO waiting list and listed with UNOS. Patients are listed according to their height and blood type. There are not statuses for lung transplant patients at present. Children receive their lung transplant on the basis of time accrued on the waiting list with reference to the appropriate height and blood type. At present, there is no acuity differentiation for children awaiting lung transplantation. Spray and Huddleston (1993) report that although it was initially thought that because of their smaller size children would wait shorter periods of time for their transplants, this has not held true. Average waiting times are 6 months to 1 year. A relatively high mortality is

associated with the wait. Again, this is probably attributable to the small number of pediatric lung donors.

During the waiting period, nutrition needs to be optimized to prevent muscle wasting and to promote wound healing in the postoperative period. Physical and occupational therapy programs are individualized to each patient to improve endurance, promote strength, and optimize oxygenation through exercise and positioning.

An ethical issue is associated with using living related donors to perform lobar transplants in children who are critically ill or have acute lung disease. The issue is the risk or presumed risk associated with removing a single lobe of lung from an otherwise healthy adult and transplanting the lobe into a critically ill recipient. Most often these types of transplants are performed on children who have been listed for a cadaveric transplant but they are deteriorating quickly and need a transplant to have any hope of survival. Many advantages and disadvantages surround this topic and far outreach the scope of this chapter. However, the one aspect of particular concern regarding living related adult lobar transplantation in a pediatric patient is the questionable pulmonary growth potential. Growth occurs if immature lungs are transplanted into pediatric recipients (Spray & Huddleston, 1993). Pulmonary growth continues until about the age of 8. However, when lobes from an adult donor are transplanted into a pediatric donor, their growth potential is essentially complete. The lobe will expand to a certain point to occupy the small chest cavity, but long-term issues regarding pulmonary function as the child grows are not well delineated.

The Donor

Potential lung donors are identified and matched according to blood type and height. Serologic testing is performed with particular attention to HIV and hepatitis. The donor needs to be free from active infectious and malignant problems. A suitable lung donor should not have a history of lung disease and should have normal lung compliance. All donors are evaluated by chest radiograph, sputum culture and Gram's stain, oxygen challenge testing, and a bronchoscopy.

The chest radiograph should be clear of any evidence of disease. Any Gram's stain that reveals fungus or heavy growth of gram-negative bacteria precludes lung donation (Franco, 1997). During the oxygen challenge test, the donor is placed on 100% inspired oxygen and an arterial blood gas analysis is obtained. A PaO_2 of greater than 300 is an acceptable value for organ donation. A bronchoscopy is performed to evaluate the endobronchial anatomy, to evaluate for gross contamination and possible foreign bodies in the endobronchial tree, and to obtain specimens for sputum cultures and Gram's stain (Franco, 1997).

Surgical Procedure

After donor lungs have been accepted, the recipient is taken to the operating room. Under general anesthesia the patient is prepped and draped in the usual fashion for open-heart surgery. Because of the small size of the child, the use of a double-lumen endotracheal tube is not always feasible. Therefore, cardiopulmonary bypass (CPB) is used. A bilateral transverse thoracosternotomy incision is made in the fourth intercostal spaces, transecting the sternum in the midline (Franco, 1997). Refer to Figure 32–3 for a diagram of the bilateral transverse thoracosternotomy incision. This type of incision is also known as a "clam shell" incision, which allows for better exposure of both lung cavities and access to the heart. The patient is then placed on CPB and the

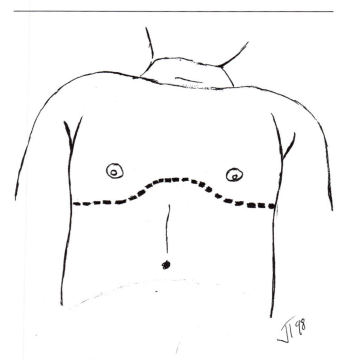

Figure 32–3 Bilateral Transverse Incision Made in the Fourth Intercostal Spaces and Crossing the Sternum Transversely in the Midline

lungs are removed. The new lungs are implanted sequentially with suture lines at the right and left bronchus, pulmonary arterial, and pulmonary venous anastomosis. The bronchial anastomosis is performed with an end-to-end anastomotic technique. This anastomosis is accomplished by suturing together the end of the donor bronchus to the end of the recipient bronchus. If substantial recipient-donor size discrepancy exists, a telescoping bronchial anastomosis of the smaller bronchus is performed (Mallory & Spray, 1997). In the hopes of maximizing growth potential in children, absorbable sutures have been used (Spray, 1996). The patient is weaned from CPB. If necessary, inotropic support is initiated and pressure-monitoring lines are secured. The chest is closed by placing stainless steel wires at the midline incision of the sternum for stability. Typically, anterior and posterior chest tubes are inserted on each side of the chest wall. This allows for adequate evacuation of the chest and accurate measurement of pleural drainage in the postoperative phase.

Ischemic times less than 6 hours have been associated with good pulmonary function in the postoperative period. However, ischemic times closer to 4 hours are desirable. Given the present state of organ shortage, accepting donors from distant locations and extending ischemic times is a reality. Through the use of bilateral sequential lung transplantation and CPB, overall ischemic times have been kept as close to 4 hours as possible.

Postoperative Care

The postoperative lung transplant recipient is cared for using the same principles as the postoperative heart transplant recipient. However, the focus is optimizing pulmonary function. These patients require the initiation of pulmonary toileting within the first few hours postoperatively. Because the lungs are denervated, patients have an absent cough reflex. There is permanent absence of the reflex from the suture line downward. Therefore, they need assistance with the mobilization and expectoration of mucus. Chest physiotherapy should be initiated within 4 hours postoperatively. Another option is the use of an intensive care bed that has the capabilities for gentle vibration. These techniques are necessary to promote the mobilization of secretions and optimization of oxygenation. This aspect of the postoperative care for the lung transplant recipient is vital. While intubated, these patients require chest physiotherapy and suctioning on a regular basis for secretion removal. Clean suction technique should be used to suction these patients. The inspired oxygen content should be decreased as quickly as possible to maintain a PaO_2 greater than 85 mm Hg or an oxygen saturation of 95% or greater. Patients are weaned from ventilatory support as soon as it can be tolerated. Once the patient is weaned extubated assistance is still required with chest physiotherapy and encouragement to cough and deep breathe.

Postoperatively, these patients can pose particular problems regarding persistent air leaks and pleural effusion. Careful attention to proper functioning and positioning of the chest tubes is necessary to drain the accumulated air or fluid. The chest tubes are inserted anteriorly and posteriorly on each side to efficiently evacuate the pleural spaces. Daily chest radiographs can evaluate the position of the chest tubes and assess the accumulation of air or fluid in the pleural spaces. However, pulmonary auscultation will alert the caregiver early in the process of potential issues if breath sounds are diminished. Removal of the chest tubes depends on the amount of fluid loss from the chest tube and whether an air leak is present. Lung transplant patients with persistent pleural effusions require adjustment in their caloric intake to manage their losses from the pleural fluid. A nutritionist's input is important.

Once these patients are extubated, they require constant reinforcement with pulmonary toilet to mobilize secretions and clear their airways. Ineffective airway clearance can lead to poor oxygenation, pooling of secretions in the small airways with alveolar collapse, and possibly the need for re-intubation.

Rejection

The diligent assessment for and timely diagnosis and treatment of graft rejection are important to posttransplant care. Generally, immunosuppressant therapy begins in the immediate postoperative period. Acute graft rejection is a common occurrence in the early postoperative phase. It manifests itself with crackles on auscultation, new infiltrates on chest radiograph, a new or persistent pleural effusion, decrease in oxygenation, and decrease in pulmonary function (Mallory, 1996). The clinical picture of acute graft rejection can be vague with subtle signs of deteriorating lung function. Most institutions use transbronchial biopsies to confirm the diagnosis of acute allograft rejection. Once the diagnosis of acute rejection is made, the patient is treated with the standard pulse dose of methylprednisolone at 10 mg/kg for a total of 3 consecutive days. Augmentation in the daily dose of prednisone may occur. Because acute rejection is confirmed microscopically as a perivascular lymphocytic process, it responds to increasing or changing the immunosuppressant medications (Mallory, 1996). Follow-up transbronchial biopsies are usually performed 2 weeks after the initial treatment of the acute rejection episode to ensure resolution.

Chronic graft rejection or bronchiolitis obliterans (BO) is an inflammatory and proliferative process that affects the small airways. This is one of the most difficult complications of lung transplantation to manage and affects approximately 50% of all transplant survivors (Mallory, 1996). Some of the signs and symptoms associated with BO are a deterioration in lung function with an obstructive-type picture, dyspnea,

cough, and a slight decrease in oxygen saturation. This process can be aggressive, occurring within the first year after transplant and showing rapid deterioration of lung function or it can have more of an insidious onset with a gradual decrease in lung function. The diagnosis of BO is difficult to confirm microscopically from a biopsy specimen. Many experts in the field of lung transplantation use a clinical definition that encompasses a decrease in lung function in the absence of any other explanation for airway obstruction as bronchiolitis obliterans syndrome (Mallory, 1996). Once the diagnosis of BO is made, changes in the immunosuppressant regimen are often undertaken with variable results. The ultimate treatment for BO is retransplantation.

Infection

Infection is another complication that occurs in the postoperative phase that has a significant impact on survival after lung transplantation. Infections appear to contribute to the lower survival rates when compared with other solid organ transplants (Mallory, 1996). In normal healthy individuals the lung can become infected with respiratory pathogens that are circulating in the air that we breathe. Because of its anatomic design, the lung comes in contact on a daily basis with particles that are potentially infective. Lung transplant recipients are already predisposed to the development of infection because of their immunosuppressed condition and the absence of their cough reflex.

Although most of the infections that lung transplant recipients encounter are bacterial, viral and fungal infections can also be fatal. The CMV infection is a serious problem for lung transplant recipients. A posttransplant infection with CMV has been associated with the development of BO (Moodie & Stillwell, 1993). Therefore, initiation of CMV prophylaxis with ganciclovir within the first 24 hours after the transplant is recommended to prevent an infection in the early postoperative period. CMV prophylaxis is discussed in detail later in the chapter.

Lung transplant recipients are cared for in a reverse-flow isolation room in an intensive care unit. There is strict adherence to good handwashing techniques. Some institutions use reverse isolation techniques when caring for lung transplant recipients. However, there is not a universal practice for caring for these patients. Isolation techniques for lung transplant recipients follow center-specific protocols. Overwhelming infections of the lung allograft still represent a significant amount of morbidity and mortality for the lung transplant recipient (Shumway & Bolman, 1997).

HEART-LUNG TRANSPLANTATION

At Stanford University Hospital in 1981, the first clinically successful heart-lung transplant was performed in a 45-

year-old man with primary pulmonary hypertension (Mankad & de Leval, 1997). Over the last several years great strides have been made in the area of pediatric heart-lung transplantation. Because of the success of lung transplantation, fewer patients with primary lung disease are requiring heart-lung transplantation. In the past, patients who were dying from cystic fibrosis were listed for heart-lung transplants. Today these patients are able to receive bilateral lung transplants only. Pediatric patients who are candidates for heart-lung transplantation have end-stage cardiac and pulmonary disease that is not amenable to medical therapy. Typically, they are extremely symptomatic and their life expectancy is less than 2 years.

The identification of potential heart-lung recipients is determined after thorough cardiac and pulmonary evaluations. Once the patients have been evaluated, they are placed on the local OPO waiting list and the UNOS list. Patients are listed according to their blood type, height, and weight. At present, there is not a status for heart-lung recipients. They are offered organs on the basis of the amount of time they have on the waiting list, along with blood type, height, and weight parameters. This type of system is similar to the lung transplant recipient with the exception that they are in need of two life-sustaining organs. Unfortunately, these patients wait a considerable amount of time before their transplant surgery. They require careful attention during the waiting period to optimize their nutritional status, maximize their medication regimens, and prevent infection. These children need to be in the best condition possible at the time of transplantation. As with lung transplant recipients, there is a considerable amount of mortality associated with the heart-lung waiting list.

According to the ISHLT the 1-year actuarial survival rate after heart-lung transplantation is 58%, with a 5-year actuarial survival of 40% (Boucek et al., 1997). The leading causes of death within the first 30 days are evenly divided between primary graft failure, infection, and hemorrhage. However, the leading cause of death within the first year after heart-lung transplant is infection (Boucek et al., 1997).

Surgical Procedure

The surgery for heart-lung transplantation is much the same for heart transplantation. The surgery is performed on CPB through a median sternotomy. Once the heart and lungs are removed, attention is focused on achieving homeostasis of the mediastinum. In children with long-standing cyanosis or children with Eisenmenger's syndrome, this can be a long tedious process (Mankad & de Leval, 1997).

The organs are prepared en bloc. An end-to-end tracheal anastomosis is performed. Anastomoses along the atrial and aortic sites are completed. Intracardiac lines are secured and temporary pacemaker wires are inserted epicardially, as well as chest tubes in both pleural spaces and the mediastinum.

Postoperative Care

The initial postoperative care of the heart-lung transplant recipient is similar to that of any open-heart surgery patient. However, attention is focused on the effects of denervation on both the heart and lungs. The use of chronotropes and inotropes to augment cardiac output and early and vigorous pulmonary toileting to promote oxygenation are important in the care of these patients. Attention to the patient's volume status is necessary to prevent volume overloading because these children are prone to noncardiogenic pulmonary edema.

Bleeding is a potential and serious problem for these patients. Routine surveillance of clotting factors and abnormalities of coagulation should be evaluated and treated quickly. If necessary, blood component replacement therapy and/or heparin reversal or the use of aprotinin should be considered. If the drug aprotinin is used during the operation, it is continued in the postoperative period in an effort to control bleeding (Mankad & de Leval, 1997). In the event that blood loss is excessive, there should be a low threshold for re-exploring the chest. This operative procedure should be undertaken because the newly transplanted lungs poorly tolerate large amounts of blood volume replacement.

Rejection

Heart-lung transplant recipients need to be monitored for signs and symptoms of both cardiac and pulmonary rejection. Refer to the separate sections on heart rejection and lung rejection for a more detailed explanation. After allograft rejection is diagnosed, a standard 3-day course of intravenous methylprednisolone at 10 mg/kg is administered. Follow-up biopsies of the organ that was being treated for rejection are performed about 1 to 2 weeks after treatment.

Heart-lung transplant patients are also at risk for developing both BO and CAD. Routine surveillance of heart and lung function is necessary to diagnose and treat rejection episodes before significant deterioration in organ function occurs. Compliance to the medical regimen of immunosuppressant medications, healthy diet, regular exercise, routine clinic visits with pulmonary function testing, ECG, echocardiograms, chest radiographs, blood testing, and surveillance biopsies of the heart and lung are extremely important to the success of heart-lung transplantation.

IMMUNOSUPPRESSION

At present, there is not one uniformly accepted and practiced immunosuppressive regimen for all transplant centers. Institutions also differ on the use of induction therapy with lymphocyte cytolytic agents such as OKT3 and Zenapax. However, most institutions use a triple-drug regimen. The immunosuppressive regimen used includes a triple-drug regimen of cyclosporine/Neoral or Prograf/Tacrolimus prednisone, and azathioprine or CellCept. Refer to Exhibit 32–1 for the immunosuppression regimen. However, in the operating room at the time of the transplant an initial dose of azathioprine of 2 to 3 mg/kg may be administered intravenously. On the patient's return to the cardiac intensive care unit an infusion of cyclosporine is started. There is an initial bolus of 0.25 to 0.5 mg/kg infused over 3 hours and then the infusion is changed to 1.5 to 2.5 mg/kg/24 hours by continuous infusion to maintain a level of 300 to 350 ng/ml. The child is switched over to the oral form of cyclosporine/Neoral or Prograf/Tacrolimus as intestinal function returns. Azathioprine, 2 to 3 mg/kg IV/PO daily, is given or CellCept, 15 mg/kg, is given orally two to three times a day in divided doses. Prednisone is administered at 1 mg/kg per day in one or two divided doses intravenously or orally. The prednisone is gradually weaned over the next 6 to 12 months with an every-other-day dosing. Again, the continued use and dosage of steroids is center specific. There may be special circumstances when the steroid needs to be discontinued as soon as possible in the postoperative period as in a patient with Becker's muscular dystrophy. However, it is not a universal practice to discontinue steroids (Kichuk et al., 1997).

Broad-spectrum antibiotic coverage is used until the chest tubes and intracardiac lines are removed. Pneumocystis pneumonia prophylaxis is started once the child is tolerating enteral feedings. Sulfamethoxazole (Bactrim) is the drug of choice administered Monday, Tuesday, and Wednesday twice a day. If the sulfamethoxazole is not tolerated, dapsone is used in a dosage of 2 mg/kg/day administered once daily. Nystatin oral suspension is the antifungal agent used at a dosage of 100,000 to 500,000 units orally by swish and swallow four times a day with gradual weaning in frequency over the next few months. Ranitidine is given for its gastrointestinal protection properties. Children taking Prograf/Tacrolimus and cyclosporine/Neoral deplete their stores of magnesium and therefore require supplementation. Calcium supplements are also recommended because chronic steroid use causes osteoporosis.

CYTOMEGALOVIRUS PROPHYLAXIS

CMV is a herpes virus that is spread through direct contact. Usually the initial infection with CMV has subclinical effects and in healthy people the virus can remain dormant with the ability to replicate and reactivate. The transplant population is at particular risk from CMV because it can be

---

Exhibit 32–1 Immunosuppression Regimen

HEART AND LUNG TRANSPLANTATION MEDICATIONS
Immunosuppressive Regimen

Azathioprine (Imuran): 2 to 3 mg/kg/day; one dose given in OR prior to transplant
OR
Mycophenolate mofetil (CellCept): 15 mg/kg PO BID started once patient taking PO
Discontinue or decrease dose for WBC <5,000

Cyclosporine: 0.25 to 0.5 mg/kg IV over 3 hours postoperatively in ICU. Then 1.5 to 2.5 mg/kg/24 hours by continuous infusion to maintain a level of 300–350 ng/ml

Change over to PO cyclosporine as intestinal function returns (oral availability in adults is 25%–75% of parenteral; absorption appears to be worse in children)

After 6 months, the level is allowed to drop to 200–300 ng/ml
OR
Tacrolimus (Prograf): 0.15 to 0.3 mg/kg/day divided PO BID. Maintain a level of 6–12 ng/ml

---

Prednisone: 1 mg/kg/day for 2 weeks after transplant IV or PO
Then decrease dose to 0.5 mg/kg/day for the next 6 months
Then decrease dose to 0.2 mg/kg/day
Then decrease to QOD

transmitted by means of the transplanted organ, blood transfusion, and contact with others in the community who may be shedding the virus. According to Waid (1994), CMV causes approximately 66% of all febrile illnesses in the transplant recipient.

Even though the CMV status of the recipient and donor is known at the time of the transplant, it is not feasible given the present organ shortage to match CMV serologic status. However, all blood products that are transfused should be CMV negative. Invasive CMV disease, if left untreated, can be fatal. Therefore, CMV titers in the posttransplant period are closely monitored. Many centers use ganciclovir in the lung and heart-lung transplant recipients as CMV prophylaxis. Ganciclovir is started preoperatively or immediately in the postoperative period and continued for a total of 6 weeks. The initial dosage is 5 mg/kg per dose every 12 hours for the first 2 weeks, then 5 mg/kg/day once daily for 4 weeks. Long-term central venous access is required for medication administration.

IMMUNIZATIONS

Infants, children, and adolescents undergoing transplants need the continued care of their primary care providers (PCP). It is the PCP who delivers the necessary and very much needed "well child" care. Immunizations are one of the aspects of care that are important in the pediatric population. All children need to be immunized. The timing of immunizations and which immunizations to give can occasionally be concerning to the PCP. The key point to remember when immunizing transplant recipients is that they cannot receive live virus vaccines. Giving live virus vaccines to the siblings of these patients is also a concern because some of these vaccines are shed for periods of time, potentially infecting the transplant recipient. Refer to Table 32–2 for the immunizations recommended for the transplant recipient and siblings. The influenza vaccine is a recommended annual immunization for the transplant recipient and the household contacts. According to a study completed by Mauch et al. (1994) influenza B virus infections can cause serious infections in the solid organ transplant recipient. They recommend routine administration of the influenza vaccine along with further study.

Most transplant recipients can resume their immunization schedule within a few months after transplantation. Typically, at this time the child has been on a consistent immunosuppressant regimen and rejection has been monitored and controlled.

COMPLIANCE

Patient and family compliance with the medical regimen is vital to the success of thoracic organ transplants. Nurses are in a key position to assess and document patient and family compliance in the pretransplant phase. Active participation of the family in the recipient's postoperative care should be encouraged and reinforced. However, if there is documented noncompliance before the referral for transplant or noncompliance with the established medical regimen during the waiting period before transplant regarding missed appointments or medication noncompliance, this should be a red flag for the medical and surgical transplant teams. These patients and families are referred to the social worker or psychologist/psychiatrist to identify issues that have an impact on their noncompliance. If absolutely necessary, these children may be placed in foster care so the medical routines can be provided for them before, during, and after their transplant. The transplant team may also decide that the patient is not a transplant candidate in light of constant noncompliance despite all attempts by the social worker and the psychiatrist/psychologist's efforts to work on the issues surrounding the noncompliance.

Kurland (1996) suggests that referring physicians and the transplant team discuss the posttransplant expectations with the potential recipients before listing them for a transplant in an attempt to ensure that the recipient would be capable of adhering to the prescribed regimen. Patient compliance is a requirement for the transplant to be successful for all parties involved. Compliance to the medical regimen before and after transplantation is the cornerstone to a successful outcome for patients and families. Therefore, the issue of compliance needs to be assessed long before the patient receives a transplant.

DIETARY ISSUES

Infants who have been on ventilators during their entire wait for a transplant or those who are tachypneic and unable

Table 32–2 Immunizations for Transplant Recipients and Their Siblings

Routine Immunizations

	Patient	Siblings
DPT/DTP/DT	Yes	Yes
HIB	Yes	Yes
Hepatitis B	Yes	Yes
OPV	**No**	**No**
IPV	Yes	Yes
MMR	**No**	Yes
Varivax	**No**	Yes
Influenza	Yes	Yes
Pneumovax	Yes	Yes

to feed by mouth provide caregivers with a challenge in the postoperative period. These infants usually require naso-gastric feedings to provide the necessary 120 to 150 kcal/kg/day to grow and thrive. Fortifying formula to increase the caloric content is almost always necessary. The introduction of solid foods is usually postponed until adequate caloric intake and weight gain is established. However, for developmental purposes the introduction of the spoon at the appropriate age is encouraged with two small feedings a day of cereal or fruit.

It is not uncommon to have a situation with a toddler or a school-age child during the preoperative waiting period who is being force fed or permitted to eat whatever it is that he or she wants to promote some weight gain. Then in the post-transplant phase after their child has received steroids, they will not eat a nutritious diet. Bad dietary habits that were formed out of a need for weight gain and sustaining life are difficult to change. It is important for the families to be supported and educated in the appropriate serving portions for a child that encourages heart-healthy eating using all the food groups with emphasis on nutritious snacks. Close monitoring of the child's weight gain along with a nutritionist's input is important to promote healthy eating and prevent obesity.

Adolescents pose a particular challenge in that their diets are almost always high in sodium and fat. This age group needs support in selecting foods that are nutritious and palatable enough to fit into their socially driven lifestyles. Education is the key along with close supervision and support as they strive to fit in with their peers. Obesity and hypertension are potentially detrimental health issues specific to this age group, which are impacted by poor dietary habits. Adolescents need to be supported and educated regarding portion size and food content. A nutritionist can assist them with making food choices that fit into their busy lifestyles that are low in fat, sodium, and calories.

RETURNING TO SCHOOL

For most children, returning to school is a symbol that they are well enough to resume normal activities with their peers. It is recommended that children return to school sometime within 3 months after transplantation. Usually at this point they have been on a steady immunosuppressant regimen and their outpatient appointments are about every month. Letters are sent to the school nurse and their teachers outlining infectious disease precautions. Particular attention is focused on the chickenpox virus. If a transplant recipient is exposed to another person with chickenpox, the transplanted child's family needs to be notified as soon as possible. The family is instructed to contact the transplant center to arrange for an injection of varicella immune globulin. Varicella immune globulin is given to immunocompromised patients to prevent

or lessen the varicella disease. For best results it should be administered within 96 hours of exposure. Refer to the package insert for dosage recommendations, which are based on weight. While children are home recovering, arrange for home tutoring to avoid lapses in academic progress.

Because some of these children may not have received the immunization against measles, mumps, and rubella (MMR), particular attention needs to be paid to these diseases and the potential exposure to the transplant recipient. MMR is a live virus vaccine, which can be extremely harmful if administered to a transplant recipient. Typically, the school needs documentation as to why the child is unable to receive the MMR vaccine.

Regular physical education classes are recommended. However, the child should be permitted rest periods whenever necessary. High-level contact sports are not permitted because of the possible deleterious effects from chest trauma that may occur after a recent sternotomy.

Thorough handwashing is encouraged and reinforced. Handwashing prevents the spread of germs that can cause serious illness in the immunocompromised person. Children need supervision with this practice in school and in the home environment. This is particularly important during the cold and flu season.

USE OF OVER-THE-COUNTER AND PRESCRIPTION MEDICATIONS

Coughs, colds, bouts of otitis media, and strep throats are just a few of the "typical" illness that afflict children. The reaction by almost all health care providers is to prescribe something to help relieve some of the symptoms or an antibiotic to fight the bacterial infection. With immunosuppressed children this practice cannot be automatic. Careful attention needs to be paid to the potential drug interactions that may occur with the immunosuppressant medications.

Particular attention should be paid to the various antibiotics that are prescribed to treat bacterial and fungal infections. For example, antibiotics in the erythromycin family increase cyclosporine and Prograf levels. This increase is reflected in an elevated BUN and creatinine along with all the side effects associated with elevated drug levels. Therefore, it is best to consult with the transplant team or a pharmacist familiar with immunosuppressant medications before prescribing or recommending over-the-counter or other medication.

CONCLUSION

Heart, lung, and heart-lung transplantation is a viable option for infants and children with end-stage heart and lung disease. However, because of the shortage of donor organs, most of these children are hospitalized for a long time awaiting their lifesaving transplant. The care that these children receive during their wait has a great impact on their postoperative course. These children need to be in the best condition possible when undergoing their transplant.

Nurses who care for this population of patients play a vital role not only in the postoperative care of the transplant patient but also in assessing compliance, exercise tolerance, nutrition, and psychological adjustment. Educating the patient and family is a large aspect of the nurse's role. Information regarding medications, infection, rejection, and follow-up care needs to be provided to the patient and family preoperatively and reinforced postoperatively. As consistent care providers who interact with both the patient and family, nursing input is crucial to the expert care provided to the cardiothoracic transplant patient.

REFERENCES

Boucek, M.M., Novick, R.J., Bennett, L.E., Fiol, B., Keck, B.M., & Hosenpud, J.D. (1997). The registry of the international society of heart and lung transplantation: First official pediatric report—1997. *The Journal of Heart and Lung Transplantation, 16*(12), 1189–1206.

Franco, K.L. (1997). Lung transplantation for pulmonary hypertension. In K.L. Franco (Ed.), *Pediatric cardiopulmonary transplantation* (pp. 303–318). Armonk, NY: Futura Publishing.

Gundry, S.R. (1997). Infant and pediatric cardiac transplantation. In K.L. Franco (Ed.), *Pediatric cardiopulmonary transplantation* (pp. 97–114). Armonk, NY: Futura Publishing.

Hosenpud, J.D., Bennett, L.E., Keck, B.M., Fiol, B., & Novick, R.J. (1997). The registry of the international society for heart and lung transplantation: Fourteenth official report—1997. *The Journal of Heart and Lung Transplantation, 16*(7), 691–712.

Kichuk, M.R., Itescu, S, Michler, R.E., & Addonizio, L.J. (1997). Transplant immunology and pediatric immunosuppression. In K.L. Franco (Ed.), *Pediatric cardiopulmonary transplantation* (pp. 1–26). Armonk, NY: Futura Publishing.

Kshettry, V.R., & Bolman, R.M. (1995). Heart-lung transplantation. In M.W. Flye (Ed.), *Atlas of organ transplantation* (pp. 279–292). Philadelphia: W.B. Saunders Company.

Kurland, G. (1996). Pediatric lung transplantation: Indications and contraindications. *Seminars in Thoracic and Cardiovascular Surgery, 8*(3), 277–285.

Mallory, G.B. (1996). Major medical complications of lung transplantation: A pediatric perspective. *Seminars in Thoracic and Cardiovascular Surgery, 8*(3), 305–312.

Mallory, G.B., & Spray, T.L. (1997). Lung transplantation for cystic fibrosis in children. In K.L. Franco (Ed.), *Pediatric cardiopulmonary transplantation* (pp. 277–301). Armonk, NY: Futura Publishing.

Mankad, P.S., & de Leval, M.R. (1997). Heart-lung transplantation. In K.L. Franco (Ed.), *Pediatric cardiopulmonary transplantation* (pp. 167–184). Armonk, NY: Futura Publishing.

Mauch, T.J., Bratton, S., Myers, T., Krane, E., Gentry, S.R., & Kashtan, C.E. (1994). Influenza B virus infection in pediatric solid organ transplant recipients. *Pediatrics, 94*(2), 225–229.

Moodie, D.S., & Stillwell, P.C. (1993). Thoracic organ transplantation in children: The state of heart, heart-lung and lung transplantation. *Clinical Pediatrics, 32*(6), 322–328.

Neuberger, S., Vincent, R.N., Doelling, N., Sullivan, K., Honeycutt, S., Kantor, K.R., & Fyfe, D. (1997). Comparison of quantitative echocardiography with endomyocardial biopsy to define myocardial rejection in pediatric patients after cardiac transplantation. *The American Journal of Cardiology, 79*, 447–450.

Shumway, S.J., & Bolman, R.M. (1997). Single lung transplantation in children. In K.L. Franco (Ed.), *Pediatric cardiopulmonary transplantation* (pp. 269–275). Armonk, NY: Futura Publishing.

Spray, T.L. (1995). Pediatric heart transplantation. In M.W. Flye (Ed.), *Atlas of organ transplantation* (pp. 259–277). Philadelphia: W.B. Saunders Company.

Spray, T.L. (1996). Lung transplantation in children with pulmonary hypertension and congenital heart disease. *Seminars in Thoracic and Cardiovascular Surgery, 8*(3), 286–295.

Spray, T.L., & Huddleston, C.B. (1993). Pediatric lung transplantation. *Chest Surgery Clinics of North America, 3*(1), 123–143.

United Network of Organ Sharing. (1999). *1998 annual report of the U.S. Scientific Registry for Transplant Recipients and the Organ Procurement and Transplantation Network: Transplant data, 1988–1997*. Richmond, VA: Author.

Waid, T.H. (1994). Preventing CMV disease with cytomegalovirus immune globulins. *Pharmacy and Therapeutics*, 760–762, 765–766, 771–773.

CHAPTER 33

The Surgical Neonate

Katherine E. Keener, Kimberly D. Knoerlein, Wendy M. McKenney, Linda Miranda McNamara, Dorothy M. Mullaney, and Susan M. Quinn

Providing for the needs of the surgical neonate requires knowledge of pathophysiology and neonatal care practices, the ability to recognize and respond to complications, and giving supportive care to the family. A multidisciplinary team approach toward the surgical neonate involves parents, neonatal nurses, nurse practitioners, neonatologists, pediatric surgeons, respiratory therapists, social workers, radiologists, and anesthesiologists who work together to provide high-quality care to ensure optimal outcomes.

The surgical neonate is a unique individual requiring specialized care and a distinct approach to his or her medical management during the preoperative, intraoperative, and postoperative period. This chapter discusses specific physiologic problems experienced by the surgical neonate involving cardiorespiratory stabilization, thermoregulation, fluid and electrolyte management, drug therapy, wound care, and nutritional support. Nursing therapies are also presented and focus on the needs of the neonate and family from admission to discharge.

PRENATAL DIAGNOSIS, PERINATAL MANAGEMENT, AND PRENATAL FAMILY COUNSELING

Approximately 2% to 3% of all infants born have a birth defect or a genetic abnormality (Plouffe & Donahue, 1994; Shaw, 1990; Shirley, Bottomley, & Robinson, 1992). Technology has advanced to the point where many congenital surgical defects are diagnosed in utero. Many defects can be palliated or corrected with surgery, often in the neonatal period. The cascade of events leading to successful neonatal surgery begins prenatally.

Prenatal diagnosis guides the decision of the neonate's delivery in view of the congenital defect and anticipated need for surgery. Full-term delivery is preferred to minimize problems with transition to extrauterine life. Unfortunately, maternal or fetal complications do not always make this possible. Early diagnosis offers guidance to the optimal mode of delivery—Caesarean section versus vaginal delivery. Some congenital defects may be amenable to in utero surgery (Duncan & Adzick, 1996). See Chapter 9 for further information regarding fetal surgery.

Several prenatal diagnostic screening techniques are available. However, not all are appropriate for every prenatal patient. Some of the common diagnostic screening techniques currently available for prenatal diagnosis of a congenital defect or genetic abnormality include ultrasonography, alpha-fetoprotein (AFP) levels, and amniocentesis.

Prenatal ultrasonography is the most commonly used method of diagnosing a congenital defect that requires surgical intervention. Screening of the fetal anatomy using ultrasonography can determine the gestational age of the fetus, monitor fetal status, and detect fetal malformations. It also evaluates amniotic fluid volume, lung development, and renal anatomy, all which may be interrelated. Routine ultrasonographic screening in a low-risk maternal population is generally obtained between 18 to 20 weeks' gestation or midtrimester (Skupski, Chervenak, & McCullough, 1994). Abnormalities detected by ultrasonography include omphalocele, gastroschisis, diaphragmatic hernia, and other serious congenital defects.

Evaluation of maternal serum levels of alpha-fetoprotein (AFP) is offered to women early in pregnancy. AFP, a major protein produced by the fetus, is excreted into the maternal amniotic fluid. Abnormal levels have been associated with anencephaly, open neural tube defects, trisomy 21 (Down syndrome), twin gestation, omphalocele, intestinal obstruction, discrepancy in fetal dating, and intrauterine growth retardation (Plouffe & Donahue, 1994; Rowe, O'Neil,

Grosfeld, Fonkalsrud, & Coran, 1995a). AFP is not an exact test and warrants further screening of abnormal results.

Amniocentesis may be performed at any time during pregnancy but is most commonly performed between 12 to 18 weeks' gestation (Plouffe & Donahue, 1994). Amniotic fluid is removed during the procedure to assess for abnormalities, either inherited or metabolic, and is also used to screen for fetal lung maturity (Duncan & Adzick, 1996). Neonates with immature lungs are at increased risk for respiratory distress syndrome (RDS). Amniocentesis analyzes fetal cells for karyotyping, and results are available approximately 2 weeks after the procedure. The ability to accurately diagnose fetal abnormalities with amniocentesis is greater than 98% (Rowe et al., 1995a).

Once a surgical abnormality has been identified prenatally, plans must be made regarding the most appropriate management. This often requires referral to a tertiary care facility that offers neonatal and pediatric surgical services. However, those neonates who are delivered unexpectedly at a local hospital require transport to the closest tertiary care facility shortly after birth for further evaluation and management of the malformation (Shirley et al., 1992). Transported neonates require a warm environment, a secured airway, and adequate vascular access. For those born with gastrointestinal abnormalities, a nasogastric tube is needed for decompression and prevention of aspiration during the transport process.

Parents should arrange for a tour of the neonatal intensive care unit (NICU) before delivery and meet with members of the surgical and neonatal teams to discuss findings and probable prognosis for their infant (Shirley et al., 1992). Information given to the family should include the natural history of the abnormality, timing of the surgery, anticipated surgical outcomes, possible long-term sequelae, and any other foreseen problems surrounding the neonate's course. Decisions in the management and treatment of the neonate require a team approach, which includes parents, nurses, obstetricians, pediatric surgeons, nurse practitioners, neonatologists, and radiologists (Duncan & Adzick, 1996; Shirley et al., 1992). Supportive services should be provided to the parents and their family members as indicated.

NEONATAL MANAGEMENT

The key to successful management of the surgical neonate is the ability to recognize rapidly changing physiologic characteristics and provide prompt treatment. Successful preoperative stabilization of the surgical neonate augments the infant's ability to survive the surgical intervention. After delivery and initial stabilization, all infants receive routine interventions such as prophylactic eye ointment with erythromycin or tetracycline and vitamin K (0.5 mg for infants <1 kg; 1 mg for infants >1 kg) as recommended by the American Academy of Pediatrics (Kenner, Amlung, &

Flandermeyer, 1998c). Newborns normally receive their first hepatitis B vaccine in the nursery just before discharge. However, surgical neonates who may require a lengthy hospital stay should get their scheduled series of immunizations once stable.

Management of the surgical neonate involves stabilization and ongoing assessment of cardiopulmonary status, thermoregulation, fluid and electrolyte balance, drug therapy, wound care, and nutritional support.

CARDIOVASCULAR AND RESPIRATORY STABILIZATION

The stabilization of the surgical neonate's cardiorespiratory function before surgery optimizes the ability of the neonate to survive anesthesia and surgery with fewer complications. Care providers must have a basic understanding of the unique pathophysiology that occurs during transition from fetal circulation to neonatal circulation because most surgical infants require repair immediately or shortly after birth.

The main organ of oxygenation changes from placenta to lungs after delivery of the neonate and clamping of the umbilical cord. Transition to extrauterine life begins with the first breath, causing the lungs to expand, systemic vascular resistance to rise, and pulmonary vascular resistance to fall. This enables blood to freely flow into the lungs, starting the process of oxygenation and removal of carbon dioxide necessary to sustain life. Fetal shunts allow blood to bypass the lungs in utero. The foramen ovale, one of the intrauterine fetal shunts, closes as a result of changes in systemic blood flow. The ductus arteriosus, another fetal shunt, normally closes within 15 to 24 hours of birth in response to increased arterial oxygen content and the effects of circulating prostaglandins (Flanagan & Fyler, 1994). However, the ductus arteriosus may reopen as a result of several contributing factors. One factor frequently seen in the neonatal period is hypoxia. Decreased oxygen to the neonate can cause a constricted ductus to reopen and reestablish intrauterine fetal circulation, which shunts blood away from the lungs. This increases pulmonary vascular resistance and leads to persistent pulmonary hypertension of the newborn. Ductal-dependent cyanotic congenital heart lesions require patency of the ductus arteriosus to maintain oxygenation and adequate perfusion in the critical newborn period. Unlike the adult, cardiac output in the neonate is largely rate dependent. The neonate compensates for a fall in cardiac output by increasing his or her heart rate. Poor cardiac output in the neonate may be a result of conditions such as congenital heart disease, sepsis, hypovolemia, and asphyxia.

Several neonatal respiratory conditions interfere with adequate ventilation and perfusion in the surgical neonate. These include respiratory distress syndrome, pneumonia, transient tachypnea of the newborn, and aspiration syndromes, which may occur from pulmonary congestion as a result of congenital heart disease. In the preoperative period the establishment of adequate ventilation, oxygenation, perfusion, and correction of acid-base status before the added stress of surgery and anesthesia optimizes the neonate's outcome. Various surgical conditions can directly impair air exchange, oxygenation, and tissue perfusion and require immediate attention. A complete history, physical examination, and laboratory data are needed to effectively evaluate and manage the surgical neonate (see Exhibit 33–1) (Adcock, Consolvo, & Berry, 1998).

Assessment of the surgical neonate immediately after birth includes observing the infant's ability to transition from intrauterine to extrauterine life. Neonates are obligate nose breathers, and those diagnosed with choanal atresia, a bony or membranous occlusion blocking the passageway between the nose and the pharynx, require the placement of an oral airway to establish adequate ventilation (Hansen & Corbet, 1998). Bag-mask ventilation is contraindicated in infants with diaphragmatic hernia and tracheoesophageal fistula because of accumulation of air within the abdomen (Kenner, Amlung, & Flandermeyer, 1998b). Any abdominal wall defect, such as omphalocele, gastroschisis, or bowel obstruction, may present with abdominal distention causing inadequate lung volumes and/or problems with lung expansion. Therefore, decompression of the stomach is needed by placing a nasogastric tube to gentle suction (Kenner et al., 1998b).

Pharmacologic support may be necessary to improve cardiac function, which in turn improves organ perfusion. Ino-

tropic agents such as dopamine and dobutamine are frequently used for this purpose. The use of prostaglandins promotes dilation of the ductus arteriosus in neonates with congenital heart disease dependent on ductal shunting for oxygenation and perfusion (Ward, 1994). Before surgery, inotropes are mixed in enough solution for infusion throughout the surgical procedure. Labeling of all drip lines is necessary to avoid inadvertent fluid bolus or disconnection of a life-sustaining drug.

Use of invasive and noninvasive monitoring can be extremely helpful. Invasive monitoring includes the use of central venous lines and umbilical catheters to monitor pressures in the right atrium and give information on fluid status, especially if large amounts of fluid loss are expected. Arterial catheterization enables monitoring of blood pressure and heart rate. It also provides easy access for blood sampling to determine respiratory or metabolic acidosis, which should be corrected immediately. Noninvasive monitoring includes the use of pulse oximetry for arterial saturation and transcutaneous end-tidal carbon dioxide monitoring, which provides information on oxygenation and ventilation.

In the postoperative period, assessment of the neonate's vital signs, color, perfusion, and urine output must be performed on return from the operating room. The clinical condition of the neonate can deteriorate more rapidly and with less warning than in any other age group. Postoperative complications seen in neonates that must be expediently corrected are respiratory distress, shock, and hemorrhage. Most infants return from the operating room on ventilatory sup-

---

Exhibit 33–1 Evaluation of the Surgical Neonate

History	Laboratory	Physical Examination	
• Obstetric	*Chest radiograph*	*Heart rate*	*General appearance*
• Perinatal	• May identify respiratory cause for acid-base disturbance	• Rhythm	Color
• Labor		• Tachycardia	• Cyanosis peripheral/central
• Neonatal	*Arterial blood gases*	• Peripheral pulses	• Pallor
• Family	• Will point to the primary acid-base derangement	• Irregularities	• Mottling
	• Compensation	*Blood pressure*	• Gray
	• Degree of hypoxemia	• High or low blood pressure	Activity
		• Wide or narrow pulse pressures	• Alert
			• Lethargic
		Respiratory effort	• Anxious
		Signs of distress	• Relaxed
		• Nasal flaring	
		• Expiratory grunting	
		• Stridor	
		• Retractions	
		• Tachypnea	

port. Ventilatory management of the neonate is influenced by underlying respiratory disease and the primary surgical condition. The intubated neonate should be closely monitored for endotracheal tube dislodgment and patency of the tube should be maintained by suctioning as needed to prevent obstruction from secretions. Auscultation of breath sounds, observing for adequate chest rise, monitoring blood gases, and following oxygen saturation assist in determining the surgical neonate's respiratory status. Assessing the infant's respiratory efforts, pulse oximetry, transcutaneous end-tidal carbon dioxide monitoring, and following blood gases is helpful in managing ventilator support.

Cardiac output should be assessed by observing the heart rate, peripheral perfusion, and urine output. An infant who is tachycardiac could be responding to pain or intravascular volume depletion. Bradycardia is more ominous and is often caused by hypoxia. When the systemic perfusion is adequate, the skin is warm and peripheral pulses are strong and easily palpated. It is important that an infant with low cardiac output be treated immediately. Ten to 20 ml/kg of 5% albumin or normal saline should be administered to infants with tachycardia, poor peripheral perfusion, and hypotension. Packed red blood cells can be used for volume replacement. Vital signs are reassessed for response and the need for further volume resuscitation. If, after several attempts with volume replacement, no improvement is noted in peripheral perfusion, heart rate, and urine output, the use of inotropes may be needed to improve cardiac output.

THERMOREGULATION

Neonates are uniquely vulnerable to cold stress and overheating. The consequences of either can be devastating if not recognized early and corrected. It is imperative that the bedside nurse monitor temperature closely and stay alert for signs of heat or cold stress. Hypothermia is common in neonates. Premature neonates with immature skin are at an even higher risk. Heat is lost in greater degrees with the smaller neonates and is inversely related to decreasing gestational age (Perlstein, 1992). Neonates are at risk for derangements in thermoregulation because of their large surface/mass ratio. Hyperthermia can occur but is more often than not caused by environmental factors. An older infant will mount a febrile response to infection, but hypothermia is more frequently seen in premature neonates who may be septic. Temperature instability may be one of the first signs of sepsis the neonate exhibits. If fever is caused by infection, the core temperature will be warmer than the skin temperature and the neonate will likely be vasoconstricted. Evaluation for sepsis is warranted.

Neonates undergoing surgery are at high risk for hypothermia. Infants can become chilled during transfer to and from the operating room (OR), on exposure to cold surfaces and fluids, with exposure of viscera during the surgical procedure, and secondary to the effects of sedation and anesthesia. Neonates, unlike older infants and adults, do not respond to heat loss by shivering. Instead, heat is generated through chemical thermogenesis and peripheral vasoconstriction. On exposure to cold, norepinephrine and thyroid hormones are released. This hormonal response induces lipolysis of brown fat stores found in the interscapular, paraspinal, and perirenal areas (Perlstein, 1992). This lipolysis and fatty acid oxidation release heat into the bloodstream. Cold stress initiates an increase in oxygen consumption, glucose use, and acid production. This further leads to depletion of glycogen stores and metabolic acidosis. Severe acidosis and hypoxia occur if steps to correct the hypothermia are not taken (Rushton, 1988).

Hyperthermia is infrequent, and most times it is due to environmental causes. Iatrogenic causes of hyperthermia include overdressing the neonate and mechanical derangements of isolettes or radiant warmers. A temperature probe that loses contact with skin induces the temperature sensor to increase the heat output in efforts to increase the neonate's temperature. An isolette placed in direct sunlight experiences solar gain and can dramatically increase the temperature inside the isolette. This induces heat-losing mechanisms in the neonate. The skin flushes as the blood vessels dilate. The skin temperature is warmer than the core temperature (Perlstein, 1992). Body temperature of 42° C can cause seizures, deranged thermoregulation, and permanent brain damage (Holtzclaw, 1990). Management is by cooling the infant and environment. Slowly decreasing body temperature is preferable because rapid changes may induce apnea, particularly in premature neonates.

The surgical neonate requires special care to maintain euthermia. During the preoperative period, the infant should be kept in a neutral thermal environment. The goal is maintenance of normal body temperature with little stress on the infant who needs to conserve energy for the stress of surgery and recovery. Use of a transport isolette during transfer to the OR is an excellent way of maintaining optimal body temperature. If an isolette is not available for transport to the OR, the neonate should wear a cap, be placed on a radiant warmer, and be covered with warmed blankets. A layer of plastic wrap over the infant and beneath the blankets provides superior protection from heat loss (Gregory, 1992). The OR should be prewarmed to a higher than normal level before the infant's arrival and a water- or air-warming blanket should be heated to 40° C.

Intraoperatively, efforts should be made to prevent heat loss. The infant should lie on the warming blanket and have only the surgical area exposed. The head covering should be left on if possible. Overhead warming lights or a servo-controlled infrared heater may be used during the procedure. Anesthetic gases should be warmed and humidified. Warming skin preparation solutions, blood, and irrigating fluids plays a large role in minimizing heat loss. If the intravenous tubing is placed beneath the warming blanket, those fluids will be near body temperature when infusing. Body temperature must be monitored continuously to detect alterations. This may be performed by having a temperature probe placed in the esophagus, skin, or rectum (Gregory, 1992).

Postoperatively, heat can be lost on the transport from the OR to the NICU. On arrival in the NICU, the surgical neonate should be kept in a neutral thermal environment with continuous temperature monitoring. The radiant warmer or incubator should be preheated to the appropriate neutral thermal temperature before the neonate arrives to reduce heat loss to the environment. The neonate's central nervous system's response to cold may be impaired by sedation and drugs used for anesthesia and pain control. Cardiovascular agents can cause vasodilation, further enhancing heat loss through radiation and convection (Holtzclaw, 1990). Dressings may become saturated and cool on exposure to air, further exacerbating heat losses. The surgical neonate's temperature should be continuously monitored to maintain the neutral thermal environment.

FLUIDS AND ELECTROLYTES

Fluid management of the surgical neonate compared with the older infant or adult needs to account for the physiologic and pathologic differences that are unique to this group of infants. The neonate's metabolic rate is double, water requirements are four to five times greater, and the excretion of sodium is only 10% of that in older children and adults (Adcock et al., 1998). Fluid requirements change rapidly during the first week of life and can be higher in the premature infant. Understanding the changing water composition of the fetus and neonate enables clinicians to provide better fluid and electrolyte management.

Gestational age is a large determinant of the percentage and distribution of total body water. Both term and preterm infants are born with excess total body water, in particular extracellular water. Newborns typically undergo a physiologic diuresis of up to 10% of body weight over the first 4 to 5 days of life to remove this excess fluid. This is important for caregivers to understand when providing fluid and electrolytes to neonates shortly after birth, especially in managing those born extremely prematurely or growth retarded. Neonates weighing less than 1,500 grams have rapidly changing fluid requirements during the first week of life and may have up to three times the fluid loss as term infants. Giving excess fluids and electrolytes during this period of natural diuresis increases the neonate's risk for patent ductus arteriosus, left ventricular failure, congestive heart failure, respiratory distress syndrome, bronchopulmonary dysplasia, and necrotizing enterocolitis (Letton & Chwals, 1997).

The kidneys play a vital role in fluid and electrolyte regulation in the neonate, although the full functional capacity of the kidney does not reach adult levels until 2 years of age. The kidney's ability to regulate fluid and electrolyte homeostasis remains limited in the term and particularly in the preterm infant. Neonates less than 34 weeks' gestation have reduced glomerular filtration rates and tubular immaturity that alters their ability to handle filtered solutes. Accurate measurements of urine output, specific gravity, and osmolarity are especially important in the surgical neonate because of the added stress of surgery and anesthesia. Urine volumes should be 1 to 2 ml/kg/hr, which will keep the specific gravity between 1.009 and 1.012 and urine osmolarity between 250 and 290 mmol/kg (Puri & Sweed, 1996).

In the preoperative period a complete and thorough evaluation of the fluid and electrolyte status of the surgical neonate is needed (see Exhibit 33–2) (Rushton, 1988). Vascular access should be obtained to provide fluid boluses, drugs, and blood products when necessary. Stabilization of an infant's fluid and electrolyte status before surgery helps the infant endure the stress of surgery with few complications. Inadequate assessment of fluid intake can lead to dehydration, depletion of intravascular volume, hypotension, poor perfusion with acidosis, and hypernatremia (Puri & Sweed, 1996). Administration of excess amounts of fluid, particularly in the preterm infant, may result in pulmonary edema, patent ductus arteriosus, bronchopulmonary dysplasia, and cerebral intraventricular hemorrhage (Puri & Sweed, 1996).

Clinical and laboratory assessment of the neonate's fluid and electrolyte status should continue intraoperatively. Losses of fluid and blood should be recorded and replaced during the procedure or shortly after surgery with packed red blood cells, normal saline, or 5% albumin. If the surgical procedure is lengthy, electrolytes and blood glucose should be monitored and corrected if abnormal (Warde, 1996). Urine output may be accurately assessed intraoperatively with placement of a catheter into the bladder. The environment must be kept warm to prevent further loss of fluid from open peritoneal surfaces.

Careful assessment and management of fluid and electrolyte status preoperatively and intraoperatively often decrease complications postoperatively. If the surgical neonate has not been kept well hydrated and has been hypotensive, transient renal failure with oliguria may occur and needs to be managed with fluid restriction and correction of electrolyte imbalances such as hyperkalemia and metabolic acidosis (Gorman, 1996). Syndrome of inappropriate secretion of antidiuretic hormone (SIADH) is common in the neonatal population and results from pain, tissue injury, hypoperfusion, and ventilation. This results in fluid retention by increasing permeability of collecting ducts and tubules of the kidney, causing increased reabsorption of water, resulting in oliguria and hyponatremia. Antidiuretic hormone (ADH)

Exhibit 33–2 Assessment of Fluid and Electrolyte Status in the Neonate

Physical Assessment	Fluid Intake and Output	Monitor Laboratory Data	Hemodynamic Monitoring
Mucous membranes	*Measurement of losses*	*Hematocrit*	*Central venous pressures*
Skin	Urine, stool/stoma, vomitus, drainage	Drops with overload	Are indicated for monitoring right heart pressures to assess venous return and blood volume
Poor turgor with hypovolemia	Weight of dressings	Elevated with dehydration	May be helpful in the infant with myocardial insufficiency, SIADH, renal tubular necrosis, or rapid fluid shifts
Dependent or pitting edema with overload	Urinary catheter for meticulous monitoring	*Serum and urine electrolytes*	Normal range 4–8 mm Hg
Eyes	External urine collection device or diaper weights	*Serum osmolality*	
Sunken in dehydration	Strict measurement	Normal 280–295 mOsm/l	
Periorbital edema with overload	*Determine adequacy of urine output*	*BUN and creatinine*	
Fontanelle	Average 1–2 ml/kg/hr	Not very helpful in first 24 hours of life	
Depressed with dehydration	*Monitor specific gravity and/or urine osmolarity*	Provides indirect data about ECF and GFR	
Bulging with overload	Neonates cannot concentrate urine below 1.015–1.020	*CO$_2$ and HCO$_2$*	
Peripheral perfusion	*Monitor weight*	Indirect measures of intravascular volume depletion	
Capillary refill time slowed with hypovolemia	Daily or BID weights using same scale	*Total protein*	
Liver size	Determine appropriate weight gain or loss	May indicate intravascular albumin depletion	
Increased with overload CHF			
Neurologic changes			
Tachycardia may indicate hypovolemia			
Hypotension is a late sign of hypovolemia			
Alterations in ECG may denote acid-base or electrolyte imbalance			

controls the concentration of sodium in the extracellular space and, when inappropriately secreted, water is conserved and sodium is excreted. Gastrointestinal drainage results in loss of additional fluids and electrolytes such as sodium and potassium. Significant fluid losses from any drainage tube or ostomy need to be replaced with additional fluid and electrolytes such as half normal saline milliliter per milliliter to keep serum levels within normal ranges.

DRUG THERAPY

The pharmacokinetics of a drug vary in the neonatal population and change with postconceptional age because of growth, development, and organ maturation. This presents a challenge in the neonate because of differences in absorption, distribution, metabolism, and excretion. Factors responsible for this difficulty in predicting a drug's action re-

late to the neonate's immature hepatic and renal function, poor perfusion that may limit absorption, delayed gastric emptying, high total body water and low body fat, illness, and decreased protein affinity for drugs. Neonatal medication doses are based on the infant's weight. Thus doses can vary tremendously in this population. Caregivers need to be knowledgeable about the drug, dosage, and delivery route to ensure the correct medication is given to the neonate. All drug dosage calculations should be double checked by two nurses before administration.

Absorption of a drug depends on the site of administration and how effectively it transfers into the circulation. The most reliable route of drug administration in the neonate is the intravenous route. Drugs are delivered directly into the bloodstream bypassing the absorption phase and rapidly reaching serum drug concentrations for an immediate drug response. Although intravenous drug therapy is ideal, several problems using this route of drug administration in neonates must be recognized. Rapid serum drug concentrations can lead to undesired and toxic reactions because adequate and equal distribution to all organs is not always guaranteed. Peak serum concentrations may be less than trough concentrations because of inadequate infusion of the entire drug.

In the neonate, absorption from the gastrointestinal tract is delayed and depends on gastrointestinal pH, gastric emptying time, enzyme activity, microbial colonization, and clinical status. Neonates have a gastric pH ranging from 6 to 8, with decreased gastric acid production during the first 30 days of life. Delayed gastric emptying time in the neonate slows passage of a drug into the intestines, resulting in a prolonged absorption phase (Ward, 1994).

Drugs given by the intramuscular route rely on adequate perfusion and muscle mass for greater absorption. In a sick or hypothermic neonate, perfusion may not be adequate causing delayed drug action. With limited amounts of muscle mass, injections may enter the subcutaneous tissue where absorption is slow and unpredictable. Multiple intramuscular injections should be avoided because of ineffective drug concentrations and potential damage to the neonate's tissues that may lead to abscesses (Ward, 1991).

Distribution is the movement of the absorbed drug to and through body fluids, organs, and tissues. An increase in total body water of the neonate, often seen after surgery, may require a larger per kilogram drug dose to achieve the desired concentration and effect (Kenner, Amlung, & Flandermeyer, 1998d). Because fluid status changes rapidly, drug monitoring is needed to ensure adequate serum levels for effective treatment in compromised neonates.

The primary site of drug metabolism is in the liver. Other organs such as the kidneys, intestines, lungs, adrenal glands, and skin are more limited but capable of this function. Many drugs require biotransformation before they can be eliminated from the body. Frequently in the sick neonate biotransformation may be accelerated or slowed because of organ damage, drug interactions, poor nutrition, or disease state. The first-pass effect occurs when a drug moves directly from the intestinal absorption site to the liver and gets metabolized and excreted before reaching target organ sites (Martin, 1993). This can alter drug availability, and, with the poor gastrointestinal motility often seen in the premature neonate, accentuated and unpredictable circulating concentration of the drug may take place.

The elimination of both metabolized and unchanged drug from the body is called excretion. The kidneys provide this function through glomerular filtration, tubular excretion, and tubular reabsorption. Other important organs of excretion are the lungs, gastrointestinal tract, and liver. Glomerular function increases steadily after birth, whereas tubular function matures more slowly, causing a glomerular and tubular imbalance. Renal function of neonates may be changed by hypoxemia, decreased perfusion, and nephrotoxic drugs such as gentamicin, indomethacin, and amphotericin B. All of these factors alter drug elimination. Normally, increased glomerular function reflects improved cardiac output, decreased renal vascular resistance, redistribution of intrarenal blood flow, and changes in basement membrane permeability (Bernhardt, 1990). This may be impaired in neonates after surgical procedures or illness, which makes dosing requirements unpredictable. Carefully individualized titration and blood level monitoring is necessary to ensure safe serum levels of renally excreted medications (Valley, 1997).

Risks of anesthesia are greater in the neonate than in the older infant and adult. This is due to multiple factors related to prematurity, underlying disease processes, and limited physiologic reserves. Problems that may present with anesthetic administration in the neonatal population include inability to maintain a patent airway, poor ventilation and oxygenation leading to respiratory arrest, hypothermia, hypotension, and fluid overload. Adequate preoperative assessment of cardiovascular and respiratory status is necessary to ensure stability during the surgical procedure. Continuous monitoring is essential during the operation to prevent complications.

Historically, systemic analgesia and sedation were rarely administered to neonates. Most believed the neonatal nervous system was not mature enough for perception of pain because of incomplete myelinization (Phillips, 1995). This information led to the undertreatment or lack of treatment of pain in neonates. Anand and colleagues studied premature infants undergoing surgery with minimal anesthesia and found a high incidence of postoperative complications and mortality rates (Franck, 1994). Other research focused on pain perception of neonates revealed that the central nervous system of a second trimester fetus possesses the anatomic and neurochemical capabilities for experiencing pain (Stevens & Franck, 1995).

The difficulty in pain management of neonates is the interpretation of physiologic and behavioral indicators, the neonate's only means of communication. Physiologic parameters that may indicate pain include increased heart and respiratory rates, elevated blood pressure, desaturation, pallor, dilated pupils, apnea, cyanosis, muscle tremors, and palmar sweating (Franck, 1994; Phillips, 1995; Stevens, 1996). In addition, behavioral parameters include localized motor activity such as facial grimacing, brow bulge, eye squeeze, nasolabial furrow, open lips, stretched mouth, lip purse, taut tongue, chin quiver, crying, agitation, and alteration of sleep state (Franck, 1994; Phillips, 1995; Stevens, 1996). It may be difficult to distinguish pain from agitation. Pain assessment measures are unreliable in neonates with low birth weights who receive mechanical ventilation and who are neurologically impaired or sedated. These infants may have a delay or lack of response to painful stimuli because of depletion of physiologic reserves that affect their response capability, thus making it difficult for caregivers to assess pain (Stevens & Franck, 1995).

Agitation can be caused by a number of factors such as environmental overstimulation, respiratory insufficiency, neurologic irritability, and a need to change position. Many problems lead to agitation in the neonate and must be distinguished from pain. Environmental stimulation such as loud noises, bright lights, or certain stimuli associated with unpleasant events may trigger the neonate to exhibit agitation. Nursery staff can minimize noxious stimuli by elimination of unnecessary noise, limiting the number of people at the bedside, and protecting the neonate's environment. Nurses caring for these infants must use their expertise in assessment to distinguish these factors from actual pain and discomfort. A goal of neonatal nurses is to provide comfort and relief of pain by effectively communicating the infant's needs to the health care team.

Two approaches to pain management in neonates are nonpharmacologic and pharmacologic (see Exhibit 33–3) (Franck, 1994; Kenner, Amlung, & Flandermeyer, 1998e; Kenner et al., 1998d; McRae, Rourke, & Imperial-Perez, 1997). Nonpharmacologic pain management techniques support the neonate's own coping mechanisms. Many noxious stimuli in the neonatal intensive care unit result from routine handling and procedures. Often nurses can minimize pain by gentle handling and quick, efficient, skilled execution of invasive procedures (Franck, 1994). Nurses can decrease aversive environmental stimuli by turning down the lights, offering time-out periods, silencing unnecessary alarms, and asking people to speak softly away from the bedside (McRae et al., 1997). Minimal handling protocols are another way in which nurses can change the neonate's environment. This prevents undue stress and allows less interruption of sleep states. Quieting techniques such as swaddling, encouraging nonnutritive sucking, and containment to prevent disorganization aid recovery from stressful procedures. Posting the infant's likes and dislikes at the bedside helps maintain consistency of care and builds trust in these developing neonates.

Postoperative pain can be anticipated in the surgical neonate. Therefore, pharmacologic agents should be instituted. Continuous drip infusions of morphine or fentanyl are frequently used in neonates postoperatively. Morphine provides better sedative effects and there is less tolerance and physical dependence when it is used for long periods of time. Monitor for adverse effects, which include decreased intestinal motility, abdominal distention, respiratory depression, urine retention, and tolerance (Glass, 1993). Fentanyl is short acting and more potent than morphine. One major problem with continuous long-term fentanyl administration is the development of tolerance and physical dependence within 3 to 5 days. Neonates should be weaned slowly off fentanyl over several days to prevent the effects of drug withdrawal. Further information regarding drug therapy can be found in Chapter 6 of this text.

WOUND CARE

The surgical neonate is vulnerable to infection during hospitalization. Thus, the nurse must provide careful wound care in an attempt to prevent infection. Wound healing follows a pattern and is consistent for humans of any age. What is unique in the neonatal population is the neonate's rapid ability to heal. There is less scar hypertrophy occurring from birth to age 1 (Vander Kolk, 1997). However, wound healing can be compromised for a number of reasons. Infection, poor nutrition, impaired circulation, hematomas, and seromas can all contribute to wound dehiscence (Rowe, O'Neill, Grosfeld, Fonkalsrud, & Coran, 1995b). Wound dehiscence is managed with wet-to-dry dressings to allow the wound to granulate and contract.

Wound infection can occur during or after the surgical procedure and can be a complicating factor. Neonates are at an immunologic disadvantage because IgA and IgM immunoglobulins do not transfer from mother to fetus in utero. However, IgG transfers across the placenta beginning at 32 weeks' gestational age. Near-term neonates receive passive immunization from their mother. Although the neonate can mount an immune response with granulocytes, there is a relative lack of complement factor and impaired neutrophil migration, which makes this response less effective. Neonates have minimal to no antigen exposure and overwhelming sepsis can develop from bacterial proliferation and overgrowth. Postoperative wound infections in the newborn may require treatment with antibiotics. Infection occurs more frequently after a "contaminated" surgery, such as an intestinal perforation, versus a "clean" surgery, such as ligation of a patent ductus arteriosus (Jankelelvich, 1998).

The first dressing change is typically performed by the surgeons. Gentle restraints or analgesia may be required if the dressing change is painful or the infant is vigorous. Nursing assessment of the surgical site is ongoing. These observations may provide the first indication of wound infection or poor healing. If any suspicion of infection exists, blood cultures should be drawn before initiating broad-spectrum antibiotics that target both aerobes and anaerobes, grampositive and gram-negative organisms. Obtaining urine and cerebral spinal fluid (CSF) needs to be considered because neonates are vulnerable to overwhelming sepsis with infection from any site.

NUTRITIONAL SUPPORT

At birth, the neonate has substantial nutritional demands because of a high metabolic rate, rapid growth, and development. Compared with older infants the neonate has limited

Exhibit 33–3 Pharmacologic and Nonpharmacologic Interventions for Pain Management in Neonates

Pharmacologic	Nonpharmacologic
Mild pain	*Environment interventions*
Acetaminophen (Tylenol)	Dim lights
Moderate to severe pain	Decrease or minimize noise
Opioids	Time out periods
Morphine	Turning off radios and unnecessary alarms
Fentanyl	Speak softly
Systemic analgesia	Conduct rounds away from bedside
Epidural (bupivacaine with an opioid	Acoustical tile
fentanyl or morphine)	Spot lighting
Local anesthetics	*Infant interventions*
Lidocaine	Provide boundaries for infants
EMLA (Eutectic mixture of local	Group together invasive procedures
anesthetics)	Pacifier-nonnutritive sucking
Agitation control	Hand-to-mouth sucking
Sedative/hypnotic	Holding during painful procedure
Lorazepam (Ativan)	Gentle handling
Midazolam (Versed)	Rest periods between procedures
Chloral hydrate	Minimal handling protocol initiated
	Swaddling/containment/nesting
	Positioning on side or prone (stomach)
	Kinesthetic motion (rhythmic, repetitive, cyclic stimulation) (i.e., waterbed, rocking)
	Tactile stimulation (i.e., massage, stroking)

caloric stores, and surgical neonates are at a much higher risk of malnutrition as a result of increased metabolic demands from surgery, nutrient losses, and sepsis (Scharil, 1996). In the neonate, the gastrointestinal tract is structurally and functionally mature by 33 to 34 weeks' gestation for adequate absorption and use of nutrients to support growth. However, several anatomic and physiologic characteristics exist that can compromise the neonate's nutrition such as poor suck-swallow coordination, absent or weak gag reflexes, and an incompetent gastroesophageal sphincter, which puts the neonate at risk for aspiration. Another characteristic of neonates that limits adequate intake is their small stomach size, with an average capacity of 30 ml (Lefrak-Okikawa & Meier, 1993). They also have delayed gastric emptying time and decreased intestinal motility, both of which become more pronounced after surgical interventions. Intestinal enzymes needed for protein digestion and carbohydrate and fat absorption are decreased because of immaturity or compromise of the gastrointestinal system affecting growth and development of all organ systems.

Early identification of the surgical neonate at risk for nutritional deficiency is the first step toward proper nutritional management. Daily caloric requirements in healthy neonates average 100 to 120 kcal/kg/day but may be as high as 150 to 180 kcal/kg/day for premature or medically compromised neonates. This intake can be achieved with total parenteral nutrition, 20 kcal per ounce formulas, or mother's breast milk, which is the preferred formula because it contains immunoglobulins and digestive enzymes and enhances gut growth (Bryan & Zlotkin, 1993; D'Garkubgyem & Bryne, 1991; Scharil, 1996). Expected weight gain for preterm neonates is approximately 20 to 30 gm/kg/day and term neonates average 10 to 15 gm/kg/day. Daily weight changes may reflect fluctuations in body water, but over several days the average indicates growth trends (Luck, 1990; Taylor, 1997).

Approximately 20% to 30% of surgically stressed neonates have increased nutritional requirements needed to promote wound healing, maintain adequate respiratory function, and resist infection (Taylor, 1997). Daily caloric requirements should be assessed on an individual basis and reassessed as the neonate's condition changes. An appropriate distribution of calories for adequate nutrition in healthy or compromised neonates should contain 8% to 12% of total caloric intake as protein, 35% to 55% as carbohydrates, and 35% to 55% as fat (Fletcher, 1994; Lefrak-Okikawa & Meier, 1993). Carbohydrates, especially glucose, are one of the neonate's main energy nutrients and are essential to the brain for normal metabolism (Luck, 1990). Premature neonates need approximately 4 to 6 mg/kg/min of glucose and term neonates need 8 to 10 mg/kg/min to maintain glucose use and stores. Protein is needed for adequate growth, synthesis of enzymes and hormones, wound healing, and increased energy. Neonates undergoing surgery need 2.5 to 3.5 gm/kg/day of protein to maintain sufficient weight gain and nitrogen balance. Fats are a major source for growth, metabolism, and muscle activity with total daily needs of 3 to 4 gm/kg/day. As a rule, no more than 60% of calories should be given as fat to allow for metabolic clearing and prevent complications of fat malabsorption (Fletcher, 1994). Surgical neonates require optimal nutritional intake preoperatively to promote successful recovery during the postoperative healing phase.

The development of total parenteral nutrition (TPN) has increased the quality and length of survival in surgically compromised neonates who would otherwise have malnutrition or die. TPN may be infused by peripheral IV, percutaneous central venous catheter, or central line access and initiated in those neonates who are without enteral intake for more than 3 days or have delayed intestinal function. Further explanation of TPN can be found in Chapter 4 of this text.

Nurses have an important task in the initiation of enteral feedings to premature or compromised neonates. Close monitoring during advancement of feedings can provide clues to intolerance. Nursing assessment for signs of feeding difficulties include bilious aspirates, vomiting, diarrhea, and abdominal distention. Stool consistency and color should also be noted and the stool checked for reducing substances indicative of carbohydrate malabsorption and blood in the stool, an early sign of necrotizing enterocolitis, a common occurrence in premature infants (Harjo & Jones, 1993; Taylor, 1997). Any of these signs warrant further investigation and should be reported immediately to the surgical team.

To facilitate tolerance of enteral feedings nurses should provide neonates the opportunity for nonnutritive sucking during gavage feedings, which accelerates maturation of the sucking reflex, decreases oxygen consumption, and improves weight gain (Kenner et al., 1998e). Prone or right side down positions during or after feedings may also be initiated to improve gastric emptying time and prevent regurgitation and aspiration. Reducing stress and stimulation before or during feedings decreases fluctuations in oxygenation that may interfere with gut perfusion and function (Estrada & Brennan-Behm, 1993).

Nurses and clinicians can evaluate individual neonates for adequate growth and nutrition by plotting anthropometric measurements of daily weight, weekly head circumference, length, fluid, and caloric intake on the bedside growth chart. The most sensitive indicator of good nutrition in neonates is the head circumference, with average increases between 0.5 cm and 1.0 cm per week. If problems are seen, adjustments can be made in the nutritional plan to ensure optimal growth.

FAMILY FOCUS, DISCHARGE, AND FOLLOW-UP

Parenting the surgical neonate is unlike parenting the normal newborn. Different approaches must be initiated by the health care team for successful parental attachment, newborn care, and discharge planning. Nurses need to focus their educational efforts on family adaptation to stresses that accompany the surgical neonate, as well as the stresses parents experience in having a newborn. Parents of premature neonates often do not immediately experience normal newborn events such as holding and feeding their infant. This is due to early stabilization of the critically ill neonate requiring immediate surgical interventions or transport to a local tertiary care facility for further evaluation and management. In some cases, parents have no preparation for their infant's surgical interventions until immediately after delivery. This can interfere with parent-infant attachment and continue for some period of time.

Parents of the surgical neonate often are unable to complete the three final steps of attachment—(1) hearing and seeing the infant, (2) touching and holding the infant, and (3) caretaking, as identified by Klaus and Kennell—for days to sometimes weeks after the birth of their infant (Klaus & Kennel, 1979). Parents often show hesitancy in accepting care responsibilities because of this delayed parent-infant attachment, which can lead to interaction deprivation. This can affect the mother's commitment to her infant, her maternal self-confidence in her ability to mother the infant, and altered behavior toward the infant in such areas as infant stimulation and skilled caregiving (Barnett, Leiderman, Grobstein, & Klaus, 1970). Parent-infant bonding can be strengthened if parents are allowed to feed, bathe, and change their newborn. Mothers who are breastfeeding should be encouraged to provide breast milk for the infant despite their feeding status. Mothers can store their expressed milk in sterile plastic bags or containers and freeze them for later use. This gives mothers the sense that they are providing something that is beneficial for their infants.

Moehn and Rossetti (1996) looked at the effects of neonatal intensive care on parental emotions and attachment. The study provided nurses with insights on how to empower parents as caregivers. The study concluded that nurses must be sensitive listeners and must acknowledge parental feelings and provide for their needs, knowing that parents experience stressors based on their infant's condition and their personal experiences. Second, nurses should identify parental stressors through interaction and communication with parents rather than through assumption and they should include parents in the everyday care of their infant to allow parents the opportunity to assume the caregiver role. Last, nurses must help prepare parents throughout the hospital course for the neonate's discharge home (Moehn & Rossetti, 1996). Maintaining daily communication with parents to keep them informed of their infant's progress is a top priority of the health care team members. Providing parents with a consistent nurturing environment eases the transition into successful parenting and facilitates the process of acceptance of their surgical neonate.

In the preoperative period, a tour of the NICU allows parents the opportunity to meet the members of the health care team and familiarize themselves with the unique NICU environment. During the tour, nurses can talk with parents about what to expect in the immediate preoperative period and throughout the neonate's stay in the hospital. This affords parents the opportunity to prepare for the birth of their child and the surgery. Parent teaching begins in the preoperative period. Initial nursing responsibilities include helping parents become familiar with intrusive medical equipment and helping parents understand the need for stabilization of their infant before surgery. Allowing parents to perform simple caregiving needs for their infant strengthens parent-infant attachments and eases the feeling of helplessness during the initial preoperative period.

Parents should be helped to cope with the stress of uncertainty. During pregnancy they fantasize their newborn to be healthy and perfect. With the birth of a sick neonate, those perceptions are shattered for the whole family, leaving them in a psychologically disorganized state in which their normal coping skills become inadequate (Seigel, Gardner, & Merenstein, 1989). Encouraging parents to verbalize their feelings and concerns is most helpful during this stressful time. Nurses can discuss with parents ways in which they can personalize their infant's bedside with pictures of their family, stuffed animals, and colorful name cards. This will give the parents an opportunity to feel like they can do something for their infant.

Most critically ill neonates are sensitive to environmental stimuli and gentle touching because of their limited energy reserves. Parents are initially unable to determine when to soothe, when to touch, and when not to touch. Parents may see their infant respond to their touch by turning away, grimacing, and crying inconsolably. This type of infant behavior is viewed by parents as negative, making it difficult for them to cope and understand. Nurses must guide parents in understanding their infant's cues to overstimulation, pain, and contentment.

"Going home" are two words that elicit joy, disbelief, anxiety, and ambivalence in the parents of the surgical neonate. While in the hospital, parents come to depend on the supportive environment of the NICU to understand and cope with the behavior and care of their infant (Kenner & Baggwell, 1994). The transition from hospital to home begins on admission. For most parents, taking home their infant is one of the most stressful times. When their infant has had surgery and has been hospitalized since birth, the stress is even greater. Nurses need to help parents become the primary caregivers for their neonate and instill in them the confidence and skills necessary to care for their infant on their own (Moehn & Rossetti, 1996). The surgical neonate may often go home needing more than just normal newborn care. Parents should be instructed in medication administration, formula preparation, use of special equipment, and emergencies that require physician input. Many resources are available to families to make the transition to home smoother. Educational pamphlets given to parents are an excellent way to educate them regarding such things as signs of infection, how to care for a gastrostomy tube, and wound care.

Before discharge, a systematic assessment to collect information about the needs of the surgical neonate and the family is warranted. This information identifies concerns in the home environment and with the parent-infant interaction and is used to evaluate areas for further interventions or referrals to other services. Nurses familiar with the infant and family play a vital role in this assessment process. Their input determines the type of services that may be needed to provide a smooth transition to the home environment for parents and their infant.

Most parents return for a postoperative surgical visit within 2 weeks of discharge. This follow-up visit provides an opportunity to assess wound healing, monitor weight gain, and reinforce discharge teaching. Encourage parents to ask questions and begin to discuss additional surgical interventions. Further follow-up appointments with their primary care provider are needed to initiate the infant's immunizations and monitor the neonate's developmental progress.

CONCLUSION

Nurses and clinicians who provide care to surgical neonates must have a thorough working knowledge and understanding of neonatal physiology and care practices that set them apart from other infants. Initiation of routine prenatal screening has allowed early detection of neonates needing surgery immediately after delivery. Prenatal counseling and referral to the closest high-risk perinatal center offering pediatric surgical services provides the neonate with the best possible chance for survival.

Considerable challenges exist in the neonate's medical and surgical management requiring immediate interventions. Stabilization of the neonate before surgery must take place to optimize the neonate's ability to withstand anesthesia and the surgical procedure with minimal complications. Neonates are at increased risk for problems with thermoregulation, fluid and electrolyte disturbances, cardiorespiratory compromise, pain, inadequate nutrition, and infection.

Family support throughout the hospital stay is the responsibility of all health care team members. Parent participation in their infant's care from admission to discharge builds confidence and provides the skills needed to care for their infant at home. Neonates require expert care from a multidisciplinary team approach and a thorough knowledge of the principles of management during the preoperative, intraoperative, and postoperative phases to ensure the best possible outcomes.

REFERENCES

Adcock, E.W., Consolvo, C.A., & Berry, D.D. (1998). Fluid and electrolyte management. In G.G. Merenstein & S.L. Garner (Eds.), *Handbook of neonatal intensive care* (4th ed., pp. 243–258). St. Louis, MO: Mosby.

Barnett, C.R., Leiderman, P.H., Grobstein, R., & Klaus, M.H. (1970). Neonatal separation: The maternal side of interactional deprivation. *Pediatrics, 45,* 197–205.

Bernhardt, J. (1990). Renal/genitourinary disorders. In P. Beachy & J. Deacon (Eds.), *Core curriculum for neonatal intensive care nursing* (pp. 365–393). Philadelphia: W.B. Saunders Company.

Bryan, H., & Zlotkin, S. (1993). Prenatal and postnatal nutrition. In J. Pomerance & C. Richardson (Eds.), *Neonatology for the clinician* (pp. 123–137). Norwalk, CT: Appleton & Lange.

D'Garkubgycm, A., & Byrne, W. (1991). Nutrition in the newborn. In H. Taeusch, R. Ballard, & M. Avery (Eds.), *Diseases of the newborn* (6th ed., pp. 709–727). Philadelphia: W.B. Saunders Company.

Duncan, B.W., & Adzick, N.S. (1996). Perinatal diagnosis of surgical diseases. In P. Puri (Ed.), *Newborn surgery* (pp. 15–23). Oxford: Butterworth-Heinemann.

Estrada, E., & Brennan-Behm, M. (1993). Neonatal nutrition. In P. Beachy & J. Deacon (Eds.), *Core curriculum for neonatal intensive care nursing* (pp. 254–280). Philadelphia: W.B. Saunders Company.

Flanagan, M., & Fyler, D. (1994). Cardiac disease. In G. Avery, M. Fletcher, & M. MacDonald (Eds.), *Neonatology: Pathophysiology and management of the newborn* (4th ed., pp. 516–559). Philadelphia: J.B. Lippincott-Raven Publishers.

Fletcher, A. (1994). Nutrition. In G. Avery, M. Fletcher, & M. MacDonald (Eds.), *Neonatology: Pathophysiology and management of the newborn* (4th ed., pp. 330–356). Philadelphia: Lippincott-Raven Publishers.

Franck, L. (1994). Identification, management, and prevention of pain in the neonate. In C. Kenner, A. Brueggemeyer, & L. Gunderson (Eds.), *Comprehensive neonatal nursing* (pp. 913–925). Philadelphia: W.B. Saunders Company.

Glass, S. (1993). Neonatal pain management. In P. Beachy & J. Deacon (Eds.), *Core curriculum for neonatal intensive care nursing* (pp. 695–697). Philadelphia: W.B. Saunders Company.

Gorman, W.A. (1996). Fluid and electrolyte balance in the newborn. In P. Puri (Ed.), *Newborn surgery* (pp. 72–81). Great Britain: The University Press.

Gregory, G. (1992). Anesthesia for premature infants. In A. Fanaroff & R. Martin (Eds.), *Neonatal-perinatal medicine: Diseases of the fetus and infant* (pp. 456–464). St. Louis, MO: Mosby.

Hansen, T., & Corbet, A. (1998). Diseases of the airways. In H. Taeusch & R. Ballard (Eds.), *Avery's diseases of the newborn* (pp. 661–667). Philadelphia: W.B. Saunders Company.

Harjo, J., & Jones, M. (1993). The surgical neonate. In C. Kenner, A. Brueggemeyer, & L. Gunderson (Eds.), *Comprehensive neonatal nursing: A physiologic perspective* (pp. 903–912). Philadelphia: W.B. Saunders Company.

Holtzclaw, B. (1990). Temperature problems in the post-operative period. *Critical Care Nursing Clinics of North America, 2*(4), 589–598.

Jankelelvich, S. (1998). Wounds, abscesses and other infections caused by anaerobic bacteria. In S. Katz, A. Gershon, & P. Hotez (Eds.), *Krugman's infectious diseases of children* (pp. 667–705). St. Louis, MO: Mosby.

Kenner, C., Amlung, S., & Flandermeyer, A. (1998a). Assessment and management of respiratory dysfunction: New care technologies. In C. Kenner, S. Amlung, & A. Flandermeyer (Eds.), *Protocols in neonatal nursing* (pp. 101–136). Philadelphia: W.B. Saunders Company.

Kenner, C., Amlung, S., & Flandermeyer, A. (1998b). Assessment and management of gastrointestinal dysfunction. In C. Kenner, S. Amlung, & A. Flandermeyer (Eds.), *Protocols in neonatal nursing* (pp. 197–257). Philadelphia: W.B. Saunders Company.

Kenner, C., Amlung, S., & Flandermeyer, A. (1998c). Assessment and management of hematologic dysfunction. In C. Kenner, S. Amlung, & A. Flandermeyer (Eds.), *Protocols in neonatal nursing* (pp. 357–396). Philadelphia: W.B. Saunders Company.

Kenner, C., Amlung, S., & Flandermeyer, A. (1998d). Principles of neonatal drug therapy. In C. Kenner, S. Amlung, & A. Flandermeyer (Eds.), *Protocols in neonatal nursing* (pp. 604–615). Philadelphia: W.B. Saunders Company.

Kenner, C., Amlung, S., & Flandermeyer, A. (1998e). Neonatal development. In C. Kenner, S. Amlung, & A. Flandermeyer (Eds.), *Protocols in neonatal nursing* (pp. 660–678). Philadelphia: W.B. Saunders Company.

Kenner, C., & Baggwell, G. (1994). Assessment and management of the transition to home. In C. Kenner, A. Brueggemeyer, & L. Gunderson (Eds.), *Comprehensive neonatal nursing: A physiologic perspective* (pp. 1134–1147). Philadelphia: W.B. Saunders Company.

Klaus, M., & Kennel, J. (1979). Care of the parents. In M. Klaus & A. Fanaroff (Eds.), *Care of the high risk neonate* (pp. 146–172). Philadelphia: W.B. Saunders Company.

Lefrak-Okikawa, L., & Meier, P. (1993). Nutrition: Physiologic basis of metabolism and management of enteral and parenteral nutrition. In C. Kenner, A. Brueggemeyer, & L. Gunderson (Eds.), *Comprehensive neonatal nursing: A physiologic perspective* (pp. 414–433). Philadelphia: W.B. Saunders Company.

Letton, R., & Chwals, W. (1997). Fluid and electrolyte management. In K. Oldham, P. Colombani, & R. Foglia (Eds.), *Surgery of infants and children: Scientific principles and practice* (pp. 83–96). Philadelphia: Lippincott-Raven Publishers.

Luck, S. (1990). Nutrition and metabolism. In J. Raffensperger (Ed.), *Swenson's pediatric surgery* (5th ed., pp. 81–90). Norwalk, CT: Appleton & Lange.

Martin, R. (1993). Pharmacology in neonatal care. In P. Beachy & J. Deacon (Eds.), *Core curriculum for neonatal intensive care nursing* (pp. 501–519). Philadelphia: W.B. Saunders Company.

McRae, M., Rourke, D., & Imperial-Perez, F. (1997). Development of a research-based standard for assessment, intervention, and evaluation of pain after neonatal and pediatric cardiac surgery. *Pediatric Nursing, 23*(3), 263–271.

Moehn, D., & Rossetti, L. (1996). The effects of neonatal care on parental emotions and attachment. *Infant-Toddler Intervention, 6*(3), 229–246.

Perlstein, P. (1992). Physical environment. In A. Fanaroff & R. Martin (Eds.), *Neonatal-perinatal medicine: Diseases of the fetus and infant* (pp. 401–419). St. Louis, MO: Mosby.

Phillips, P. (1995). Neonatal pain management: A call to action. *Pediatric Nursing, 21*(2), 195–199.

Plouffe, L., & Donahue, J. (1994). Techniques for early diagnosis of the abnormal fetus. *Clinics in Perinatology, 21,* 723–741.

Puri, P., & Sweed, Y. (1996). Preoperative assessment. In P. Puri (Ed.), *Newborn surgery* (pp. 41–51). Great Britain: The University Press.

Rowe, M., O'Neil, J., Grosfeld, J., Fonkalsrud, E., & Coran, A. (1995a). Prenatal diagnosis and fetal surgery. *Essentials of pediatric surgery* (pp. 15–23). St. Louis, MO: Mosby.

Rowe, M., O'Neill, J., Grosfeld, J., Fonkalsrud, E., & Coran, A. (1995b). Nutritional support of the pediatric surgical patient. *Essentials of pediatric surgery* (pp. 76–93). St. Louis, MO: Mosby.

Rushton, C. (1988). The surgical neonate: Principles of nursing management. *Pediatric Nursing, 14*(2), 141–151.

Scharil, A. (1996). Nutrition. In P. Puri (Ed.), *Newborn surgery* (pp. 82–94). Great Britain: The University Press.

Seigel, R., Gardner, S., & Merenstein, G. (1989). Families in crisis: Theoretical and practical considerations. In G. Merenstein & S. Gardner (Eds.), *Handbook of neonatal intensive care* (2nd ed., pp. 565–592). St. Louis, MO: Mosby.

Shaw, N. (1990). Common surgical problems in the newborn. *Journal of Perinatal Neonatal Nursing, 3,* 50–65.

Shirley, I., Bottomley, F., & Robinson, V. (1992). Routine radiographer screening for fetal abnormalities by ultrasound in an unselected low risk population. *The British Journal of Radiology, 65,* 565–569.

Skupski, D., Chervenak, F., & McCullough, L. (1994). Is routine ultrasound screening for all patients? *Clinics in Perinatology, 21,* 707–721.

Stevens, B. (1996). Pain management in newborns: How far have we progressed in research and practice? *Birth, 23*(4), 229–235.

Stevens, B., & Franck, L. (1995). Special needs of preterm infants in the management of pain and discomfort. *Journal of Obstetric and Gynecologic Neonatal Nursing, 24*(9), 856–862.

Taylor, L. (1997). Nutrition and central venous access. In D. Nakayama, C. Bose, N. Chescheir, & R. Valley (Eds.), *Critical care of the surgical newborn* (pp. 125–153). New York: Futura Publishing.

Valley, R. (1997). Anesthesia and postoperative pain management. In D. Nakayama, C. Bose, N. Chescheir, & R. Valley (Eds.), *Critical care of the surgical newborn* (pp. 125–153). New York: Futura Publishing.

Vander Kolk, C. (1997). Plastic and reconstructive surgery. In K. Oldham, P. Colombani, & R. Foglia (Eds.), *Surgery of infants and children* (pp. 1633–1645). Philadelphia: Lippincott-Raven Publishers.

Ward, R. (1991). Pharmacologic principles and practicalities. In H. Taeusch, R. Ballard, & M. Avery (Eds.), *Shaffer and Avery's: Diseases of the newborn* (6th ed., pp. 285–292). Philadelphia: W.B. Saunders Company.

Ward, R. (1994). The use of therapeutic drugs. In G. Avery, M. Fletcher, & M. MacDonald (Eds.), *Neonatology: Pathophysiology and management of the newborn* (4th ed., pp. 1271–1299). Philadelphia: Lippincott-Raven Publishers.

Warde, D. (1996). Anaesthesia. In P. Puri (Ed.), *Newborn surgery* (pp. 52–61). Great Britain: The University Press.

PART VII

Nursing Care of the Injured Child

CHAPTER 34

Pediatric Trauma

Pam Pieper

INTRODUCTION

Injuries, often preventable, occur in seconds and have the potential to kill or permanently change the life of a child. The goal of those involved in pediatric trauma is to prevent its occurrence and treat those affected so as to maximize their potential for recovery. This chapter presents an overview of the nursing care required by the pediatric trauma patient.

Epidemiology

Approximately 16 million injured children are seen in emergency departments annually in the United States, with about 600,000 requiring hospitalization. Trauma is the number one killer of children older than the age of 1. Thirty-nine percent of the deaths of children younger than 14 in 1995 (5,695 children) were caused by injuries (Tepas, 2000). The number of children estimated to have a permanent impairment as a result of trauma is more than 50,000/year (Schafermeyer, 1993). Local injury data should be reviewed to develop prevention strategies.

Host Factors

Common mechanisms of injury vary with the developmental level, usually correlating with the age of the child. Other host factors that affect injury rates are gender and race. By the age of 1, boys are injured more often than girls, and by adolescence their injury rate is twice that of girls (Wesson & Hu, 1995). Male homicide rates are approximately triple those of females (Li et al., 1996) and approximately one half of homicide victims are black. Although suicide rates are higher for males than females, females attempt suicide three times more often than males. The suicide rate for whites is twice the rate of nonwhites (Wesson & Hu, 1995).

Environmental Factors

The most significant environmental factor affecting injury patterns in children is their socioeconomic status. Children who live in poverty die 2.6 times more often than those who do not (Nersesian, Petit, Shaper, Lemieux, & Naor, 1985). Risk factor exposure is higher in impoverished children; for example, they are less likely to be restrained in a motor vehicle or to wear a helmet when bicycle riding.

Intentional injuries include child abuse, interpersonal violence, and suicide. The actual rate of child abuse, which includes physical, emotional, and sexual abuse, is unknown (Durch & Lohr, 1993). In 1994, 48 states had a total of more than 1 million cases of reported child abuse and neglect, and 1,111 of those children died (Hennes, 1998).

Injury Prevention

Injury prevention is by far the most effective and cost-efficient method to address the issue of pediatric trauma. Primary care nurses have an important opportunity to provide developmentally appropriate anticipatory guidance at each well-child visit. Unfortunately, many nurses' first contact is after the child has already been injured. The child and family should be educated about injury prevention specifically related to the child's situation during the hospitalization and before discharge.

The most cost-effective, and therefore the highest priority, injury prevention strategy involves automatic protection and elimination of environmental hazards (Maier, 1993). Airbags and automatic seat belts are two examples of design changes that provide automatic protection. Another strategy is legislative change that requires alteration in risk-taking behavior, such as bicycle helmet laws. The least effective strategy is education because it requires an audience motivated to change its behavior (Shafi et al., 1998). Programs are most effective (1) with significant local involvement and (2) when they are aimed at a specific problem occurring within a defined high-risk population. Injury prevention strategies others have found to be successful include those published by Birkland (1993), Martin, Langley, and Coffman (1995), and Stylianos and Eichelberger (1993).

CLINICAL PRESENTATION

Prehospital Triage

Triage protocols are most important for those children with serious brain, internal, and skeletal injuries to avoid preventable death and disability. The survival rate in those children who are taken to pediatric trauma centers is approximately 10 times greater than if they were treated elsewhere (Cooper et al., 1993). One method to determine which children require treatment at a pediatric trauma center is by using triage criteria such as the Pediatric Trauma Score (PTS) (see Table 34–1 for a modified version of the PTS) (Tepas, Mollitt, Talbert, & Bryant, 1987). The purpose of this scoring system is rapid assessment of the severity of a child's injury by prehospital providers in the midst of an often chaotic situation. A more detailed "Field Triage Decision Scheme" is presented in *Resources for Optimal Care of the Injured Patient: 1999* (Committee on Trauma, American College of Surgeons, 1998).

Primary Survey

The primary survey includes evaluation of the child's airway with cervical spine immobilization, breathing and ventilation, circulation with hemorrhage control, disability in terms of neurologic status, and exposure with thorough examination for any obvious injuries (Silverman, 1993). Although the assessment and treatment priorities are the same in children and adults, there are a number of anatomic differences that must be taken into consideration (American College of Surgeons Committee on Trauma, 1997).

Airway

The anatomy of the child's airway is different from that of an adult's (see Exhibit 34–1). In a child without a possible neck injury, placing the child in the sniffing position easily opens the airway. If there is any possibility of a neck injury, the jaw thrust is used to open the airway while maintaining the cervical spine in neutral position (Silverman, 1993). Any obstructing material should be suctioned from the oropharynx and also the nares in neonates because they are obligate nasal breathers. An oropharyngeal or nasopharyngeal airway may be needed to maintain a patent airway. A nasopharyn-

geal airway should be used in conscious and semiconscious children because an oropharyngeal airway may elicit the gag reflex and stimulate vomiting in these patients (Chameides & Hazinski, 1997).

Oxygen should be provided at 100% by means of blow-by, mask, or nasal cannula in children with questionable airway reliability. Endotracheal intubation is indicated for children with a Glasgow Coma Score (GCS) of ≤8 (see Exhibit 34–2), who are unable to maintain an adequate airway, or who are hypovolemic to the extent that operative intervention is required (American College of Surgeons Committee on Trauma, 1997). Orotracheal intubation is recommended for children because it is technically easier (Chameides & Hazinski, 1997; American College of Surgeons Committee on Trauma, 1997). The most accurate method for determining the appropriate sized endotracheal tube (ETT) needed is the length-based Broselow tape (Luten et al., 1992). If this tape is not available, an ETT with an outside diameter approximating the diameter of the child's little finger or external nares or the formula ETT mm internal diameter = (age in years/4) + 4 for children older than 2 years of age may be used. An uncuffed ETT should be used in children younger than 8 to 10 years of age. A natural seal is formed at the narrowest portion of the airway, the cricoid ring. Figure 34–1 shows a protocol used for emergency intubation called rapid sequence intubation or induction (RSI). The most frequent complication of endotracheal intubation is right mainstem bronchial intubation. This occurs more frequently in infants and children because of the short length of their tracheas. Breath sounds and the quality of chest rise should be assessed frequently after intubation.

Breathing

Normal vital signs for infants and children are presented in Table 34–2. Because they are diaphragmatic breathers, infants and young children have compromised ventilation any time full diaphragmatic excursion is impaired. The most common reason for this is gastric distention caused by the swallowing of air when the child is crying or assisted ventilation with a face mask. Gastric distention is relieved by passing a nasogastric or orogastric tube.

Pulse oximetry is useful in assessing oxygenation as long as there is adequate peripheral perfusion. Carbon dioxide measurements may be followed in intubated patients with an end tidal CO_2 monitor. These readings are correlated with the $PaCO_2$ from an arterial blood gas. A tension pneumothorax is suspected in an intubated child on positive-pressure ventilation whose respiratory status acutely deteriorates (see Figure 34–2 and Table 34–5). Treatment of acidosis with sodium bicarbonate before the establishment of adequate ventilation and perfusion is contraindicated because it leads to increased hypercarbia and acidosis (American College of Surgeons Committee on Trauma, 1997).

Table 34–1 Color Coded Pediatric Trauma Score

Component	+2		+1		−1	
Size	Orange, green[a] >20 kg (44+ lb)	G	Yellow, white, blue[a] 10–20 kg (22–43 lb)	G	Red, purple[a] <10 kg (<22 lb)	B
Airway	Normal	G	Adjunct (e.g., O₂, mask, cannula, oral/ nasal airway)	G	Assisted or intubated (BVM, ETT, EOA, Cric)	R
Consciousness	Awake	G	Amnesia or any reliable history of loss of consciousness	B	Altered mental status (drowsy/lethargic/ unresponsive) or paralysis or suspected spinal cord fracture	R
Circulation	Good peripheral pulses/ perfusion; SBP >90 mm Hg	G	Carotid/femoral pulses palpable; SBP 50–90 mm Hg	B	Weak or no palpable pulses; SBP <50 mm Hg	R
Fracture	None seen or suspected	G	Single closed fracture anywhere	B	Any open long bone fracture or multiple fractures	R
Cutaneous	No visible injury	G	Contusion, abrasion, or laceration <3"	G	Laceration >3" or any penetrating injury to head, neck, or torso or amputation/tissue loss or 2°/3° burns to >10% TBSA	R

R = any one (1)—transport to trauma center
B = any two (2)—transport to trauma center
G = follow local protocols

[a] Colors listed relate to those found on Broselow tape.

Exhibit 34–1 Airway and Breathing Differences in Children

Airway	Pediatric airway more likely to become obstructed
	Diameter and length smaller[a]
	Tongue relatively larger in oropharynx[a]
	Head to body ratio larger → neck flexion[b]
	Narrowest portion of airway at the cricoid carti-
	lage (<10 years old)[a]
	Larynx funnel shaped[a]
Breathing	Infants and young children are diaphragmatic
	breathers
	Compromised ventilation with impairment of
	diaphragmatic excursion[a]
	Gastric distention most common reason
	Swallow air when crying
	Assisted ventilation with face mask
	Relieved with nasogastric or orogastric tube

[a]Chameides & Hazinski, 1997. [b]Tobias, 1996.

Circulation

Reflex tachycardia and peripheral vasoconstriction in children allow them to present with normal blood pressures until they have lost approximately 25% (20 ml/kg) of their total blood volume (American College of Surgeons Committee on Trauma, 1997; Chameides & Hazinski, 1997). However, tachycardia is caused not only by hypovolemia but also by pain and fear, both of which frequently occur in injured children. The use of capillary refill as an indicator of hypovolemia should be avoided because of the effect ambient temperature has on capillary refill (Baraff, 1993; Gorlick, Shaw, & Baker, 1993). Systemic responses of children to hypovolemia are presented in Table 34–3. When a source of ongoing blood loss is visible, direct pressure and elevation usually stop the bleeding (Graneto & Soglin, 1993; Silverman, 1993).

Two large-bore peripheral intravenous (IV) lines are inserted, preferably in the upper extremities, to facilitate rapid infusion of fluids to restore circulating volume. If it is not possible to start an IV within a few minutes, intraosseus (IO)

Exhibit 34–2 Pediatric Coma Scale

Eye Opening			
<1 Year		*>1 Year*	*Score*
Spontaneously		Spontaneously	4
To shout		To verbal command	3
To pain		To pain	2
No response		No response	1
Best Verbal Response			
0–23 Months	*2 to 5 Years*	*>5 Years*	5
Smiles, coos appropriately	Appropriate words/phrases	Oriented and converses	4
Cries, consolable	Inappropriate words	Disoriented and converses	3
Persistent inappropriate crying and/ or screaming	Persistent crying and screaming	Inappropriate words	
			2
Grunts, agitated, restless	Grunts	Incomprehensible sounds	1
No response	No response	No response	
Best Motor Response			
<1 Year		*>1 Year*	
Spontaneous		Obeys	6
Localized pain		Localizes pain	5
Flexion-withdrawal		Flexion-withdrawal	4
Flexion-abnormal (decorticate rigidity)		Flexion-abnormal (decorticate rigidity)	3
			2
Extension (decerebrate)		Extension (decerebrate rigidity)	1
No response		No response	

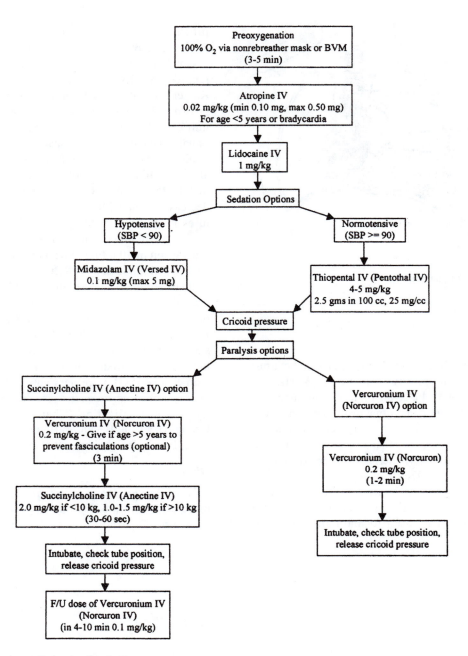

Figure 34–1 Rapid Sequence Induction/Intubation

Table 34–2 Normal Pediatric Vital Signs: Upper Limits of Heart and Respiratory Rates, Lower Limits of Systolic Blood Pressure

Age Group	Heart Rate (beats minute)	Systolic Blood Pressure (mm Hg)	Respiratory Rate (breaths/minute)
Birth to 6 mo	180–160	60–80	60
Infant	160	80	40
Preschool	120	90	30
Adolescent	100	100	20

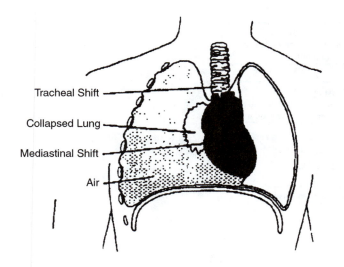

Figure 34–2 Tension Pneumothorax

Tracheal Shift

Collapsed Lung

Mediastinal Shift

Air

access allows drugs, fluids, and blood products to be infused directly into the bone marrow (Chameides & Hazinski, 1997; Silverman, 1993). Place an IO in the proximal tibial plateau, the distal femur, distal tibia, or the sternum (Tepas, 2000). It should not be placed in an injured extremity. Although it is generally suggested that an IO only be attempted in children ≤6 years of age (American College of Surgeons Committee on Trauma, 1997; Chameides & Hazinski, 1997). Guy, Haley, and Zuspan (1993) determined that an IO can easily be inserted in older children. They suggest that pressure infusion devices be used to maintain flow of the

infusate. Central venous lines and peripheral venous cutdowns may be attempted by experienced practitioners.

Any child who is suspected of being hypovolemic should receive an initial IV bolus of warmed normal saline or Ringer's lactate in addition to maintenance IV fluids. Approximately 3 ml of crystalloid is required to replace each milliliter of blood lost because the infused fluid does not all remain in the intravascular space. This is known as the "3 for 1 rule." The estimated blood volume in an infant is 80 ml/kg, and in a child it is 75 ml/kg. Children must lose approximately 25% of their blood volume before demonstrating a decrease in their blood pressure; therefore crystalloid boluses are given in 20 ml/kg (25% of 80 ml/kg) increments. If there is no improvement by the second bolus, a third bolus or transfusion of 10 ml/kg O-negative or type-specific warmed packed red blood cells (PRBCs) should be considered. Abnormal hemodynamic status after PRBC transfusion indicates the need for operative intervention (American College of Surgeons Committee on Trauma, 1997; Chameides & Hazinski, 1997). Closely monitor the child's hemodynamic status until there is no longer any possibility of significant bleeding (Silverman, 1993). Use of pneumatic antishock garments (PASG) or military antishock trousers (MAST) is no longer recommended because they reduce neither mortality nor hospitalization (Chameides & Hazinski, 1997; Chang, Harrison, Beech, & Helmer, 1995; Mattox, Bickell, Pepe, Burch, & Feliciano, 1989).

Disability

Head injuries are the most frequent cause of death and morbidity in injured children (DiScala, 1998). Repeated evaluations of the child's neurologic status using the

Table 34–3 Systemic Responses to Blood Loss in the Pediatric Patient

System	<25% Blood Volume Loss	25%–45% Blood Volume Loss	>45% Blood Volume Loss
Cardiac	Weak, thready pulse; increased heart rate	Increased heart rate	Hypotension, tachycardia to bradycardia
Central nervous system (CNS)	Lethargic, irritable, confused	Change in level of consciousness, dulled response to pain	Comatose
Skin	Cool, clammy	Cyanotic, decreased capillary refill, cold extremities	Pale, cold
Kidneys	Minimal decrease in urine output; increased specific gravity	Minimal urine output	No urine output

Glasgow Coma Scale (GCS) should be performed and recorded (Exhibit 34–2). In addition, pupillary size, responsiveness to light, and position should be documented. It is essential to record a baseline evaluation of the child's neurologic status with frequent re-evaluations.

Exposure

The final aspect of the primary survey requires complete exposure of the child to evaluate for any visible injuries. In the infant and child, care should be taken to prevent hypothermia. Complications of hypothermia include metabolic acidosis and a shift in the oxygen hemoglobin dissociation curve to the left so that O_2 is bound more tightly to hemoglobin, leading to tissue hypoxia (Rasmussen & Grande, 1994). Methods to prevent or treat hypothermia include heated blankets; warming lights; and warmed IV fluids, blood, and inhaled gases (Bernardo, Henker, Bove, & Sereika, 1997). Temperatures should be periodically assessed and recorded during the resuscitation. Although rectal temperatures are generally considered to be the most accurate, Bernardo et al. (1996) found that aural infrared temperatures were adequate for screening in children with moderate to severe injuries.

Secondary Survey

Following initial stabilization, a secondary systematic total body survey is performed. The child's vital signs and level of consciousness require frequent reassessment and recording during this time. All systems should be evaluated. However, the order in which the survey is done varies depending on the child's suspected injuries.

History

The prehospital care of providers provide valuable information regarding the injury mechanism and prehospital events. A complete history and the child's allergies, medications, and immunization status, particularly tetanus, should be obtained from the family.

Brain Injuries

Incidence. Ninety-seven percent of children under the age of 14 who die have an intracranial injury; one third have an isolated brain injury (Lescohier & DiScala, 1993). Fortunately, minor brain injuries constitute the vast majority of brain injuries in children.

Primary and Secondary Injuries. Primary brain injuries occur at the time of the traumatic event and include scalp, skull, blood vessel, and brain injuries (Silverman, 1993). Secondary injuries are precipitated by the damage caused by the traumatic event and include injuries from hypoxia, hypercarbia, increased intracranial pressure (ICP), and hypotension. These injuries are potentially avoidable and man-

date that the ABCs (airway, breathing, and circulation) be adequately assessed and addressed in the brain-injured child. Hypotension within 24 hours of injury is the single most damaging secondary injury in terms of mortality, poor neurologic and functional outcomes, and length of hospital stay (Kokoska, Smith, Pittman, & Weber, 1998; Pigula, Wald, Shackford, & Vane, 1993). Hypoxia ($PaO_2 \leq 60$ mm Hg) has not been found to statistically worsen the outcome (Pigula et al., 1993).

Pathophysiology. The brain, cerebrospinal fluid (CSF), and blood fill the fixed intracranial vault. The intracranial pressure (ICP) is normally maintained at ≤ 10 mm Hg by minor volume variations in these three elements. When a child's brain is injured, it swells and displaces the CSF into the spinal subarachnoid space. If the swelling continues, eventually the ventricles become compressed or even obliterated. Hyperventilation causes cerebral vasoconstriction, thus decreasing cerebral blood flow and thereby decreasing ICP. Despite this, current recommendations discourage prophylactic or prolonged hyperventilation ($PaCO_2 \leq 35$ mm Hg) during the first 24 hours postinjury because cerebral blood flow is already decreased to <50% of normal in patients with severe traumatic brain injury (TBI) during that time. If the child is hyperventilated to a $PaCO_2 < 30$ mm Hg, there is significant risk of causing cerebral ischemia. The risk of cerebral edema developing continues for 3 to 5 days postinjury. Prevention and early treatment of intracranial hypertension include normothermia, volume resuscitation, seizure prophylaxis, raising the head of the bed 30 degrees, prevention of jugular venous drainage obstruction, sedation with possible pharmacologic paralysis, and maintenance of a $PaO_2 > 60$ mm Hg. An algorithm for intracranial hypertension is found in Figure 34–3. ICP monitoring should be initiated in children with a GCS of ≤ 8 or if cerebral edema, intracranial bleeding, or compressed basilar cisterns are found on the head computerized tomography (CT). The ICP relates directly to the cerebral perfusion pressure (CPP) by way of the equation: MAP (mean arterial pressure) − ICP = CPP. CPP is a more accurate predictor of outcome than the ICP and should be maintained at ≥ 70 mm Hg to decrease the incidence of further intracerebral injury (Bullock et al., 1995).

Evaluation: Glasgow Coma Scale. The GCS was developed to evaluate the level of consciousness in adults (Jennett & Teasdale, 1977). Modifications to this scale have been made so that it is applicable for use in infants and young children (see Exhibit 34–2) (James & Trauner, 1985; Raimondi & Hirschauer, 1984; Simpson & Reilly, 1982). Children whose GCS on admission is ≤ 8 are considered to have a major TBI (Ghajar & Hariri, 1992). However, a very low GCS (3 to 5) is not always an accurate prognostic indicator in children (Lieh-Lai et al., 1992).

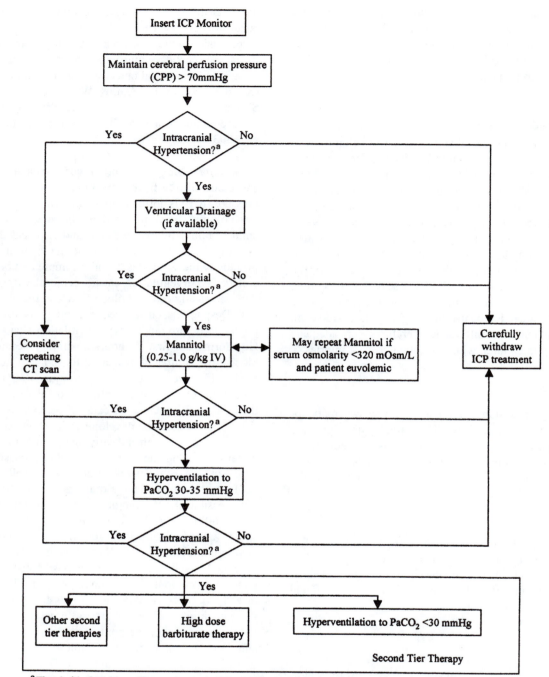

Figure 34–3 Critical Pathway for Treatment of Intracranial Hypertension in the Patient with Severe Head Injury (Treatment Option)

Evaluation: Physical Examination. The GCS evaluations and pupillary reflexes are serially documented to provide an ongoing record of the child's mental status. Results of inspection and gentle palpation of the head are also recorded (Silverman, 1993). Any infant with a bulging fontanel should have a neurosurgical consultation, even if the infant is awake and alert, because sudden deterioration may occur (American College of Surgeons Committee on Trauma, 1997).

Evaluation: Radiologic Evaluation. The head CT is the standard method of evaluating for intracranial injuries (ICI).

A neurosurgical consult is obtained for those children in whom the head CT demonstrates a neurosurgical lesion.

In this era of cost containment, the routine observation in the hospital of children with minor brain injuries is being re-addressed. Discharge criteria for children with a minor head injury include a normal head CT, a GCS of 15 (although they may have had a brief loss of consciousness), and a history of only minor trauma. In addition, there must be reliable parents, telephone and transportation access, and a home within a "reasonable distance" of medical care (Dahl-Grove, Chande, & Barnoski, 1995; Mitchell et al., 1994; Schunk, Rodgerson, & Woodward, 1996). Written and verbal recommendations should be provided before discharge and a follow-up telephone call should be made within 48 hours.

Specific Injuries. Table 34–4 provides a list of specific brain injuries, their signs and symptoms, treatments, and complications.

Increased Intracranial Pressure. The most accurate and reliable method for monitoring ICP is a ventricular catheter attached to an external strain gauge or catheter tip pressure transducer. In addition, these catheters allow for therapeutic CSF drainage. An ICP monitor is placed by the neurosurgeon at the bedside or in the operating room. Elevated ICP is related to the potential for cerebral herniation. However, as the importance of the CPP has become better understood, it has become evident that there is no particular ICP for which treatment should be initiated. The guidelines at present recommend treatment of ICP when it reaches 20 to 25 mm Hg. However, a portion of the brain may abnormally protrude, or herniate, through an opening in the skull at lower ICPs than that, depending on where the lesion is located. A higher ICP may be tolerated as long as the CPP is at least 70 mm Hg (Bullock et al., 1995).

An algorithm for the treatment of intracranial hypertension is seen in Figure 34–3. Glucocorticoids are not recommended for patients with severe TBI to decrease ICP or improve outcome. Because hyperthermia increases cerebral metabolism and therefore ICP, it needs to be controlled with acetaminophen and a cooling blanket. If ventricular drainage is not available or does not decrease the ICP sufficiently, the osmotic diuretic mannitol may be used. It raises the serum osmolality, thus pulling water into the bloodstream from the intracellular and interstitial spaces. However, once the serum osmolarity reaches 320 mOsm/L, mannitol should be stopped to prevent renal failure, and hyperventilation to a $PaCO_2$ of 30 to 35 mm Hg is initiated to attempt to control an elevated ICP. If the ICP continues to remain elevated at this point, second tier therapies such as high-dose barbiturate-induced coma or craniotomy (removal of a portion of the skull) must be considered (Bullock et al., 1995).

Strict urine output is monitored in children with TBI by means of an indwelling urinary catheter. Evaluation of the urine indicates whether two common complications of TBI, diabetes insipidus (DI) and the syndrome of inappropriate antidiuretic hormone secretion (SIADH), occur. In DI there is copious dilute urine output, whereas in SIADH there is an excess reabsorption of water, leading to decreased, concentrated urine output (Bullock et al., 1995).

Thoracic Injuries

Incidence and Pathophysiology. Serious intrathoracic trauma may be present in children without external or skeletal evidence of the significant energy that was transmitted causing the injury. This is due to the increased flexibility of their highly cartilaginous chest walls (Beaver & Laschinger, 1992; Manson, Babyn, Palder, & Bergman, 1993). Thoracic trauma is the second most common cause of death from pediatric injury (Cooper, 1995; Cooper, Barlow, DiScala, & String, 1994). Six percent of the 25,301 patients entered into the National Pediatric Trauma Registry (NPTR) between 1985 and 1991 had thoracic injuries, 86% of which were caused by blunt mechanisms. The automobile was involved in 74% of blunt thoracic trauma and gunshot wounds (GSW) caused 60% of penetrating thoracic trauma. The most common intrathoracic injuries are pulmonary contusions and lacerations (48%), pneumothoraces and hemothoraces (41%), and rib fractures (30%) (Cooper et al., 1994).

Evaluation. Evaluation for possible thoracic injuries includes inspection for external signs of trauma, such as contusions and abrasions from shoulder seat belt injuries or penetrating wounds from GSW. The child's pulse oximetry and respiratory status should be continually re-evaluated. On percussion, the normally resonant sound heard over the lung changes to dullness over a hemothorax or atelectasis and becomes hyperresonant over a pneumothorax. Auscultation of breath sounds may demonstrate hemothoraces or pneumothoraces or atelectasis by absent or decreased breath sounds over the affected area (Bates, Bickley, & Hoekelman, 1995). Plain chest radiographs are frequently taken with a portable machine in the trauma center during resuscitation. They allow visualization of chest injuries in need of immediate attention, as well as trauma to the thoracic skeleton (Cooper, 1995). An electrocardiogram (ECG) may be indicated to evaluate for a possible myocardial contusion if the child received a significant impact to the chest.

Specific Injuries. Table 34–5 provides a list of specific thoracic injuries, their signs and symptoms, treatments, and complications.

Abdominal Injuries

Incidence and Pathophysiology. Blunt mechanisms cause 86% of abdominal injuries in children, most of which involve motor vehicles (Cooper et al., 1994). Although abdominal injuries occur slightly more frequently than thoracic

Table 34–4 Specific Head Injuries

Injury	Diagnostics/Description	Treatment	Comments/Complications
Concussion	Brief loss of neurologic function ± loss of consciousness or amnesia[d]	Supportive care[d] May need head computed tomography (CT)[d]	If no persistent symptoms and reliable caregiver, may be observed at home[d]
Scalp injuries Laceration	Inspection	Irrigation and gentle debridement Sutures/staples as needed, remove in 5–7 days Thin layer of topical antibiotic ointment	If associated with open depressed skull fracture, laceration is a potential source of intracranial infection[a]
Subgaleal hematomas	Inspection, palpation Injury to tissue external to the skull	None, reabsorb spontaneously Avoid aspiration (risk of infection)	
Skull fractures	Head CT with bone windows		
Linear	Fine line visible on radiographs (CT or skull radiographs)[d]	If not depressed or diastatic (traumatic separation through cranial suture lines), not treated	Most common skull fracture, usually insignificant[d]
Depressed	Depression of bone visible on CT	If depressed ≥thickness of skull, elevated in the operating room[d]	Increased chance of postinjury seizures
Basilar	On inspection may have CSF rhinorrhea or otorrhea[a,d] Battle's sign: posterior auricular ecchymosis[d] Raccoon eyes: periorbital ecchymosis[d] Pneumocephalus on CT[a]	Serial neurologic examinations Examinations of cranial nerves VII (facial) and VIII (acoustic)	May not be visible radiographically[d] Possible complications: Seventh nerve palsy Hearing deficit Meningitis (if CSF leak)
Hematomas	Noncontrast enhanced head CT		
Epidural (extradural) hematoma (EDH)	Tearing of meningeal blood vessels[a] May have brief loss of consciousness, a lucid interval and then deterioration[b]	Evacuation of large or rapidly expanding EDHs[b] Surgical intervention also indicated for deteriorating LOC[b]	Often rapid, marked recovery after evacuation w/minimal sequelae

continues

Table 34–4 continued

Injury	Diagnostics/Description	Treatment	Comments/Complications
Hematomas (continued)			
Subdural hematoma (SDH)	Rupture of bridging cerebral veins[b]	PICU observation with supportive care[b] Craniotomy and evacuation of clot if symptomatic with significant lesion, decreasing LOC, or enlarging lesion on repeat CT[b] Possible intracranial pressure monitor[b]	Most common intracranial injury in infant victims of intentional trauma[a] May have ipsilateral hemiparesis and oculomotor palsy[b]
Subarachnoid hemorrhages (SAH)	Bleeding of microvessels within the subarachnoid space[b] (where the CSF circulates)	Observation for 24–48 hours[b]	Possible complication: Hydrocephalus[b] May require shunt if hydrocephalus is severe[b]
Intracerebral hematoma/ cerebral contusion	Bleeding within the cerebral parenchyma[b] Coup = at impact site[a] Contracoup = opposite impact site[a]	Supportive care May rarely require operative intervention for large focal lesions[b]	May cause increased ICP from edema and bleeding[b] May have significant morbidity depending on where lesion located[b]
Diffuse axonal injury (DAI)	Head CT[c] MRI of head provides better visualization of DAI than CT[c] Diffuse shearing injury at gray/white matter boundary[c]	See section on increased intracranial pressure in text	Most common cause of vegetative state and severe disability[a]

Note: CSF = cerebral spinal fluid; LOC = level of consciousness; MRI = magnetic resonance imaging.
[a] Graham, 1996. [b] Lowe & Northrup, 1996. [c] Prow, Cole, Yeakley, Diaz-Marchan, & Hayman, 1996. [d] Soud, Saum, & Pikulski, 1998.

injuries (8% versus 6%), their mortality is approximately half that of children who have intrathoracic injuries. Factors contributing to abdominal trauma in children include less adipose tissue and less developed abdominal wall musculature. In addition, the costal margin in a young child does not extend as far caudally, thus providing the liver and spleen less protection than those of an adolescent or adult (Schafermeyer, 1993; Tepas, 2000).

Evaluation. A detailed history of the mechanism of injury is extremely helpful in the initial evaluation of a child with abdominal trauma. Careful serial monitoring and recording of vital signs and repeated physical examinations are extremely important in determining hemodynamic stability in the child who may have an ongoing blood loss from an intra-abdominal organ injury. Inspection of the abdomen may demonstrate such visible injuries as lapbelt abrasions or contusions across the lower abdomen, the distinctive circular contusion from the end of a bicycle handlebar, or the site of a penetrating injury. These visible injuries provide clues to potential intra-abdominal organ injuries. Gastric distention occurs frequently in young children who have gulped air while crying, have had an esophageal intubation, or who have received bag-valve-mask ventilation. Gastric distention is relieved by placement of an orogastric tube. Interpretation of a child's response to abdominal palpation is likely to be more difficult than an adult's in that they are often crying and frightened and state it hurts anywhere they are touched.

To screen for peritoneal and pericardial fluid, focused abdominal sonography for trauma (FAST) is often now being

Table 34–5 Specific Thoracic Injuries

Injury	Signs and Symptoms	Treatment	Complications
Pulmonary contusion (bruise of lung)	Respiratory distress,[d] may not appear for several hours	Pain management Respiratory support to maintain normal oxygen saturation[b] Avoid fluid overloading[a] Generally resolve in 7–10 days[a]	Pneumonia[b] Adult respiratory distress syndrome (ARDS)[b]
Pneumothoraces (air in pleural space)	Visible on chest radiograph (CXR)[d]	Respiratory support to maintain normal oxygen saturation[b]	
Simple	Tachypnea[d] Increased respiratory effort[d] Decreased or absent breath sounds on affected side[a] Hyperresonance on percussion[a]	If comprises <15% total lung volume and no respiratory distress, may just observe[c] Chest tube[a]	Respiratory distress
Tension (see Figure 34–2)	Sudden respiratory deterioration Most often related to mechanical ventilation[a]	Immediate large-bore needle thoracostomy (rush of air out when needle reaches trapped air) One-way valve or underwater seal to needle until replaced with chest tube Chest tube[a]	Decreased venous return to heart Decreased cardiac output
Open	Visible open sucking chest wound	Cover open wound and surrounding area with sterile occlusive dressing and tape securely on three sides Chest tube	Tension pneumothorax
Hemothorax (blood in pleural space)	Decreased breath sounds on affected side[d] Dullness on percussion[d] Elevation of hemidiaphragm or blunting of costophrenic angle on upright CXR[a] Re-evaluate on serial radiographs	Chest tube if increasing hemothorax on serial CXRs[a] Transfusion if hypovolemic shock Thoracotomy for Blood loss >2–4 ml/kg/hr from chest tube[b] Massive air leak[b]	Shock[a] Respiratory distress
Rib fractures	Tachypnea[d] Shallow respirations[d] Rib fractures on serial CXR	Pain management[a] Prevention of atelectasis (forceful exhalation, e.g., blowing bubbles or a pinwheel)	Atelectasis and pneumonia[a,d] Respiratory failure[d]
Traumatic asphyxia	Visibly striking petechia and cyanosis on face, neck, and chest Retinal and subconjunctival hemorrhages	Supportive care[b] Gradual spontaneous resolution	
Myocardial contusion (bruise of cardiac muscle)	Arrhythmias such as premature ventricular contractions (PVCs) and tachycardia[a]	12-lead electrocardiogram (ECG)[a] Cardiac monitor and close observation for arrhythmias[a] Most require no therapeutic intervention[b]	Sudden dysrhythmias[a]
Cardiac tamponade (blood in pericardial sac)	Hypotensive in spite of appropriate fluid resuscitation Positive ultrasound[d]	Aspiration of nonclotting blood on pericardiocentesis is diagnostic and initial treatment[a] Thoracotomy and repair of injury[a]	Decreased cardiac output secondary to restriction of ventricular filling[d]

[a] Beaver & Laschinger, 1992. [b] Cooper, 1995. [c] Schafermeyer, 1993. [d] Zander & Hazinski, 1992.

performed in the trauma center either by radiologists or surgeons trained in this procedure (Bode, Niezen, van Vugt, & Schipper, 1993; Forster, Pillasch, Zielke, Malewski, & Rothmund, 1993; Luks et al., 1993; Rothlin et al., 1993; Rozycki, Ochsner, Jaffin, & Champion, 1993). The results of these studies may demonstrate the presence of free fluid, which is indicative of a possible solid organ injury. However, these studies are operator dependent. If FAST is performed immediately on arrival in the emergency department, sufficient blood may not have accumulated to be visible on FAST (Thourani, Pettitt, Schmidt, Cooper, & Rozycki, 1998). If there is continuing suspicion of an abdominal organ injury, the FAST should be repeated or an abdominal CT obtained to identify solid organ injury.

Abdominal CT is generally accepted as the mode of choice for diagnosis of solid organ injuries in hemodynamically stable patients (Esposito & Gamelli, 1996). In addition to the presence or absence of free peritoneal fluid, the CT demonstrates the presence of free air in unusual places and the anatomic configuration of the solid organs and bowel loops (Tepas, 2000). Diagnostic peritoneal lavage (DPL) indicates the presence of blood or intestinal contents in the peritoneal fluid. DPL was used before the wide availability of sophisticated CTs. It is used only rarely now, such as when the child requires general anesthesia for other injuries, has a neurologic injury, or is obtunded (Tepas, 2000).

At present, the decision to operate on a child with intra-abdominal solid organ injury is based on hemodynamic instability of the child despite 40 ml/kg crystalloid resuscitation with normal saline or Ringer's lactate (see Figure 34–4) (Haller, Papa, Drugas, & Colombani, 1994). Serial hemoglobin and hematocrits (H & H) correlate with solid and hollow abdominal organ injuries. The decision to transfuse a child with decreasing H & H is made on the basis of the presence of abnormal tissue perfusion and vital signs. Hemodynamically stable children with hemoglobin levels ≥7 gm/dl do not require a blood transfusion (Umali, Andrews, & White, 1992).

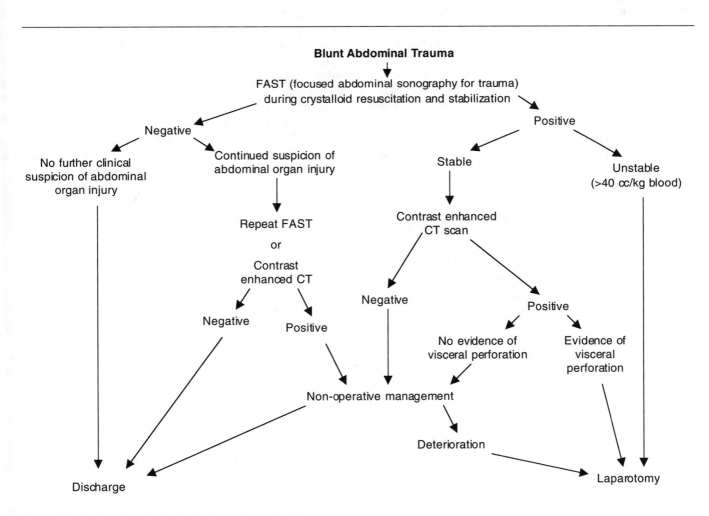

Figure 34–4 Algorithm for Pediatric Blunt Abdominal Trauma

Specific Injuries. Blunt abdominal trauma in children most commonly injures the spleen, liver, and kidney, with an occurrence rate of 28% to 30% in each category. In contrast, 70% of children with penetrating injuries have damage to the intestinal tract. The liver is the second most frequently injured intra-abdominal organ in penetrating trauma, occurring 27% of the time (Cooper et al., 1994).

Splenic Injuries. Children with splenic injuries have pain and guarding in the left upper abdomen. The pain may radiate to the left shoulder. King and Shumacker (1952) reported an "increased susceptibility to infection" in young infants in whom the spleen had been removed. Francke and Neu (1981) found that the complete removal of a child's spleen subjected the child to an 85 times greater risk of developing overwhelming postsplenectomy infection (OPSI). The mortality rate of OPSI is approximately 50% (Tepas, 2000). Upadhyaya and Simpson (1968) were the first to advocate nonoperative management of hemodynamically stable children with splenic rupture. They found children who had isolated splenic injuries often had almost stopped bleeding from the injury by the time a laparotomy was undertaken. Today conservative management of children with most splenic injuries is the standard of care. The requirements for nonoperative management of a splenic injury include close monitoring of the child by the surgical team able to intervene if that becomes necessary and immediate availability of both blood for transfusion and a fully staffed operating room. The presence of a brain injury should not affect the decision to conservatively manage a child's splenic injury (Keller, Sartorelli, & Vane, 1996). A protocol for care of children with blunt abdominal trauma is seen in Figure 34–4.

In this era of cost containment, children with nonoperatively managed splenic injuries no longer remain in the hospital for 7 to 10 days. Lynch, Ford, Gardner, and Weiner (1993) determined that in their population of 53 children with mildly to moderately injured spleens, stable hematocrits were achieved by day 2.06 and that the children could have gone home on day 4. They also found that these patients did not require ICU monitoring. See Appendix 34–A for a caremap developed for children with isolated splenic injuries grades I to III. Before discharge, the family should be instructed in the importance of restricting the child's activity at home. Follow-up care for children with splenic injuries is not well defined. Some authors advocate a CT or nuclear scan 1 week postinjury because of a small chance of a delayed rupture of a splenic hematoma or increase in size of the damage (Tepas, 2000). Others do not radiographically re-evaluate the child's abdomen for 6 weeks or at all (Pranikoff, Hirschl, Schlesinger, Polley, & Coran, 1994). Lynch, Meza, Newman, Gardner, and Albanese (1997) determined the length of time to radiographic evidence of a healed splenic injury was directly related to how significant the injury was.

When the child may return to full activity is important to the child and family. Recommendations range from 8 weeks to 6 months postinjury with and without radiologic evaluation (Lynch et al., 1997; Morse & Garcia, 1994; Pranikoff et al., 1994; Tepas, 2000).

Hepatic Injuries. Richie and Fonkalsrud (1972) first published the idea of nonoperative management of subcapsular liver hematomas in 1972. At present, the same criteria used for surgical intervention for splenic injury (see Figure 34–4) may also be applied for those hepatic injuries that do not involve damage to the hepatic veins, portal vein, or suprarenal inferior vena cava (Tepas, 2000). There are different hepatic injury classifications, including those from the Organ Injury Scaling Committee of the American Association for the Surgery of Trauma (Moore et al., 1995). Hemodynamically unstable children with liver injuries involving these major vessels or who have massive liver damage are at significant risk for exsanguination and require immediate operative intervention. Operative management is also indicated for children with a penetrating liver injury. A delayed hemorrhage is more common in children who have hepatic rather than splenic injuries (Moulton et al., 1992), possibly because of intraparenchymal vascular injuries (Tepas, 1993). This typically occurs on postinjury day 3 to 5; therefore strict bed rest is recommended for 5 to 7 days after the injury occurred (Cooper, 1992), although some institutions allow children with minor hepatic injuries to go home as early as day 3 (Bulas, Eichelberger, Sivit, Wright, & Gotschall, 1993).

The most common long-term complication from liver injuries is bile leakage (Cooper, 1992; Moulton, Downey, Anderson, & Lynch, 1993). The length of time required for complete healing of a liver injury depends on the extent of the injury. Bulas et al. (1993) recommend a follow-up CT in 3 months for a mild injury, 3 to 6 months for moderate injuries, and 9 months for severe injuries to document complete resolution of the injury before allowing the child to resume full activity.

Pancreatic Injuries. The most common cause of pediatric pancreatic injuries is bicycle handlebars (Arkovitz, Johnson, & Garcia, 1997), with compression of the pancreas against the spine causing injury to the body or neck of the pancreas (Shilyansky et al., 1998). Arkovitz et al. (1997) recommend that children who present with abdominal pain, a history of a handlebar injury, and an elevated serum amylase have a double contrast abdominal (intravenous and oral) CT and be admitted. Oral contrast improves the diagnostic value of the CT scan. Treatment decisions are determined by the grade of the pancreatic injury and the child's clinical status (Keller, Stafford, & Vane, 1997). If there is no major ductal injury (grades I and II) and the child remains clinically stable, most pancreatic trauma may be managed nonoperatively (Keller et al., 1997; Moore et al., 1990). Nonoperative treatment for pancreatic injuries includes making the child NPO and initiating total parenteral nutrition (TPN) until the elevated serum amylase levels approach normal and there is resolution of the abdominal pain. Shilyansky et al. (1998) reported on nonoperative management of pancreatic injury and found that the average length of time to symptom resolution was 15 days. The most common complication of pancreatic injuries is a pancreatic pseudocyst (40%), some of which require percutaneous drainage; others resolve spontaneously (Shilyansky et al., 1998).

Intestinal Injuries. Fourteen percent of children with intra-abdominal injuries from blunt mechanisms have damage to the gastrointestinal tract, involving the small bowel (64%) or the colon and rectum (21%) (Cooper et al., 1994). The most common of these mechanisms involves lapbelts, where the child's torso is suddenly flexed at the hips and then thrown backwards against the seat during rapid deceleration. The abdominal contents are compressed between the lapbelt and the child's spine (Moss & Musemeche, 1996). Chance fractures, burst fractures of lumbar vertebrae, are often associated with intestinal injuries caused by this mechanism (Kurkchubasche, Fendya, Tracy, Silen, & Weber, 1997). Seventy percent of intra-abdominal injuries from penetrating trauma have damage to the gastrointestinal tract involving the small bowel (40%) or the colon and rectum (39%) (Cooper et al., 1994).

Prompt diagnosis of small bowel injuries remains problematic. Abdominal CT scans inconsistently demonstrate small bowel injuries. Extravasation of enteral contrast or pneumoperitoneum indicates the presence of an intestinal injury. Other nonspecific findings on CT include bowel wall thickening, free intraperitoneal fluid without the presence of solid organ injury, and evidence of an ileus (Kurkchubasche et al., 1997). Laboratory tests, including amylase levels, are nonspecific and do not aid in the diagnosis of small bowel injuries (Isaacman et al., 1993). Moss and Musemeche (1996) found that serial abdominal physical examinations in conscious patients were 100% diagnostic for small bowel injuries requiring operative intervention. All of them had abdominal tenderness on arrival. Jerby, Attorri, and Morton (1997) noted that the children in their study who had diffuse abdominal tenderness were found to have major intestinal injuries at the time of surgery in contradistinction to those with localized tenderness who had minor intestinal injuries.

Duodenal hematomas push the submucosa into the lumen of the duodenum, causing symptoms of a partial small bowel obstruction. The diagnosis is made when a filling defect is seen on an upper gastrointestinal contrast study. Treatment includes gastric decompression and TPN (Tepas, 2000). If the hematoma has still not resolved after 2 or 3 weeks, surgical drainage may be necessary (Newman, 1993).

Renal Injuries. Renal injuries occur in 28% of children injured by blunt mechanisms and 10% by penetrating mechanisms. Ninety-five percent of renal injuries recorded in NPTR-2 were blunt injuries (Cooper et al., 1994). Children are more likely to have renal injuries than adults because of the larger relative size of their kidneys and the general lack of protection of abdominal organs noted at the beginning of this section in addition to children having less perirenal fat (Allshouse & Bett, 1993). The severity of the renal injury does not correlate to the degree of hematuria present (Angus et al., 1993; Zander & Hazinski, 1992). Children with clinical findings of abdominal or flank tenderness, blood at the urethral meatus, or pelvic instability should be further evaluated for genitourinary injuries regardless of the degree of hematuria (Abou-Jaoude, Sugarman, Fallat, & Casale, 1996).

Most children with renal injuries are hemodynamically stable and are managed nonoperatively. A CT scan of the abdomen in children with blunt trauma allows visualization of renal injuries while also evaluating for other intra-abdominal organ injuries. Before surgery, an intravenous pyelogram (IVP) should be obtained in children who are hemodynamically unstable secondary to gross renal pedicle disruption to demonstrate a functioning second kidney and for baseline renal perfusion (Tepas, 2000). Children with penetrating injuries are evaluated with plain films and an IVP (Angus et al., 1993). Nonoperative management of renal injuries includes bed rest until gross hematuria clears and restricted activity until microscopic hematuria resolves (Allshouse & Bett, 1993). The potential for late-onset posttraumatic hypertension necessitates blood pressure evaluation every 6 months for at least 1 to 2 years after the injury (Pieper, 1994).

Extremity Fractures

Incidence and Pathophysiology. Fifty-seven percent of the more than 31,000 pediatric trauma patients included in the NPTR-3 had a least one fracture, 2% of which were isolated extremity fractures. Of the 40% who had functional limitations at the time of discharge, 47% of those with 1 to 3 and 25% of those with ≥4 functional limitations had a fracture (DiScala, 1999). A significant impact is required to break a bone and the most common mechanisms involve motor vehicle crashes, with the patient either inside the vehicle or being struck by the vehicle, and falls.

Evaluation. Evaluation of suspected extremity fractures includes the "five Ps": pain, pallor, pulses, paresthesias, and paralysis (Emergency Nurses Association, 1995). Obvious or suspected fractures may be revealed by inspection. The bone may protrude through the skin, the extremity may have an abnormal bend or rotation when compared with the uninjured extremity, or there may be swelling or discoloration over suspected fracture sites. In addition, complaints of extremity pain should prompt further evaluation, including palpation of proximal and distal pulses and evaluation of sensation and movement distal to the area. A splint should be applied to the extremity, including the joints above and below the injury. The splint stabilizes the fracture and prevents further neurovascular and soft tissue damage, decreases pain, and prevents a closed fracture from becoming an open one (Alonso, 1993). There is the potential for significant blood loss into the dead space surrounding fracture sites (Tepas, 2000). A sterile dressing should be applied if there is an open wound present. Once in the trauma center, all extremities are evaluated, starting distally. Full gentle range of motion of joints in extremities without obvious fractures is performed and injuries to soft tissues are recorded in addition to findings of the neurovascular examination of each limb.

Anteroposterior and lateral radiographs of any suspected fracture sites, including the joints above and below, are taken (Alonso, 1993). Children have active growth plates and a significant amount of cartilaginous tissue in their skeletons, making the interpretation of their radiographs significantly more difficult than those of an adult. The growth plate is involved in up to one third of pediatric fractures. In 1963, Salter and Harris classified growth plate fractures as I to V. Included among possible long-term consequences of growth plate fractures are progressive angular deformity, limb length discrepancy, joint incongruity, and a greater chance of refracture of the growth plate. Other fractures seen in children that are not found in adults include greenstick fractures, traumatic bowing, and torus or buckle fractures (Thomas, 1993).

Specific Injuries. Table 34–6 provides a list of specific extremity injuries, their signs and symptoms, treatments, and complications.

PSYCHOSOCIAL ISSUES

Care of the Child

Developmentally appropriate explanations of pending procedures should be provided to injured children, including those with a decreased level of consciousness. General pediatric nursing textbooks include information on developmental stages. Wong (1982) provides a concise review of developmentally appropriate nursing interventions specifically related to pediatric trauma patients. Child life therapists render a tremendous service by helping to make the hospital a less threatening place and by decreasing the boredom. Regression and behaviors not usually exhibited at home are not uncommon among hospitalized children. Trauma or pediatric psychologists help the child and the family adapt to the stresses surrounding the child's injury, as well as providing significant support to the staff.

Care of the Family

Families of injured children are often initially distraught. One of the most precious things in their lives has been hurt, and they frequently express feelings of guilt, "If only I had ____, this wouldn't have happened." It is important to encourage families to make use of pre-established support systems in addition to making them aware of services provided in the hospital, including pastoral care, social services, and the trauma psychologist. Particularly when a child is critically injured, they often cannot bring themselves to leave the premises for the first several days. They should be encouraged to have friends bring them food and clean clothes and to take care of things at home such as other children or pets. The family needs to understand that the nursing staff will take care of their child, but only they can take care of their own personal needs, such as sleeping, eating, and showering. They need a great deal of energy to endure their child's hospital stay, even without any setbacks. The family may feel as if they are on an uncontrolled roller coaster ride. Tired parents are less capable of tolerating the situation. Parents should be encouraged to participate in their child's care and asked to share information about how the child has coped in the past. Families often want to share stories and pictures of their child before the injury, which helps the staff to better understand the dichotomy the family is attempting to reconcile.

Families often repeat the same questions. Let them know that their stress levels are so high that you do not expect them to remember all that they are told. They should be encouraged to ask if they do not understand something. The nurse should try to be present when physicians are talking to the family both to be sure that the family understands the explanation and so that the nursing staff can reinforce what was said. When families have questions that a particular physician or service needs to answer, suggest that the family write them down so the questions are not forgotten when the appropriate person is available.

Families need to be told about hospital and unit policies regarding visitors, including sibling visitation, food in the child's room, cellular phones, and to whom information regarding the child's status will be given over the telephone. Written information about the unit that includes these policies is helpful to families. It is important that policies are consistently enforced across all shifts.

DISCHARGE PLANNING

Discharge planning for trauma patients ranges anywhere from making sure the child has a safe ride home (appropriate car seat or restraint device) to calling the organ procurement organization. Priorities for discharge planning must be set quickly as length of hospital stays continue to decrease. Be-

Table 34–6 Specific Extremity Fractures

Bone Fractured	Common Injury Mechanisms	Treatment Modalities	Potential Complications
Humerus	Backwards fall onto outstretched hand Most often SH I & II fractures	Immobilization Possible percutaneous pinning if extreme abduction needed to reduce Open or closed reduction, may require general anesthesia	Distal fractures Brachial artery injuries Compartment syndrome Radial or median nerve damage Malunion
Radius and ulna	Fall forward onto outstretched hand Most often shaft, torus, and SH I & II fractures of the distal radius	Immobilization Open or closed reduction, may require general anesthesia	Complications uncommon
Femur	Child hit by motor vehicle	Traction splint in field Intramedullary rodding Intermediate spica cast Traction with delayed spica cast	Significant blood loss, not usually cause of shock
Tibia and fibula	Motor vehicle crashes Falls	Torus or nondisplaced fractures: Short or long leg cast Observed in hospital overnight if at risk for compartment syndrome Displaced fractures: Knee and ankle immobilization in long leg splint Ice packs for 48 hours Elevation about heart Open fractures: May require external fixation	Compartment syndrome Neurovascular injuries Leg length discrepancy Malunion Angular deformity Premature closure of upper tibial physis

Note: SH = Salter Harris.

fore discharge, future problems that may occur as a result of the child's injuries should be discussed. Many children who have survived brain injuries have difficulties transitioning back to school (Bowen et al., 1997). Parents need to know that if their child starts having difficulties at home or school, the child may need to have a neuropsychological evaluation performed. The names and office telephone numbers of health care providers involved in their child's care should be provided to the parents. In this era of managed care, ensuring that the child's health plan allows follow-up visits with the involved physicians is a real issue. Generally, the insurance companies have a case manager who will help with discharge arrangements for home equipment, supplies, nursing, physical/occupational/speech therapies, and outpatient appointments. Arrangements for home tutoring should be made according to local guidelines.

Optimal rehabilitation for injured children allows them to reach their maximum potential. Unfortunately, not all children who could benefit from rehabilitation are given that option (Osberg & Unsworth, 1997). A referral to an appropriate rehabilitation hospital should be made shortly after admission on any moderately to severely brain-injured child to prevent delay in transfer.

In some instances, children with severe brain injuries are candidates for organ donation. The organ procurement organization (OPO) should be notified according to state and institutional guidelines. A cerebral perfusion scan that demonstrates no blood flow is presently considered the best brain death confirmatory study because the neurons cannot survive without oxygen carried by the blood (Dorr, 1997). However, brain death determination must be made according to state regulations. The family should be told of that determination before the OPO discusses organ donation with the family unless the family requests to speak with them earlier. Many families are extremely grateful to have the opportunity to have something positive come from the death of their child.

CURRENT AND POTENTIAL RESEARCH

There is a tremendous amount of epidemiologic data that has been collected regarding pediatric injuries, the largest repository of which is the National Pediatric Trauma Registry (NPTR). These types of data are valuable in determining local and national directions for and effectiveness of injury prevention programs.

Advances in neuronal physiology research made in the laboratory will lead to advances in clinical management of increased ICP. Other researchers are involved in studies of patients with adult respiratory distress syndrome and sepsis, attempting to improve patient outcomes from these potential

secondary insults to trauma patients. The role of nutrition in the injured patient is another area of ongoing research.

Changes in the child's environment, such as the development of safer cars, have a significant impact on the severity of injuries. Research in "social engineering" is investigating methods to modify the behavior of society to provide a safer environment for children and adults (Hall, 1994).

CONCLUSION

Nurses who care for injured children need to be fully cognizant of pediatric anatomic and physiologic characteristics and to appreciate the differences in children who are of varying ages, developmental levels, and sizes. It is also necessary to anticipate what those differences will mean with respect to any given child's response to a traumatic injury and the treatments that follow. The most effective method to decrease the morbidity and mortality associated with pediatric trauma continues to be injury prevention.

REFERENCES

Abou-Jaude, W.A., Sugarman, J.M., Fallat, M.E., & Casale, A.J. (1996). Indicators of genitourinary tract injury or anomaly in cases of pediatric blunt trauma. *Journal of Pediatric Surgery, 31*, 86–90.

Allshouse, M.J., & Bett, J.M. (1993). Genitourinary injury. In M.R. Eichelberger (Ed.), *Pediatric trauma: Prevention, acute care, rehabilitation* (pp. 503–520). St. Louis, MO: Mosby.

Alonso, J.E. (1993). Musculoskeletal injuries. In D.G. MacEwen, J.R. Kasser, & S.D. Heinrich (Eds.), *Pediatric fractures: A practical approach to assessment and treatment* (pp. 30–37). Baltimore: Williams & Wilkins.

American College of Surgeons Committee on Trauma. (1997). *ATLS: Advanced trauma life support for doctors, student course manual* (6th ed.). Chicago: American College of Surgeons.

Angus, L.D.G., Tachmes, L., Kahn, S., Gulmi, F., Gintautas, J., & Shaftan, G.W. (1993). Surgical management of pediatric renal trauma: An urban experience. *The American Surgeon, 59*, 388–394.

Arkovitz, M.S., Johnson, N., & Garcia, V.F. (1997). Pancreatic trauma in children: Mechanisms of injury. *Journal of Trauma, 42*, 49–53.

Baraff, L.J. (1993). Capillary refill: Is it a useful sign? [Commentary]. *Pediatrics, 92*, 723–724.

Bates, B., Bickley, L.S., & Hoekelman, R.A. (1995). *Physical examination and history taking* (6th ed.). Philadelphia: Lippincott-Raven Publishers.

Beaver, B.L., & Laschinger, J.C. (1992). Pediatric thoracic trauma. *Seminars in Thoracic and Cardiovascular Surgery, 4*, 255–262.

Bernardo, L.M., Clemence, B., Henker, R., Hogue, B., Schenkel, K., & Walters, P. (1996). A comparison of aural and rectal temperature measurements in children with moderate and severe injuries. *Journal of Emergency Nursing, 22*, 403–408.

Bernardo, L.M., Henker, R., Bove, M., & Sereika, S. (1997). The effect of administered crystalloid fluid temperature on aural temperature of moderately and severely injured children. *Journal of Emergency Nursing, 23*, 105–111.

Birkland, P. (1993). International update: Two successful Canadian pro-

grams teach teenagers trauma prevention. *Journal of Emergency Nursing, 19*, 35A–36A.

Bode, P.J., Niezen, R.A., van Vugt, A.B., & Schipper, J. (1993). Abdominal ultrasound as a reliable indicator for conclusive laparotomy in blunt abdominal trauma. *Journal of Trauma, 34*, 27–31.

Bond, S.J., Eichelberger, M.R., Gotschall, C.S., Sivit, C.J., & Randolph, J.G. (1996). Nonoperative management of blunt hepatic and splenic injury in children. *Annals of Surgery, 223*, 286–289.

Bowen, J.M., Clark, E., Bigler, E.D., Gardner, M., Nilsson, D., Gooch, J., & Pompa, J. (1997). Childhood traumatic brain injury: Neuropsychological status at the time of hospital discharge. *Developmental Medicine and Child Neurology, 39*, 17–25.

Bulas, D.I., Eichelberger, M.R., Sivit, C.J., Wright, C.J., & Gotschall, C.S. (1993). Hepatic injury from blunt trauma in children: Follow-up evaluation with CT. *American Journal of Roentgenology, 160*, 347–351.

Bullock, R., Chestnut, R.M., Clifton, G., Ghajar, J., Marion, D.W., Narayan, R.K., Newell, D.W., Pitts, L.H., Rosner, M.J., & Wilberger, J.E. (1995). *Guidelines for the management of severe head injury.* A Joint Initiative of The Brain Trauma Foundation, The American Association of Neurological Surgeons, & The Joint Section on Neurotrauma and Critical Care.

Chameides, L, & Hazinski, M.F. (Eds.). (1997). *Pediatric advanced life support.* Dallas, TX: American Heart Association.

Chang, F.C., Harrison, P.B., Beech, R.R., & Helmer, S.D. (1995). PASG: Does it help in the management of traumatic shock? *Journal of Trauma, 39*, 453–456.

Committee on Trauma, American College of Surgeons. (1998). *Resources for optimal care of the injured patient: 1999.* Chicago: American College of Surgeons.

Cooper, A. (1992). Liver injuries in children: Treatments tried, lessons learned. *Seminars in Pediatric Surgery, 1*, 152–161.

Cooper, A. (1995). Thoracic injuries. *Seminars in Pediatric Surgery, 4*, 109–115.

Cooper, A., Barlow, B., DiScala C., & String, D. (1994). Mortality and truncal injury: The pediatric perspective. *Journal of Pediatric Surgery, 29,* 33–38.

Cooper, A., Barlow, B., DiScala, C., String, D., Ray, K., & Mottley, L. (1993). Efficacy of pediatric trauma care: Results of a population based study. *Journal of Pediatric Surgery, 28,* 299–305.

Dahl-Grove, D.L., Chande, V.T., & Barnoski, A. (1995). Closed head injuries in children: Is hospital admission always necessary? *Pediatric Emergency Care, 11,* 86–88.

DiScala, C. (1999). *National pediatric trauma registry biannual report, October 1999.* Boston: Research and Training Center at Tufts University School of Medicine New England Medical Center and the American Pediatric Surgical Association.

Dorr, P. (1997). Outcomes manager: Brain death criteria in the pediatric patient. *Critical Care Nursing Quarterly, 20,* 14–21.

Durch, J.S., & Lohr, K.N. (Eds.). (1993). Risking our children's health: A need for emergency care. In *Emergency medical services for children* (pp. 38–65). Washington, DC: National Academy Press.

Emergency Nurses Association. (1995). *TNCC: Trauma nursing core course provider manual* (4th ed.). Park Ridge, IL: Author.

Esposito, T.J., & Gamelli, R.L. (1996). Injury to the spleen. In D.V. Feliciano, E.E. Moore, & K.L. Mattox (Eds.), *Trauma* (3rd ed., pp. 525–550). Stamford, CT: Appleton & Lange.

Forster, F., Pillasch, J., Zielke, A., Malewski, U., & Rothmund, M. (1993). Ultrasonography in blunt abdominal trauma: Influence of the investigators' experience. *Journal of Trauma, 34,* 264–269.

Francke, E.L., & Neu, H.C. (1981). Postsplenectomy infection. *Surgical Clinics of North America, 61,* 135–155.

Ghajar, J., & Hariri, R.J. (1992). Management of pediatric head injury. *Pediatric Clinics of North America, 39,* 1093–1125.

Gorelick, M.H., Shaw, K.N., & Baker, M.D. (1993). Effect of ambient temperature on capillary refill in healthy children. *Pediatrics, 92,* 699–702.

Graham, D.I. (1996). Neuropathy of head injury. In R.K. Narayan, J.E. Wilberger, & J.T. Povlishock (Eds.), *Neurotrauma* (pp. 44–52). New York: McGraw-Hill.

Graneto, J.W., & Soglin, D.F. (1993). Transport and stabilization of the pediatric trauma patient. *Pediatric Clinics of North America, 40,* 365–380.

Guy, J., Haley, K., & Zuspan, S.J. (1993). Use of intraosseous infusion in the pediatric trauma patient. *Journal of Pediatric Surgery, 28,* 158–161.

Hall, S.C. (1994). Pediatric trauma in the 90s: An overview. *International Anesthesiology Clinics, 32,* 1–9.

Haller, J.A., Papa, P., Drugas, G., & Colombani, P. (1994). Nonoperative management of solid organ injuries in children: Is it safe? *Annals of Surgery, 219,* 625–628.

Hennes, H. (1998). A review of violence statistics among children and adolescents in the United States. *Pediatric Clinics of North America, 45,* 269–280.

Isaacman, D.J., Scarfone, R.J., Kost, S.I., Gochman, R.F., Davis, H.W., Bernardo, L.M., & Nakayama, D.K. (1993). Utility of routine laboratory testing for detecting intra-abdominal injury in the pediatric trauma patient. *Pediatrics, 92,* 691–694.

James, H.E., & Trauner, D.A. (1985). The Glasgow coma scale. In H.E. James, N.G. Anas, & R.M. Perkin (Eds.), *Brain insults in infants and children: Pathophysiology and management* (pp. 183–186). Orlando, FL: Harcourt Brace & Company.

Jennett, B., & Teasdale, G. (1977). Aspects of coma after severe head injury. *The Lancet, 8017,* 878–881.

Jerby, B.L., Attorri, R.J., & Morton, D., Jr. (1997). Blunt intestinal injury in children: The role of the physical examination. *Journal of Pediatric Surgery, 32,* 580–584.

Keller, M.S., Sartorelli, K.H., & Vane, D.W. (1996). Associated head injury should not prevent nonoperative management of spleen or liver injury in children. *Journal of Trauma, 41,* 471–475.

Keller, M.S., Stafford, P.W., & Vane, D.W. (1997). Conservative management of pancreatic trauma in children. *Journal of Trauma, 42,* 1097–1100.

King, H., & Shumacker, H.B. (1952). Splenic studies. *Annals of Surgery, 136,* 239–242.

Kokoska, E.R., Smith, G.S., Pittman, T., & Weber, T.R. (1998). Early hypotension worsens neurological outcome in pediatric patients with moderately severe head trauma. *Journal of Pediatric Surgery, 33,* 333–338.

Kurkchubasche, A.G., Fendya, D.G., Tracy, T.F., Silen, M.L., & Weber, T.R. (1997). Blunt intestinal injury in children: Diagnostic and therapeutic considerations. *Archives of Surgery, 132,* 652–657.

Lescohier, I., & DiScala, C. (1993). Blunt trauma in children: Causes and outcomes of head versus extracranial injury. *Pediatrics, 91,* 721–725.

Li, G., Baker, S.P., DiScala, C., Fowler, C., Ling, J., & Kelen, G.D. (1996). Factors associated with the intent of firearm-related injuries in pediatric trauma patients. *Archives of Pediatric and Adolescent Medicine, 150,* 1160–1165.

Lieh-Lai, M.W., Theodorou, A.A., Sarnaik, A.P., Meert, K.L., Moylan, P.M., & Canaday, A.I. (1992). Limitations of the Glasgow coma scale in predicting outcome in children with traumatic brain injury. *Journal of Pediatrics, 120,* 195–199.

Lowe, J.G., & Northrup, B.E. (1996). Traumatic intracranial hemorrhage. In R.W. Evans (Ed.), *Neurology and trauma* (pp. 140–147). Philadelphia: W.B. Saunders Company.

Luks, F.I., Lemire, A., St.-Vil, D., DiLorenzo, M., Filaitrault, D., & Ouimet, A. (1993). Blunt abdominal trauma in children: The practical value of ultrasonography. *Journal of Trauma, 34,* 607–611.

Luten, R.C., Wears, R.L., Broselow, J., Zaritsky, A., Barnett, T.M., Lee, T., Bailey, A., Vally, R., Brown, R., & Rosenthal, B. (1992). Length-based endotracheal tube and emergency equipment in pediatrics. *Annals of Emergency Medicine, 21,* 900–904.

Lynch, J.M., Ford, H., Gardner, M.J., & Weiner, E.S. (1993). Is early discharge following isolated splenic injury in the hemodynamically stable child possible? *Journal of Pediatric Surgery, 28,* 1403–1407.

Lynch, J.M., Meza, M.P., Newman, B., Gardner, M.J., & Albanese, C.T. (1997). Computed tomography grade of splenic injury is predictive of the time required for radiographic healing. *Journal of Pediatric Surgery, 32,* 1093–1096.

Maier, R.V. (1993). Injury prevention and control. In Committee on Trauma, American College of Surgeons, *Resources for optimal care of the injured patient: 1993* (pp. 13–15). Chicago: American College of Surgeons.

Manson, D., Babyn, P.S., Palder, S., & Bergman, K. (1993). CT of blunt chest trauma in children. *Pediatric Radiology, 23,* 1–5.

Martin, V., Langley, B., & Coffman, S. (1995). Patterns of injury in pediatric patients in one Florida community and implications for prevention programs. *Journal of Emergency Nursing, 21,* 12–16.

Mattox, K.L., Bickell, W., Pepe, P.E., Burch, J., & Feliciano, D. (1989). Prospective MAST study in 911 patients. *Journal of Trauma, 29,* 1104–1112.

McSwain, N.E., Butman, A.M., McConnell, W.K., & Vomacka, R.W. (Eds.). (1990). Thoracic trauma. *In PHTLS: Basic and advanced prehospital life support* (2nd ed.). Akron, OH: Emergency Training.

Mitchell, K.A., Fallat, M.W., Raque, G.H., Hardwick, V.G., Groff, D.B., & Nagaraj, H.S. (1994). Evaluation of minor head injury in children. *Journal of Pediatric Surgery, 29,* 851–854.

Moore, E.E., Cogbill, T.H., Malangoni, M.A., Jurkovich, G.J., Champion, H.R., Gennarelli, T.A., McAninch, J.W., Pachter, H.L., Shackford, S.R., & Trafton, P.G. (1990). Organ injury scaling, II: Pancreas, duodenum, small bowel, colon, and rectum. *Journal of Trauma, 30,* 1427–1429.

Moore, E.E., Cogbill, T.H., Jurkovich, G.J., Shackford, S.R., Malangoni, M.A., & Champion, H.R. (1995). Organ injury scaling: spleen and liver (1994 revisions). *Journal of Trauma, 38,* 323–324.

Morse, M.A., & Garcia, V.F. (1994). Selective nonoperative management of pediatric blunt splenic trauma: Risk of missed associated injuries. *Journal of Pediatric Surgery, 29,* 23–27.

Moss, R.L., & Musemeche, C.A. (1996). Clinical judgement is superior to diagnostic tests in the management of pediatric small bowel injury. *Journal of Pediatric Surgery, 31,* 1178–1182.

Moulton, S.L., Downey, E.C., Anderson, D.S, & Lynch, F.P. (1993). Blunt bile duct injuries in children. *Journal of Pediatric Surgery, 28,* 795–797.

Moulton, S.L., Lynch, F.P., Hoyt, D.B., Kitchen, L., Pinckney, L., Canty, T.G., & Collins, D.L. (1992). Operative intervention for pediatric liver injuries: Avoiding delay in treatment. *Journal of Pediatric Surgery, 27,* 958–963.

Nersesian, W.S., Petit, W.R., Shaper, R., Lemieux, D., & Naor, E. (1985). Childhood death and poverty: A study of all childhood deaths in Maine, 1976 to 1980. *Pediatrics, 75,* 41–50.

Newman, K.D. (1993). Gastric and intestinal injury. In M.R. Eichelberger (Ed.), *Pediatric trauma: Prevention, acute care, rehabilitation* (pp. 475–481). St. Louis, MO: Mosby.

Osberg, J.S., & Unsworth, C.A. (1997). Trauma-rehabilitation connections: Discharge and admission decisions for children. *Pediatric Rehabilitation, 1,* 131–146.

Pieper, P. (1994). Pediatric trauma: An overview. *Nursing Clinics of North America, 29,* 563–584.

Pigula, F.A., Wald, S.L., Shackford, S.R., & Vane, D.W. (1993). The effect of hypotension and hypoxia on children with severe head injuries. *Journal of Pediatric Surgery, 28,* 310–316.

Pranikoff, T., Hirschl, R.B., Schlesinger, A.E., Polley, T.Z., & Coran, A.G. (1994). Resolution of splenic injury after nonoperative management. *Journal of Pediatric Surgery, 29,* 1336–1369.

Prow, H.W., Cole, J.W., Yeakley, J., Diaz-Marchan, P.J., & Hayman, L.A. (1996). Non-invasive neuroimaging in closed head trauma. In R.W. Evans (Ed.), *Neurology and trauma* (pp. 43–44). Philadelphia: W.B. Saunders Company.

Raimondi, A.J., & Hirschauer, J. (1984). Head injury in the infant and toddler: Coma scoring and outcome scale. *Child's Brain, 11,* 12–35.

Rasmussen, G.E., & Grande, C.M. (1994). Blood, fluids, and electrolytes in the pediatric trauma patient. *International Anesthesiology Clinics, 32,* 79–101.

Richie, J.P., & Fonkalsrud, E.W. (1972). Subcapsular hematoma of the liver: Nonoperative management. *Archives of Surgery, 104,* 781–784.

Rothlin, M.A., Naf, R., Amgwerd, M., Candinas, D., Frick, T., & Trentz, O. (1993). Ultrasound in blunt abdominal and thoracic trauma. *Journal of Trauma, 34,* 488–495.

Rozycki, G.S., Ochsner, M.G., Jaffin, J.H., & Champion, H.R. (1993). Prospective evaluation of surgeons' use of ultrasound in the evaluation of trauma patients. *Journal of Trauma, 34,* 516–527.

Salter, R.B., & Harris, W.R. (1963). Injuries involving the epiphyseal plate. *Journal of Bone and Joint Surgery, 45-A,* 587–622.

Schafermeyer, R. (1993). Pediatric trauma. *Emergency Medicine Clinics of North America, 11,* 187–205.

Schunk, J.E., Rodgerson, J.D., & Woodward., G.A. (1996). The utility of head computed tomographic scanning in pediatric patients with normal neurologic examination in the emergency department. *Pediatric Emergency Care, 12,* 160–165.

Shafi, S., Gilbert, J.C., Loghmanee, F., Allen, J.E., Caty, M.G., Glick, P.L., Carden, S., & Azizkhan, R.G. (1998). Impact of bicycle helmet safety legislation on children admitted to a regional pediatric trauma center. *Journal of Pediatric Surgery, 33,* 317–321.

Shilyansky, J., Sena, L.M., Kreller, M., Chait, P., Babyn, P.S., Filler, R.M., & Pearl, R.H. (1998). Nonoperative management of pancreatic injuries in children. *Journal of Pediatric Surgery, 33,* 343–349.

Silverman, B.K. (Ed.). (1993). *APLS: The pediatric emergency medicine course* (2nd ed.). Elk Grove Village, IL: American Academy of Pediatrics and America College of Emergency Physicians.

Simpson, D., & Reilly, P. (1982). Pediatric coma scale [Letter to the editor]. *Lancet, 8295,* 450.

Soud, T., Saum, P.D., & Pikulski, S. (1998). Trauma—Selected systems. In T.E. Soud & J.S. Rogers (Eds.), *Manual of pediatric emergency nursing* (pp. 511–539). St. Louis, MO: Mosby.

Stylianos, S., & Eichelberger, M.R. (1993). Pediatric trauma: Prevention strategies. *Pediatric Clinics of North America, 40,* 1359–1368.

Tepas, J.J., III. (1993). Blunt abdominal trauma in children. *Current Opinions in Pediatrics, 5,* 317–324.

Tepas, J.J., III. (2000). Pediatric trauma. In K.L. Mattox, D.V. Feliciano, & E.E. Moore (Eds.), *Trauma* (4th ed., pp. 1075–1096). Stamford, CT: Appleton & Lange.

Tepas, J.J., III, Mollitt, D.L., Talbert, J.L., & Bryant, M. (1987). The pediatric trauma score as a predictor of injury severity in the injured child. *Journal of Pediatric Surgery, 22,* 14–18.

Thomas, M.D. (1993). Musculoskeletal injury. In M.R. Eichelberger (Ed.), *Pediatric trauma: prevention, acute care, rehabilitation* (pp. 533–547). St. Louis, MO: Mosby.

Thourani, V.H., Pettitt, B.J., Schmidt, J.A., Cooper, W.A., & Rozycki, G.S. (1998). Validation of surgeon-performed emergency abdominal ultrasonography in pediatric trauma patients. *Journal of Pediatric Surgery, 33,* 322–328.

Tobias, J.D. (1996). Airway management for pediatric emergencies. *Pediatric Annals, 25,* 317–320, 323–324, 326–328.

Umali, E., Andrews, H.G., & White, J.J. (1992). A critical analysis of blood transfusion requirements in children with blunt abdominal trauma. *The American Surgeon, 58,* 736–739.

Upadhyaya, P., & Simpson, J.S. (1968). Splenic trauma in children. *Surgery, Gynecology and Obstetrics, 126,* 781–790.

Wesson, D., & Hu, X. (1995). The real incidence of pediatric trauma. *Seminars in Pediatric Surgery, 4,* 83–87.

Wong, D.L. (1982). Childhood trauma: Its developmental aspects and nursing interventions. *Critical Care Quarterly, 5,* 47–60.

Zander, J., & Hazinski, M.F. (1992). Pulmonary disorders. In M.F. Hazinski (Ed.), *Nursing care of the critically ill child* (2nd ed., pp. 395–497). St. Louis, MO: Mosby.

Appendix 34–A

Caremap for Isolated Splenic Injury (AAST Grades I, II, and III as Determined by Initial CT)

	Injury Day	*POD 1*	*POD 2*	*POD 3*	*POD 4*
Treatments	NGT to LCS (optional) Incentive spirometry (optional) IVF: NS at 100% maintenance NPO	DC NGT IVF: D5 1/4 NS w/20 mEq KCl/1	PO liquids DC IVF when tolerating PO liquids	Regular diet	→
Medications	MSO$_4$ 0.05–0.1 mg/kg IV q2–4h PRN pain	→	DC MSO$_4$ Acetaminophen PRN pain Ibuprofen PRN pain	→	→
Assessment and monitoring	Initial assessment VS q2h x8 PSD on monitor Serial exams	VS q4h	Transfer to floor		DC home
Activity	Strict bedrest	BRP with assistance	OOB to chair	Playroom	
Consults	Social services Trauma psychologist Child life		→	→	
Tests	H&H q12h If Hct <30, type and cross 2 units PRBCs	H&H am		H&H am	
Education	Orientation to room/unit		Orientation to room/floor	Review home activities	
Discharge planning	Limited activity at home				F/U appt in ~10 days Consider F/U abd CT in 6–8 wks

Note: It is essential that original note include AAST grade.
Source: Copyright © 2000, J.J. Tepas, III, and P. Pieper.

CHAPTER 35

Burn Care of Children

Robin Moushey and Lisa Meadows

INTRODUCTION TO PEDIATRIC BURN CARE

Burns constitute the second most common cause of accidental death in children less than 5 years of age in the United States (Grayck, Specer, & Munster, 1996). The burn insult is a devastating life event. The physical and psychological stability of the child is destroyed, disrupting the family and impacting caregivers. Improved management of burn patients, including such areas as fluid resuscitation, nutrition, and infection control, has resulted in a decline in burn mortality. A multidisciplinary approach is integral to the care of the burned child.

The skin is the largest organ in the body, making up 15% of total body weight (Sharp, 1993). The skin functions to protect from injury and infection, prevent loss of body fluids, regulate body temperature, and provide sensory contact with the environment, all of which are crucial to survival. Children's curious nature, their inability to protect themselves, and their thin epidermis are a perfect setup for significant burn injuries. The stressors of the trauma surrounding children are many. They suffer the painful and frightening occurrence of the trauma itself, and multiple family members may be involved. Often children feel guilty for the cause of the accident and for the failure in saving the lives of others. Loss of siblings and/or parents compounds the grief that children experience. Younger children are at higher risk for a significant burn because of the larger body surface area per pound of weight than adults. Their epidermis is thinner, causing deeper injuries at shorter heat exposures (see Table 35–1).

Burn injuries result from accidental or intentional events. The child should be carefully assessed and questions should be asked to determine the circumstances of the injury. Social work involvement is integral in the initial burn assessment. One should keep an open mind and provide support for the family throughout the child's hospitalization.

Many principles in this chapter can be used in caring for children with other devastating skin or tissue loss. This chapter discusses the following aspects of pediatric burn management: assessment of burn acuity and initial care, children's risk for airway obstruction, fluid requirements, assessment of body surface area and burn depth, pain management, burn wound management, nutrition, infection, and the multidisciplinary approach to care.

ASSESSING BURN ACUITY

Prehospital care for burns includes all the components of trauma stabilization, including assessment and support of airway, breathing, and circulation. Prehospital interventions specific to burn care include the removal or extinguishing of the heat source followed by application of clean, dry materials to prevent hypothermia. Moist coverings cause hypothermia and hypoperfusion to tissues and should be avoided. The body surface area burn (BSAB) should be estimated.

Assessing the burn wound percentage is a dynamic process. Various assessment methods exist. The rule of nines, which divides the body into areas of 9% is used with adults but can result in dangerously high BSAB estimates in children because it does not incorporate the increased BSA of the head. The Lund and Browder chart, which divides each body part into a percentage, considers changes in body surface area that occur during childhood development (see Figure 35–1). The palmar method allows a quick assessment to be made by using the palm of the child's hand to equal 1% of the child's total body surface area. Field personnel without access to the Lund and Browder chart should use the palmar method or simply describe the injury to the receiving hospital (e.g., half of the arm).

Field personnel contact the burn center with the necessary information to prioritize care of the child in the acute man-

Table 35–1 Time/Temperature/Burn Chart

Temperature (°F)	Seconds To Produce Partial-Thickness Burn in Children (sec)[a]
120	150
125	30–60
130	15
135	5
140	2.50
145	1.50
150	.75
155	.50

[a]Note: It takes twice as long to produce the same burn in an adult.
Source: Adapted from "Scald Burn Prevention Strategy," 1990, *Children's National Medical Center*, p. 67.

agement phase. These critical variables include age of the child, airway involvement, BSAB, location of the burn, burning agent, and time the burn occurred.

On admission to the hospital unit, the burn care team examines the child after removing all clothing, jewelry, and coverings used in transport. The burn is covered immediately with a warm dry sheet or blanket. The child should not be exposed unnecessarily. Overhead warming lights or other exogenous heat sources should be used to maintain body temperature. The child's state of consciousness should be evaluated and the presence of other injuries should be assessed. See Exhibit 35–1 for a checklist of the initial assessment of the child with burns.

Children who fulfill one or more of the American Burn Association criteria adapted for the pediatric population are candidates for admission to a burn center (see Exhibit 35–2).

One advantage to a pediatric burn center is the ability to provide for intensive care monitoring. See Exhibit 35–3 for suggested admission criteria to a burn intensive care unit.

AIRWAY MANAGEMENT

All children with burn injuries should be immediately assessed for airway patency. Edema formation from third spacing and inflammation can compromise the airway in children with burns several hours after injury, so they should be reassessed continuously. Children with the following categories of burn injuries are at high risk for airway compromise: house fires; isolated confined area surrounded by flames (e.g., crib); burns covering the face, neck, or chest; electrical burns; and BSAB greater than 20%.

The child with a major burn should be placed on a pulse oximeter and 100% oxygen (O_2) administered. Blood gases and carboxyhemoglobin levels should be obtained as indi-

AREA	1 YR.	1–4 YRS.	5–9 YRS.	10–14 YRS.	15 YRS.	ADULT	2°	3°
Head	19	17	13	11	9	7		
Neck	2	2	2	2	2	2		
Anterior trunk	13	13	13	13	13	13		
Posterior trunk	13	13	13	13	13	13		
Right buttock	2½	2½	2½	2½	2½	2½		
Left buttock	2½	2½	2½	2½	2½	2½		
Genitalia	1	1	1	1	1	1		
Right upper arm	4	4	4	4	4	4		
Left upper arm	4	4	4	4	4	4		
Right lower arm	3	3	3	3	3	3		
Left lower arm	3	3	3	3	3	3		
Right hand	2½	2½	2½	2½	2½	2½		
Left hand	2½	2½	2½	2½	2½	2½		
Right thigh	5½	6½	8	8½	9	9½		
Left thigh	5½	6½	8	8½	9	9½		
Right leg	5	5	5½	6	6½	7		
Left leg	5	5	5½	6	6½	8		
Right foot	3½	3½	3½	3½	3½	3½		
Left foot	3½	3½	3½	3½	3½	3½		
TOTAL								

Rule of Nines

Head	9%
Anterior Trunk	18%
Posterior Trunk	18%
Right Upper Extremity	9%
Left Upper Extremity	9%
Right Lower Extremity	18%
Left Lower Extremity	18%
Perineum	1%

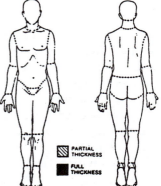

PARTIAL THICKNESS

FULL THICKNESS

Figure 35–1 Lund and Browder Chart

Exhibit 35–1 Checklist for Initial Assessment of the Child with Burns

Airway	Circulation	Secondary Survey

Assess for the following:
  Facial/neck burns
  Perioral burns (nose, lips, mouth, or throat)
  Singed nasal hairs, eyebrows, facial soot
  Carbon particles in the mouth or sputum
  Circumferential burns of the chest
Observe for patency of airway:
  Stridor/wheezing
  Difficulty swallowing
  Hoarseness
  Chest excursion
  Respiratory rate, depth, rhythm
	Cut clothing off and remove all watches, rings, other jewelry.
	Cover child with warm blankets.
	Place patient on cardiorespiratory monitor.
	Assess for signs of adequate cardiac output every 15 minutes:
	  Quality, rate, and rhythm of central and peripheral pulses
	  Color
	  Capillary refill
	  BP
	  Level of consciousness
	Children with 10% but less than 15% BSA burn: Maintenance IV fluid rate
	Children with 15%–20% BSA burn, start 2 large-bore IVs.
	Maintenance IV fluid rate.
	  +
	Resuscitative fluid requirements: 4 ml lactated Ringer's x Kg B.W. x % BSAB
	  1/2 total volume in first 8 hours (calculate based on time of initial burn injury)
	  Remainder 1/2 to be infused over 16 hr (hr 9–24)
	Use fluid warmer to deliver IV fluids.
	Maintain UO 1–2 ml/kg/hr
	Laboratory tests: CBC, comprehensive metabolic panel, type and cross-match if coexisting trauma is present.
		Weigh the patient.
		Assist in assessment of BSAB.
		Insert Foley catheter with 15%–20% BSA burn
		Insert NG tube in children with 20% BSAB. Monitor for nausea, vomiting, and presence of ileus secondary to decreased GI circulation.
		Observe for circumferential full-thickness burns of the extremities.
		Observe for any open wounds that might indicate open fractures, related to the mechanism of injury or trauma.
		Elevate injured extremities.
		Make baseline assessment of all affected extremities and reassess every 15–30 minutes:
		  Peripheral pulses (brachial, radial, popliteal, pedal), Doppler as needed
		  Extremity temp, color, and capillary refill, pain or paresthesia
		Prepare for possibility of escharotomy.
		Obtain urinalysis.

Breathing

Place patient on 100% humidified O_2 + oximeter if at risk for compromised airway.

Evaluate respiratory rate, depth, rhythm, and breath sounds.

Obtain ABGs and carboxyhemoglobin as indicated.

Assess for signs of CO poisoning; report of decreased respirations or apnea at scene.
  Cherry red normal skin
  Confusion/coma
  Increased carboxyhemoglobin

Assist with intubation procedure if patient is not breathing effectively or obstruction is possible.

Observe for circumferential full-thickness burns of the thorax that might decrease chest expansion. Assist with escharotomy, if necessary.

cated. The young child with a small airway diameter does not need circumferential burns around the neck or chest to have impaired ventilation. Early blood gases may have satisfactory results, but if airway edema progresses, hypercapnia results and respiratory acidosis develops.

The extent of smoke inhalation injury is the prime determination for burn outcomes (Herndon, Rutan, Alison, & Cox, 1993). Children caught in a house fire will often hide rather than escape. Obvious signs of smoke inhalation are facial burns, soot in airways, singed hair, hoarseness, and dysphagia. History obtained from the scene includes altered level of consciousness and apnea.

Damage to the airway comes from varied factors. Although fire surrounds the child with intense heat, dry air reaching the carina is cooled to 50° (Sharp, 1993), and there is usually not heat exposure below the epiglottis. Toxins from combustion can be absorbed systemically or cause direct injury to the tracheobronchial lining. Carbon monoxide (CO) and cyanide are absorbed systemically, whereas direct injury is caused by exposure to aldehydes, hydrochloride, chlorine, and ammonia (Sharp, 1993).

Carbon monoxide poisoning occurs when carbon monoxide has been inhaled and absorbed by the pulmonary circulation, displacing oxygen from the red blood cells and decreas-

Exhibit 35–2 Burn Center Admission Criteria

Second- and Third-Degree Burns
- BSA > 10%
    - Age < 10
    - Age > 50
- BSA > 20%
    - All other ages

Third-Degree Burns
- BSA > 5%
- Face-Hands-Feet-Genitalia-Perineum-Major Joints
- Electric injury
- Chemical injury
- Inhalation injury
- Circumferential burns of an extremity/chest

---

ing the capacity of the blood to carry oxygen to the cells in the body. The carbon monoxide binds with the hemoglobin 200 to 250 times more readily than oxygen does and is then converted to carboxyhemoglobin. Oxygen levels decrease and hypoxemia develops.

Normal carboxyhemoglobin levels are 5% to 10%, with the half-life of carboxyhemoglobin being 5 hours on room air and 1 hour on 100% O_2 (Walker, 1996). Therefore, the carboxyhemoglobin level obtained in the emergency department may be lower than the level obtained in the field. Scherb (1990) states that "COHgb levels are not accurate indicators of the degree of poisoning. The signs and symptoms exhibited by the patient, especially the level of consciousness, are more important when determining the severity of poisoning" (p. 144).

Symptoms of CO poisoning include nausea and vomiting, headache, irritability, confusion, decreased consciousness, and respiratory failure. These symptoms may be confused with pain, hypoxia, head injury, electrolyte abnormalities, anxiety, or separation from parents. Cherry red discoloration may be detected in mucous membranes but is difficult to assess because of irritation and inflammation from the injury itself. Once a child has been diagnosed with CO poisoning,

---

Exhibit 35–3 Requirements for Intensive Care Monitoring

Intensive care monitoring is required for:

- Children < 2 yr old with BSAB > 15%
- Children > 2 yr old with BSAB > 20%
- Electrical burns
- Inhalation injuries
- Burns covering face/neck with potential airway obstruction

---

humidified oxygen should be supplied at 100% by means of a tight-fitting nonrebreather mask. The oxygen saturation may appear normal or falsely elevated in smoke inhalation because the hemoglobin molecule carrying carbon monoxide and/or oxygen is recognized by the pulse oximetry. Respiratory rate, depth, rhythm, and breath sounds should continue to be assessed and arterial blood gases and carboxyhemoglobin levels should be followed.

A difficult decision is whether to intubate a child who initially is breathing on his or her own. When in doubt, intubate. Early intubation saves the child considerable airway trauma. The goal is to perform an intubation in a controlled setting with the child adequately sedated rather than as an emergency procedure. It is essential for physicians, nurses, and respiratory therapists to work together to maintain airway integrity. See Exhibit 35–4 for suggestions for securing an endotracheal tube in a child with facial burns.

With a circumferential full-thickness chest burn, if blood gases are not satisfactory or chest excursion is limited after intubation, chest escharotomies may be warranted to allow sufficient pulmonary expansion and oxygenation (see "Wound Assessment" later in this chapter).

INTRAVENOUS FLUID GUIDELINES

The goals of burn fluid resuscitation are to restore vascular volume, perfuse the kidneys, and replace sodium losses. Loss of plasma and interstitial fluid from damaged skin and capillaries has an impact on the child's precarious water and electrolyte balance. Serotonins, histamines, and prostaglandins are some of the vasoactive mediators released in response to bodily stress (Sharp, 1993). These mediators cause an increase in capillary permeability in both burned and unburned tissues. Sodium and protein molecules leave the capillaries and enter the interstitial space raising oncotic pressure. This increase in oncotic pressure pulls water from the capillaries, causing a fluid shift from vascular to interstitial compartments otherwise known as third spacing. This process continues for approximately 24 hours after injury until capillary healing begins.

Other factors contribute to the complexity of fluid management in the patient with burns. Cardiac output is decreased in major burns by the release of a myocardial depressant factor. The release of antidiuretic hormone conserves water while aldosterone retains sodium with accompanying water retention. Both actions restrict urine output. Kidney perfusion and urine output can be severely disrupted 24 hours after burn injury unless fluid loss is replaced and hydration is maintained. Clinically, the child may have edematous interstitial tissue but a decreased vascular fluid volume.

Obtaining and maintaining adequate hydration of the child with burns requires careful assessment and ongoing re-evaluation. Overhydration can cause increasing tissue edema

Exhibit 35–4 Suggestions for Securing Endotracheal Tube on Child with Facial Burns

Securing the endotracheal tube (ET) on children with burns on the face and neck is challenging. The following interventions are helpful:

- Use trach ties to secure the ET tube around the head. These ties are larger than umbilical tape and less likely to cause pressure points on edematous tissue.
- Suture the ET tube. One suture is placed inside the mouth and a second suture is inserted under the chin through the mandible. The ties are brought up and tied around the ET tube. Circummandibular stabilization causes less damage to nares; it may be performed immediately after intubation, and it secures the airway.
- Wire ET tube to dental plate. Although this provides adequate security, it usually cannot be done immediately.
- Place isolation masks backward on the child and use the ties to secure the ET tube. This is a short-term temporary intervention.
- Use protective skin barriers on unburned skin when possible to secure ties or tape.
- There are various commercial products to secure ET tubes, but these may prove to be less beneficial for the young child.

compromising perfusion to body tissues. Insufficient fluid replacement decreases the flow of oxygen to the tissues compromising kidney function. Adequate tissue perfusion enhances the oxygenation of both burned and unburned tissue, which is essential for optimal outcomes (Carvajal, 1994).

Controversy exists regarding the composition and quantity of IV fluids and the most accurate assessment of satisfactory clinical outcomes for the child (Carvajal, 1994). For simplicity of this chapter, the pediatric resuscitative guidelines of the *American Burn Life Support Manual* (1994) are used.

Calculate fluid resuscitation from the time of initial burn injury—not the time the child arrived at the emergency department. An accurate weight is determined and the BSAB recalculated to ensure an accurate estimation for fluid resuscitation.

IV replacement fluids are calculated at 3 to 4 ml/kg/hr × percent BSAB (Advanced Burn Life Support Manual, 1994). One half of the total volume is given over the first 8 hours and the remainder is given over the next 16 hours. The maintenance fluid volume for each child is added separately to the IV fluid replacement orders (see Table 35–2).

The composition of lactated Ringer's (LR) solution is close to normal body fluids and is a commonly used resuscitation IV fluid (275 mOsm/L; Na 130; K 4; Ca 3; Cl 109; lactate 28). Albumin is administered specific to each burn

center's guidelines; however, it is usually not administered in the first 24 hours. Once initial fluid resuscitation orders are completed, IV fluids should be monitored and adjusted. Ongoing assessment of fluid status of the burn patient includes monitoring vital signs, physical examination, serial hematocrit, BUN, specific gravity, and adjusting for ongoing fluid losses. Urine output should be maintained at 1 to 2 ml/kg/hr.

As capillary and lymphatic function begins to return to the preburn state, kidney perfusion increases and diuresis occurs. Intravenous fluid composition and rates are adjusted to the child's response to therapy.

WOUND ASSESSMENT

Skin exposure to a hot source can destroy the epidermis and the dermis containing glands and hair follicles. Intense and prolonged heat exposure can damage subcutaneous and adipose tissue. The depth of tissue damage caused by fire and electrical sources may be evident immediately. However, burns occurring from grease, contact, and scalds can take 24 to 72 hours before the actual depth is manifested. Overall goals for wound management include debriding, cleaning, and protecting the wound; minimizing infection; and maximizing function. The wound should be accurately described rather than labeling the depth of the burn (see Exhibit 35–5).

Full-thickness and partial-thickness injuries can occur simultaneously in a burn wound. Sensation and capillary refill should be assessed by gentle palpation only. Appearance of intact hair follicles during immediate wound assessment does not rule out the possibility of a full-thickness injury.

When edema is present in full-thickness injury, circumferential eschar prevents further expansion of tissues. Blood vessels become compressed and ischemia develops. Although it is difficult to assess in a burned patient, the hallmark signs and symptoms of diminished circulation are cool, pale, painful, or tingling extremities, and/or pulselessness with immobile digits and poor capillary refill. Full-thickness circumferential burn injuries that result in vascular compromise require escharotomy. An escharotomy is indicated to allow blood flow to distal extremities or to enhance compliance of chest wall ventilation. By definition, a full-thickness burn is anesthetic; however, the child's state of consciousness and level of anxiety will require pharmacologic intervention before an escharotomy.

An escharotomy is performed with a scalpel or electrocautery and consists of making a longitudinal incision through both ends of the circumferential burn eschar. Minimal blood loss occurs. The incision should be deep enough to penetrate the eschar. As tissues release occurs, the subcutaneous fat bulges through the incision, tension is relieved, and effective blood flow returns. Once the initial incision is made, pulses

Table 35–2 General IV Guidelines According to BSA Burned

	<10%	10% ≤ 15%	>15%
Location of IV	Peripheral	Peripheral	Peripheral Difficult access: cutdown, central line, intraosseous infusion
Purpose	Hydration for child with limited PO intake	Hydration for child with limited PO intake	Resuscitation related to size of burn wound; hydration for child with limited PO intake or NPO status
	Pain medication administration	Pain medication administration	Pain medication administration
IVF rate	Maintenance	Maintenance	Maintenance fluid rate: + resuscitative: 3–4 ml LR × KGBW[a] × BSAB 1/2 total volume over first 8 hr Remainder given over next 16 hr

[a] KGBW = Body weight in kilograms.
Note: See text for IV formula reference.

should be reassessed. If they are nonpalpable, one should consider extending the incision to ensure that the incision extends through the entire eschar. Persistent signs of ischemia or children with fourth-degree injuries (e.g., involvement of muscle, bone, electrical injury) may be at risk for compartment syndrome, necessitating fasciotomies. The wounds may be covered with Silvadene or wet-to-dry dressings once the procedure is complete.

Exhibit 35–5 Classification of Depth of Burn Injury

Superficial (first degree)	Erythema; mild edema and pain; blanches with pressure
Partial thickness (second degree)	Pink to red; moist; moderate edema; extremely painful; vesicles
Full thickness (third degree)	Waxy-white to black; dry leathery; thrombosed vessels; edema; painless
(fourth degree)	Dry; leathery; black; painless; possible exposed bones, tendons, muscles

PAIN IN CHILDREN WITH BURNS

Children who are burned require appropriate pain management. Pain is a symptom of traumatic loss of body tissue and should be treated accordingly. Some burn dressing changes require general anesthesia to adequately manage the pain. A common mistake made in the pain management of a child with a burn is testing the child's tolerance to the initial procedure before increasing pain medication. Children enter a shocklike state after injury that can mask their expressive ability during the first burn dressing. Although it is difficult to predict the most effective pain management plan for a child with new burns, providing a dose that gives the maximum coverage for pain and anxiety is optimal. The initial experience of the child sets the stage for behavioral consequences the rest of the hospitalization and after discharge.

Initial assessment criteria for appropriate pain management include the child's age and realistic behavioral expectations; BSAB, age of burn, burning agent, and depth; child's previous experiences and coping mechanisms; and medical history. Corollary issues are the response of the child and family, time necessary for debridement and whirlpool, nutritional concerns, and difficulty in maintaining IV access.

It is helpful to look at wound and pain management in three phases. The acute phase is usually 24 to 72 hours after injury. The goal during this period is aggressive pain control and wound debridement. Decisions regarding surgical debridement and/or skin grafting and application of alternative dressings are made. A combination of oxycodone (0.15 to 0.4 mg/kg PO) and midazolam (Versed) (0.5 to 1 mg/kg PO) decreases pain and anxiety in children when administered 30 minutes before the procedure. Nurses can administer these dosages safely by monitoring the child's vital signs and oxygen saturation every 15 minutes from the time the medications are given until 30 minutes after the debridement is complete. If the child is sleeping, vital signs are taken every 30 minutes and the child should remain on the pulse oximeter until awake. Children may require supplemental IV medications (e.g., ketamine, morphine, propofol, fentanyl) or nitrous oxide to obtain adequate pain control. These agents should be given by trained personnel and monitored per hospital protocol.

The transition phase follows the acute phase when the switch is made from IV medications to oral pain medications or a combination of both. Children can participate more actively in wound care after their acute pain has been addressed. The exact timing of this phase depends on the treatment plan and the child's previous response to care. Antianxiety medication such as midazolam may still be required in addition to the narcotic analgesics. If the child displays uncontrollable irritability from the midazolam, the agent can be reversed with IV flumazenil (Romazicon) and the symptoms can be alleviated with IV morphine, acetaminophen with codeine, or diphenhydramine (Benadryl). Place the child in a non-stimulating environment.

Once most of the wound is epithelialized or grafted, the child enters the healing phase. Medications such as acetaminophen with codeine, combinations of acetaminophen and oxycodone, and/or diphenhydramine are used during the healing phase in the hospital and at home. Children with severe burns who have received narcotics for pain relief for an extended period require a plan to wean them carefully and methodically off the narcotics. Otherwise signs and symptoms of withdrawal become evident.

Because there are tremendous variations in pain management methods, the side effects and the child's individual response to the medications should be continually assessed. Possible side effects of any sedative are respiratory depression, nausea, vomiting, and irritability. If the child with respiratory compromise responds quickly to oxygen and airway positioning, the medication should be resumed the following day. If the child does not respond quickly to the preceding measures, the daily medications should be changed or taking the child to the operating room for future dressing changes and pain management should be considered.

To help alleviate the pain, the use of play, distraction, music and video therapy, toys, stories, and especially the child's participation with wound care is highly valued. A child as young as 18 months can press gauze between the toes or hold the tape to participate in wound care. Blowing bubbles is an optimal form of play and distraction for chil-

dren. The pain service supports the acute phase with aggressive pain management during wound debridement. The transitional stage is a collaborative shift from pain management by the pain service to more psychological supportive efforts by child life service. These efforts are continued during the child's healing phase.

WOUND CARE

The objective of wound care is to keep the burned area clean and moist. Epithelial cells survive better in a moist environment. To cover a scabbed wound, epithelial cells are forced to exert more energy to burrow under the scar and lay down new cells (David, 1987). Wound exudate consists of serum, colonizing bacteria, and dead leukocytes. Mechanical, chemical, or surgical debridement that decreases the accumulation of eschar is needed before healing takes place. This allows the effective use of topical ointments and/or the early use of alternative dressings.

Consistency is essential in burn care to assess the wound and evaluate the effectiveness of any treatment plan and dressing application. Wound care approaches are based on the stage of burn progression. Once-a-day dressing changes are adequate for debridement when a child is appropriately sedated. Wound treatment plans, although chosen for effectiveness and ease of use, should always consider patient comfort.

On initial debridement, all blisters should be removed, except those on the palms of the hands and the soles of the feet (Sharp, 1993). Large blisters on the palms of the hands may require debridement if range of motion is restricted. Although intact blisters serve as a biologic dressing, clinical experience shows they usually do not remain intact.

One percent silver sulfadiazine is the most commonly used primary topical agent on burn wounds. It provides moisture and has an antimicrobial effect. Silver sulfadiazine cream, 1/16 to 1/8 inch thick, is applied to the wound before wrapping with gauze. A side effect of silver sulfadiazine is leukopenia. The leukopenia may not be a true allergic reaction but rather the bone marrow's response to the stress of the burn. If a skin rash develops after reapplication of the silver sulfadiazine, the child may have an allergy to products with sulfa. A product without sulfa such as polymixin B (Polysporin) should then be tried. Combining nystatin with topical agents may decrease a *Candida* superinfection and is used in some centers (Rose & Herndon, 1997).

Another dressing used on burn wounds is Biobrane-L (light adherence), a synthetic substance that can be applied to a partial-thickness burn wound once it is cleaned and debrided. Biobrane consists of a layer of collagen, silicone, and nylon and allows visibility of the wound. It is available in different sheet sizes or gloves. The Biobrane is stretched over a clean wound and the edges are adhered onto non-burned areas with adhesive strips. This facilitates drainage to pass through the pores of the Biobrane instead of accumulating on the wound. A bulky dressing is wrapped over the Biobrane and it is covered with an Ace wrap to provide additional pressure. To ensure Biobrane's adherence, movement and range of motion exercises are minimized 24 to 48 hours after application. Daily wound debridement is eliminated because Biobrane is left on the wound until it is healed.

Small burn injuries can be managed in the primary care setting. The same principles are used as in the inpatient management of burn wounds, including obtaining a history of the burn, evaluating the extent of the wound, and using pain management strategies. Families should be offered suggestions about burn wound management materials to avoid excessive costs. The list of options in wound management increases each year, and references to many of these are in the Wound Care Product Glossary in Appendix 35–B. Wounds can be wrapped with a white 100% cotton T-shirt, pillow case, or sheet that has been cut up and rewashed for a cost-saving method. Tube socks can be cut and used over arms/legs. Panty liners without deodorant can be used for gauze.

Deep partial or full-thickness wounds that require an extended period of time to heal usually require excision and grafting in the operating room. Excisions may be tangential or fascial. In tangential excisions, thin layers of necrotic tissue are excised until bleeding tissue is reached. In fascial excision, all necrotic burn and subcutaneous tissue is removed until the superficial fascia is visualized (Sadowski, 1992). The choice of excision method depends on the depth of burn and the surgeon's preference for the optimal graft bed.

Autografts are obtained from the child's own body and may be split thickness or full thickness. Split-thickness grafts consist of epithelium and part of dermis. These grafts are applied as either sheet grafts or mesh grafts, depending on the location of the burn and the surgeon's preference. A sheet graft is skin taken from a donor site and directly placed over the burn bed. A mesh graft is skin taken from a donor site and placed through a mesher that stretches the skin two to three times its size. If the child does not have adequate skin for autografting, donor skin is used. Allografts or homografts are tissue from same species (i.e., cadaver skin), whereas xenografts or heterografts are tissue from different species (e.g., pigskin).

Nursing considerations regarding postgraft care are described in Appendix 35–A. Leaving the donor site open to air in children is not recommended. Children scratch the area, causing damage to budding tissue. Even when children are medicated for itching, protecting the donor site remains a problem in pediatric care.

NUTRITION

The metabolic needs of children with burn injuries increase with tissue destruction, daily nitrogen losses, and postburn hypermetabolism (Sadowski, 1992; Sharp; 1993). The hypermetabolic state is 1.5 to 2 times the norm for the child and lasts until the wound is epithelialized or grafted (Sadowski, 1992). The patient should be assessed for an ileus and monitored for nausea and vomiting for 24 to 48 hours. A nasogastric tube (NG) is placed for decompression in any child with greater than 20% BSAB. Children with less than 15% BSAB should receive a high-calorie and high-protein diet with snacks or supplemental nutrition formulas. A feeding tube is placed in children with greater than 15% to 20% BSAB for continuous 12- to 24-hour enteral feedings with supplemental calorie intake to meet calorie needs. Caloric needs are adjusted on the basis of the percent of burn, activity level, and stress level (e.g., physical therapy, dressing changes, infection, fever, and operating room visits). Although they are able to consume an oral diet, few children are able to take in adequate calories. Often nasogastric or nasojejunal feedings are needed to supplement oral intake. Early enteral feedings promote gut motility and prevent intestinal ischemia (Sadowski, 1992).

Translocation of the gastrointestinal flora, which is the release of gram-negative bacteria and endotoxins from the bowel lumen, contributes to the development of sepsis in the burned patient. Central venous total parental nutrition (TPN) should only be used on those children who cannot tolerate NG feedings. When administering NG feedings, the following are helpful hints in securing NG tube position. Stomahesive wafers/DuoDerm and transparent dressings are helpful when used on intact skin or the NG may be tied or secured to the endotracheal tube or around the head. The area under the ties should always be assessed for undue pressure caused by edema formation. Utilize arm cuffs when necessary to ensure that tube stays properly placed. Refer to Chapter 4 for further information on nutrition in the child with burns.

INFECTION

One of the major risk factors for mortality in children with burn injuries is infection. The primary barrier to infection is lost when the body loses the skin's protective covering. The burn wound colonizes with organisms within 24 hours of exposure to the environment. The initial contaminant comes from the child's own skin flora. Additionally, many children admitted with burns may have a preexisting upper respiratory infection that is exacerbated with the trauma of the burn.

To heal the child, health care providers perform many procedural interventions that increase the risk of infection. Intubation, blood gas monitoring, IV access, Foley catheters, and NG tubes are key risk factors. The use of systemic antibiotics has increased burn wound survival. However, the control of gram-negative/positive flora by broad-spectrum antibiotics may result in burn wounds becoming colonized by opportunistic yeast fungi. For this reason, antibiotics are used judiciously for treatment of infections. Early surgical debridement and grafting allows for faster wound closure, establishing a new barrier to infection. Providing adequate nutrition stimulates the gastrointestinal tract and reduces the risk of translocation of organisms and provides nutrients to heal (Periti & Donati, 1995).

Children who have been burned initially have difficulty maintaining body temperature. However, they soon enter a hypermetabolic state in which their hypothalamus "resets," and it is usual for them to run a low-grade temperature. Initial temperature spikes to 39° C are common, but when seen 48 hours after the burn, the child should be assessed for sepsis and other signs of common childhood infections (e.g., otitis media, influenza). White blood cell changes, the child's activity and appetite, and the appearance of the wound or grafts are all variables to be considered. The child should be assessed, not the temperature. Children who have an unusual fever, hypothermia, anorexia, and/or change in sensorium or vital signs should be evaluated for development of sepsis. Blood cultures should be drawn after a careful patient assessment is made.

THE MULTIDISCIPLINARY APPROACH TO CARE

Burn treatment progresses through three major components of care and requires a multitude of team members. The physiologic impact of burn trauma is addressed throughout the acute management phase. Optimal wound care during this time is facilitated by aggressive treatment of pain and anxiety. Children may express thoughts concerning survival and death. Guilt feelings may be heightened if children have played with matches and caused harm to family members and/or belongings. The burn team should work closely together to maximize family and child support.

The transitional phase evolves when the plan of care is established. Focus is on wound care, nutrition, and infection control. It is normal that children and families initially reject the sight of the burn injury. Acceptance is accomplished over time with support and patience. In the hospital, mirrors can be covered with cards and greetings until facial swelling decreases. However, whenever children request to look, they should be accommodated. A mirror should be available during treatment. When explaining grafts to children and families, it is important to focus on the value of covering the skin first and cosmesis later. Discuss how skin color returns and make a game for the child to find signs of new skin budding. Pain medications can be adjusted to allow children to participate in burn care routines. This gives the child and family some mastery and control of care in the hospital, which can continue at home.

The healing phase coordinates efforts for full functional recovery of both physiological and psychological domains. Transition to home is optimized by minimizing contractions, providing as "near-normal" appearance as possible, maximizing the child's coping ability and personal strengths, and alleviating the anxiety and painful memories of burn treatment. Physical and occupational therapists are key members of the team during this phase.

The multidisciplinary team addresses all these patient needs from admission to postdischarge. Relationships formed from this collaborative process stimulate and support the team to foster successful patient outcomes.

CONCLUSION

Burns in children can result in devastating injuries to the child and significant emotional trauma to the child and family. Appropriate management of the child with a burn requires knowledgeable and skilled caregivers from the prehospital phase and initial resuscitation, throughout the hospitalization, to rehabilitation and return to the home, school, and community. In addition to management of the burn wound itself, airway and nutritional support, fluid and pain management, and prevention of infection are also particularly important. A multidisciplinary team aids in the provision of comprehensive medical, psychosocial, and rehabilitative care to the child and family.

REFERENCES

Advanced Burn Life Support Course. (1994). *Pediatric thermal injury* (pp. 63–70). National Burn Institute.

American Burn Life Support Course. (1994*). Shock and fluid resuscitation* (pp. 25–38). National Burn Institute.

American Burn Association. (1988, March). Hospital and prehospital resources for optimal care of patients with burn injury: Guidelines for development and operation of burn centers. *Journal of Burn Care and Rehabilitation,* 98–104.

Carvajal, H. (1994). Fluid resuscitation of pediatric burn victims: A critical approach. *Pediatric Nephrology, 8,* 357–366.

David, J. (1987). Tissue damage and repair. In Smith & Martin, *Wound Management* (pp. 1–21). United Kingdom: Martin & Dunitz.

Grayck, E., Specer, R., & Munster, A. (1996). Burns, inhalational injury, and electrical injury. In M. Rogers & D. Nichols (Eds.), *Textbook of pediatric intensive care* (pp. 1521–1542). Baltimore: Williams & Wilkins.

Herndon, D., Rutan, R., Alison, W., & Cox, C. (1993). Management of burn injuries. In M. Eichelberger (Ed.), *Pediatric trauma: Prevention, acute care, rehabilitation* (pp. 568–590). St. Louis, MO: Mosby.

Periti, P., & Donati, L. (1995). Survival and therapy of burn patients at the threshold of the twenty-first century: A review. *Journal of Chemotherapy, 7*(6), 475–502.

Rose, J.K., & Herndon, D.N. (1997, March). Advances in the treatment of burn patients. *Burns, 23*(1), 519–526.

Sadowski, D. (1992). Care the child with burns. In M.F. Helsinki (Ed.), *Nursing care of the critically ill child* (pp. 875–927). St. Louis, MO: Mosby-Year Book.

Scherb, B.J. (1990). Carbon monoxide poisoning: Hyperbaric oxygenation preparations. *Dimensions of Critical Care Nursing, 9*(3), 143–149.

Sharp, R. (1993). Burns. In K. Ashcroft & T. Holder (Eds.), *Pediatric surgery burns* (pp. 89–102). Philadelphia: W.B. Saunders Company.

Walker, A. (1996). Emergency department management of house fire burns and carbon monoxide poisoning in children. *Current Opinion in Pediatrics, 8*(3), 239–242.

SUGGESTED READINGS

Alexander, J., Marshall, E., & Hambright, F. (1991). Would you recognize this toxic emergency? *RN, 54*(1), 26–31.

Asburn, M.A. (1995, May/June). Burn pain: The management of procedure-related pain. *Journal of Burn Care and Rehabilitation,* 365–371.

Attorri, R., Randolph, J., & Troku, O. (1993). Burn in children. In P. Holbrook (Ed.), *Textbook of pediatric critical care* (pp. 1092–1101). Philadelphia: W.B. Saunders Company.

Beushausen, T., & Mucke, K. (1997). Anesthesia and pain management in pediatric burn patients. *Pediatric Surgery International, 12,* 327–333.

Bonham, A. (1996). Managing procedural pain in children with burns: Part 1. Assessment of pain in children. *International Journal of Trauma Nursing, 2,* 68–73.

Bonham, A. (1996). Managing procedural pain in children with burns: Part 2. Nursing management of children in pain. *International Journal of Trauma Nursing, 3,* 74–77.

Carvajal, J., & Griffith, J. (1992). Burn and inhalation injuries. In B. Fuhrman & J. Zimmerman (Eds.), *Pediatric critical care* (pp. 1209–1222). St. Louis, MO: Mosby.

Cass, D.L., Meuli, M., & Adzick, N.S. (1997). Scar war: Implications of fetal wound healing for the pediatric burn patient. *Pediatric Surgery Interview, 12,* 484–489.

Cortiella, J., & Marvin, J. (1997). Management of the pediatric burn patient. *Burn Management Nursing Clinics of North America, 32*(2), 311–329.

Doctor, M.E. (1994). Parent participation during painful wound care procedures. *Journal of Burn Care and Rehabilitation.* 288–292.

Foglia, R., & Moushey, R. (1994). *Burn care resource manual.* St. Louis, MO: St. Louis Children's Hospital.

Germann, G., Cedidi, C., & Hartmann, B. (1997). Post burn reconstruction during growth and development. *Pediatric Surgery International, 12,* 321–326.

Gordon, M., & Goodwin, C. (1997). Initial assessment, management, and stabilization. *Burn Management Nursing Clinics of North America, 32*(2), 237–249.

Kavanaugh, C. (1983). Psychological intervention with the severely burned child: Report of an experimental comparison of two approaches and their effects on psychological sequelae. *Journal of the American Academy of Child and Adolescent Psychiatry, 22*(2), 145–156.

Kavanaugh, C., & Freeman, R. (1984, May). Should children participate in burn care? *American Journal of Nursing,* 64.

Kavanaugh, C., Lasoff, E., Eide, Y., Freeman, R., McEttrick, M., Dar, R., Helgerson, R., Remensynder, J., & Kalin, N. (1991). Learned helplessness and the pediatric burn patient: Dressing change behavior and serum cortisol and B-endorphin. *Advances in pediatrics* (pp. 335–363). St. Louis, MO: Mosby.

Kuehn, C., Ahrenholz, D., & Jolem, L. (1989). Care of the burn wound. *Trauma Quarterly, 5*(4), 33–42.

Meagher, J. (1990). Burns. In J. Raffensperger (Ed.), *Swenson's pediatric surgery* (pp. 317–337). Stamford, CT: Appleton & Lange.

National Safe Kids Campaign. (1990). *Scald burn prevention strategy.* Washington, DC: Author.

Parsons, L. (1997). Office management of minor burns. *Lippincott's Primary Care Practice, 1*(1), 40–49.

Sheridan, R., & Tompkins, R. (1997). Burns. In K. Oldham, P. Colombani, & R. Foglia (Eds.), *Scientific principles of pediatric surgery* (pp. 517–533). Philadelphia: Lippincott-Raven Publishers.

Sittig, K., & Deitch, E. (1989). Principles and practices in the fluid resuscitation of thermally injured patients. *Trauma Quarterly, 5*(4), 7–18.

Watkins, P. (1993). This one's for Billy. *Journal of Burn Care and Rehabilitation, 14*(1), 58–64.

Wolf, S.E., Debroy, M., & Herndon, D.N. (1997). The cornerstones and directions of pediatric burn care. *Pediatric Surgery International, 12,* 312–320.

Appendix 35–A

Caremap for Postgraft Burns

| ✓ complete |
| • variance |

Signature: _____

_____

Title: Burns: Post-Graft Care _____

_____

Allergies: _____

_____   _____

Record orders in appropriate section.

Clinical Problem	OR Day _____ (date)	POD 1 _____ (date)	POD 2 _____ (date)
Pain/Irritability	__ Morphine IV prn or MSO4 gtt __ TC III __ Benadryl .5–1 mg/kg every 4–6 hours	__ Morphine IV prn or MSO4 gtt __ TC III __ Benadryl .5–1 mg/kg every 4–6 hours	__ Morphine IV prn or MSO4 gtt __ TC III __ Benadryl .5–1 mg/kg every 4–6 hours
Infection	__ Outer dressings protected from soiling	__ Trim and replace soiled outer dressings as needed	__ Trim and replace soiled outer dressings as needed
Temperature regulation	__ Maintain temperature every 4 hours, unless fever—then every 1 hour __ If blood/fluid loss, monitor temperature for post complications	__ Maintain temperature every 4 hours, unless fever—then every 1 hour __ If blood/fluid loss, monitor temperature for post complications	__ Maintain temperature every 4 hours, unless fever—then every 1 hour __ If blood/fluid loss, monitor temperature for post complications
Nutrition hydration	__ NPO prior to OR __ Advance diet as tolerated __ Resume NG feeds when awake and alert __ IVF until po well	__ HL IV fluid __ If po well when awake and alert, encourage high protein and high calorie diet __ Resume NG feeds	__ Resume NG feeds
Activity	__ Position for comfort and protection of wound __ TC and DB every 2 hours __ Bedrest __ 1S every 1 hour x 10 when awake	__ Bedrest	__ Bedrest
Assessment/interventions Grafted areas	__ Upper and lower extremities circulation check with vital signs __ Check weeping, soiling __ CBC pre-op if elevated temperature	__ CBC if blood loss during surgery	
Assessment/interventions Donor sites	__ Reinforce donor sites as needed __ Cover thigh dressings with Ace wrap/transparent dressing __ CBC pre-op if elevated temperature	__ If increased bleeding, take off outer wraps and place new kerlix __ CBC if blood loss during surgery	

Courtesy of St. Louis Children's Hospital, St. Louis, Missouri.

POD 3 _____ (date)	POD 4 _____ (date)	POD 5 _____ (date)	POD 6 _____ (date)	POD 7 _____ (date)
__ Morphine IV prn or MSO4 gtt __ TC III __ Benadryl .5–1 mg/kg every 4–6 hours	__ Morphine IV prn or MSO4 gtt __ TC III __ Benadryl .5–1 mg/kg every 4–6 hours	__ Morphine IV prn or MSO4 gtt __ TC III __ Benadryl .5–1 mg/kg every 4–6 hours	__ Morphine IV prn or MSO4 gtt __ TC III __ Benadryl .5–1 mg/kg every 4–6 hours	__ Morphine IV prn or MSO4 gtt __ TC III __ Benadryl .5–1 mg/kg every 4–6 hours
__ Wound culture if wound looks infected __ Blood culture if temperature above 38.5				__ No infection __ Normal temperature
__ Maintain temperature every 8 hours __ Heat lamp and warm blankets with dressing change		__ Heat lamp and warm blankets with dressing change		__ Maintains temperature
__ Resume NG feeds	__ Resume NG feeds	__ D/C NG feeds		__ IV fluids with staple removal
__ Up in wheelchair or wagon with affected extremity secured and elevated	__ Up in wheelchair or wagon with affected extremity secured and elevated	__ Start physical therapy/ occupational therapy for active and passive range of motion __ Increase activity	__ Increase activity	__ Active range of motion __ Increased participation in burn care
__ Soak in whirlpool tub without turning on agitators __ Re-wrap with Xeroform/ gauze __ Roll grafts with sterile Q-tip if fluid collection appears __ Wound culture if wound looks infected __ Blood culture for temperature above 38.5	__ Hold dressing if wounds look clean on day 3; reinforce as needed __ Wound culture if wound looks infected __ Blood culture for temperature above 38.5	__ Place in whirlpool with agitators on __ Wound culture if wound looks infected __ Blood culture for temperature above 38.5	__ Place in whirlpool with agitators on __ Wound culture if wound looks infected __ Blood culture for temperature above 38.5	__ Staples or sutures removed with whirlpool __ Check all lab work for final results __ Trim loose graft edges as needed
__ Soak in whirlpool without agitators __ Wound culture if wound looks infected __ Blood culture for temperature above 38.5	__ Wound culture if wound looks infected __ Blood culture for temperature above 38.5	__ Wound culture if wound looks infected __ Blood culture for temperature above 38.5 __ Trim donor dressing if scarlet red, Xeroform	__ Wound culture if wound looks infected __ Blood culture for temperature above 38.5 __ Trim donor dressing if scarlet red, Xeroform	__ Remove donor dressings when appropriate __ Adaptive for home __ Check all lab work for final results

continues

Appendix 35–A continued

| ✓ complete |
| • variance |

Title: Burns: Post-Graft Care

Signature: _____

_____

_____

_____   _____

_____   _____

Allergies: _____

Record orders in appropriate section.

Clinical Problem	OR Day _____ (date)	POD 1 _____ (date)	POD 2 _____ (date)
Dressing change medications			
IVs	__ D5½ Normal Saline with 20 KCL __ D5 Lactated Ringers → at maintenance rate or replacement rate for blood loss & NPO times		__ Hold therapy __ Contact Pain Service for Day 3
Consults	__ Physical Therapy/Occupational Therapy may see prior to OR __ Child Life Services __ Psychology __ Nutrition		
Equipment	__ IVAC pump for IV fluids __ Medinfusion if antibiotics __ PCA or IVAC pump if narcotic drip	__ O₂ if sats below 93% __ Splints	
Discharge planning/teaching	__ Home Health alerted __ Make sure Burn Care Booklet given		

POD 3 _____ (date)	POD 4 _____ (date)	POD 5 _____ (date)	POD 6 _____ (date)	POD 7 _____ (date)
__ po Versed/Oxycodone (Valium) .5–1 mg/kg 15–30 minutes before procedure __ Back-up MSO4 or Fentanyl		__ po Versed/Oxycodone __ Back-up IV meds __ Back-up MSO4 or Fentanyl and/or Nitrous Oxide before procedure	__ po Versed/Oxycodone, TC III, or Percocet	__ If staples, po Versed/ Oxycodone __ Back-up Morphine or Nitrous Oxide
__ EN75 for use with meds if needed __ HL IV post change				__ Discontinue heplock after staples taken out
__ Call House Officer __ Call Surgical Attending	__ Contact Pain Service for day 5 and 7			__ Complete discharge teaching __ Home Care nursing
__ Pulse oximeter with dressing change __ Anesthesia cart __ Bain airway circuit		__ Dressing—Xeroform over grafts __ Dressing—Adaptic over donor if SR	__ Dressing—Xeroform over grafts __ Dressing—Adaptic over donor if SR	__ Home care supplies obtained __ Anesthesia cart __ Bain airway circuit
__ Have guardian see wound if possible		__ Have guardian participate, if possible, with dressing change __ Encourage child to help	__ Have guardian participate, if possible, with dressing change __ Encourage child to help	__ May go home if no staples and if: • wound intact • no infection • ROM good • ambulating well • home resources ok • clinic appointment • OT/PT appointment

Appendix 35–B

Wound Care Product Glossary

Product	Phase	Description/Use
Adaptic	Transitional Healing	Protective sterile dressing with a light petroleum coating. May be used to keep healing wound or donor site moist and clean; used in combination with Polysporin for small open areas and healed wounds that have been abraded.
Allevyn	Healing	Absorbent hydrophilic polyurethane dressing containing three layers: (1) nonadherent contact layer; (2) highly absorbent central layer (10 times more absorptive than 4x4s); and (3) waterproof outer layer. Placed on wound pink side up and generally used with IntraSite gel to calm granulation tissue.
Alloderm		Human dermal graft that can be applied to a debrided wound. It is then covered by an ultra-thin wide meshed skin graft.
Biobrane	Acute Transitional	An ultra-thin semipermeable silicone membrane mechanically bonded to a flexible knitted nylon fabric—incorporates peptides and porcine collagen. Used over partial-thickness burns and sometimes over donor sites. Often used in conjunction with whirlpooling and occasionally with Silvadene. The large bore sheets are used to facilitate wound drainage. It is a comfortable dressing because it protects nerve endings, so they are not irritated when the wound is cleaned. Decreases wound healing time and does not have to be changed after first application.
Calcium Algonate Dressing	Transitional Healing	Generally used to control bleeding and absorb exudate. Promotes moist wound healing; may leave fibers in the wound. May be used over donor sites and leaking tubes.
Cultured Epithelial Autografts	Acute	Epithelial cells are harvested from the child's own skin to foster growth of epithelial cells and are used to cover large BSAB.
Elastogel	Healing	Gel-like substance used to soften scar areas and diminish keloid formation. May use under Jobst stocking.
Exudry	Acute Transitional	Permeable outer layer that allows wound to breathe; a cellulose layer used to promote moist wound healing environment; a high absorbent layer draws exudate and retains fluid; two nonadherent layers to prevent shearing of grafts. Used for burns draining large amounts, or large BSAB. Comes in sheets, pads, jackets, and gloves. Jacket application decreases endotracheal tube dislocation during dressing change.
Hyginet	Any	Elastic netting used to secure dressings, especially on scalp burns after wrapping with gauze.

Product	Phase	Description/Use
Hypafix Tape	Any	Cloth-like tape that may be used to secure dressings. Works well on areas that are difficult to secure and when tape will not stick due to excessive sweating or moisture.
Integra		A bilayer skin replacement system. It contains a dermal replacement layer and an epidermal substitute layer (ESL). The ESL is eventually removed and covered with an autograft.
IntraSite Gel	Acute Transitional	Provides moist wound healing. Contains a starch substance that draws fluids out of the wound. Cleans and debrides the wound. Generally used on clean wounds with granulation tissue formation to help flatten tissue. Used on escharotomy/fasciotomy or avulsed wounds until closure can be performed.
Jobst Garment	Healing	Provides maximum pressure on a healed burn to minimize scar formation; fits tightly like a girdle. A positive pressure system measured to fit each area.
N-Terface	Transitional Healing	Thin gossamerlike gauze dressing used in conjunction with Polysporin, Silvadene, or wet-to-dry dressing. Either surface may be placed next to the wound. It provides a protective covering and allows exudate away from the wound. Because it is protective, it allows some relief of discomfort. It may become adherent to the wound and may be left on for several days if wound is clean underneath. Use on wounds where no progression has been seen for several days, wounds with an angry red appearance, or in conjunction with Polysporin on open areas on healed wounds.
Scarlet Red	Transitional	Fine mesh, absorbent gauze impregnated with 5% scarlet red in a nonmedicinal blend of lanolin, olive oil, and petrolatum. Helps promote epithelial cell growth. Used to cover donor sites. Left in place under gauze dressing.
Transparent Dressing	Healing	Used over pink, clean burn wounds and to anchor Biobrane. Allows for easy visualization of wounds. Works better when wound is less weepy.
Tubigrip	Healing	Minimal support dressing used as an interim dressing pre-Jobst placement to help minimize keloid formation.
Xeroform	Transitional Healing	Petroleum-based antimicrobial dressing. Generally used as a moist protective dressing over skin grafts or as a donor site dressing.

CHAPTER 36

Clinical Nursing Research

Elaine Stashinko

With the advent of managed care, rapid changes in health care delivery systems, and brief hospitalizations, children requiring surgery often have complex health problems with limited access to professional nursing resources. Health professionals are challenged to help the child and parents through the procedure effectively, with minimal distress, and efficiently (Brennan, 1994). Therefore, early intervention with children at risk for poor surgical outcomes or children who fall off the proposed critical pathway or caremap is imperative. It is equally important to validate the relevance of the protocols within critical pathways and the role of nursing in their implementation. Research is an important tool for describing, validating and improving nursing care.

"Research is a systematic, formal, rigorous and precise process employed to gain solutions to problems and/or to discover and interpret new facts and relationships" (Waltz & Bausell, 1981, p. 1). Nursing research has been defined broadly as " a systematic search for knowledge about issues of importance to the nursing profession" (Polit and Hungler, 1995, p. 3). Providing direct patient care; developing critical pathways, protocols, or policies; evaluating new products, equipment, or quality outcomes; and providing education are all components of nursing that require a research base (Smith, 1998). Clinical nursing research involves both making nursing practice a focus for research and increasing the application of research findings to practice. Therefore, this chapter describes both the conduct of clinical nursing research and strategies for integrating research within practice.

NURSING SCIENCE

Nursing is characterized by great diversity. This diversity has enabled nurses to study human behavior in wellness and illness from a variety of philosophical perspectives (Jacox, Suppe, Campbell, & Stashinko, 1999). These approaches may be categorized as post-positivist, interpretive/humanistic, and critical/emancipatory.

Post-positivism is the dominant philosophical approach in contemporary science. The ultimate goal of post-positivist science is to explain, predict, and control phenomena. Emphasis is placed on observable data, experimental control, and reduction of bias.

The interpretive/humanistic approach focuses on understanding the meaning of events or experiences within different contexts. Individual's subjective experiences or stories are valued within this perspective, and the conduct of research is with qualitative methods in natural settings (i.e., a child's home).

The critical/emancipatory approach encompasses critical theory, feminist research, Afrocentric research, and action or participatory research (Jacox et al., 1999). Emancipatory research challenges the validity of assumptions made by the dominant culture, such as concepts of normality and risk, and exposes power imbalances. The uniqueness of the emancipatory paradigm lies in going beyond individual transformation to include nursing action changing the community and/or health care system (Immelt, Coyne, Stashinko, Campbell, 1998).

Because nursing is a science and an art, both the ability to generalize and individualize care are important and necessary within practice. The problem of providing standardized care in most situations while simultaneously acknowledging the child's/family's unique perspective and need for individualized care is a challenge for clinical nurses in every setting. Meeting this research challenge requires knowledge and application of a variety of research theories, designs, and methods.

CONDUCTING CLINICAL NURSING RESEARCH

The steps of the research process are flexible and vary depending on the level of scientific inquiry and type of study. However, the general sequence of actions for the conduct of a clinical nursing research study are outlined in Figure 36–1 and described within this section.

Identify a Nursing Research Problem

The first step in the research process is identifying a research problem. According to Diers (1979), a research problem is a *nursing* research problem when nurses have access to and control over the phenomenon being studied, and the phenomenon is relevant and important to real-world nursing problems and decisions. To generate a researchable topic important to clinical nursing, think and reflect on everyday practice.

- Note inconsistencies among nurses, the way nurses practice, and nursing outcomes. Ask questions such as "What's the best way to *do this dressing change*?" "I wonder if sending home this preadmission preparation video helps/works most of the time?"
- Note inconsistencies between standards of care and reality. Ask questions such as, "What could we do to make *the transition after surgery to home care* easier?"
- Question traditional methods of practice. "Why do we always *take temperatures every 4 hours during the night*?"
- Note clinical indicators: events with a high frequency of occurrence (i.e., falls and medication errors).
- Note variances in patient outcomes. Observe and consider what factors predispose children to poor and excellent outcomes. Think broadly; child development, family, and cultural factors are as important to consider as pathophysiology and medical history.
- Question the cost-effectiveness of equally desirable interventions. Investigate creative and innovative ways to intervene more cost-effectively.

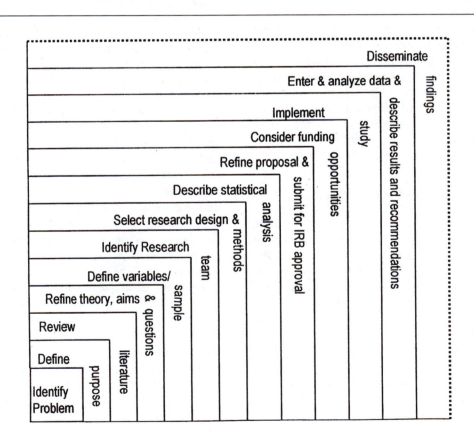

Figure 36–1 The Clinical Research Process

Define the Purpose of the Research

Scientific research can be categorized in terms of goals or methods. The broad goals of research may be prediction and control, comprehension and understanding, or emancipation (Immelt et al., 1998). Articulate the specific aims and goals of the research. The specific aim should reflect the research problem, the nature of the inquiry, the study variables, and the study population.

State the significance of this research to nursing and the health care of children. Ask, "Why do this research?" "So what will it mean for the nursing care of children and families experiencing surgery?"

Review the Literature

Review the theoretical and research literature pertinent to the identified research problem. Search the Cumulative Index to Nursing and Allied Health Literature (CINAHL) and MEDLINE online databases for current research and descriptive literature. Review any relevant theories that pertain to the area of concern.

Critique the research germane to the problem. What are the gaps in the literature? Does the literature support the assessment of the problem and its significance? What relationships do the theories reviewed pose and how does this fit with the proposed study? What additional variables do the relevant theories direct you to measure? If a research study of the problem is reported in the literature, critique it closely. What were the limitations of this study? Isolated studies can almost never provide an adequate justification for making changes in nursing practice (Polit & Hungler, 1995). By replicating this study with your sample in your setting, how would you further contribute to the knowledge of this problem?

Refine the Theory, Aims, and Research Question(s)

Refine the aims and formulate research questions and/or hypotheses. A research question is the problem statement in an interrogative form. The research question identifies the variables of interest, their possible interrelationships, and the study population. A hypothesis states a predicted relationship between two or more variables and is testable.

Carefully choose the verbs you use in the specific aim and research questions. The verbs communicate information about the theoretical approach and the nature of the study design. For example, a study that *explores* some phenomenon or process is likely to be a descriptive, qualitative study whose goal is increased understanding or discovery of knowledge. A study that seeks to *test* the effectiveness of a new technology or *compare* two interventions suggests an experimental or quasi-experimental design (Polit & Hungler, 1995).

Define Study Variables

Identify the major study variables. Identify child, nurse, and context-related variables that may have an impact on the study variables.

Child-related variables may include demographics such as age, gender, ethnicity, and severity of illness, as well as other individual child characteristics. Nurse-related variables may include education, professional experience, and staffing. Examples of context-related variables are time since surgery, parental presence, and absence or presence of preoperative preparation.

Define Target Sample

Define who you want to include in your study. Sampling refers to the process of selecting a pool of study participants that is representative or matches key characteristics of the population for whom the results are generalizable. Specifically define the age range of the potential subjects, gender, race and ethnicity, clinical diagnoses, and study site. Specify eligibility inclusion criteria and exclusion criteria. For example, you may choose to exclude individuals who are not English-speaking. Be prepared to justify your sampling decisions with rationale and literature support.

Identify the potential number of subjects you hope to recruit in your study. Statistical methods such as power analysis are available for developing sample size estimates. Beginning nurse researchers should consider the nature of the investigation, the homogeneity of the population (the more similar, the smaller the sample size), and anticipate attrition when estimating sample size. Sample attrition or dropout rates from studies of 20% are not uncommon in longitudinal studies with vulnerable populations or hard-to-track families (Polit & Hungler, 1995). Attrition is problematic because child participants who are unwilling or unable to continue study participation because of death, deteriorating health, or early discharge may differ in important respects from individuals who continue to participate, resulting in potential biases to the results. In general, the larger the sample, the more representative of the population it is likely to be.

Sampling techniques include probability and nonprobability sampling. Probability sampling involves some form of random selection in choosing the sample. In nonprobability sampling, participants are selected by nonrandom methods such as convenience sampling, using the most conveniently available persons as study participants.

Think practically and scientifically about sampling decisions. How many children meet this criteria at this site during a 1-month period? How long will it take to recruit the number you need for this study? If the study is burdensome or has more than one data collection period, oversample to allow for attrition. Do you have the time, energy, and re-

Table 36–1 A Descriptive Design in Nursing Research

Type of Design	Purpose of Study	Sample
Descriptive/correlational	The purposes of this study were to: 1. "identify and record pain behaviors manifest by children and adolescents during the first 3 days after surgery, 2. document the reported pain intensities, and 3. examine the relationship between behaviors manifest and pain scores reported." (Tesler, Holzemer, & Savedra, 1998, p. 41)	(*n* = 37), self-selected, multiethnic, 18 boys and 19 girls 8 to 17 years old. Surgical procedures included 19% orthopedic, 16% thoracic, 13% genitourinary, 38% other surgeries.

sources to recruit this sample? How can you maximize your resources and support to make this study feasible?

Identify the Research Team

Identify who should be on your research team. Assess your level of expertise in conducting research. Are you a novice or experienced researcher? Have you coordinated research projects before? Identify people who can act as research mentors, consultants, statisticians, and data collectors and managers. Experienced researchers can be found through networking with schools of nursing, larger academic medical centers, professional organizations such as Sigma Theta Tau International Honor Society of Nursing (STT), and the research committees of pediatric nursing specialty organizations (Smith, 1998). Barter for research resources. Nursing students and novice staff nurses are often willing to conduct study interviews or retrieve medical record data for the research experience and inclusion in a poster presentation or published paper.

Select the Research Design

Research involves "critical investigation of natural phenomena guided by theory and hypotheses about the presumed relations among such phenomena" (Kerlinger, 1986, p. 10). The theory and research question drives the design.

A research design is a roadmap or blueprint for study organization. Research designs may be classified by purpose. Types of research designs include exploratory, historical, descriptive, explanatory, experimental or quasi-experimental, and methodological.

The purpose of an exploratory research design is to name or give an in-depth description of a phenomenon. Exploratory research often uses a qualitative approach to capture the essence of the phenomenon or to generate or extend theory related to the phenomenon.

Historical research seeks to explain the present or to anticipate the future on the basis of a systematic collection and critical evaluation and interpretation of data that already exist (Wilson, 1987). Data evidence are derived from historical sources such as diaries, letters, past hospital records, and newspaper and journal articles.

"Descriptive designs are used when the primary purpose of the study is to name, characterize, or thoroughly describe a phenomenon" (Mateo & Kirchhoff, 1991, p. 171). Correlational research investigates the relationships among variables and may be descriptive or explanatory. In Table 36–1, an example of a descriptive-correlational design to investigate children's postsurgical pain behaviors is outlined.

Experimental and quasi-experimental studies test hypotheses about cause-effect relationships. In a true experimental study design, the investigator manipulates the "causative" or independent variable, and subjects are randomly assigned to experimental or comparison/control groups.

Methodological studies develop or refine a new research technique or procedure. Testing the reliability and validity of a pain behavior scale developed for toddlers on infants is an example of a methodological study.

Design decisions include the selection and assignment of subjects to one or more comparison groups, the type and number of observations needed, the number of data collection times, and the perspective of the study with regard to time. A study may be prospective (includes plan for data to be collected) with regard to time or retrospective (data already collected, such as review of existing medical records).

Clarify the Methods and Data Collection Tools

Identify the sources of data, methods, and measurement tools.

The source of data may be a person (e.g., child or parent), a medical record, historical records, or even an animal cell line.

A variety of data collection methods are used by nurse researchers. However, the approaches used most frequently include written or verbal self-reports, observation, and biophysiologic measures (e.g., blood pressure, laboratory values).

Factors to consider when selecting the method of tool administration include characteristics of the child and family participants, complexity of the instructions or task, and anticipated response rate (Wilson, 1987). Estimate the age, developmental stage, and reading level of your target sample. The selected measurement tools should not only be reliable and valid for your sample but should also reflect an appropriate reading level.

Timing of administration and the severity and limitations of the illness are also important considerations in the researcher's decision to read or self-administer an instrument. A child who is 3 hours postoperative may be too tired and weak to reliably answer a questionnaire that takes 1 hour to complete. Options for this scenario include substituting a shorter questionnaire, leaving the instrument with the parents with a stamped, self-addressed envelope for mail-in return, or calling the child/family at home for a telephone interview.

The study response rate is defined as the number of people who consent to participate in the study relative to the number of people sampled (Polit and Hungler, 1995). A response rate greater than 50% is probably sufficient for surveys, but the higher the return rate, the better the chances of getting representative, valid results. Suggestions for increasing survey results include: (1) whenever possible, make the questionnaire brief, easy to read, and easy to complete; (2) personalize administration (generally the response rate is higher when participants are recruited and data are collected through direct contact rather than mailing); (3) reward participation (Rewards may range from verbal or written expressions of appreciation to stickers, food, or financial renumeration. It is essential that rewards do not unduly influence a subject's participation or represent a form of coercion.); (4) enhance ease of return (Surveys that are personally distributed may be picked up by the administrator. A large, well-marked box or folder may be provided in a central place on the unit or office to facilitate staff survey returns. If questionnaires are mailed, provide stamped addressed return envelopes.); and (5) follow-up mailings (Follow-up mailings [flyers, postcards] or telephone reminders done at approximately 1 and 3 weeks after the initial survey promote participation.).

Describe the Statistical Analysis

Describe the statistical methods to address each study research question or hypotheses. Consult with a statistician or expert clinical researcher who is knowledgeable about your research design, statistical tests, and computer programs and resources. A statistician can help you prepare the data collection tools to facilitate coding and computer entry, select statistical tests for data analysis, and suggest computer programs or personnel for data entry and analysis.

Refine the Research Proposal

The research proposal should reflect a clear and concise picture of the research plan. The research proposal ought to summarize the study's specific aims (including research questions and/or hypotheses), significance, background or review of literature, and methods. The method section includes sample and setting, design, variables, data collection procedures, informed consent or animal protection procedures, data analyses plan, and time frames for study implementation. Actual copies of research instruments or results of preliminary studies may be attached in appendixes.

Before final revision, submit the research proposal for peer review by clinical and research experts. Persons who know the topic and have clinical experience with this phenomenon or this target population may provide insight not available in the literature. Professional colleagues may suggest additional confounding variables that may have an impact on the outcome or predict weaknesses in the data collection process and suggest alternatives. Persons with research expertise can critique the validity and congruence of the research aims, design, methods, and plan of analysis. Revisions ought to reflect thoughtful consideration of reviewers' critique and feedback and, hopefully, result in a more clear, organized, and persuasive proposal.

Submit the Proposal for Institutional Review Board (IRB) Approvals

Review the criteria and process for human studies committee approval in your institution and any institution where you plan to collect the data. Research funded by federal money or conducted at institutions supported by federal dollars must comply with federal ethics guidelines. Federal regulations define children as persons who have not attained the legal age for consent under the laws of the jurisdiction in which the research is conducted (DHHS, 1983). Although in most states children become adults on their 18th birthday, some variation still exits among states on the age of autonomous consent (Conrad & Horner, 1997; Thurber, Deatrick, & Grey, 1992). Therefore, unless a child qualifies as a mature or emancipated minor, parental (or legal guardian) permission and child assent are required for participation in research.

Child assent refers to "a child's informed agreement to the conditions of participation" (Conrad & Horner, 1997). Although individual review boards are responsible for determining when a child is old enough to provide assent for participation in research (DHHS, 1983; OPRR, 1993), the usual age of assent is approximately 7 years. The child's refusal to assent overrides a parent's permission for the child's participation, unless participation may provide direct therapeutic benefit to the child that would otherwise be unavailable (Weithorn & Scherer, 1994).

Research involving children requires "a conscientious effort to envision children's understanding of events, their potential reactions, and the possible immediate and long-term consequences" (Conrad & Horner, 1997, p. 163). Describe the potential risks and benefits of this research for the child participants. Anticipate any psychological, as well as physical, burdens to the child and his or her family. Describe any measures that will be taken to minimize and deal with risks.

Consider Funding Opportunities

Calculate the projected costs of the study. Take into account the costs of purchasing instruments and manuals, xeroxing consents and instruments, postage for mailings, data entry, and statistical consultation.

Small research grant opportunities are available through many professional nursing organizations such as Sigma Theta Tau International Honor Society of Nursing (STT), the American Nurses Association (ANA), and Society of Pediatric Nurses, and specialty journals such as *Pediatric Nursing*.

Implement the Study

Study implementation involves collecting and managing the data according to the research plan. A pilot study to determine the feasibility of the design or the reliability and validity of chosen tools with the population may be an initial step. Contact key personnel at the study site and orient staff before study implementation.

Enter and Analyze the Study Data

Before data analysis, data are coded, entered into a computer, and cleaned or verified. For most studies, statistical software packages available for a home or office personal computer are used by researchers to analyze data. Examples of frequently used statistical software packages include SPSSX and SAS for quantitative analyses and Ethnograph for qualitative data analyses.

Describe the Study Results, Conclusions, and Recommendations

Describe the study outcomes and congruence with the literature and stated hypotheses (if applicable). Consider both the statistical and clinical significance of the study results. A discussion section follows the results and offers the researcher's interpretation of the results and implications for future research and clinical practice. Discuss the study limitations and the generalizability of the study findings.

Disseminate Research Findings

Share study results with child, family, and/or staff participants as soon as possible after completion.

Communicate the study conclusions and practice implications to the nursing and interdisciplinary community. Present a paper or poster at a relevant conference, emphasizing the study and its conclusions. Consider your target audience in publishing the study results.

For a more in-depth review of the nursing research process, refer to Mateo and Kirchhoff's (1991) text, *Conducting and Using Nursing Research in the Clinical Setting*, Hinshaw's (1999) *Handbook of Clinical Nursing Research*, or a general textbook on nursing research such as Polit and Hungler's (1995) *Nursing Research: Principles and Methods*.

INTEGRATING RESEARCH IN CLINICAL PRACTICE

"Evidence-based nursing deemphasizes ritual, isolated and unsystematic clinical experiences, ungrounded opinions and tradition as a basis for nursing practices . . . and stresses instead the use of research findings and, as appropriate, quality improvement data, other operational and evaluation data, the consensus of recognized experts and affirmed experience to substantiate practice" (Stetler et al., 1998, pp. 48–49). Two strategies for achieving evidence-based nursing practice include application of (1) research-based clinical practice guidelines, and (2) research utilization models.

An increasing number of research-based practice guidelines can be readily integrated into clinical practice. The Agency for Health Care Policy Research (AHCPR), the Association for Care of Children's Health (ACCH), the American Academy of Pediatrics (AAP), and the Society of Pediatric Nurses (SPN) have all developed and published pediatric-specific clinical practice guidelines. Clinically relevant pediatric guideline topics range from assessment and management of acute pain in children (Acute Pain Management Guideline Panel, 1992) to family-centered care (SPN, 1998). Most of these clinical practice guidelines are available via the Internet at the organization's web site.

Research utilization involves translating scientific research findings into evidence-based nursing practice (Keefe, 1993). Several models for translating research findings into practice decisions have been developed. One useful model for research utilization is the Stetler model. This model is a prescriptive, practitioner-oriented framework involving six phases (Stetler, 1994).

In discussing nursing scholarship, Gebbie (1997) states, "We have not shown well *how* we make a difference in the efficiency, effectiveness, and quality of care. This century we will, or we will lose the privilege of providing care" (p. 119). Conducting and using nursing research to advance nursing science and practice and to respond to health care changes is no longer a luxury; it is a necessity.

REFERENCES

Acute Pain Management Guideline Panel. (1992). *Acute pain management in infants, children, and adolescents: Operative and medical procedures. Quick reference guide for clinicians.* (AHCPR Pub. No. 92-0020). Rockville, MD: Agency for Health Care Policy and Research, Public Health Service, U.S. Department of Health and Human Services.

Brennan, A. (1994). Caring for children during procedures: A review of the literature. *Pediatric Nursing, 20*(5), 451–458.

Conrad, B., & Horner, S. (1997). Issues in pediatric research: Safeguarding the children. *Journal of the Society of Pediatric Nurses, 2*(4), 163–171.

Department of Health and Human Services (DHHS). (March 8, 1983). Additional protection for children involved as subjects in research. *48 Federal Register 9818*; codified in 45 CFR 46 Subpart D.

Diers, D. (1979). *Research in nursing practice.* Philadelphia: Lippincott-Raven Publishers.

Gebbie, K. (1997). Future of nursing scholarship: Disciplinary, interdisciplinary. *Image: Journal of Nursing Scholarship, 29*(2), 119.

Hinshaw, A.S., Feetham, S., & Shaver, J. (Eds.) (1999). *Handbook of clinical nursing research.* Thousand Oaks, CA: Sage Publications.

Immelt, S., Coyne, K., Stashinko, E., & Campbell, J. (1998). The paradigm mosaic. Unpublished manuscript.

Jacox, A., Suppe, F., Campbell, J., & Stashinko, E. (1999). Diversity in philosophical approaches. In A. Hinshaw, S. Feetham, & J. Shaver. (Eds.), *Handbook for clinical nursing research.* Thousand Oaks, CA: Sage Publications.

Keefe, M. (1993). An integrated approach to incorporating research findings into practice. *MCN, American Journal of Maternal Child Nursing 18*, 65–70.

Kerlinger, F.N. (1986). *Foundations of behavioral research* (3rd ed.). Orlando, FL: Holt, Rinehart and Winston.

Mateo, M.A., & Kirchhoff, K.T. (1991). *Conducting and using nursing research in the clinical setting.* Baltimore: Williams & Wilkins.

Office for the Protection from Research Risks (OPRR), Department of Health and Human Services, National Institutes of Health. (1993). *Protecting human research subjects: Institutional review board guidebook.* Washington, DC: U.S. Government Printing Office.

Polit, D., & Hungler, B. (1995). *Nursing research: Principles and methods* (5th ed.). Philadelphia: Lippincott-Raven Publishers.

Smith, S. (1998). Getting nursing research going in a community hospital with limited resources. *Journal of the Society of Pediatric Nurses, 3*(1), 47–49.

Society of Pediatric Nurses (SPN). (1998). Family-centered care: Putting it into action.

Stetler, C. (1994, Jan./Feb.). Refinement of the Stetler-Marram model for application of research findings to practice. *Nursing Outlook, 42*, 15–25.

Stetler, C., Brunell, M., Giuliano, K., Morsi, D., Prince, L., & Newell-Stokes, V. (1998). Evidence-based practice and the role of nursing leadership. *Journal of Nursing Administration, 28*(7/8), 45–53.

Tesler, M., Holzemer, W., & Savedra, M. (1998). Pain behaviors: Postsurgical responses of children and adolescents. *Journal of Pediatric Nursing, 13*(1), 41–46.

Thurber, F., Deatrick, J., & Grey, M. (1992). Children's participation in research: Their right to consent. *Journal of Pediatric Nursing, 7*, 165–170.

Waltz, C., & Bausell, R.B. (1981). *Nursing research: Design, statistics and computer analysis.* Philadelphia: F.A. Davis.

Weithorn, L., & Scherer, D. (1994). Children's involvement in research participation decisions: Psychological considerations. In M. Grodin & L. Glantz (Eds.), *Children as research subjects: Science, ethics and law.* New York: Oxford University Press.

Wilson, H.S. (1987). *Introducing research in nursing.* Reading, MA: Addison-Wesley Publishing Co.

Resources

ABDC News (newsletter)
Association of Birth Defect Children
827 Irma St.
Orlando, FL 32803
800-313-2232; 407-245-7035
Birth defect registry and database that matches families

Air Life Line
50 Fullerton Ct., Suite 200
Sacramento, CA 95825
800-446-1231; (fax) 916-641-0600
staff@airlifeline.org

American Cancer Society
National Headquarters
1599 Clifton Rd., NE
Atlanta, GA 30329
800-ACS-2345

American Heart Association
7272 Greenville Ave.
Dallas, TX 75231-4596
800-AHA-USA1

American Hirschsprung's Disease Association
22½ Spruce St.
Battleboro, VT 05301
802-257-0603

American Pseudo-Obstruction and Hirschsprung's Disease Society
P.O. Box 772
158 Pleasant St.
North Hanover, MA 01845
978-685-4477; (fax) 978-685-4484
Materials also in Spanish

Association for Bladder Exstrophy Children
The ABC Update (newsletter)
21 West Colony Pl., Suite 150
Durham, NC 27705
191-403-1463
Newsletter and support group for bladder exstrophy families; also has directory of members and their last procedure

Biliary Atresia & Liver Transplant Network
BALT
3835 Richmond Ave.
Box 190
Staten Island, NY 10312-3828
http://livertx.org

Brain Injury Association
105 North Alfred St.
Alexandria, VA 22314
703-236-6000
www.biausa.org

Candlelighter's Childhood Cancer Foundation
7910 Woodmont Ave., Suite 460
Bethesda, MD 20814
301-657-8401; 800-366-CCCF

The Center for Children with Chronic Illness and Disability (newsletter)
University of Minnesota, Box 721
UMHC
420 Delaware St., SE
Minneapolis, MN 55455
612-626-4032; (voice) 612-624-3939; (tty) 612-626-2134
Newsletter, videos, referrals, advocacy

Courtesy of St. Louis Children's Hospital, St. Louis, Missouri.

Cherubs Association
P.O. Box 1150
Oxford, NC 27522
919-693-8158
cherubs@gloryroad.net
Information and support for families of children with
congenital diaphragmatic hernia

Children's Hospice International
2202 Mt. Vernon Ave.
Suite 3C
Alexandria, VA 22301
www.chionline.org
800-24-CHILD

Children's Liver Association for Support Services
CLASS
2644 Emerald Dove Dr.
Valencia, CA 91355
www.transweb.org/class

Children's Organ Transplant Association, Inc. (COTA)
2501 COTA Dr.
Bloomington, IN 47403
800-366-2682; (fax) 812-336-8885

Children's Wish Foundation
P.O. Box 28785
8615 Roswell Rd.
Atlanta, GA 30358
800-323-WISH; (fax) 770-393-0683

Compassionate Friends
P.O. Box 3696
Oak Brook, IL 60522-3696
630-990-0010
www.compassionatefriends.com

EA/TEF Child & Family Support Connection, Inc.
111 W. Jackson Blvd., Suite 1145
Chicago, IL 60604-3502
312-987-9085; (fax) 312-987-9086
eatef2@aol.com

Family Voices
P.O. Box 769
Algondes, NM 87001
505-867-2368; (fax) 505-867-6517
www.familyvoices.com
famv01rw@wonder.em.cdc.gov

Grief Recovery Institute
8306 Wilshire Blvd., #21-A
Los Angeles, CA 90211
323-650-1234

The Inside Edition (newsletter)
Schremer
106 Goodwin Rd.
Eliot, ME 03903
207-439-1792
Newsletter, information, and support for families living
with bladder exstrophy and cloacal anomalies

**International Polyposis & Peutz-Jeghers Syndrome
Support Group**
c/o Jill D. Bresinger
Johns Hopkins Hospital
550 N. Broadway, Suite 108
Baltimore, MD 21205
410-614-4038; (fax) 410-614-9544

**International Society for Heart and Lung
Transplantation**
14673 Midway Rd., Suite 108
Dallas, TX 75244
972-490-9495; (fax) 972-490-9499

Latex Allergy Information Service
176 Roosevelt Ave.
Torrington, CT 06790
203-482-6869; (fax) 203-482-7640
Information, newsletter, registry

Mothers United for Moral Support (MUMS)
c/o Julie Gordon
150 Custer St.
Green Bay, WI 54301-1243
414-336-5333; (fax) 414-339-0995

**National Association of Pediatric Home and Community
Care**
21 North Quinsigamond Ave.
Shrewsbury, MA 01545
508-856-1908

**National Information Center for Children and Youth
with Disabilities**
P.O. Box 1492
Washington, DC 20013
800-695-0285
www.nichcy.org

National Kidney Foundation
30 East 33rd St.
New York, NY 10016
800-622-9010

National Rehabilitation Information Center
1010 Wayne Ave., #800
Silver Spring, MD 20910
800-346-2742; 301-562-2400
www.naric.com/naric

National Spinal Cord Injury Association
8701 Georgia Ave.
Suite 500
Silver Spring, MD 20910
800-962-9629
www.spinalcord.org

National Transplant Assistance Program
P.O. Box 258
6 Bryn Mawr Ave.
Bryn Mawr, PA 19010
800-642-8399
NTAF@transplantfund.org

NCI Cancer Information Service
Office of Cancer Communication
National Cancer Institute
Bethesda, MD 20892
800-4-CANCER

Pediatric Crohn's and Colitis Association
P.O. Box 188
Newton, MA 02168
617-489-5854; (voice and fax) 617-290-0902

Pediatric Home Care Association of America
228 Seventh St., SE
Washington, DC 20003
202-547-7424; (fax) 202-547-3540

Pediatric Ileitis & Colitis Foundation
P.O. Box 188
Newton, MA 02168
508-358-5147

The Pull-Thru Network
Greater New York Chapter of UOA
4 Woody Ln.
Westport, CT 06880
203-221-7530 Karen and Scott Brownlow
Newsletter and support for anorectal malformations, pull-through surgery, and bowel management

Ronald McDonald Houses
Ronald McDonald House Coordinator
c/o Ronald McDonald Corporation
1 Kroc Dr.
Oak Brook, IL 60521
312-836-7100

Second Wind Lung Transplant Association, Inc.
9030 West Lakeview Ct.
Crystal River, FL 34428
888-222-2690
Secondwind@xtalwind.net

Spina Bifida Association of America
4590 MacArthur Blvd., NW, #250
Washington, DC 20007-4226
800-621-3141; 202-944-3285; (fax) 202-944-3295

TEF/Vater International Support Network
c/o Jeff and Terri Burke
15301 Grey Fox Rd.
Upper Marlboro, MD 20772
301-952-6837

United Ostomy Association
19772 MacArthur Blvd., Suite 200
Irvine, CA 92612-2405
800-826-0826
Youth Committee, Parents of Ostomy Children Committee, Youth Rally

Glossary

Abscess—A localized collection of pus in a tissue or body part resulting from the invasion of pyogenic bacteria.

Acholic—Absence of bile pigments in the stool.

Acidosis—An actual or relative increase in the acidity of the blood due to an increase in acid or a decrease in bicarbonate; low pH; high hydrogen ion concentration.

Acute tubular necrosis—Acute damage to the renal tubules frequently due to ischemia resulting from shock.

Adhesions—A fibrous band holding parts together that are normally separated. Adhesions in the abdomen usually involve the intestines and are caused by inflammation or trauma, such as from previous surgery.

Aganglionosis—The absence of ganglion cells (Hirschsprung's disease).

Allograft—Transplant tissue obtained from the same species.

Amniocentesis—The removal of amniotic fluid from the amniotic sac using a needle and syringe under ultrasound guidance.

Ampulla of Vater—Where the common bile duct merges with the pancreatic duct, forming a dilated portion in the common channel just before opening into the small intestine.

Anastomosis—A surgical formation of a connection between two previously distinct structures.

Anencephaly—Congenital absence of the brain.

Anlage—The beginning of an organized tissue, organ, or part in the developing embryo.

Anthropometric—Measurement of the size, weight, and proportions of the human body.

Aplastic kidney—Extreme form of dysplastic kidney; involved kidney is a "nubbin."

Arteriovenous malformation—Tumor caused by abnormal collection of arteries and veins; characterized by a bruit or thrill.

Ascites—Abnormal accumulation of fluid in the peritoneal cavity; characterized by distention of the abdomen. Initial treatment involves sodium restriction and diuretics.

Atelectasis—Collapsed or airless condition of the alveoli of the lung caused by obstruction of the bronchus; usual symptoms include dyspnea and cyanosis.

Atresia—Congenital absence or closure of a normal body opening or tubular structure.

Autograft—A graft transferred from one part of a patient's body to another.

Balanitis—Inflammation of the skin covering the glans penis.

Barrett's esophagus—Inflammation and possible ulceration of the lower part of the esophagus caused by gastroesophageal reflux or by mucosal damage secondary to chemotherapy.

Biliary dyskinesia—Difficult flow of bile from the gallbladder.

Bronchiolitis obliterans—Inflammation of the bronchioles in which the bronchioles are partially or completely obliterated by nodular masses containing granulation and fibrotic tissue.

Catabolism—A destructive process in which complex substances such as living cells are broken down into more simple compounds.

Celiotomy—Opening the abdominal cavity through an incision in the abdominal wall; see laparotomy.

Cellular immunity—The regulatory and cytotoxic activity of the T-cells during the specific immune response.

Cholangitis—Bile stasis with bacterial flora; usually occurs in the jejunal limb and presents with fever, leukocytosis, and elevated liver enzymes; most commonly occurs after a Kasai portoenterostomy.

Colostomy—Cutting of an artificial opening in the bowel to provide diversion of the fecal stream; decompresses a portion of the bowel.

Colicky pain—Pain caused by spasm in any hollow or tubular organ.

Columnar epithelium—Epithelium composed of cylindrical cells.

Contralateral—On the opposite side.

Crepitus—A dry crackling sound.

Critical pathway—A flow or process outlining the expected clinical course for a designated disease process or procedure.

Conoidal epithelium—Epithelium composed of cone-shaped cells.

Cystic hygroma—Lymphangioma; caused by a random accidental failure of the normal development of the lymphatic system. The mass is characterized by a collection of fluid-filled spaces from lymphatic vessels; 75% occur in the cervical region.

Decannulation—Removal of the tracheostomy tube.

Deglutition—The act of swallowing.

Dehiscence—Separation of the edges of a previously approximated wound.

Diagnosis related groups (DRG)—System designed to standardize prospective payment for medical care. The reimbursement for treating all individuals within the same DRG is identical regardless of actual cost to the health care facility.

Diverticulum—Vestigial remnant of the omphalomesenteric duct (Meckel's diverticulum), a blind pouch or structure leading from a larger canal.

Dumping syndrome—Syndrome characterized by sweating and weakness after eating. There is rapid emptying of the contents of the stomach into the small intestine associated with the symptoms.

D-xylose tolerance test—Metabolic assessment of intestinal absorption of simple sugars; used in evaluation of children for small bowel transplantation.

Dysplastic kidney—Abnormal kidney development with primitive structures (histologic diagnosis); may involve cystic formation and may be associated with absent ureter or renal pelvis or stenotic ureter; accompanies hypoplasia.

Dysuria—Difficult or painful urination.

Echodense—On ultrasound, an area of increased reflection of sound waves that appears as a dark area, indicating a more solid structure.

Echocardiogram—The graphic record produced by using sound waves to visualize internal cardiac structures.

Echogenic—On ultrasound, an area of decreased reflection of sound waves that appears as a light area, indicating a more solid structure.

Ectopic—Occurring in an abnormal position.

Eisenmenger's syndrome—Congenital cyanotic cardiac defect consisting of ventricular septal defect, dextroposition of the aorta, pulmonary hypertension with pulmonary artery enlargement, and hypertrophy of the right ventricle.

Enterocolitis—Inflammation of the small intestine and colon caused by an incomplete functional obstruction of the rectum with proximal dilation, stasis, and bacterial overgrowth; leads to infection, epithelial destruction, ulceration, and bacterial invasion and may lead to death.

Epidural catheter—Spinal catheter placed under sterile conditions that lies outside of the dura for the purpose of instilling medications.

ERCP (endoscopic retrograde cholangiopancreatography)—Diagnostic or therapeutic procedure that involves a radiograph of the pancreatic duct and the biliary tree. An endoscope is used to identify the caliber of the ducts, stones, or tumors.

Escharotomy—Removal of the eschar and underlying tissue of a severely burned patient.

Evisceration—Edges of the wound part and the intestines protrude.

Exteriorization—A part of the body, such as a portion of the intestine, that is surgically exposed or brought outside the body.

Fasciotomy—Surgical incision and division of the fibrous membrane covering the muscle.

Fecalith—A stone or concretion of feces.

Fistula—An abnormal tubelike passage that connects two body tissues; may result from a congenital abnormality or injury.

Ganglion cells—Nerve tissue composed primarily of nerve bodies located outside the brain or spinal cord. Abdominal ganglion cells innervate the bowel and allow peristalsis to occur.

Gangrene—The necrosis of tissue generally resulting from an absent or deficient blood supply.

Gas bloat—Distention subsequent to abnormal gaseous accumulation in the abdominal cavity.

Gastric decompression—Removal of pressure in the stomach, usually by use of a nasogastric or gastrostomy tube connected to intermittent or constant suction; removes air and stomach contents.

Gastric outlet obstruction—Blockage at the end of the stomach.

Gavage—Feeding by a tube passed into the stomach.

Glomerular filtrate rate (GFR)—The rate at which the fluid passes from the blood through the capillary walls of the glomeruli of the kidney. GFR is estimated using the creatinine clearance rate in a 24-hour urine collection.

Hartmann's pouch—Oversewn proximal end of the intestine taken out of the circuit by the creation of an ileostomy or colostomy.

Health maintenance organization (HMO)—A prepaid health care program of a group practice. The program provides comprehensive medical care with the emphasis on maintaining health and preventing disease.

Hemangioma—Benign tumor composed of dilated blood vessels.

Hematemesis—Vomiting of blood.

Hepatomegaly—Enlargement of the liver.

Heterograft—A surgical graft of tissue from one individual/animal of one species to an individual of another species.

Human lymphocyte antigen (HLA)—Major histocompatibility antigens defined and typed by the mixed lymphocyte reaction. An individual's immune response is governed by the genes of the HLA complex.

Humoral immunity—Immunity mediated by antibodies found in body fluids such as lymph and plasma. Antibodies are secreted by B-cells, which protect the body from infection and re-infection by common organisms.

Hypercarbia—An increased concentration of carbon dioxide in the blood.

Hyperlucent—Increased ability to allow x-rays to pass through; a dark area will appear on the radiograph.

Hyperplasia—The proliferation of normal cells within normal tissue; an overgrowth of normal cells.

Hypoplastic kidney—Kidney with less than normal number of cells or nephrons.

Hypoxemia—Decreased oxygen tension (concentration) into the blood, measured by arterial oxygen partial pressure values.

Icteric—Affected with jaundice; a rough indication of bilirubin in the serum; indicates liver function.

Ileocecal junction—The anatomic location in the bowel where the ileum (the final portion of the small bowel) and the cecum (first portion of the large bowel, often a lead point for injury) join.

Ileostomy—A surgically created opening into the third potion of the small intestine (ileum).

Ileus—An intestinal obstruction; the cause of an ileus may be a functional or mechanical obstruction.

Imbricated—The overlapping of the flat fibrous sheet of connecting tissue during abdominal surgery.

Immunity—See *cellular immunity* and *humoral immunity.*

Inotropic—Affecting the force of muscle contraction, vasoactive drugs used to maximize cardiac output and improve blood flow to vital organs.

Intraosseus—Within the bone; an intraosseus needle is used to administer medications and fluids directly into the bone marrow for patients with inadequate vascular access; may be used in an emergency situation.

Ischemia—Contracted blood vessel; deficiency of blood in a body part.

Jaundice—Characterized by yellow color of the skin and eyes, usually evidence of an obstructive process in the liver.

KUB—An anteroposterior abdominal x-ray showing the kidneys, ureters, and bladder.

Laparotomy—The surgical opening of the abdomen.

Laparoscopic—Surgical procedure of exploring the abdomen using an endoscope called a laparoscope.

Laryngomalacia—A softening of the larynx.

Leukocytosis—Increase in the number of leukocytes ($> 10,000/mm^3$) in the blood caused by the presence of infection, usually transient. Other causes include hemorrhage, extensive surgery, pregnancy, toxemia, or malignant growth.

Ligament of Treitz—The suspensory band of tissue (ligament) of the duodenum; in the normal anatomic position of the small intestine the Ligament of Treitz fixes the small bowel in such a way that the duodenal-jejunal junction is in the left upper quadrant and the cecum is in the right lower quadrant; in malrotation the Ligament of Treitz is thought to be abnormal.

Lithotripsy—The use of shock waves produced by a physical external source used to crush a calculus (stone) in the bladder or urethra.

Lymphangioma—A tumor composed of lymph spaces and channels.

Managed care—A variety of methods used to finance and organize the delivery of health care in which costs are contained by controlling the provision of services. Hospitals, physicians, and other health care organizations accept a predetermined monthly payment for providing services to those patients enrolled in a managed care plan.

McBurney's point—A point 1 to 2 inches above the anterosuperior spine of the ilium, on a line between the ilium and umbilicus, where pressure produces point tenderness during acute appendicitis.

Mesenteric adenitis—Inflammation of the lymph nodes found within the peritoneal fold that surrounds and anchors the small intestine and other abdominal organs.

Mittelschmerz—Abdominal pain occurring between menstrual periods at the time of ovulation.

Mucosal layer—Covered with epithelium lining that communicates with the exterior of the body.

Multivisceral—Pertaining to or including many organs within a body cavity, particularly the abdominal organs.

Myotomy—Surgical division or anatomical dissection of muscles.

Neural tube defect—Abnormal development of the spinal cord; consistent with multifactorial inheritance.

Nosocomial—Occurring within the hospital, as in infection.

Nonimmune hydrops—Edema due to heart failure, secondary to severe anemia; may cause intrauterine death.

Obturator sign—Pain on inward rotation of the hip caused by stretching of the obturator internus muscle. This sign may be present with acute appendicitis.

Ostomy—A surgically created opening.

Paracentesis—A procedure performed to remove excess fluid from the abdominal cavity, usually a diagnostic procedure; remove fluid slowly to avoid problems with hypotension, oliguria, or hyponatremia.

Paraphimosis—Retraction of an inflamed or narrowed foreskin causing strangulation of the glans penis.

Passy-Muir speaking valve—A device used to adapt the passage of air around a tracheostomy tube so that the patient may speak.

Pelvic inflamatory disease (PID)—Infection of the uterus, fallopian tubes, and adjacent pelvic structures that is not related to pregnancy or associated with surgery.

Perforation—A hole made through a substance, organ, or body part.

Peristomal—The fringe around the stoma.

Peritonitis—Inflammation of the peritoneum characterized by exudations in the serous membrane lining the walls of the abdominal and pelvic cavities composed of serum, fibrin cells, and pus.

Phimosis—Foreskin that cannot be retracted over the glans penis due to narrowing or stenosis of the preputial orifice.

Pleural effusion—The presence of fluid in the space lining the outside of the lung (pleural space).

Pneumoperitoneum—Air in the peritoneal cavity; indicates the position of the diaphragm.

Pneumatosis intestinalis—Air or gas in the wall of the intestine.

Polyhydramnios—Excess fluid in the amniotic sac during pregnancy.

Prolapse—Falling down or out of an organ, as in a stoma.

Pruritus—Intense itching caused by elevated bilirubin levels or serum bile acids levels.

Pseudocyst—An abnormal or dilated space resembling a cyst.

Radiolucent—Allowing penetration by x-rays; a dark area appears on the radiograph.

Replogle Tube—A small double lumen nasogastric tube that is used to remove gastric secretions or rest the gastrointestinal tract. One lumen is an air vent that protects the gastric mucosa from damage. The holes are at the tip, so the tube is positioned in the stomach.

Resection—Surgical removal of a portion of an organ.

Retraction—Capable of drawing back, as in retractile testes.

Rovsing's sign—Pain in the appendiceal area when pressure is applied to the opposite side of the abdomen.

Salem sump tube—A double lumen nasogastric tube that is used to remove gastric secretions or rest the gastrointestinal tract. One lumen is an air vent that protects the gastric mucosa from damage.

Sandifer's syndrome—Voluntary contortions of the head, neck, and sometimes trunk associated with reflux esophagitis. This dystonic movement has been shown to improve peristalsis in the lower esophagus.

Sclerotherapy—Treatment by injection of a thickening or hardening agent that causes an intense inflammatory reaction to create fibrosis; used to close the lumen of esophageal or gastric varices to prevent bleeding or rupture of lymphangiomas.

Serosal layer—The outside layer of the gastrointestinal tract; extends from the stomach to the mesentery and contains nerves, lymphatics, and the blood vessels.

Short gut syndrome—Inadequate length of intestine to sustain life with enteral feedings. Exact amount of bowel required is controversial.

Splenomegaly—Enlargement of the spleen.

Suppurative—Associated with the generation of or producing pus.

Stenosis—Narrowing or contraction of a body passage.

Sternal cleft—A longitudinal opening or fissure of the sternum.

Stricturoplasty—The surgical opening of a stricture.

Third spacing—Internal redistribution of intracellular and intravascular fluid into the nonfunctional extravascular compartment, especially the peritoneum or bowel wall.

Thoracotomy—Surgical incision of the chest wall.

Thrombocytopenia—Abnormal decrease in the number of the blood platelets.

Thyroglossal duct cyst—Fluid-filled midline structure caused by abnormal development of the thyroid gland.

Torticollis—A contracted muscle that results in a palpable mass, usually found in the cervical muscles, producing a twisting of the neck and an unnatural position of the head.

Toxoplasmosis—A disease caused by infection with the protozoan *Toxoplasma gondii.*

Urinary diversion—A surgical procedure that creates a route for urine to exit the body.

Variance—A statistical indicator of the degree to which measurements in a data set are different from each other or deviate from the mean.

Varices—Dilated veins found in the submucosa of the esophagus with extension into the stomach; caused by portal hypertension. Hemorrhage may result from ruptured varices.

Xenograft—A surgical graft of tissue from an individual/animal of one species to an individual of a different species.

List of Sources

CHAPTER 1

Table 1–2 Reprinted from *Pediatric Nursing*, 1984, Volume 10, Number 1, pp. 25–28. Reprinted with permission of the publisher, Jannetti Publications, Inc., East Holly Avenue Box 56, Pitman, NJ 08071–0056; Phone (609) 256–2300; FAX (609) 589–7463. For a sample copy of the journal, please contact the publisher.

Table 1–6 Data from C.J. Coté, I.D. Todres, and J.F. Ryan, Preoperative Evaluation of Pediatric Patients, in *A Practice of Anesthesia for Infants and Children*, C.J. Coté, I.D. Todres, and N.G. Goudsouzian, eds., pp. 39–54, © 1993, W.B. Saunders Co.; S. Phillips, A.K. Daborn, and D.J. Hatch, Preoperative Fasting for Paediatric Anaesthesia, *British Journal of Anaethesia*, Vol. 73, pp. 529–536, © 1994; D.J. Steward, New Thoughts on Preparation and Premedication of Children, *Current Reviews for Post Anesthesia Care Nurses*, Vol. 17, No. 2, pp. 11–15, © 1995; American Academy of Pediatrics, Section on Anesthesiology, Evaluation and Preparation of Pediatric Patients Undergoing Anesthesia, *Pediatrics*, Vol. 98, No. 3, pp. 502–508, © 1996; E.E. Gleghorn, Preoperative Fasting: You Don't Have to Be Cruel to Be Kind, *Journal of Pediatrics*, Vol. 131, No. 1, pp. 12–13, © 1997; and M.F. Watcha, Anesthesia, in *Essentials of Pediatric Intensive Care*, 2nd ed, D.L. Levin and F.C. Morris, eds., pp. 587–603, © 1997, Churchill Livingstone Inc.

CHAPTER 2

Table 2–1 Reprinted with permission from *Master Latex List*, March 1998, © Children's Hospital of Wisconsin.

Table 2–2 Reprinted with permission from *Master Latex List*, March 1998, © Children's Hospital of Wisconsin.

CHAPTER 3

Table 3–1 Reprinted with permission from D. O'Donnell and J. Lathrop, *Pediatric Fluids and Electrolytes*, © 1993, Maxishare.

Table 3–2 Reprinted with permission from D. O'Donnell and J. Lathrop, *Pediatric Fluids and Electrolytes*, © 1993, Maxishare.

Table 3–3 Reprinted with permission from D. O'Donnell and J. Lathrop, *Pediatric Fluids and Electrolytes*, © 1993, Maxishare.

Table 3–4 Reprinted with permission from D. O'Donnell and J. Lathrop, *Pediatric Fluids and Electrolytes*, © 1993, Maxishare.

CHAPTER 4

Exhibit 4–1 Adapted with permission from D. Wilmore, *The Metabolic Management of the Critically Ill*, p. 36, © 1977, Plenum Publishing Corp.

Exhibit 4–2 Courtesy of Johns Hopkins Children's Center, Baltimore, Maryland.

Exhibit 4–3 Adapted with permission from M.A. Hildreth, D.N. Herndon, M.H. Desai, and L.D. Broemeling, Current Treatment Reduces Calories Required to Maintain Weight in Pediatric Patients with Burns, *Journal of Burn Care Rehabilitation*, Vol. 11, p. 408, © 1990, Mosby Inc.

Exhibit 4–4 Adapted from *Nutrition*, Vol. 13, M.N. Novy and K.B. Schwarz, Nutritional Considerations and Management of the Child with Liver Disease, pp. 177–184, © 1997, with permission from Elsevier Science Ltd.

Table 4–1 Adapted with permission from WHO, Energy and Protein Requirements, *FAO/WHO/UNU Expert Consultation Technical Report Series 724*, p. 71, © 1985, World Health Organization.

Table 4–2 Adapted with permission from National Research Council, *Recommended Dietary Allowances*, 10th ed., © 1989, National Academy of Sciences. Courtesy of the National Academy Press, Washington, D.C.

Table 4–4 Adapted from A. Davis, Indications and Techniques for Enteral Feedings, in *Pediatric Enteral Nutrition*, Baker, Baker, and Davis, eds., p. 82, © 1994, Aspen Publishers, Inc.

Table 4–5 Adapted with permission from M.M. Gottschlich and G.D. Warden, Vitamin Supplementation in the Pediatric Patient with Burns, *Journal of Burn Care and Rehabilitation*, Vol. 11, No. 3, p. 277, © 1990, Mosby Inc.

Table 4–6 Adapted from *Nutrition*, Vol. 13, M.N. Novy and K.B. Schwarz, Nutritional Considerations and Management of the Child with Liver Disease, pp. 177–184, © 1997, with permission from Elsevier Science Ltd.

CHAPTER 5

Figure 5–1 Copyright © 1999, T.J. Kenney.
Figure 5–2 Copyright © 1999, T.J. Kenney.
Figure 5–3 Copyright © 1999, T.J. Kenney.
Figure 5–4 Copyright © 1999, T.J. Kenney.
Figure 5–5 Copyright © 1999, T.J. Kenney.

CHAPTER 6

Exhibit 6–2 Reprinted with permission of the Association for the Care of Children's Health, 19 Mantua Road, Mt. Royal, NJ 08061 from Gaynard et al., Preparing Children and Families for Health Care Experiences, *Psychosocial Care of Children in Hospitals: A Clinical Practice Manual from the Child Life Research Projects*, p. 95, © 1990.
Table 6–1 Reprinted with permission from B. Stevens, Nursing Management of Pain in Children, in *Family-Centered Nursing Care of Children*, R. Foster, M. Hunsberger, and J. Anderson, eds., © 1989, W.B. Saunders Co.
Table 6–2 Copyright © 1998, L. Gaines.

CHAPTER 7

Exhibit 7–1 Adapted with permission from P. Kahn, *When Your Child is Technology Assisted: A Home Care Guide for Families*, © 1998, L & A Publishing.
Exhibit 7–2 Data from M. Burns and C. Thornam, Broadening the Scope of Nursing Practice: Federal Programs for Children, *Pediatric Nursing*, Vol. 19, No. 6, pp. 546–553, © 1993, W.B. Saunders Co.
Exhibit 7–3 Adapted with permission from E. Wells, Assisting Parents When a Child Dies in the ICU, *Critical Care Nurse*, Vol. 16, No. 1, pp. 58–62, © 1996, Critical Care Nurse.
Exhibit 7–4 Adapted with permission from P. Kahn, *When Your Child is Technology Assisted: A Home Care Guide for Families*, © 1998, L & A Publishing.

CHAPTER 8

Exhibit 8–1 Reprinted with permission from A. Goldman, Home Care of the Dying Child, *Journal of Palliative Care*, Vol. 12, No. 3, pp. 16–19, © 1996, Centre for Bioethics, Clinical Research Institute of Montreal.
Exhibit 8–2 Data from E. Stewart, Family-Centered Care for the Bereaved, *Pediatric Nursing*, Vol. 21, No. 2, pp. 181–184, 187, © 1995.

CHAPTER 9

Figure 9–1 Courtesy of The Children's Hospital of Philadelphia, Philadelphia, Pennsylvania.
Figure 9–2 Reprinted with permission from N.S. Adzick, Fetal Thoracic Lesions, *Seminars in Pediatric Surgery*, Vol. 2, No. 2, pp. 103–108, © 1999, W.B. Saunders Co.
Figure 9–3 Courtesy of The Children's Hospital of Philadelphia, Philadelphia, Pennsylvania.
Figure 9–4 Courtesy of The Children's Hospital of Philadelphia, Philadelphia, Pennsylvania.
Figure 9–5A Courtesy of Dr. Beverly Coleman, University of Pennsylvania.
Figure 9–5B Courtesy of Dr. Anne Hubbard, The Children's Hospital of Philadelphia.
Figure 9–6 Reprinted with permission from L.J. Howell, M.R. Harrison, N.S. Adzick, The Fetal Treatment Center, *Seminars in Pediatric Surgery*, Vol. 2, No. 2, pp. 143–146, © 1993, W.B Saunders Co.
Figure 9–7 Courtesy of The Children's Hospital of Philadelphia, Philadelphia, Pennsylvania.

CHAPTER 10

Figure 10–1 Courtesy of Amy Hyland.
Table 10–1 Adapted with permission from N.J. Tkacz, Pediatric Laparoscopy and Thorascoscopy, *Nursing Clinics of North America*, Vol. 29, No. 4, p. 67, © 1994, W.B. Saunders Co.

CHAPTER 11

Figure 11–1 Courtesy of Dr. E. Ide Smith.
Figure 11–2 Courtesy of Dr. E. Ide Smith.
Figure 11–3 Courtesy of Dr. E. Ide Smith.
Figure 11–4 Courtesy of M. Elizabeth Foster, RN.
Figure 11–5 Courtesy of Dr. E. Ide Smith.
Figure 11–6 Courtesy of Dr. Phillip C. Guzzetta, Jr.
Figure 11–7 Courtesy of Dr. Phillip C. Guzzetta, Jr.
Figure 11–8 Courtesy of Dr. E. Ide Smith.
Figure 11–9 Courtesy of Dr. Phillip C. Guzzetta, Jr.
Figure 11–10 Courtesy of Dr. Barry A. Hicks.
Figure 11–11 Courtesy of Dr. Barry A. Hicks.
Figure 11–12 Courtesy of Dr. Phillip C. Guzzetta, Jr.
Figure 11–13 Courtesy of Dr. E. Ide Smith.
Table 11–2 Data from B.M. Gates, *A Guide to Physical Examination*, 3rd ed., pp. 370–427, © 1983.

CHAPTER 12

Exhibit 12–2 Courtesy of Cardinal Glennon Children's Hospital, St. Louis, Missouri.
Figure 12–1 Courtesy of St. Louis University, St. Louis, Missouri.
Figure 12–2 Courtesy of St. Louis University, St. Louis, Missouri.
Figure 12–4 Courtesy of St. Louis University, St. Louis, Missouri.
Figure 12–5 Courtesy of Cardinal Glennon Children's Hospital, St. Louis, Missouri.
Figure 12–7 Courtesy of St. Louis University, St. Louis, Missouri.

CHAPTER 13

Figure 13–4 Reprinted with permission from K.J. Welch et al., Esophageal Atresia and Congenital Stenosis, *Pediatric Surgery*, 4th ed., p. 685, © 1986, Mosby Inc.
Figure 13–7 Reprinted with permission from K.W. Ashcraft and T.M. Holder, The Esophagus, *Pediatric Surgery*, 2nd ed., p. 239, © 1993, W.B. Saunders Co.
Figure 13–8A Reprinted with permission from K.W. Ashcraft and T.M. Holder, The Esophagus, *Pediatric Surgery*, 2nd ed., p. 241, © 1993, W.B. Saunders Co.
Figure 13–8B Reprinted with permission from K.W. Ashcraft and T.M. Holder, The Esophagus, *Pediatric Surgery*, 2nd ed., p. 241, © 1993, W.B. Saunders Co.
Figure 13–9 Reprinted with permission from Gastric Replacement of the Esophagus, *Rob & Smiths Operative*

Surgery–Pediatric Surgery, 5th ed., L. Spitz and A. Coran, eds., p. 157, © 1995, Lippincott-Raven Publishers.

Figure 13–10 Reprinted with permission from E.L. Cusick, A.A.G. Batchelor, and R.D. Spicer, Development of a Technique for Jejunal Interposition in Long-Gap Esophageal Atresia, *Journal of Pediatric Surgery*, Vol. 28, No. 8, p. 991, © 1993, W.B. Saunders.

CHAPTER 14

Figure 14–1 Reprinted with permission from K. Moore and T. Persound, *The Developing Human: Clinically Oriented Embryology*, 5th ed., p. 230, © 1993, W.B. Saunders Co.

Figure 14–2 Reprinted with permission from B. Othersen Jr., Pulmonary and Bronchial Malformation, in *Pediatric Surgery*, 2nd ed., K. Ashcraft and T. Holder, eds., p. 178, © 1993, W.B. Saunders Co.

Figure 14–3 Reprinted with permission from S. Luck, M. Reynolds, and J. Rafensburger, Congenital Bronchopulmonary Malformations, *Current Problems in Surgery*, Vol. 23, No. 4, p. 269, © 1986, Mosby Inc.

CHAPTER 15

Figure 15–1 Copyright © 2000, K. Wise.
Figure 15–2 Copyright © 2000, K. Wise.

CHAPTER 16

Figure 16–2 Courtesy of The Children's Hospital, Denver, Colorado.

Figure 16–4A Courtesy of Bard Interventional Products Division, a division of C.R. Bard, Inc., Billerica, Massachusetts.

Figure 16–4B Courtesy of Ballard Corporation.

Figure 16–4C Courtesy of Bard Interventional Products Division, a division of C.R. Bard, Inc., Billerica, Massachusetts. Genie is a trademark of C.R. Bard, Inc. or an affiliate.

Figure 16–5 Courtesy of The Children's Hospital, Denver, Colorado.

Table 16–2 Data from J.M. Sondheimer, Gastroesophageal Reflux in Children: Clinical Presentation and Diagnostic Management, *Gastrointestinal Endoscopy Clinics of North America*, Vol. 4, No. 1, pp. 55–74, © 1994.

CHAPTER 17

Figure 17–3 Reprinted with permission from J.C. Langer, *Journal of Pediatric Surgery*, Vol. 5, No. 2, p. 126, © 1998, W.B. Saunders Co.

CHAPTER 18

Figure 18–1 Reprinted with permission from J.L. Grosfeld, T.V.N. Ballantine, and R. Shoemaker, Operative Management of Intestinal Atresia and Stenosis Based on Pathologic Findings, *Journal of Pediatric Surgery*, Vol. 14, p. 368, © 1979, W.B. Saunders Co.

Figure 18–2 Reprinted with permission from J.A. O'Neil et al., *Pediatric Surgery,* 5th ed., Vol. I & II, p. 1142, © 1998, Mosby Inc.

Figure 18–3 Reprinted with permission from J.A. O'Neil et al., *Pediatric Surgery*, 5th ed., Vol. I & II, p. 1141, © 1998, Mosby Inc.

Figure 18–4 Reprinted with permission from J.A. O'Neil et al., *Pediatric Surgery*, 5th ed., Vol. I & II, p. 1141, © 1998, Mosby Inc.

Figure 18–5 Reprinted with permission from J.A. O'Neil et al., *Pediatric Surgery*, 5th ed., Vol. I & II, p. 1142, © 1998, Mosby Inc.

Figure 18–6 Reprinted with permission from J.A. O'Neil et al., *Pediatric Surgery*, 5th ed., Vol. I & II, p. 1153, © 1998, Mosby Inc.

Figure 18–7 Reprinted with permission from J.A. O'Neil et al., *Pediatric Surgery*, 5th ed., Vol. I & II, p. 1153, © 1998, Mosby Inc.

Figure 18–8 Reprinted with permission from J.A. O'Neil et al., *Pediatric Surgery*, 5th ed., Vol. I & II, p. 1153, © 1998, Mosby Inc.

Figure 18–9 Reprinted with permission from F.J. Rescorla and J.L. Grosfeld, Contemporary Management of Meconium Ileus, *World Journal of Surgery*, Vol. 17, p. 318, © 1993, Springer-Verlag New York, Inc.

Figure 18–10 Reprinted with permission from F.J. Rescorla and J.L. Grosfeld, Contemporary Management of Meconium Ileus, *World Journal of Surgery*, Vol. 17, p. 318, © 1993, Springer-Verlag New York, Inc.

Table 18–2 Reprinted with permission from J.J. Templeton, Gastrointestinal Obstruction in the Neonate, *Resident Series Lecture*, May 1995, © 1995, The Children's Hospital of Philadelphia.

CHAPTER 20

Figure 20–1 Reprinted with permission from A. Peña, *Atlas of the Surgical Management of Anorectal Malformations*, © 1990, Springer-Verlag New York, Inc.; Lois Barnes, illustrator.

Figure 20–3 Reprinted with permission from A. Peña, *Atlas of the Surgical Management of Anorectal Malformations*, © 1990, Springer-Verlag New York, Inc.; Lois Barnes, illustrator.

Figure 20–4 Reprinted with permission from A. Peña, *Atlas of the Surgical Management of Anorectal Malformations*, © 1990, Springer-Verlag New York, Inc.; Lois Barnes, illustrator.

Figure 20–5 Reprinted with permission from A. Peña, *Atlas of the Surgical Management of Anorectal Malformations*, © 1990, Springer-Verlag New York, Inc.; Lois Barnes, illustrator.

Figure 20–6 Reprinted with permission from A. Peña, *Atlas of the Surgical Management of Anorectal Malformations*, © 1990, Springer-Verlag New York, Inc.

Figure 20–7 Reprinted with permission from A. Peña, *Atlas of the Surgical Management of Anorectal Malformations*, © 1990, Springer-Verlag New York, Inc.; Lois Barnes, illustrator.

Table 20–1 Courtesy of Alberto Peña, MD, New Hyde Park, New York.

Table 20–2 Courtesy of Alberto Peña, MD, New Hyde Park, New York.

Table 20–3 Courtesy of Alberto Peña, MD, New Hyde Park, New York.

CHAPTER 21

Exhibit 21–1 Data from D.C. Broadwell and B.S. Jackson, *Principles of Ostomy Care*, © 1982, Mosby Inc.

Exhibit 21–2 Courtesy of Children's Hospital Oakland, Oakland, California.

Table 21–1 Reprinted from G. Garvin, *Critical Care Nursing Quarterly*, Vol. 20, No. 1, p. 66, © 1997, Aspen Publishers, Inc.

CHAPTER 22

Figure 22–1 Courtesy of University of Maryland, Department of Surgery, Baltimore, Maryland.

Figure 22–2 Courtesy of University of Maryland, Department of Surgery, Baltimore, Maryland.

Figure 22–3 Courtesy of University of Maryland, Department of Surgery, Baltimore, Maryland.

Figure 22–4 Courtesy of University of Maryland, Department of Surgery, Baltimore, Maryland.

CHAPTER 23

Figure 23–1 Courtesy of Erik Skarsgard, MD, Lucile Salter Packard Children's Hospital, Palo Alto, California.

Figure 23–2 Courtesy of Erik Skarsgard, MD, Lucile Salter Packard Children's Hospital, Palo Alto, California.

Figure 23–3 Courtesy of Department of Radiology, University of California San Francisco, 1998, Stanford Health Services, Palo Alto, California.

Figure 23–4 Courtesy of Department of Radiology, University of California San Francisco, 1998, Stanford Health Services, Palo Alto, California.

Figure 23–5 Courtesy of Erik Skarsgard, MD, Lucile Salter Packard Children's Hospital, Palo Alto, California.

Figure 23–6 Courtesy of Erik Skarsgard, MD, Lucile Salter Packard Children's Hospital, Palo Alto, California.

CHAPTER 25

Figure 25–1 Reprinted with permission from K.T. Oldham, P.M. Colombani, and R.P. Foglia, *Surgery of Infants and Children: Scientific Principles and Practice*, p. 1154, © 1997, Lippincott Williams & Wilkins.

Figure 25–2 Reprinted with permission from K.T. Oldham, P.M. Colombani, and R.P. Foglia, *Surgery of Infants and Children: Scientific Principles and Practice*, p. 1155, © 1997, Lippincott Williams & Wilkins.

CHAPTER 26

Figure 26–1 Courtesy of Nicholas A. Shorter, MD, Children's Hospital at Dartmouth, Lebanon, New Hampshire.

Figure 26–2 Courtesy of Nicholas A. Shorter, MD, Children's Hospital at Dartmouth, Lebanon, New Hampshire.

Figure 26–3 Courtesy of Nicholas A. Shorter, MD, Children's Hospital at Dartmouth, Lebanon, New Hampshire.

CHAPTER 27

Table 27–1 Data from K.W. Ashcraft and T.M. Holder, *Pediatric Surgery*, 2nd ed., p. 470, © 1993, W.B. Saunders Co.

CHAPTER 28

Figure 28–1 Reprinted with permission from K.W. Ashcraft, *Atlas of Pediatric Surgery*, pp. 118–119, © 1994, W.B. Saunders.

Figure 28–2A Reprinted with permission from K.W. Ashcraft, *Atlas of Pediatric Surgery*, pp. 118–119, © 1994, W.B. Saunders.

Figure 28–2B Reprinted with permission from K.W. Ashcraft, *Atlas of Pediatric Surgery*, pp. 118–119, © 1994, W.B. Saunders.

Figure 28–2C Reprinted with permission from K.W. Ashcraft, *Atlas of Pediatric Surgery*, pp. 118–119, © 1994, W.B. Saunders.

Figure 28–3 Reprinted with permission from P.G. Janu, D.A. Rogers, and T.E. Lobe, A Comparison of Laparoscopic and Traditional Open Splenectomy in Childhood, *Journal of Pediatric Surgery*, Vol. 31, pp. 109–114, © 1996, W.B. Saunders.

Figure 28–4 Reprinted with permission from P.G. Janu, D.A. Rogers, and T.E. Lobe, A Comparison of Laparoscopic and Traditional Open Splenectomy in Childhood, *Journal of Pediatric Surgery*, Vol. 31, pp. 109–114, © 1996, W.B. Saunders.

Figure 28–5 Reprinted with permission from A.W. Flake, Disorders of the Gallbladder and Biliary Tract, in *Surgery of Infants and Children: Scientific Principles and Practice*, K.T. Oldham, P.M. Colombani, and R.P. Foglia, eds., p. 1412, © 1997, Lippincott Williams & Wilkins.

Figure 28–6 Courtesy of Cedric J. Priebe, Jr., MD, University Hospital and Medical Center, State University of New York at Stony Brook.

Figure 28–7 Courtesy of Cedric J. Priebe, Jr., MD, University Hospital and Medical Center, State University of New York at Stony Brook.

CHAPTER 29

Table 29–1 Data from A.C. Guyton, *Textbook of Medical Physiology*, 8th ed., © W.B. Saunders Co.

CHAPTER 30

Exhibit 30–1 Reprinted with permission from D.M. Green et al., *Principles and Practice of Pediatric Oncology,* p. 744, © 1997, Lippincott-Raven Publishers.

Figure 30–1 Courtesy of Memorial Sloan Kettering Cancer Center, New York, New York.

Figure 30–2 Courtesy of Memorial Sloan Kettering Cancer Center, New York, New York.

Figure 30–3 Courtesy of Memorial Sloan Kettering Cancer Center, New York, New York.

Figure 30–4 Courtesy of Memorial Sloan Kettering Cancer Center, New York, New York.

Figure 30–5 Courtesy of Memorial Sloan Kettering Cancer Center, New York, New York.

Figure 30–6 Courtesy of Memorial Sloan Kettering Cancer Center, New York, New York.

Figure 30–7 Reprinted with permission from P.A. Pizzo and D.G. Poplack, *Principles and Practice of Pediatric Oncology,* p. 803, © 1997, Lippincott-Raven Publishers.

Figure 30–8 Courtesy of Memorial Sloan Kettering Cancer Center, New York, New York.

Figure 30–9 Courtesy of Memorial Sloan Kettering Cancer Center, New York, New York.

Figure 30–10 Courtesy of Memorial Sloan Kettering Cancer Center, New York, New York.

Figure 30–11 Courtesy of Memorial Sloan Kettering Cancer Center, New York, New York.

Figure 30–12 Courtesy of Memorial Sloan Kettering Cancer Center, New York, New York.

Table 30–1 Data from G.M. Brodeur and R.P. Castleberry, Neuroblastoma, in

Principles and Practice of Pediatric Oncology, 3rd ed., P.A. Pizzo and D.G. Poplack, eds., pp. 761-797, © 1997, Lippincott-Raven Publishers; J.G. Gurney, R.K. Severson, S. Davis, and L.L Robinson, *Incidence of Cancer in Children in the United States*, © 1994; P. Lanzkowsky, *Manual of Pediatric Hematology and Oncology*, pp. 419-475, © 1995, Churchill Livingstone, Inc.; Y. Ni et al., Hepatocellular Carcinoma in Childhood: Clinical Manifestations and Prognosis, *Cancer*, Vol. 68, p. 1737, © 1991; P.A. Pizzo and D.G. Poplack, *Principles and Practice of Pediatric Oncology*, p. 803, © 1997, Lippincott-Raven Publishers; and J.L. Young and R.W. Miller, Incidence of Malignant Tumors in U.S. Children, *Journal of Pediatrics*, Vol. 86, p. 254, © 1975.

Table 30–2 Data from A.E. Brodeur and G.M. Brodeur, Abdominal Masses in Children: Neuroblastoma, Wilms Tumor, and Other Considerations, *Pediatrics in Review*, Vol. 12, No. 7, pp. 197–206, © 1991; G.M. Brodeur and R.P. Castleberry, Neuroblastoma, in *Principles and Practice of Pediatric Oncology*, 3rd ed., P.A. Pizzo and D.G. Poplack, eds., pp. 761–797, © 1997, Lippincott-Raven Publishers; and M.P. LaQuaglia, Childhood Tumors, in *Surgery: Scientific Principles and Practice*, L.J. Greenfield et al, eds., pp. 2118–2140, © 1997, Lippincott-Raven Publishers.

Table 30–3 Data from A.E. Brodeur and G.M. Brodeur, Abdominal Masses in Children: Neuroblastoma, Wilms Tumor, and Other Considerations, *Pediatrics in Review*, Vol. 12, No. 7, pp. 197–206, © 1991; and International Neuroblastoma Staging System.

Table 30–4 Reprinted with permission from G.M. Brodeur and R.P. Castleberry, *Principles and Practice of Pediatric Oncology*, p. 777, © 1997, Lippincott-Raven Publishers.

Table 30–5 Data from D.M. Green et al., Wilms Tumor, in *Principles and Practice of Pediatric Oncology*, 3rd ed., P.A. Pizzo and D.G. Poplack, eds., pp. 761–797, © 1997, Lippincott-Raven Publishers; S. Federici et al., Wilms' Tumor Involving the Inferior Vena Cava: Preoperative Evaluation and Management, *Medical and Pediatric Oncology*,

Vol. 22, pp. 39–44, © 1994; and National Wilms Tumor Study Group.

Table 30–6 Reprinted with permission from M. Greenberg and R.M. Filler, *Principles and Practice of Pediatric Oncology*, p. 723, © 1997, Lippincott-Raven Publishers.

Table 30–7 Data from M. Greenberg and R.M. Filler, Hepatic Tumors, in *Principles and Practice of Pediatric Oncology*, 3rd ed., P.A. Pizzo and D.G. Poplack, eds., pp. 717–732, © 1997, Lippincott-Raven Publishers; and M.P. LaQuaglia, Childhood Tumors, in *Surgery: Scientific Principles and Practice*, L.J. Greenfield et al., eds., pp. 2118–2140, © 1997, Lippincott-Raven Publishers.

Table 30–8 Reprinted with permission from M. Greenberg and R.M. Filler, *Principles and Practice of Pediatric Oncology*, p. 724, © 1997, Lippincott-Raven Publishers.

Table 30–9 Data from P. Lanzkowsky, *Manual of Pediatric Hematology and Oncology*, pp. 419–475, © 1995, Churchill Livingstone, Inc.; M.P. LaQuaglia, Childhood Tumors, in *Surgery: Scientific Principles and Practice*, L.J. Greenfield et al., eds., pp. 2118–2140, © 1997, Lippincott-Raven Publishers; P.A. Pizzo and D.G. Poplack, *Principles and Practice of Pediatric Oncology*, p. 803, © 1997, Lippincott-Raven Publishers; and M.I. Rowe et al., *Essentials of Pediatric Surgery*, pp. 249–285, © 1995, Mosby Inc.

Table 30–10 Reprinted with permission from M.P. LaQuaglia, *Surgery: Scientific Principles and Practice*, p. 2126, © 1997, Lippincott-Raven Publishers.

Table 30–11 Reprinted with permission from P.A. Pizzo and D.G. Poplack, *Principles and Practice of Pediatric Oncology*, p. 809, © 1997, Lippincott-Raven Publishers.

Table 30–12 Data from P. Lanzkowsky, *Manual of Pediatric Hematology and Oncology*, pp. 419–475, © 1995, Churchill Livingstone, Inc.; M.P. LaQuaglia, Childhood Tumors, in *Surgery: Scientific Principles and Practice*, L.J. Greenfield et al., eds., pp. 2118–2140, © 1997, Lippincott-Raven Publishers; P.A. Pizzo and D.G. Poplack, *Principles and Practice of Pediatric*

Oncology, p. 803, © 1997, Lippincott-Raven Publishers; and M.I. Rowe et al., *Essentials of Pediatric Surgery*, pp. 249–285, © 1995, Mosby Inc.

CHAPTER 31

Exhibit 31–1 Adapted with permission from E. McNamara et al., *Organ Transplants*, in Primary Care of the Child with a Chronic Condition, J. Vessey and P. Jackson, eds., p.599, © 1996, Mosby.

Exhibit 31–2 Adapted with permission from E. McNamara et al., *Organ Transplants*, in Primary Care of the Child with a Chronic Condition, J. Vessey and P. Jackson, eds., p. 601, © 1996, Mosby.

Exhibit 31–4 Reprinted from UNOS Annual Report, *The U.S. Scientific Registry of Transplant Recipients and the Organ Procurement and Transplantation Network, Transplant Data 1988–1994*, U.S. Department of Health and Human Services, Health Resources and Services Administration.

Figure 31–1 Reprinted with permission from A.C. Guyton, *Textbook of Medical Physiology*, 8th ed., © W.B. Saunders Co.

Figure 31–2 Reprinted with permission from Brollsch, Liver Transplantation in Children from Living Related Donors, *Annals of Surgery*, October 1991, p. 432, © 1991, Lippincott-Williams & Wilkins.

Figure 31–3A Reprinted with permission from J. Reyes et al., Current Status of Intestinal Transplantation in Children, *Journal of Pediatric Surgery*, Vol. 33, No. 2, pp. 243–251, © 1993, W.B. Saunders Co.

Figure 31–3B Reprinted with permission from J. Reyes et al., Current Status of Intestinal Transplantation in Children, *Journal of Pediatric Surgery*, Vol. 33, No. 2, pp. 243–251, © 1993, W.B. Saunders Co.

Figure 31–4 Originally published in J.A. Tami, The Immune System, *American Journal of Hospital Pharmacy*, Vol. 43, No. 10, pp. 2483–2493, © 1986, American Society of Health System Pharmacists, Inc. All rights reserved. Reprinted with permission. (R2006)

Table 31–2 Reprinted from UNOS Annual Report, *The U.S. Scientific Registry of Transplant Recipients and the Organ Procurement and Transplantation*

Network, Transplant Data 1988–1994, U.S. Department of Health and Human Services, Health Resources and Services Administration.

CHAPTER 32

Exhibit 32–1 Adapted from Immunosuppression Protocol, The Children's Hospital of Philadelphia.

CHAPTER 33

Exhibit 33–1 Adapted with permission from E. Adcock, C. Consolvo, and D. Berry, in Handbook of Neonatal Intensive Care, G. Merenstein and S. Gardner, eds., p. 171, © 1998, Mosby Inc.

Exhibit 33–2 Adapted from *Pediatric Nursing,* 1988, Volume 14, Number 2, p. 149. Reprinted with permission of the publisher, Jannetti Publications, Inc., East Holly Avenue Box 56, Pitman, NJ 08071–0056; Phone (609) 256–2300; FAX (609) 589–7463. For a sample copy of the journal, please contact the publisher.

Exhibit 33–3 Data from C. Kenner, S. Amlung, and A. Flandermeyer, *Protocols in Neonatal Nursing,* pp. 589–603, 660–678, © 1998, W.B. Saunders Co.; J. Arnold and K. Anand, in *Neonatology: Pathophysiology and Management of the Newborn,* G. Avery, M. Fletcher, and M.

MacDonald, eds., pp. 1334–1345, © 1994, J.B. Lippincott Company; M. McRae, D. Rourke, and F. Imperial-Perez, *Pediatric Nursing,* Vol. 23, No. 3, pp. 263–271; and L. Franck, in *Comprehensive Neonatal Nursing,* C. Kenner, A. Brueggemeyer, and L. Gunderson, eds., pp. 913–925, © 1994, W.B. Saunders Co.

CHAPTER 34

Exhibit 34–2 Reprinted with permission from J. Simon and A. Goldberg, *Prehospital Pediatric Life Support,* p.11, © 1989, Mosby Inc.

Figure 34–1 Courtesy of Jacksonville Pediatric Injury Control System, Jacksonville, Florida.

Figure 34–2 Reprinted with permission from N.E. McSwain, Jr., *Pre-Hospital Trauma Life Support,* 2nd ed., p. 134, © 1990, W.B. Saunders Co.

Figure 34–3 Reprinted with permission from R. Bullock et al., *Guidelines for the Management of Severe Head Injury,* A Joint Initiative of The Brain Trauma Foundation, The American Association of Neurological Surgeons, and the Joint Section on Neurotrauma and Critical Care, Copyright © 1995, The Brain Trauma Foundation.

Table 34–1 Adapted with permission from J.J. Tepas et al., *Journal of Pediatric Surgery,* Vol. 22, No. 1, p. 15, © 1987, Grune & Stratton, Inc.

Table 34–2 Reprinted with permission from ACS Committee on Trauma, *Advanced Trauma Life Support® Student Manual,* 1997 ed., p. 297, © 1997, American College of Surgeons.

Table 34–3 Reprinted with permission from ACS Committee on Trauma, *Advanced Trauma Life Support® Student Manual,* 1997 ed., p. 297, © 1997, American College of Surgeons.

Table 34–6 Data from M.D. Thomas, Musculoskeletal Injury, in *Pediatric Trauma: Prevention, Acute Care, Rehabilitation,* M.R. Eichelberger, ed., p. 540–545, © 1993, Mosby Inc.

CHAPTER 35

Exhibit 35–1 Reprinted from St. Louis Children's Hospital Burn Manual, © 1994, St. Louis Children's Hospital.

Exhibit 35–2 Courtesy of American Burn Association, Chicago, Illinois.

Exhibit 35–3 Courtesy of American Burn Association, Chicago, Illinois.

Exhibit 35–5 Reprinted with permission from D. Sadowski, Care of the Child with Burns, in *Nursing Care of the Critically Ill Child,* M.F. Hazinski, ed., pp. 875–927, © 1992, W.B. Saunders Co.

Table 35–1 Adapted with permission from *Scald Burn Prevention Strategy,* p. 67, © 1990, Children's National Medical Center.

Index